HOW TO USE THIS BOOK

WHEN YOU GET THIS BOOK:

Read the **Table of Contents** at the beginning. This tells what each chapter is about, and gives the page numbers for the different subjects discussed.

TO LOOK UP A DISEASE OR OTHER ANIMAL HEALTH SUBJECT:

1. The **Index** starting on page 393 lists, in the order of the alphabet, all the subjects in this book. Also, if you look up a particular problem in the book, you will often see, "See page." This means you should turn to that page also, and you will find more information about that particular problem. Or....

2. Check the list of the **Table of Contents**. Then turn to the page listed there. This book is organized according to the systems of the body. So for instance, if the problem is associated with the digestive system (for example, diarrhea) then this topic will be covered in the digestive system chapter.

IF YOU DO NOT UNDERSTAND THE MEANING OF SOME OF THE WORDS IN THIS BOOK:

Look for the word in the **Vocabulary** which starts on page 385.

BEFORE USING ANY MEDICINE:

Always look for information on uses, dosage, precautions, and withdrawal times in the list of **Common Medicines and Their Doses,** starting on page 352.

TO BE READY FOR EMERGENCIES:

Study this book before it is needed, especially **Chapter 5, First Aid**. At the front of Chapter 5 (page 77) there is a list of common emergencies found in livestock, with a page number listed next to it. Turn to this page number for more information regarding the emergency you are facing.

TO KEEP YOUR LIVESTOCK HEALTHY:

Study especially Chapter 6 on prevention and control of infectious diseases. Study also both Chapter 7, Nutrition; and Chapter 25, the Nutrition Appendix, which give more details regarding good nutrition and health.

Where There Is No Animal Doctor

by

Maureen Birmingham and Peter N. Quesenberry

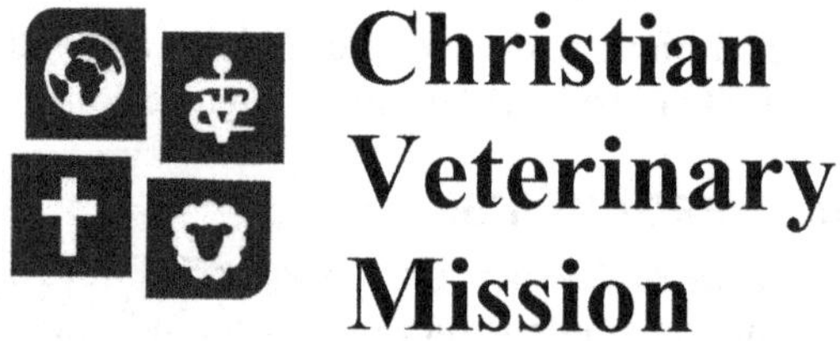

Christian Veterinary Mission

A publication of Christian Veterinary Mission

Email – vetbooks@cvm.org

www.cvm.org

Library of Congress Cataloging-in-Publishing Data

Birmingham, Maureen
  Where there is no animal doctor / by Maureen Birmingham and Peter Quesenberry. p. cm.
1. Veterinary medicine—Developing countries. 2. Animal health—Developing countries.
3. Domestic animals—Diseases—Developing countries. 4. Care of sick animals—Developing countries. I. Quesenberry, Peter N. II. Christian Veterinary Mission. III. Title.

SF755.B57 2007
636.089'091724--dc22 2006103396
Revised Edition 2016 ISBN 978-1-886532-45-8

Dedication

This book is dedicated to two groups of people:

> **farmers** throughout the
> world and **our families**.

1. To the women, men and families throughout the world who are farmers, we want to say thank you for all you have taught us through the years. You work hard every day to provide the necessities of life for your families, and for those of us who do not produce our own food. You live with the uncertainties of nature; and even when production is good you are still affected by the increasing uncertainties of world markets. Yet you still move-on with diligence and dedication. We thank you, and we pray that this book will prove useful to many of you.

2. To our families we also say thank you and dedicate this book to you.

From Pete to Mary, Nat, Cheri and Wynn – thank you. Your encouragement, prayers and patience through the years have contributed not only to this book but also to other books and other curricula that are being used in many different places.

From Maureen to Dan, Erika, Evelyn and Zoe who have provided encouragement and inspiration and also endured my absences and distracted presence while working on this book.

Thanks

First of all, we thank our two main editors:

Dr. David Ramse (BS Agriculture, MS Entomology, EdD) has worked for 24 years in international development. He has experience in Tanzania and British Guyana as an agriculturalist, and in Nepal as a project manager and a vocational education trainer. David has not only helped to edit the manuscript but has also encouraged us to keep working through the years. David is currently on faculty at Wartburg Theological Seminary where he teaches development principles to graduate students.

Dr. Paul Coe, DVM, MPVM spent 8 years following graduation from veterinary college in private food animal practice. He joined the Department of Large Animal Clinical Sciences of the College of Veterinary Medicine at Michigan State University in 1981. He teaches in both theory and clinical courses in the veterinary curriculum and commits a major portion of his time to extension, working primarily with beef producers. Dr. Coe reviews manuscripts for several journals including J.A.V.M.A., The Compendium and Theriogenology. He has helped extensively with the editing of this manuscript.

In addition, we want to thank Dr. Leroy Dorminy of Christian Vet Missions and Mr. Paul Kennel of World Concern for their un-ending encouragement and support throughout the years of this project.

A special thanks goes to David Hadrill, Veterinary Surgeon, for special input with the organization of the book in the beginning, and with ideas which helped to get the whole project started.

Thank you also to Dr. Paul Brand who encouraged Peter to begin the process in earnest.

Dr. Marion Hammerland edited the Poultry Section for technical points; and Dr. Edward L. Roberson (retired professor from the University of Georgia) edited the external parasite sections.

We thank the following for permission to use their drawings: Mrs. Ashta Uprety from the DCP in Nepal, Dr. Todd Cooney (who also designed and drew the cover for the book), Dr. Wade Bradshaw, Mrs. Margreet Korstanje, Mr. Harish Chand Sapkota, Mr. Chaiyun Panthsen, various artists from the RDC in Nepal, and Mr. Max Arratia. In addition we thank Ms. Sunida Sorwiset for helping with typing.

Finally, we especially thank Mary, Nat and Cheri Quesenberry for editing, typing, re-doing drawings, and helping to complete the index. Without their input, the book would not have been finished.

Disclaimer

This book was prepared according to the current veterinary literature available. It is developed by people in the veterinary mission field, as a service to farmers, technicians and veterinary practitioners working in areas where livestock still play a very important role in village life. The editors, authors, co-authors, and contributors to this volume, as well as Christian Veterinary Mission and World Concern, assume no responsibility for and make no warranty with respect to the results that may be obtained from the uses, procedures, withdrawal periods, or dosages listed and do not necessarily endorse them.

Furthermore, the editors, authors, co-authors, and contributors to this volume, as well as Christian Veterinary Mission and World Concern, shall not be liable to anyone whatsoever for any damage resulting from reliance on any information contained in this work. This applies to drugs and their usage and to any veterinary procedures outlined.

Since this book will enjoy worldwide distribution the veterinary procedures, drugs, doses, indications, and withdrawal periods detailed herein do not and cannot comply with all the laws of each sovereign country. Before performing any procedure, giving veterinary advice or using any animal drugs the reader must become familiar with the local laws and regulations that apply to the practice of veterinary medicine and drug use in animals and practice strict adherence to those laws. Similarly, this book is not intended to substitute for the complete prescribing information prepared by each manufacturer for each drug. The package insert and directions for use of every drug product should be read, understood and followed before any drug is administered or prescribed.

Raising Healthy Animals Series

Every year, thousands of people around the world struggle to survive because they don't have the right knowledge, skills and resources to care for their animals. Christian Veterinary Mission (CVM) sends veterinary professionals to live and work alongside many of these people to encourage them and provide them with not only much needed veterinary expertise, but also the hope that is only found in Christ. CVM veterinarians build lasting relationships with individuals and communities, helping them be transformed through Christ's love.

CVM, in its effort to be meaningfully involved in work in the developing world, quickly found there was little appropriate educational material available. CVM set about developing basic resource materials in animal husbandry for farmers and agricultural workers. Apparently, they met a real need, as these books have been accepted throughout the developing nations of the world.

The series of books published by Christian Veterinary Mission includes the following in order of publication:

Raising Healthy Pigs	Drugs and Their Usage
* Raising Healthy Rabbits	**Where There Is No Animal Doctor
* Raising Healthy Fish	Raising Healthy Horses
Raising Healthy Cattle	Zoonoses: Animal Diseases That Affect Humans
Raising Healthy Poultry*+	Raising Healthy Honey Bees
Raising Healthy Goats	Slaughter and Preservation of Meat
* Raising Healthy Sheep	Disease and Parasite Prevention in Farm Animals

Also available in: * Spanish + French **Spanish, Myanmar, Tamil, Thai, Chinese

CVM fieldworkers have also developed specific training materials for the countries in which they work.

All of these books have been put together by Christian men and women; in a labor of love and service, for people in need throughout the world. It demonstrates dedication to their profession, service to humanity and a witness to their faith. We hope that they are a help to you in developing an appropriate livestock program to meet your needs. We pray God's blessing on their use.

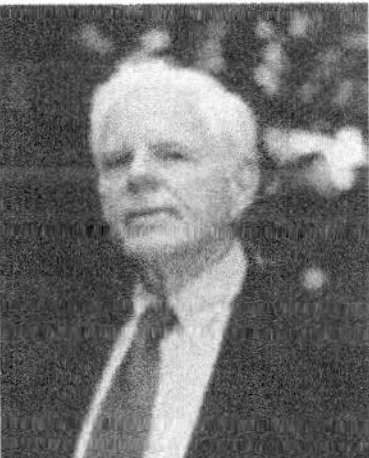

Leroy Dorminy
CVM Founder

Christian Veterinary Mission (Publisher of this book)

Our vision is to see
Christ's love expressed through veterinary medicine.

Our mission is to
challenge, empower and facilitate veterinarians to serve through their profession, living out their Christian faith.

CVM also provides education and encouragement for those who desire to minister through service, prayer, relationship building, and modeling Christ's love.

About CVM

Christian Veterinary Mission (CVM) is a registered non- profit Christian Service Organization 501(c)(3) based in Washington, U.S.A.

CVM was founded in 1976 by Dr. Leroy Dorminy who came to realize the impact that veterinarians could have by integrating their faith with their practice, both locally and around the world. In 2008, CVM had nearly 30 veterinary professionals serving full-time internationally and over 200 veterinary professionals and student volunteers serve on short- term cross-cultural mission trips annually. CVM sponsors fellowship & prayer breakfasts at over 20 U.S. veterinary meetings each year and reaches out to veterinary students through Christian Veterinary Fellowship (CVF) groups in every veterinary school in the U.S. by encouraging them in spiritual growth and professional development.

There are over 3,500 veterinarians affiliated with CVM in the U.S. CVM also partners with organizations and networks in other countries that are focused on empowering Christian veterinarians. CVM has a volunteer advisory board of veterinarians who guide its vision, mission, and programming.

CVM books and the free International Animal Health Newsletter were written with small farmers, veterinarians, and agricultural development workers in mind. Our desire is that they would help individuals and groups develop an appropriate livestock program to meet community needs. CVM's Endowment Fund was started in the early years of the organization's life. The fund provides for meaningful programs that could not be funded by the regular budgeting process.

Introduction
WHY THIS BOOK?

The idea for a book "Where There is No Vet" was conceived years ago. Work was officially started in 1985 by the late Dr. Bill Baker who worked as a veterinarian in Haiti for eight years. Dr. Baker recognized the important role of livestock in the lives of most rural people in the world. He wanted to develop a useful book for people living in areas "where there is no veterinarian." This book expands that original vision and is written for _anyone interested in livestock health, regardless of whether they own livestock themselves._ In this book such workers are called _"Animal Health Agents"_ _(AHAs)._

Many components of animal husbandry and health are necessary for proper and profitable livestock production. These include the following components:

**Good hygiene &
 sanitation (cleanliness)**

**Proper shelter
 & environment**

**Adequate quantities of
good drinking water**

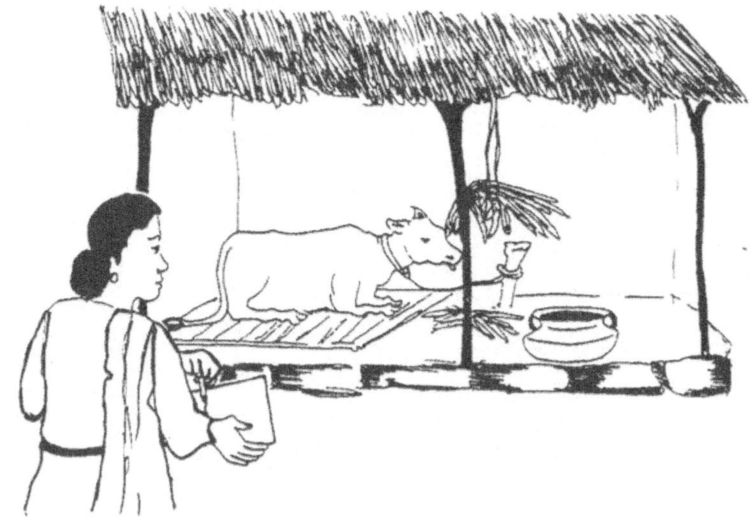

Proper nutrition

**Proper selection of
breeding animals**

**Prevention, control
& treatment of diseases**

**Well-kept records with
breeding dates, etc.**

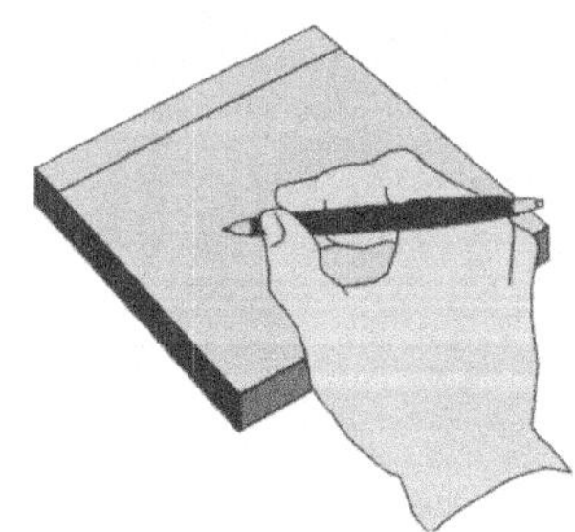

**Good daily observation,
management & decision-making**

**A means of marketing livestock
& livestock products**

This book is primarily concerned with issues of animal health or "veterinary medicine."

Our Definition of Veterinary Medicine:

Veterinary medicine is the science and practice of:

*- disease **prevention, control, & treatment** in animals and*
*- **promoting** good animal nutrition and health.*

WHO IS AN ANIMAL HEALTH AGENT (AHA)?

This book is written for workers, both male and female, whom we call **AHA**s (Animal Health Agents). An **AHA** is any person working to improve the health of livestock. An AHA will usually fit into one of three categories:

1. **Trained Farmers**: These are farmers who have received some training (formal or informal) and are actively treating the most common animal health problems in their communities. More importantly, these farmers might also participate in disease prevention activities, such as vaccinations and parasite control.

2. **Technicians:** These people generally have at least a middle-school education and one or two years of specific training in the area of agriculture or livestock production. Animal health technicians may be self-employed or employed by the government a non-governmental organization or a livestock producers' group.

3. **Community leaders/development workers:** These are community development workers or leaders working with communities interested in livestock health.

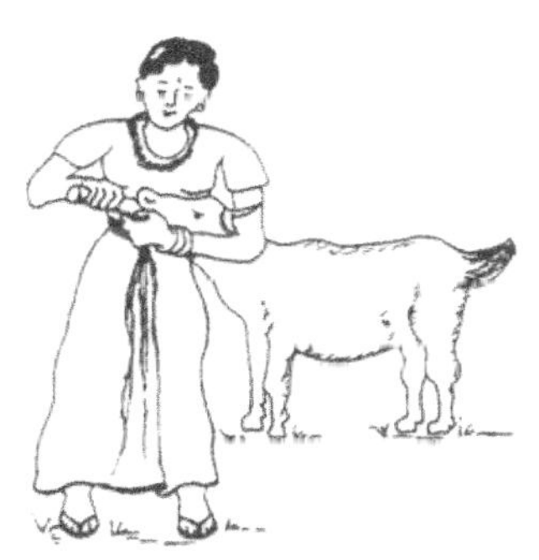 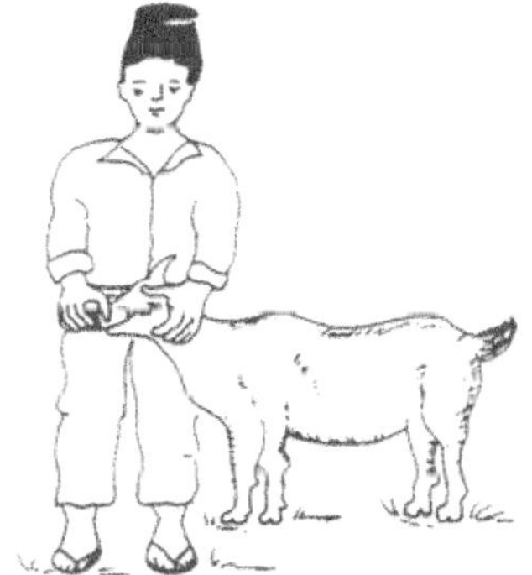

WHAT YOU NEED TO USE THIS BOOK

Special equipment and special vocabulary are not necessary to improve the health of livestock. Since animals cannot speak to indicate when, where, and for how long they are sick, we must use our senses and available information to identify and treat the problem. The following "equipment" and abilities are needed:

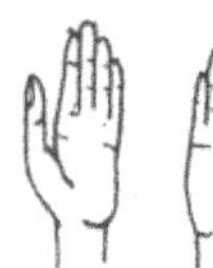 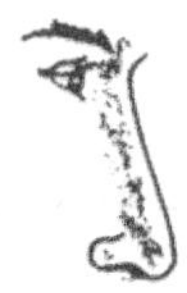 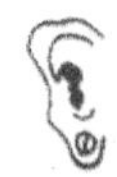

good **hands**, **eyes**, **ears**, & **nose** to examine the animal & its environment;

respect for farmers, and the **ability to listen** to their thoughts & observations regarding their own animals;

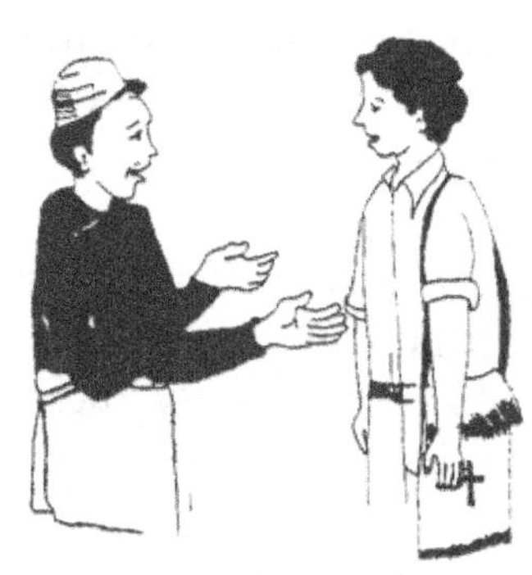

common sense, **patience**, & **appreciation** for livestock & livestock production;

a genuine desire to **learn** and to **improve the quality of life** in a community.

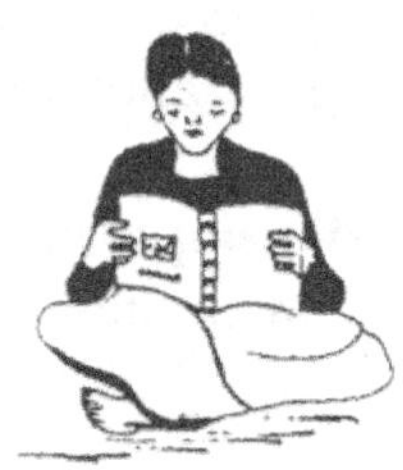

Specifically, this book will address the following issues:

* **Case History:** Asking the right questions to diagnose the problem.

* **Physical Examination:** Using sight, sound, touch, & smell to examine animals.

* **Diagnosis:** Determining what disease is affecting the animal's body.

* **Treatment:** Treating the disease and using, whenever possible, local equipment & medicines.

* **Prevention/Control:** Preventing potential problems.

HOW TO USE THIS BOOK

The book is organized in the same order that an AHA should approach a sick animal;

- know the basics about disease (e.g. infectious/non-infectious, chronic/acute);
- know the basics about the body systems;
- properly restrain and handle livestock;
- take a history and examine the animal and the environment;
- determine whether the animal is sick;
- identify the system(s) of the body affected;
- identify the disease affecting that system;
- treat, control, and prevent the disease.

Thus, the book is primarily organized by systems and the diseases most commonly affecting those systems. By using the table of contents at the beginning of the book, one can turn to the system affected or the disease within that system.

An index at the end lists any subject covered in this book.

The last chapter of the book describes specific medicines and their doses. Brand names are listed in *italics*.

An attempt was made to write in simple (but not childish) English. Nevertheless, some technical words are used and are included in a list of definitions located just before the index. In addition, both the female and male pronouns, "she" and "he" are used alternately from chapter to chapter. In the introduction chapter the pronoun "she" is used. In the first chapter the pronoun, "he" is used, and so on through the book.

Perhaps it is impossible to try to provide useful information for most livestock species of the world! It is important that the information in this book be adapted to the local situation by persons who understand the local customs, language, beliefs, and felt needs - as well as the indigenous knowledge, practices, and medicines available for livestock health.

We (the authors) encourage those persons wishing to use, adapt, and/or translate parts or all of this book for local use to do so, provided it is done not-for-profit. Permission is not necessary. However, we would simply appreciate knowing about it and receiving a copy of your production at the following address: World Concern/Christian Veterinary Mission, 19303 Fremont Avenue North, Seattle, WA 98133.

We would also like to learn from <u>you</u> and enthusiastically welcome any suggestions on how to improve this book.

HEALTHY, PRODUCTIVE ANIMALS - WHOSE RESPONSIBILITY ARE THEY?

Livestock owners and village-based **Animal Health Agents** (AHAs) must take responsibility for the health of their own livestock. No government can do this for them. However, livestock owners and AHAs cannot handle all livestock health problems alone. Some problems require assistance from specially-trained people, such as government extension agents, veterinary technicians, or veterinary doctors. Successful farmers and animal health workers know when to treat a sick animal themselves and when to ask for help.

Know your limits!

Every person working with animals, especially in remote areas, should learn when to treat an animal themselves; and when to ask for help.

EXISTING ANIMAL HEALTH SERVICES

Livestock owners in some areas do not have access to adequate animal health services or supplies, making livestock production difficult and risky. Other factors affecting livestock production include political and environmental instability, as well as inadequate infrastructure. These factors are beyond the control of most local farmers.

Factors Affecting Livestock Production

Inadequate Supplies
- Feed
- Grazing Land
- Equipment, Medicines & Vaccines
- Good Water
- Seeds

Inadequate Infrastructure
- Roads & Transport
- Slaughter facilities
- Meat processing facilities
- Storage Facilities
- Marketing outlets

Instability / Unpredictability
- Political
- Grazing / water laws, rights
- Environmental
- Market Prices

Inadequate Technical Support
- Animal nutritionists
- Forage specialists
- Animal scientists
- Veterinarians

Nevertheless, most countries deliver some level of animal health services to farmers. Countries should also have enforced regulations related to animal production, disease control, and safety of animal products such as meat and milk.

> **Livestock Need Two Kinds of Health Care**
>
> 1. **Curative Care** which is the treatment of sick animals. This usually occurs at a local level.
>
> 2. **Preventive Care** which consists of disease control & prevention activities such as vaccination, worming, dipping, and vitamin & mineral supplementation. This should happen at both the local and national levels.

AHAs and farmers should try to understand the animal health system in their own country and <u>how to access existing services</u>.

Services include **curative care** by which sick animals are treated and **preventive care** by which diseases are prevented or controlled. Preventive care includes vaccinations, parasite control, as well as vitamin and mineral supplementation.

Services may be private or public (i.e. provided by the government). Sometimes farmers organize themselves into cooperatives to pool resources and have a louder voice in the market place and in the government. Even in remote rural areas, services can be developed for the most common animal diseases, especially if these services are integrated into community activities and development programs. **The real challenge is to make services available to <u>all</u> farmers**.

Small-Scale & Remote Farmers Are Often Neglected

Even with adequate resources, good plans, and dedicated AHAs, small-scale farmers or farmers in remote areas may not receive the help they need for various reasons:

1. Farmers may have limited cash, making it difficult for them to purchase medicines or supplies or to support local animal health workers.

2. Services may not reach remote areas due to poor communication, migrating herds, poor transportation, political/economic instability, & natural disasters.

3. Professional workers may prefer to work in or near population centers where they earn more money and life is more convenient.

4. Wealthy or large-scale farmers may control various sectors of the livestock industry such as feed, medicines, marketing outlets, or market prices. This makes it difficult for small-scale farmers to compete.

5. Importation of food aid, food animal products, or by-products may seriously and suddenly alter local market prices.

6. The community or key community leaders may not be sufficiently involved in the planning process for livestock development. Instead, plans are made at more central levels without local input. This results in poor motivation and participation by local, small-scale farmers.

1.0   HEALTH & DISEASE
1.1 HEALTH & DISEASE DEFINED

Which is better?
A cow that gives milk, babies and manure, or a cow that gives only some manure?

Most people prefer manure, milk, and babies! The manure can be used for fuel or spread on the fields to enrich the soil, and the milk used for home consumption or sold for cash. The babies can be sold or raised to pull a plow, carry a load, accumulate wealth, or sold for needed cash. A stronger, healthier animal will produce more work, or sell for more money.

> **Most people want their livestock to provide as many benefits as possible!**

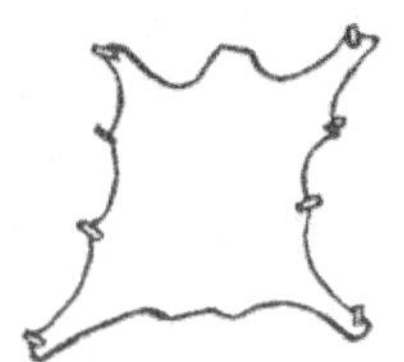

Leather

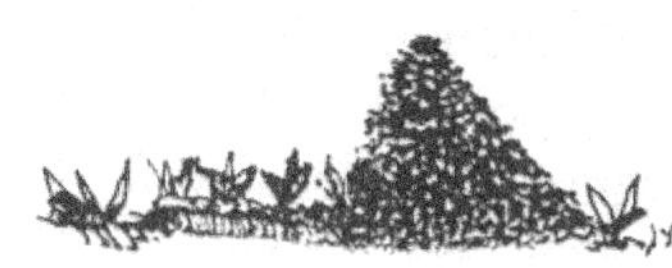

Wool   **Manure for fuel & fertilizer**

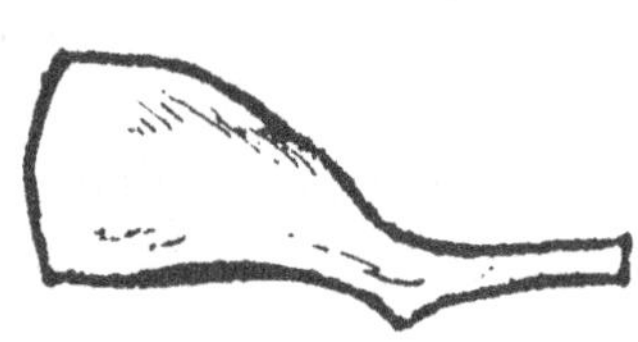

Meat

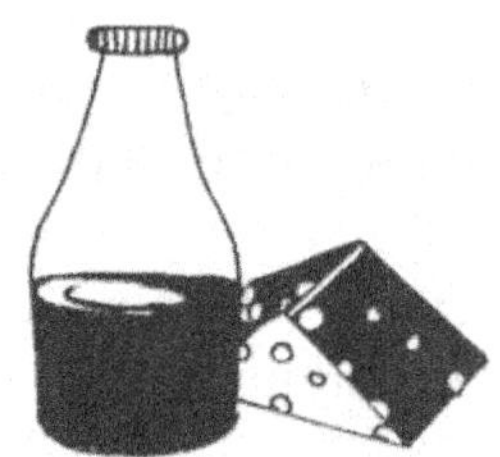

Milk & Cheese

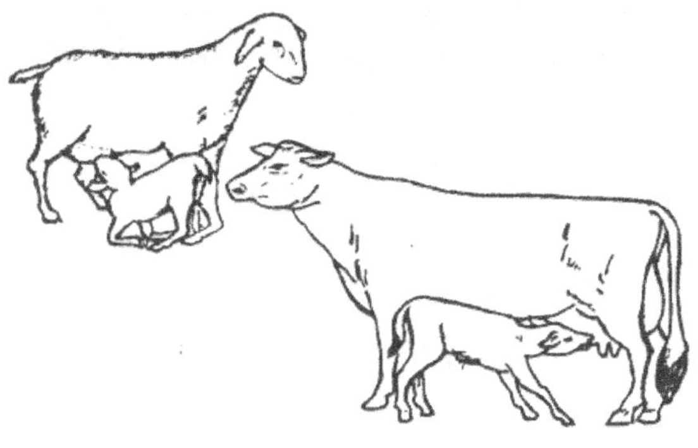

Babies

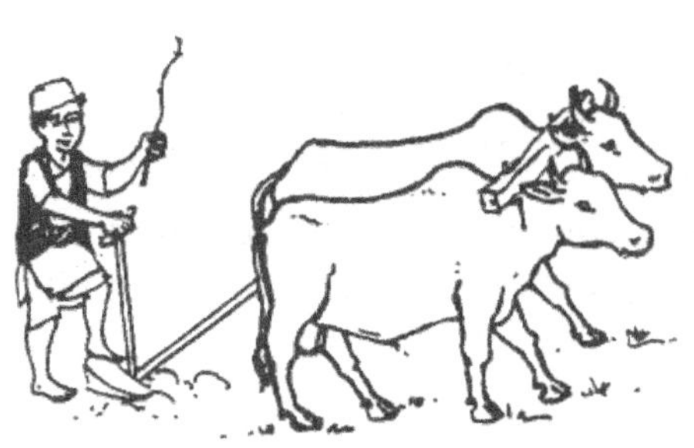

Work

WHAT IS A HEALTHY ANIMAL???

A healthy animal is one that is not sick <u>and</u> brings as much benefit as possible to its owner.

WHAT IS A DISEASED ANIMAL???

A diseased animal is one that is not giving its owner as many benefits as normal.

An animal health agent is concerned with:

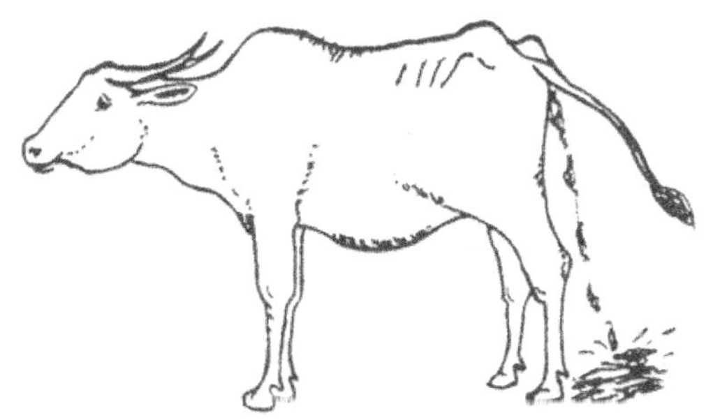

TREATING SICK ANIMALS

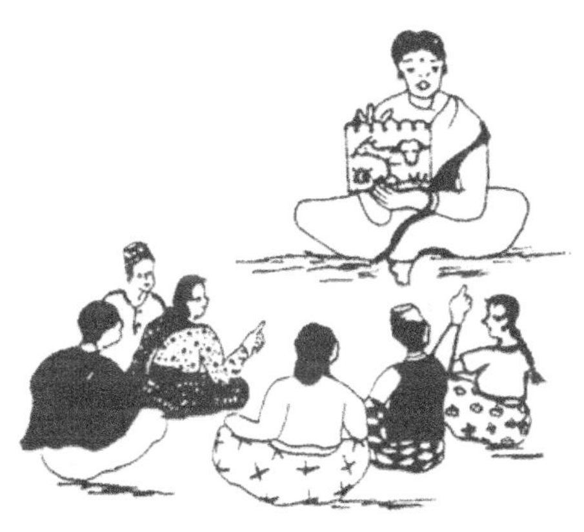

PROMOTING ANIMAL HEALTH

PREVENTING DISEASE

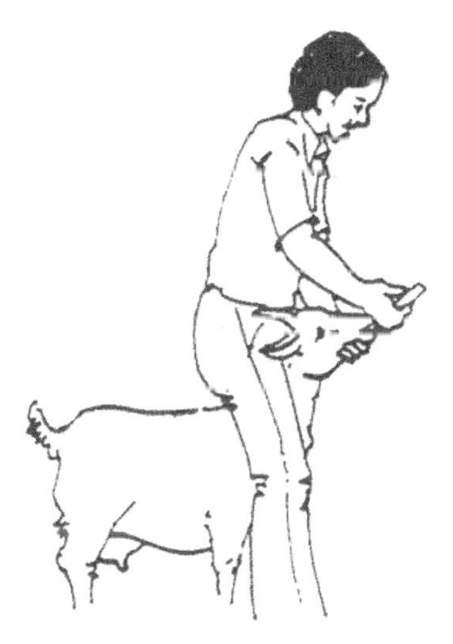

1.2   PREVENTION IS BETTER THAN CURE!

Why?

A sick animal is unable to produce as much meat, milk, manure, or draft power. The lost production plus the expense of treatment cost much more than preventing the disease.

Diseases often slow growth and reduce milk production even after the animal is cured.

Diseases may leave permanent damage.

Diseases may kill the animal and cause a total loss.

Some animal diseases may spread to humans.

Nevertheless, even with the best disease prevention program, **there will always be some sick animals**. Because of this, it is important to also be able to both <u>treat and prevent</u> the most common diseases.

Start with treatment: When starting animal health programs, communities are usually interested <u>more in treatment</u> than prevention. If an AHA can properly treat sick animals, he establishes credibility and the community becomes more receptive to issues of disease prevention! This process takes time. As the community gradually learns more about livestock health, they come to realize that <u>prevention</u> is most important.

Take opportunities to promote prevention: A good animal health agent knows when to quietly treat a sick animal and when to take opportunities to discuss prevention. For instance, while treating a buffalo calf with worms, it is good to discuss parasite control in the farmer's other animals. When treating tetanus in a horse, a good AHA can mention that other horses should be vaccinated against tetanus. A good AHA can even explain to a farmer that children should also receive worm medicine and vaccines, and send the farmer with his children to the nearest human health worker.

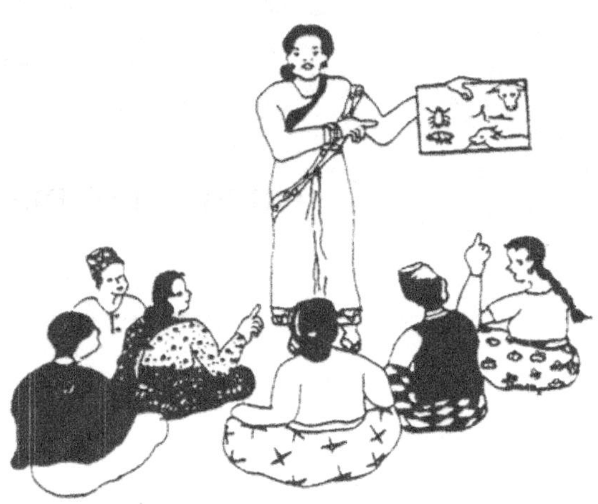

Disease is anything that causes an animal to be less productive than normal.

But what causes disease?

A calf begins to breathe with difficulty and cannot stand up. Why does this happen?

The **local people** say it is because the owner has done something wrong, and the traditional healer must drive out an evil spirit from the calf.

The **livestock advisor** says it is because the calf is kept in a dark, damp pen and does not have fresh air to breathe.

The **veterinary doctor** says it is because the calf has a lung infection.

A **community development Worker** say it is because there is no public grazing land and the calf does not get enough to eat.

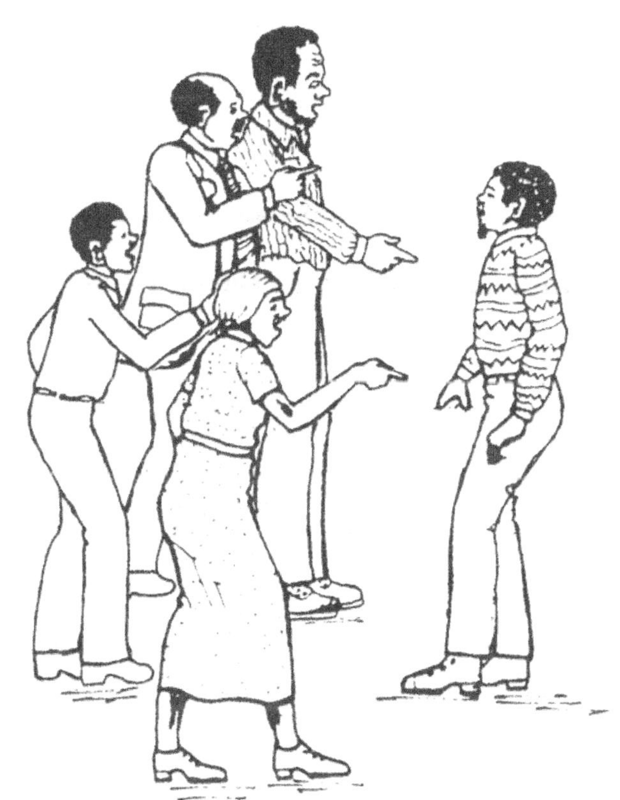

People with different backgrounds and training may have different points of view.

So who is correct? Indeed, several factors were causing sickness in this calf. The calf was sick because it had a lung infection. The calf was probably more prone to getting the lung infection because it was kept in a dark, damp pen with no fresh air and was not getting enough to eat.

> **Remember: Sickness often results from a combination of factors.**

To make good and safe use of this book, please read on....

To make good use of this book, and to safely use the recommended medicines, please read this chapter to help understand some basic principles about disease and their causes.

> Diseases can be divided into groups according to:
>
> the **DURATION** of the disease,
>
> the **SYSTEM** that the disease affects,
>
> and the **CAUSE**.

1.3.1 Distinguishing Diseases Based Upon Their Duration

Duration refers to how quickly the animal became sick, and how long the illness lasts.

Acute Diseases

An acute disease is one that begins <u>rapidly</u> and generally does not last for a long time. Animals with acute diseases should be restored rapidly to health whenever possible; otherwise, the disease may become chronic.

Examples of acute diseases are *Hemorrhagic Septicemia (HS)*, *Erysipelas*, *Anthrax*, and *Foot and Mouth Disease (FMD)*. FMD can also become a chronic disease if the animal is not treated properly and if the feet become infected. The feet may take more than one year to heal.

Chronic Diseases

Chronic diseases last a long time. An animal with a chronic disease fails to produce or grow as it should. Instead it slowly deteriorates until it either dies or slowly recovers, sometimes due to treatment and sometimes on its own. Animals with a chronic disease are weakened and more prone to getting other diseases. Examples of chronic diseases are malnutrition and internal parasites.

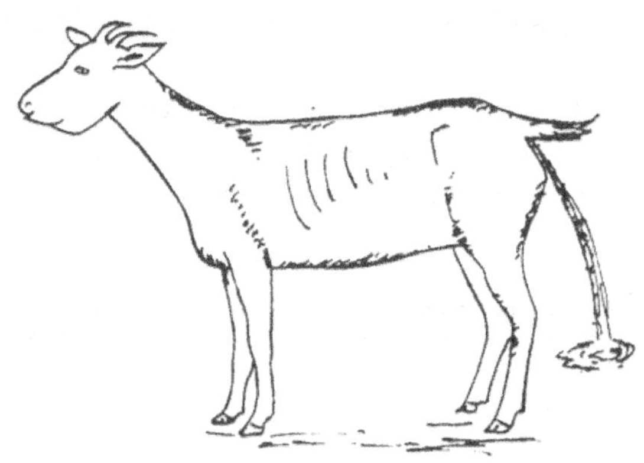

Acute diseases cause financial losses through death of animals, abortions and loss of meat and milk production.

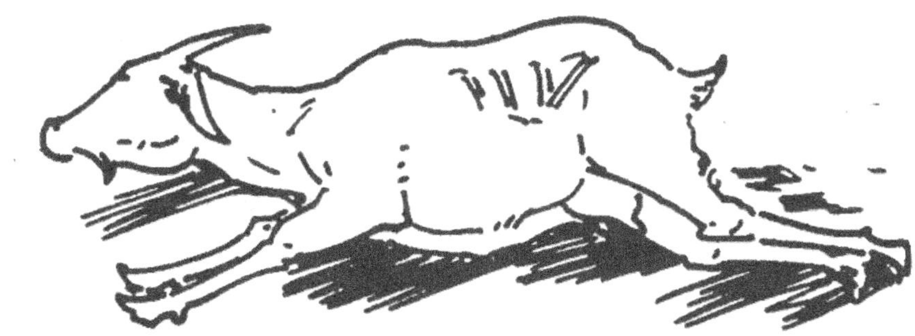

Chronic diseases cause financial loss through a slow, more hidden process of reduced productivity. Less milk is given, the animals grow more slowly and produce less meat, many animals are unable to reproduce, working animals are too weak to work properly, and animals don't live as long as healthy animals do.

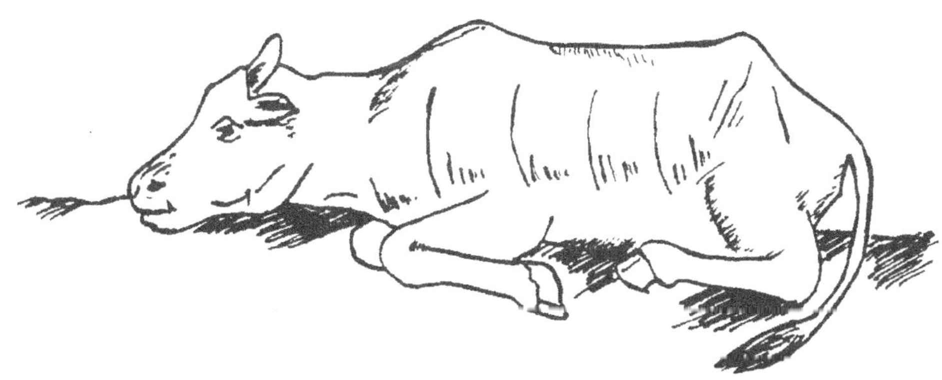

1.3.2 Distinguishing Diseases Based Upon
Which Body System They Affect

An important first step in treating a sick animal is to identify the body system(s) affected. For instance:

This animal has diarrhea. Diarrhea is usually caused by diseases which affect the digestive system. Therefore, the AHA should concentrate on diseases that attack the digestive system.

This animal has fluids running from its nose and it is breathing abnormally. It probably has a disease in its respiratory system. Therefore, the AHA should concentrate on those diseases that attack the respiratory system.

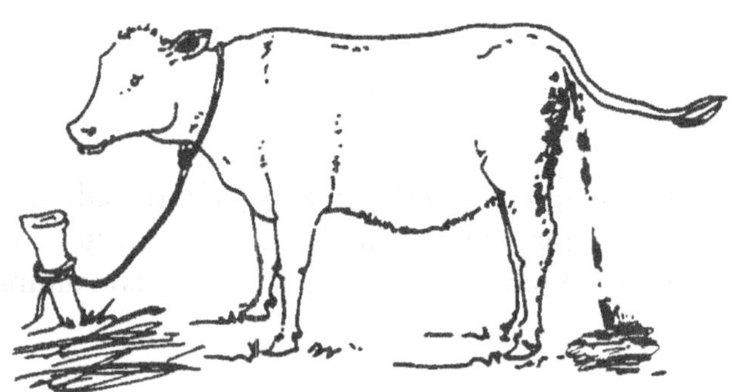 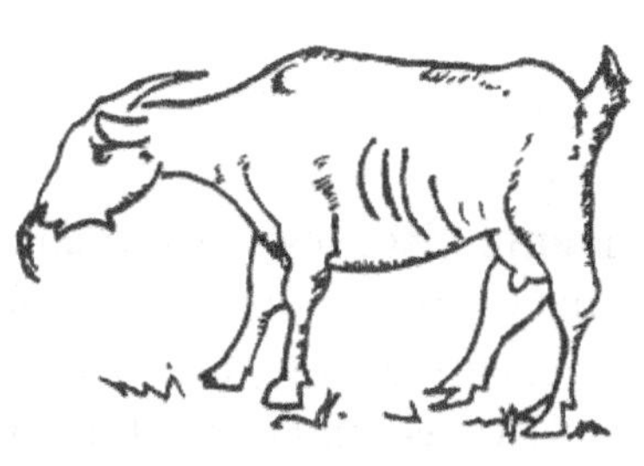

But remember:

Some diseases affect more than one system at a time!

Some animals suffer from more than one disease at a time!

For example, an ox is thin and has diarrhea. It may be suffering from both malnutrition <u>and</u> internal parasites, and must therefore, be treated for both.

For this reason, it is important to thoroughly examine the animal, to try to detect and treat all of its ailments!

1.3.3 Distinguishing Diseases Based Upon Their Cause

Based upon the cause diseases can be divided into two main categories, infectious and non-infectious. Infectious diseases can be divided further into contagious and non-contagious diseases.

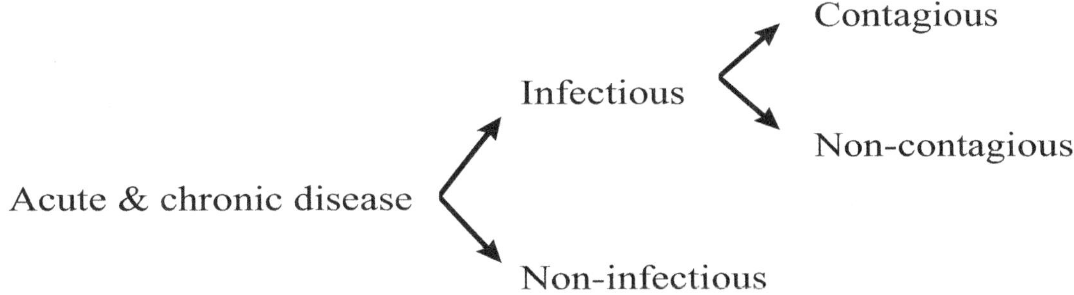

Infectious Diseases

Infectious diseases are caused by living organisms such as bacteria, viruses, and parasites. The living organisms enter the body through the skin or a body opening and cause damage. An animal with an infectious disease is said to have an **infection**.

Some infectious diseases are spread <u>directly</u> from animal to animal. These are called **"contagious"** diseases. Other infectious diseases are not spread <u>directly</u> from animal to animal, and are therefore **"non-contagious"** infectious diseases.

Examples of <u>contagious</u> diseases:
Rinderpest spreads directly from one animal to another through the saliva.
Hemorrhagic Septicemia is spread through the saliva and nasal discharge.
Mange Mites are often spread directly by physical contact.

Examples of non-contagious diseases:
The **tetanus** organism is found in the soil and animal manure. If soil or manure containing this organism gets into a wound, then tetanus may result.
A **liver fluke** must first pass through a snail before it can infect a new animal.

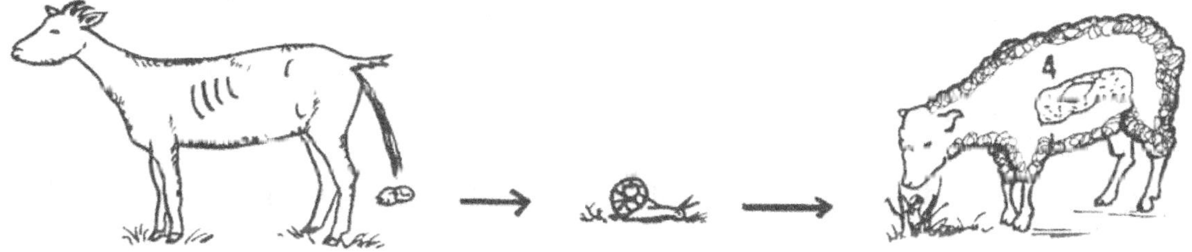

Zoonotic Diseases are infectious diseases (contagious or non-contagious) that infect both man and animals (e.g. rabies)

Non-infectious Diseases

Non-infectious diseases are <u>not</u> caused by living organisms and do not spread from one animal to another.

Examples of non-infectious diseases:
Malnutrition
Malfunction of body parts (such as heart problems, cancer, ulcers, arthritis)
Injuries or inflammation (broken bones, wounds, ulcers, arthritis)
Allergies
Toxins (poisons)

Why is it important to distinguish between infectious and non-infectious?
Many villagers demand an injection for their sick animal, regardless of the cause. However, it is useless to treat a non-infectious disease like poor nutrition with an expensive injection that is made for infectious diseases. An AHA must gently explain and persuade villagers that it is a waste of money and medicine, both of which may be in short supply!

> An AHA must know the difference between infectious and non-infectious diseases to properly treat sick animals!!

Summary of this chapter

Classification of Diseases

Decide if a disease is *chronic or acute*
Remember:
Chronic diseases last a long time and often require a long time for recovery.
Acute diseases begin rapidly and result in rapid recovery, death or chronic disease.

Decide *which body system* is affected
Remember:
More than one body system can be affected simultaneously, so do a <u>thorough</u> examination!

Determine whether the disease is *infectious or non-infectious*.
Remember:
Acute and chronic disease can be either <u>infectious</u> or <u>non-infectious</u>.
Infectious diseases can be <u>contagious</u> or <u>non-contagious</u>.
A <u>zoonotic disease</u> is an infectious disease (contagious or non-contagious) which people and animals share.

2.0　Restraint & Handling, Aging and Weight
2.1 RESTRAINT & HANDLING OF LIVESTOCK

Working with livestock can be dangerous. However, livestock that are treated gently and handled frequently from the time they are babies are usually more tame.

> **CAUTION!**
> **Any animal can be dangerous when it is frightened, excited, hungry or in pain.**
>
> **Be especially careful around mothers with babies and adult males during mating season.**

There are many local methods of holding and tying livestock. This chapter explains some of the most common methods.

How to Tie a Fixed Knot:

Tying knots around the necks of animals can be dangerous. If the knot becomes tight and the animal begins to struggle, it may be impossible to untie the knot quickly, and the animal may suffocate. The following knot, called a "bowline," can be tied quickly and is a fixed knot so it will not tighten when it is pulled.

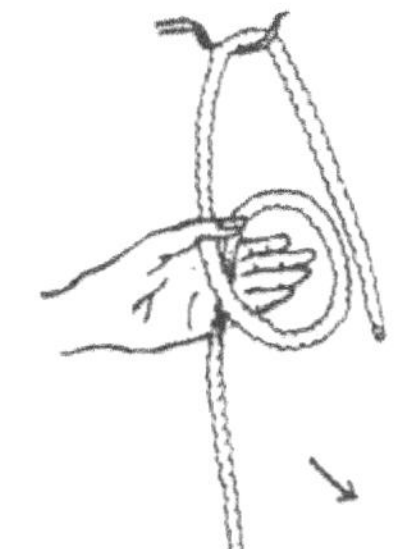 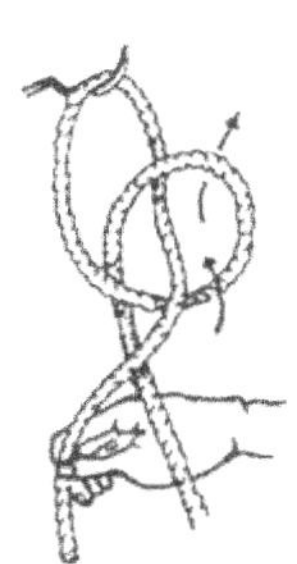 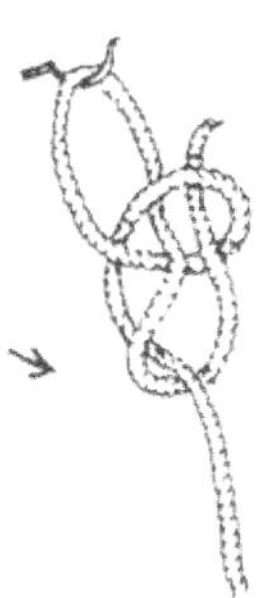 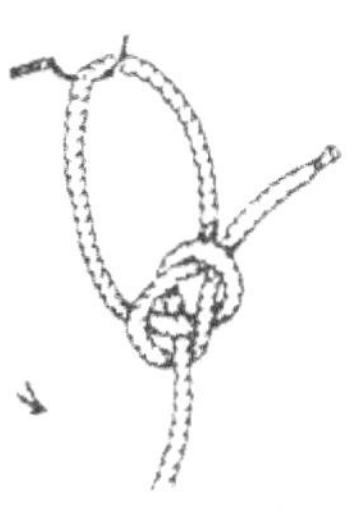

How to Tie a Quick Release Knot:

A quick release knot is one that can be quickly untied if an animal struggles or becomes tangled.

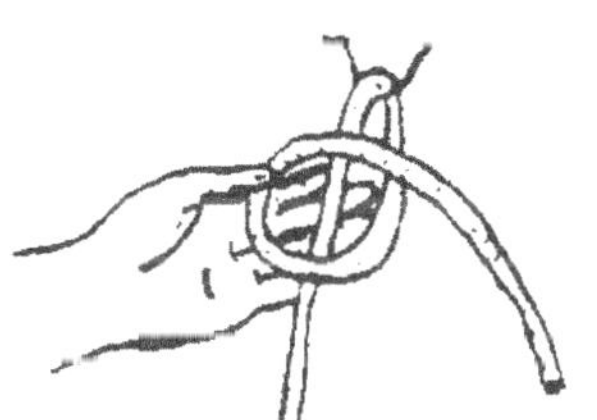 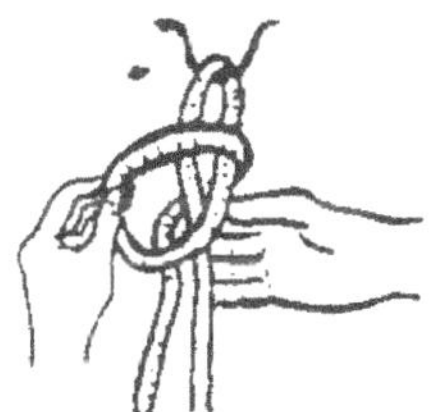 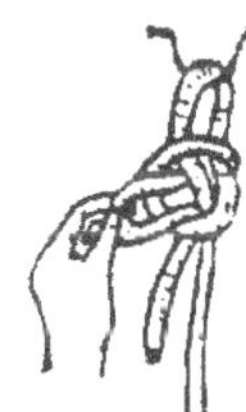

CATTLE AND BUFFALO

A person is more likely to become injured when treating a large, strong animal in a small space. It is better to treat animals in open areas where there is light to see and enough room to avoid being kicked or hit.

Making a halter

- Tie a fixed knot on the animal's neck.
- Make a loop in the free end, pass this loop through the neck loop and slip it over the muzzle.

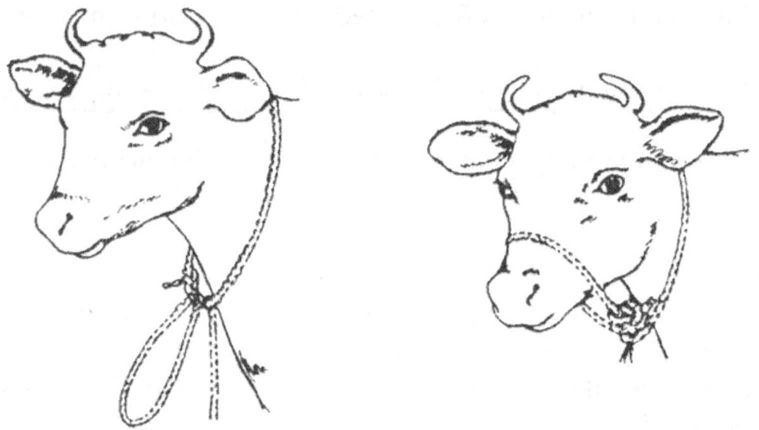

Making a tail tie

Tail ties are useful, especially when working alone, to hold the tail out of the way.

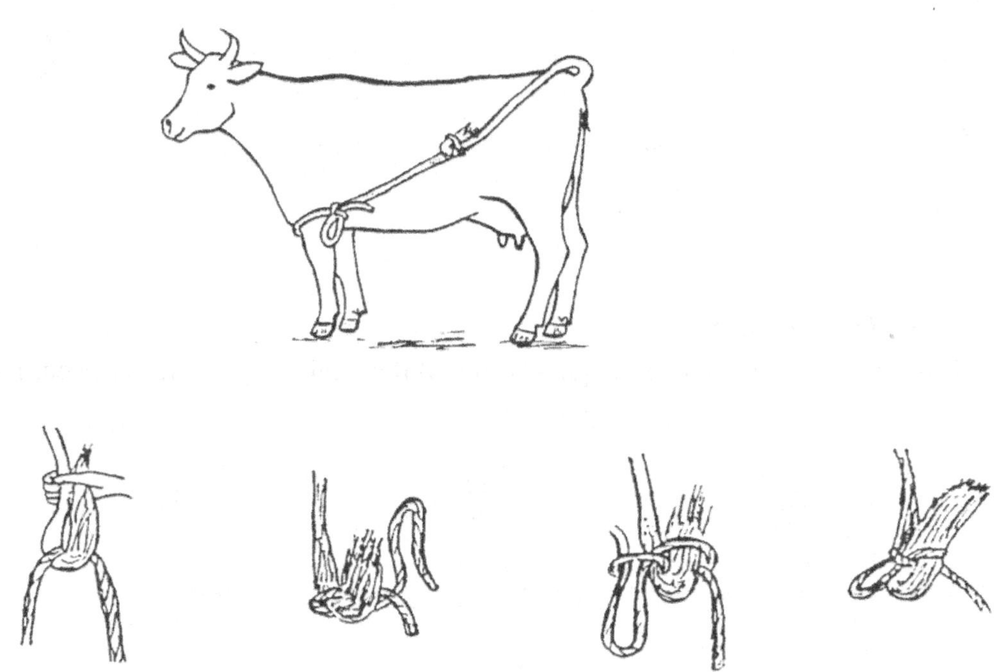

Control by the Nose

Since the noses of cattle and buffalo are sensitive, these animals can be restrained by controlling their nose.

Nose Rings

When a hole is made in the nose and a metal or rope ring is put through the hole, the animal can be restrained by grabbing the nose ring or attaching other ropes, chains or sticks to it.

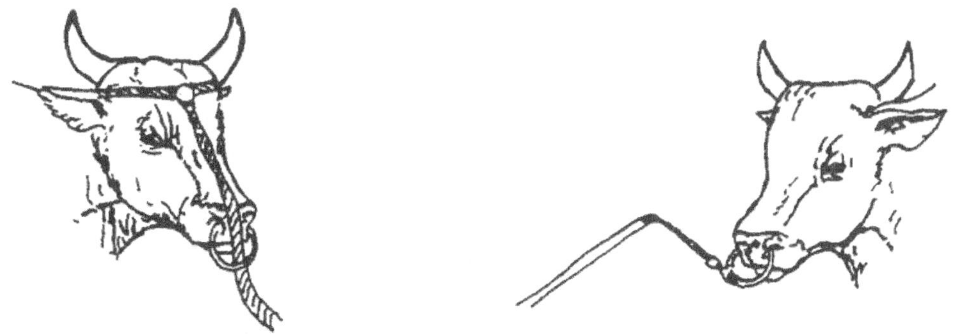

Grabbing the nose with fingers or nose holders

The nose can also be grabbed by hand or with special nose holders. Additional restraint is achieved by lifting the tail up.

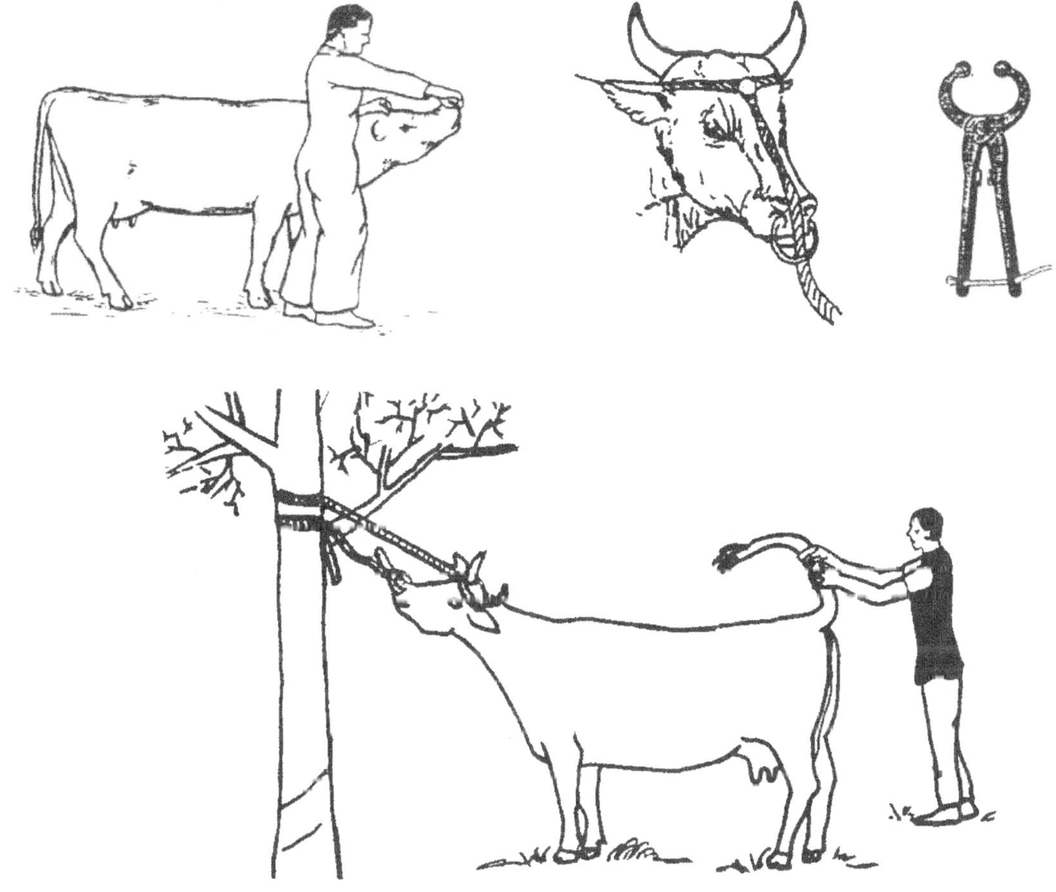

If animals are to be examined, treated, and vaccinated regularly in one place; then it is worthwhile to build a simple crate. A crate should be built on dry, flat ground using local materials such as bamboo or wood. If there is any gradient, animals should enter the crate going <u>uphill</u>. There should be space around the crate for examining all parts of the animal.

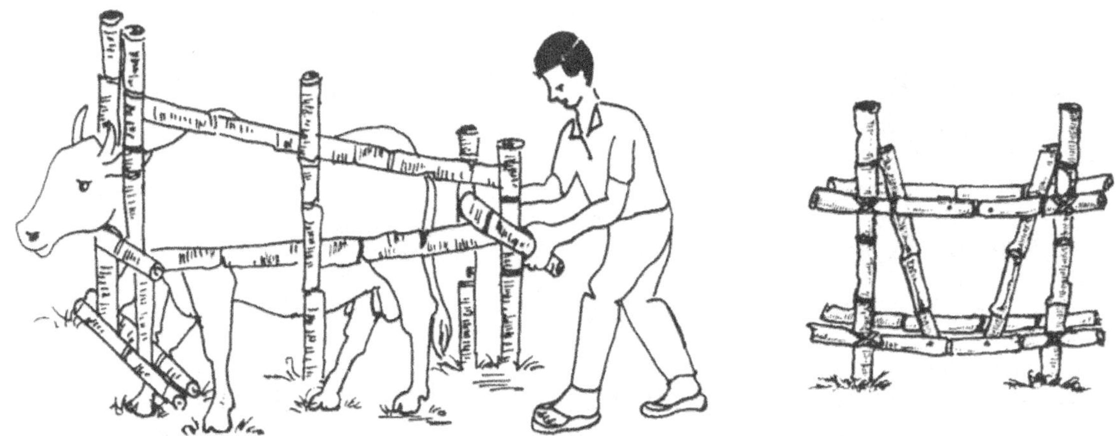

Note: The posts should be sunk <u>at least</u> 60 cm into the ground and preferably one meter to withstand a big, strong animal. If the crate is only for cows or oxen, it can be smaller in size. If it is only for buffalo, it should be bigger in size.

If no crate is available, cattle and buffalo can be tied between two strong posts or trees placed three feet apart. Tie the ropes low to the ground.

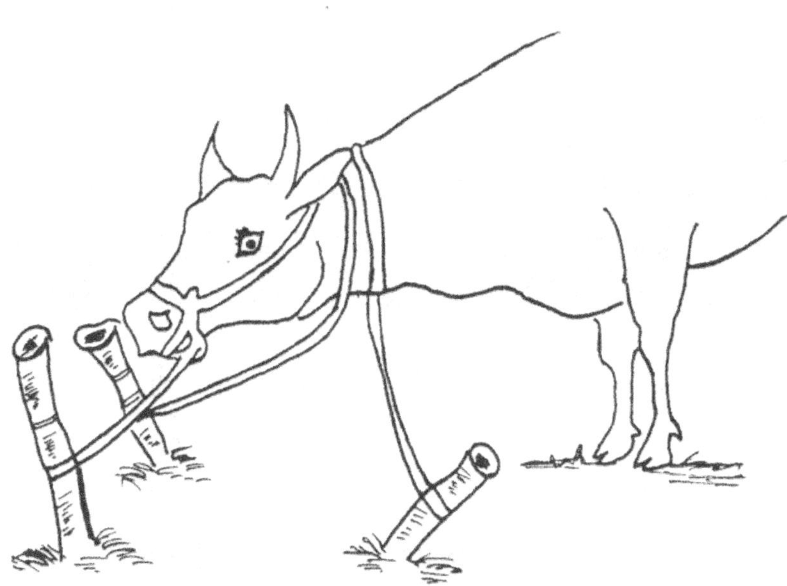

To prevent kicking

Cattle tend to hit with their heads and to kick, particularly to the side, whereas buffalo tend to hit only with their heads. There are many methods of tying cattle legs and feet, to keep them from kicking.

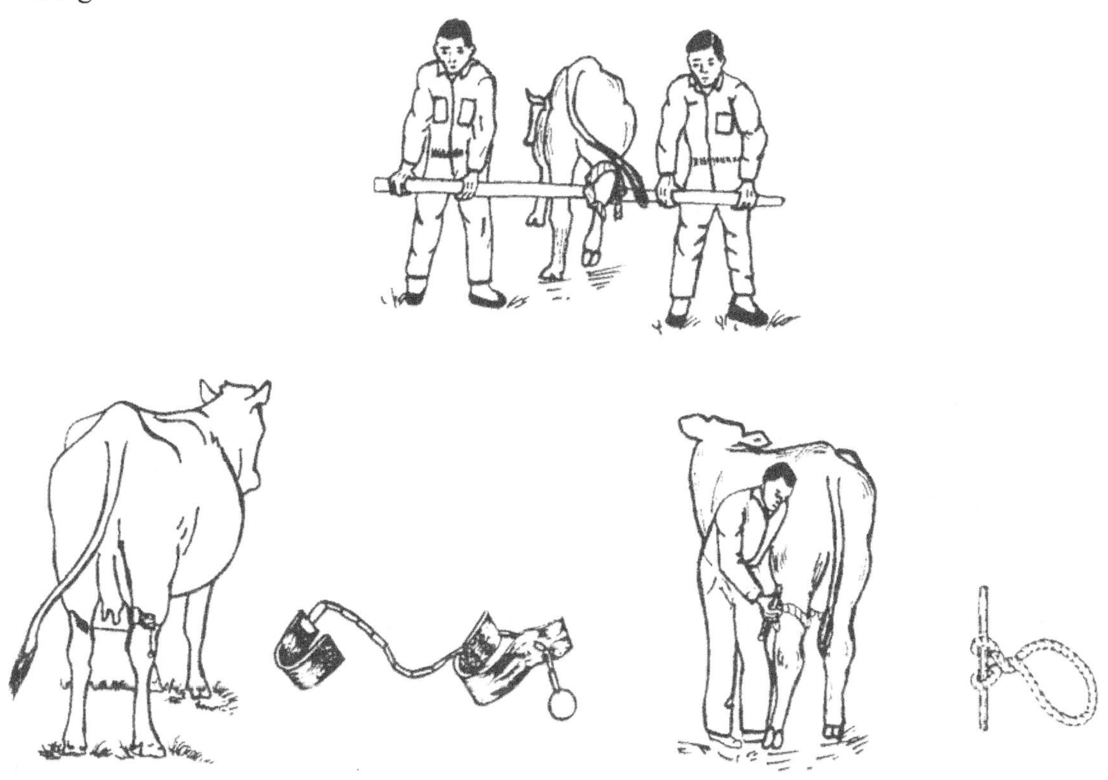

To lift a leg

There are several clever ways to lift front and back legs, in order to prevent kicking.

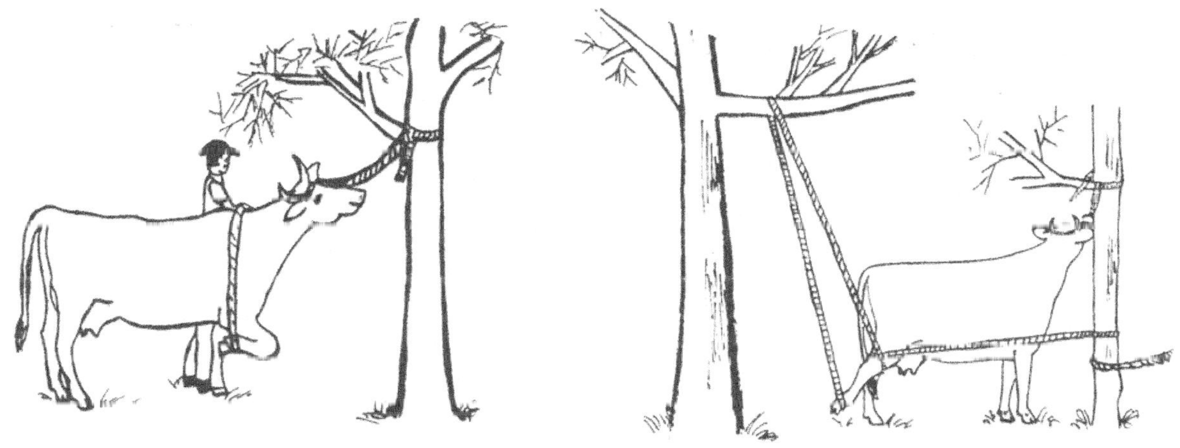

If no crate is available and/or an animal is difficult to control, the animal should be forced to lie down using ropes. This process is called "casting." Regardless of the method, you will need the following to cast an animal:

- The ground should be fairly level and soft - without rocks or sticks that could injure an animal when it falls down.

- A short rope or halter is needed to hold the head.

- A soft rope is also needed which is at least 12-15 meters long (35 feet). The rope should be at least the width of your finger. Nylon ropes, although strong, are not ideal because they can wound the skin. Cotton ropes are ideal.

- At least two to three people are needed. One person will be needed to jump on the animal as soon as it lies down, and hold down its head. At least one strong person (preferably two or three) will be needed to pull on the rope.

The Two-Loop Method for Adult Cattle and Buffalo

1. Using the short rope and a fixed knot, tie the animal's head or horns to a strong post or tree. The rope should be tied at the base of the post or tree - i.e. near the ground, otherwise you will "hang" the animal.

2. Pass a long rope around the animal's neck and tie a bowline knot - i.e. a knot that does not tighten once it is tied.

3. A person standing on the left side of the animal should pass the free end of the rope over the back of the animal, to another person standing on the right side of the animal. This second person should pass the rope back under the animal's body to the person on the left hand side, completing a loop around the animal's chest (just behind the front legs).

4. Pass the rope around the animal's body again and back over the top to make a second loop around the body, just in front of the hip bones.

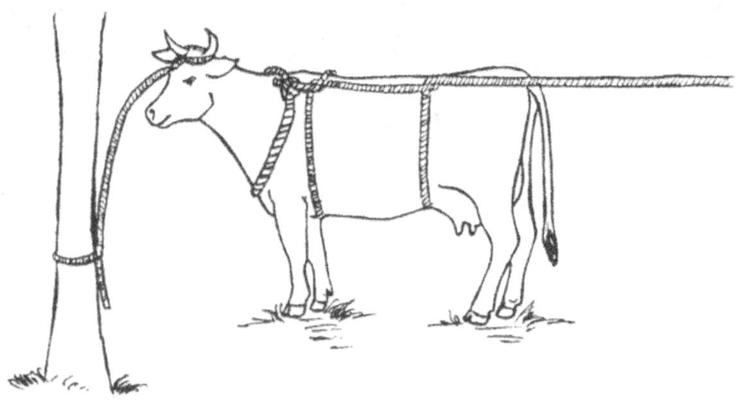

5.   Have one or two people pull on the free end of the rope and the animal should lie down.

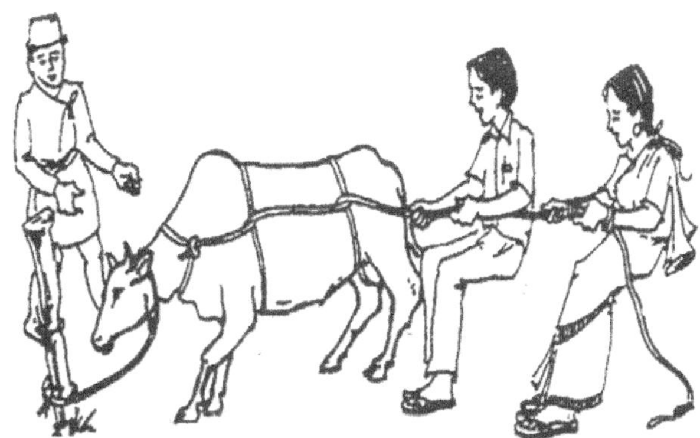

6.   Once on the ground, the animal's head and neck must be held firmly to the ground.
        If its head is held firmly, the animal cannot stand up and will usually stop struggling.

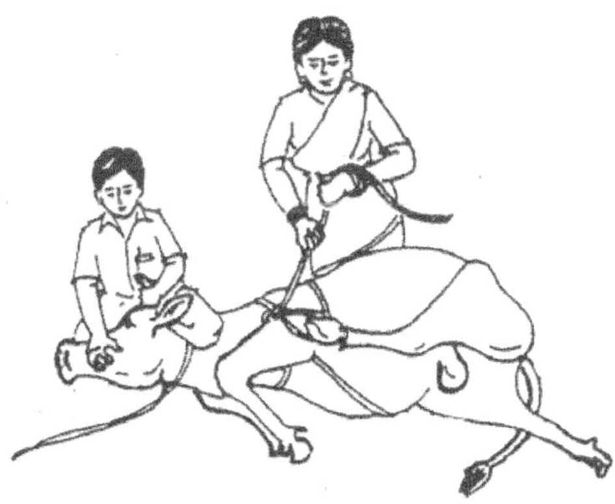

7.   Once the animal is lying down, the legs can be tied together using several methods.
        This will prevent kicking and will make castration or examination of the udder much
        easier.

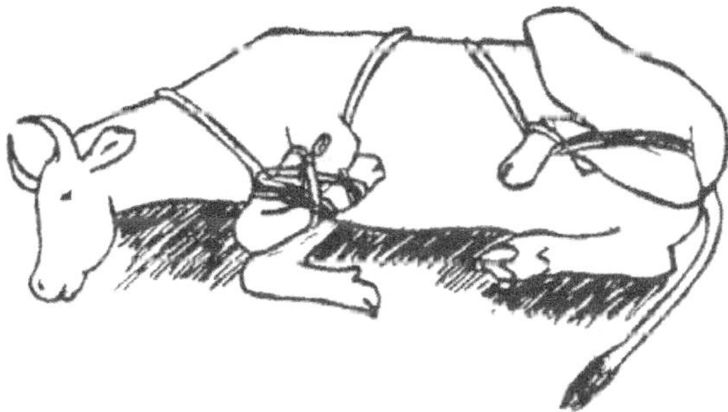

Method for tying large cattle

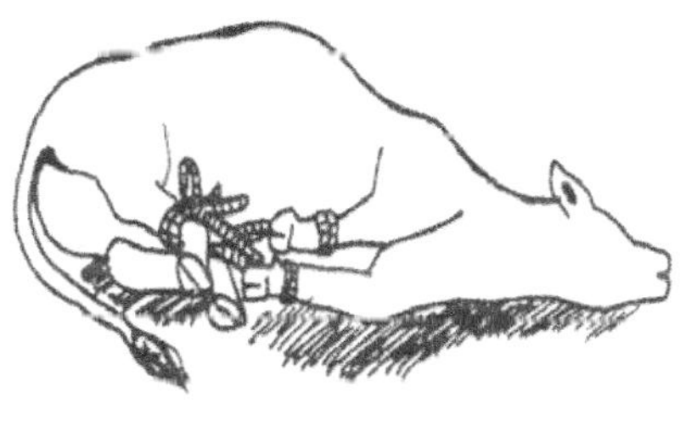

Method for tying a calf

The Criss-Cross Method for Adult Cattle and Buffalo
For some cattle, this method works better because it does not pinch either the udder or the penis of the animal. Using the short rope, tie the animal's head as described above.

1.	Fold the long rope in half.

2.	Place the middle of the rope over the neck.

3.	Cross the ends under the neck.

4.	Pass the ends of the rope back inside the front legs, up over the back and cross them again.

5.	Pass both ends of the rope down the sides of the animal and inside (between) the back legs.

6.	Pull both ends of the rope to force the animal to lie down.
7.	Once again, it is important to tie the legs securely to prevent the animal from kicking and attempting to get up.

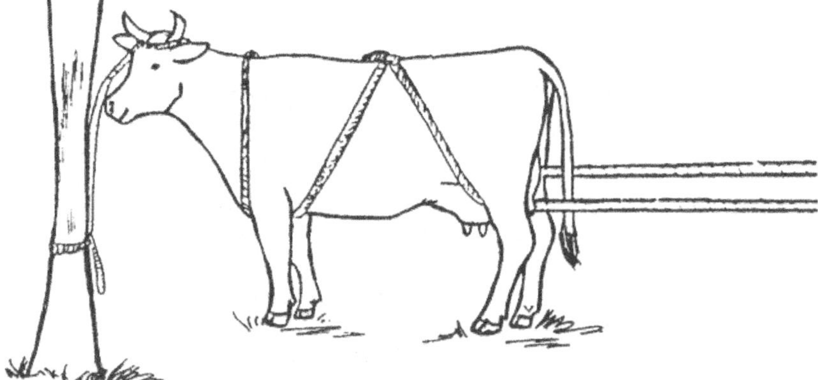

CALVES

Calves which are light enough to lift off the ground can be easily laid on their side.

1.	Stand on the left side of the calf.
2.	Hold it under the throat with your left hand.
3.	Hold the skin in front of the hind leg with your right hand.
4.	Lift the calf using your right knee and right arm.
5.	Slide it to the ground down your right leg.
6.	Kneel firmly on its neck with your left knee just behind its ear.

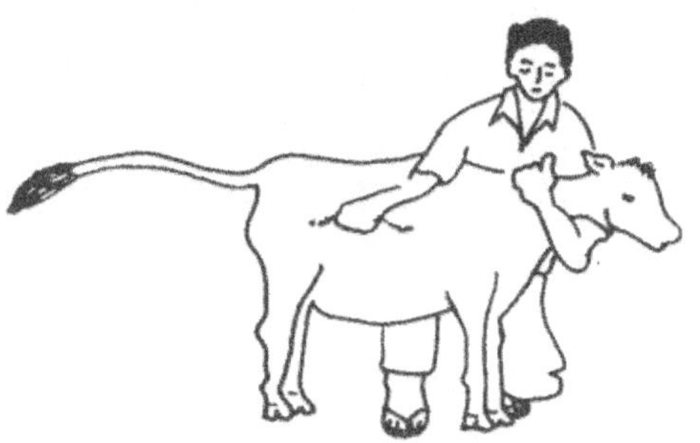

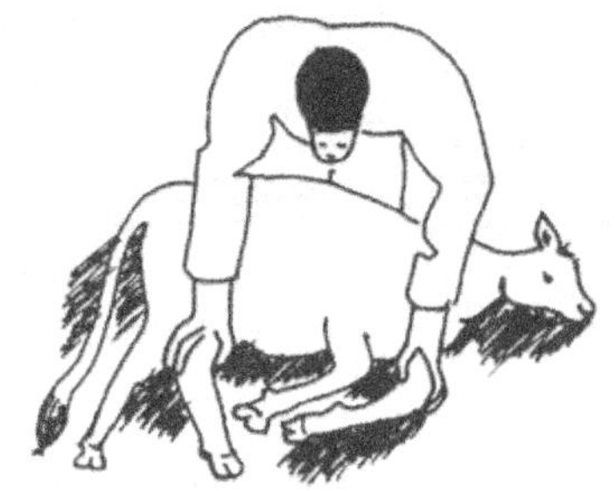

HORSES, MULES, & BURROS

Horses, mules and burros can seriously injure people who are unaccustomed to handling them or are not careful. Unlike cows, they can **strike with both front and hind feet**. Whereas cows usually kick to the side, horses usually kick straight back with their hind feet.

It is better to handle horses, mules and burros in an open area instead of a crate since they are more prone to panic and struggle. The key to handling horses is to make slow, deliberate movements around them and avoid surprising them with sudden noises or gestures, or by suddenly approaching or poking them. Horses do not see well, particularly straight in front of them, so approach them from the side. Talk quietly while working so they know where you are at all times.

Halter

Gentle horses, mules and burros can be restrained using a halter <u>with a rope attached to it</u> to control the animal's head.

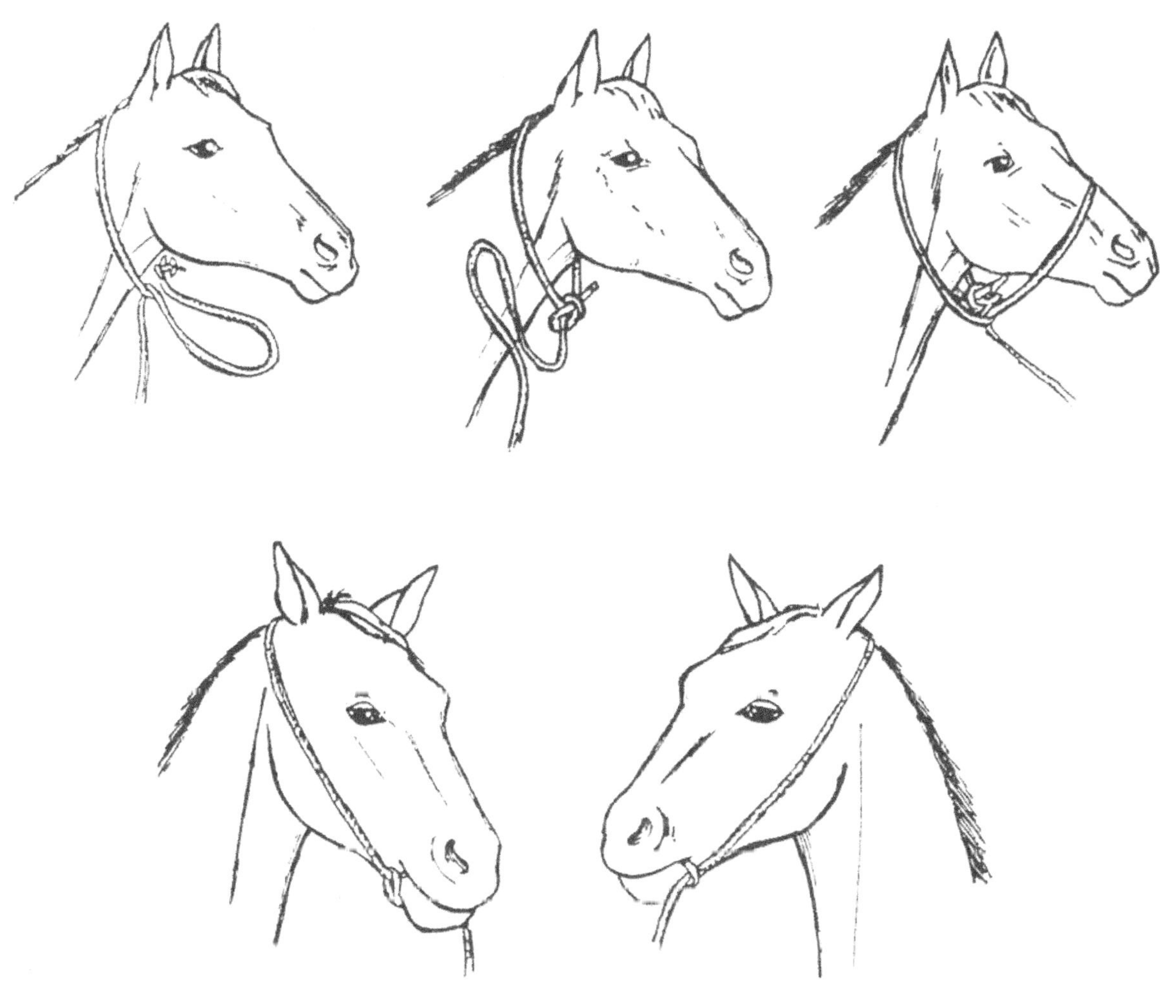

Twitching

Horses, mules or burros that are nervous, which will not hold still or are likely to react during a certain procedure or treatment, can be restrained using a "twitch." A twitch can be made with small loop, made of rope or chain, attached to the end of a stick. When placing a twitch on a horse, mule or burro, <u>always</u> stand to the side of the animal's head <u>and never directly in front of it</u> to avoid being struck by its front feet. Place the loop around the upper lip and twist the stick until the loop tightens. Do this slowly and deliberately to minimize a bad reaction. Once it is tight, the horse, mule or burro is usually well restrained. Stay to the side of the animal at all times while using the twitch.

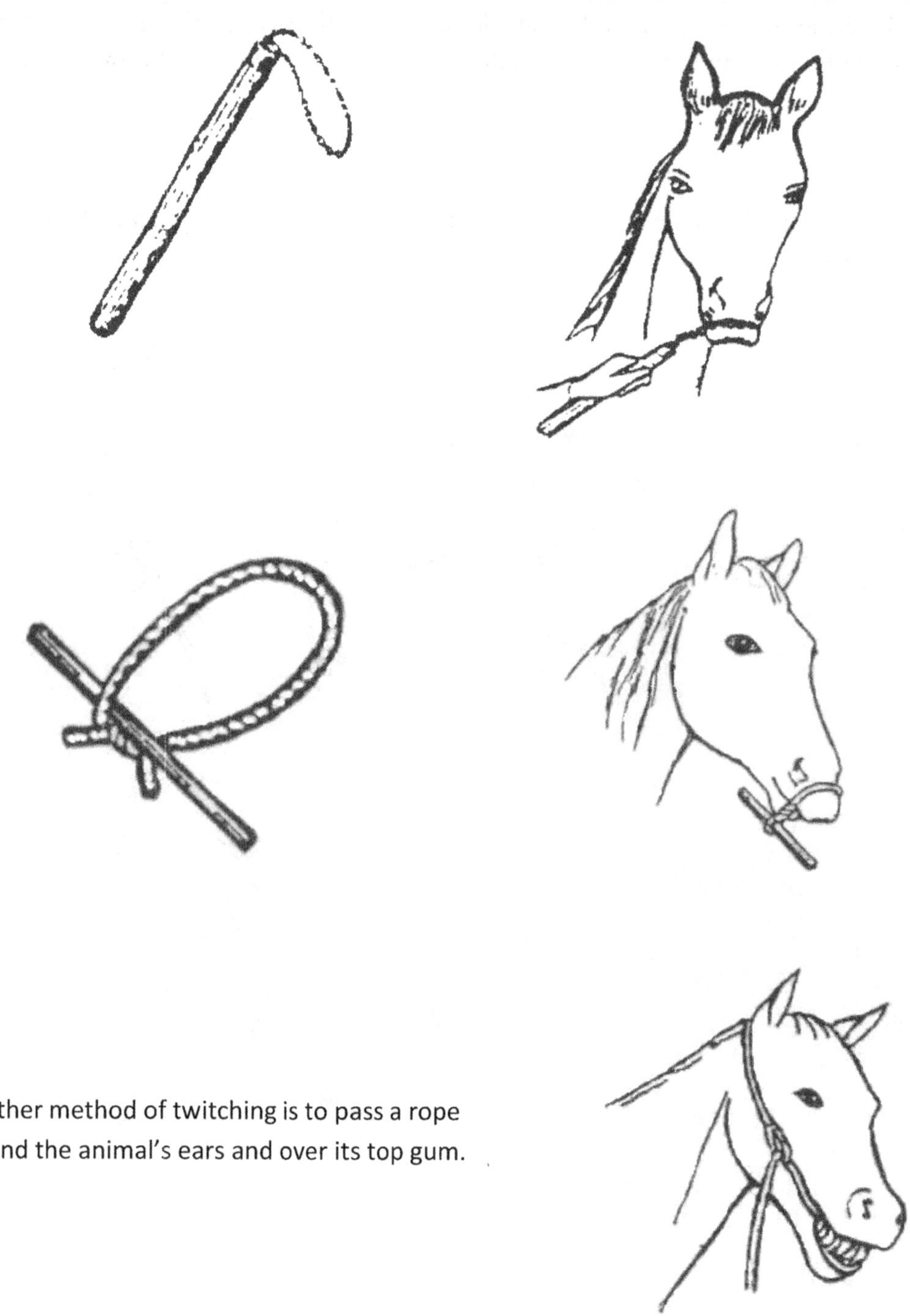

Another method of twitching is to pass a rope
behind the animal's ears and over its top gum.

Casting A Horse

For some procedures, like castrations, it is necessary to cast a horse and tie its legs. Use a soft cotton rope (if possible) at least 15 meters long and one finger-width in diameter.

1. Tie the horse to a strong post with a short rope attached to its halter or around its neck using a bowline (i.e. non-slip) knot. Tie the rope low on the post, near the ground.

2. Take the long rope and tie the middle portion of the rope around the neck of the horse, using a non-slip knot. The rope should be fairly low on the neck, near the chest.

3. Pass each of the two free-ends of the rope along the sides of the horse's body.

4. Pass these ends on towards the back of the horse and make a loop around each hind leg, just above the hoof. Some owners prefer to wrap a rag, towel or leather band around the back legs before casting to avoid rope burns.

5. Pass the free ends of the rope up alongside the body, and then slip the ends of the rope under the rope that is around the neck.

6. Pass the ends of the rope towards the back of the animal.

7. Have two or more people pull on the ropes until the horse "sits down." Then roll the horse onto one side.

8. Have another strong person immediately grab the head and hold it firmly against the ground. The horse cannot stand up when its head is held on the ground.

9. The rear legs of the horse should be tied firmly in place, wrapping the ropes thoroughly around the hock (knee) and fetlock (ankle). The rear legs can be pulled forward along the horse's side or tied to the front legs.

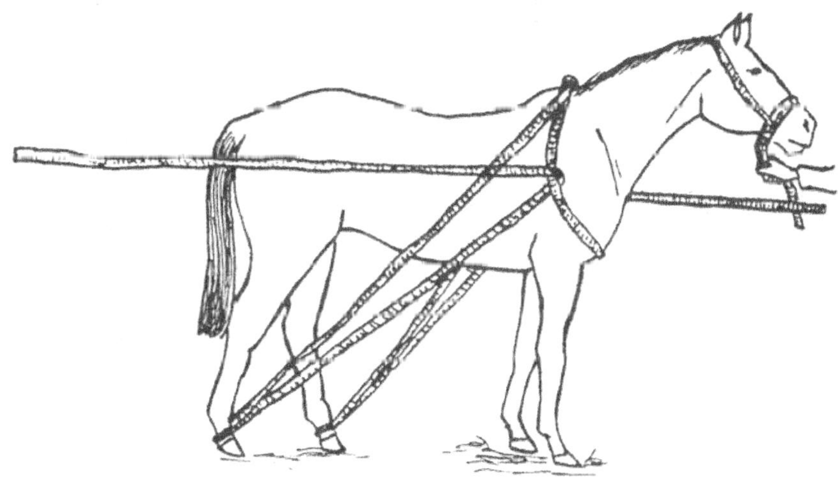

SHEEP AND GOATS

Sheep and goats are easier to handle due to their smaller size. As with other animals, sheep and goats should be handled as gently as possible. Too much stress from rough handling can kill a goat or sheep.

Feeding medicine to sheep, goats, & small calves

1. Hold on to the head, and back the sheep, goat or calf into a corner.

2. Continue holding the head and straddle the animal's neck such that the back of your knees are in front of the sheep's shoulders. Once your legs are blocking the animal's shoulders (so it can't move forward), your hands are free to work.

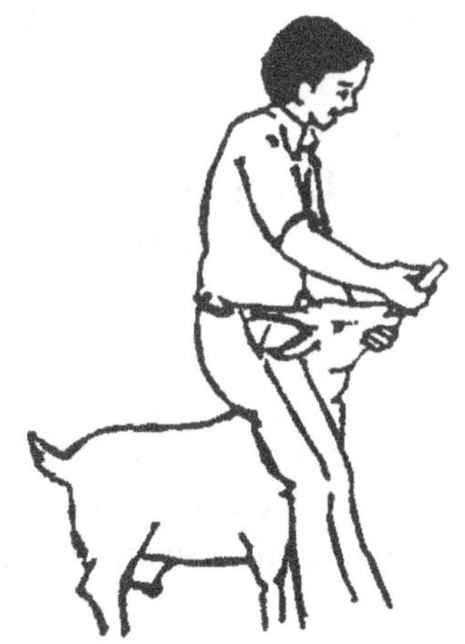

Another method of restraining sheep and small goats
(This method is not for large goats).

1. While on the left side of the sheep, place your left hand under the jaw of the sheep and your right hand behind the sheep to keep it from going backwards.

2. With your right hand, grasp the fold of skin directly in front of the rear leg.

3. Lift the front of the sheep off the ground, mostly with your left arm, and, with the help of your right arm, place the sheep's rump in a sitting position on the ground.

4. Hold the sheep between your legs in a sitting position. As long as it cannot place its feet firmly on the ground, it cannot get up and it usually will not struggle to get up.

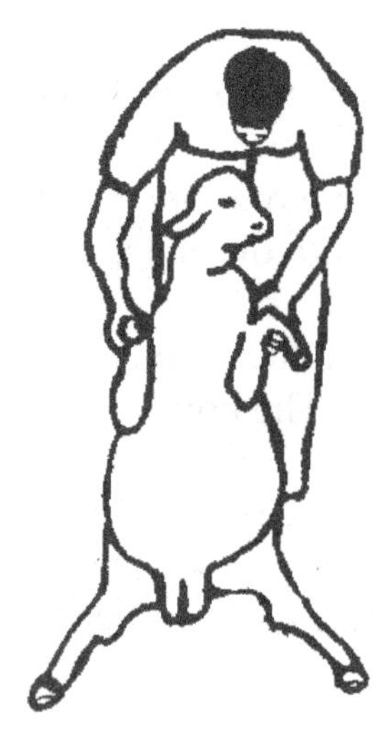

Note: For fat-tailed sheep, lean them to one side.

For large, gentle goats
Larger goats, particularly dairy goats that are accustomed to being handled, can often be restrained by simply holding their head firmly. Sometimes lifting one of their front legs also helps to restrain them.

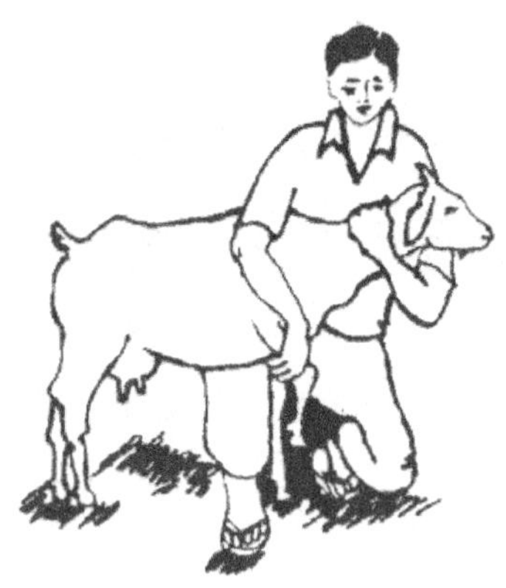

PIGS

Mother pigs (sows with babies) and adult males (boars) are unpredictable and often dangerous since they may attack and bite when they are upset or protecting their babies.

Handle pigs as gently as possible, particularly in hot weather. Pigs of all ages can overheat if they struggle, and can even die from heat stress. If boars overheat, they can be sterile for several months. Sows easily overheat when giving birth. In hot weather, pigs should be handled during the coolest parts of the day, that is, early morning or evening.

Small and Medium-Sized Pigs: (for castration)

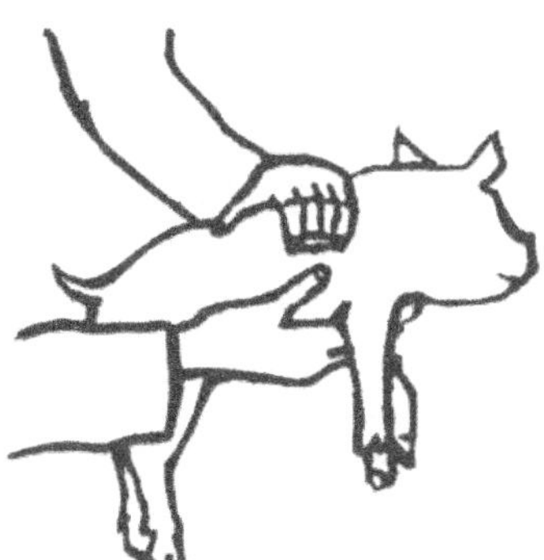

1. While standing behind the pig, grab one or both hind legs, or with both hands grab the pig just behind the shoulders.
2. Hold it by its hind legs so that it hangs down with its belly facing away from you.
3. Steady the pig by holding its shoulders between your knees. See castration, page 173.

Restraining Big Pigs Using a Rope or Snare

Ropes and snares are used for larger pigs. A snare keeps the pig more at a distance. When using a rope, it must be at least ten feet long and the diameter of your finger. The rope should have an "eye" on one end, and the free end of the rope should be passed through the eye to make a loop. Approach the pig from behind and place the loop over the pig's snout and into its mouth. Move the rope behind the large canine teeth and tighten the loop. Tie the rope securely to a tree or post. For maximum restraint, tie the rope to the root of a tree, or low down, so the pig's snout is touching the ground. A snare can be used in the same manner except that it cannot be tied to a tree or post.

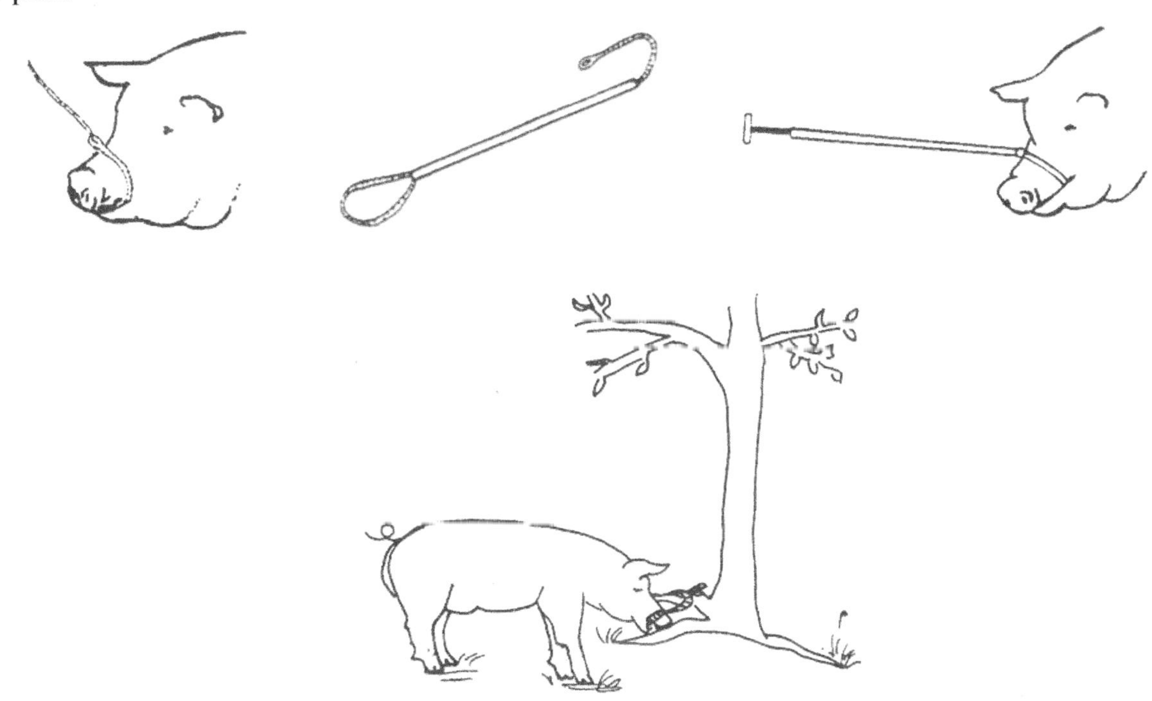

Method of moving a large pig using a bucket:
Pigs will usually back up when they cannot see ahead. Place a bucket on their head and guide them by pulling on their tail.

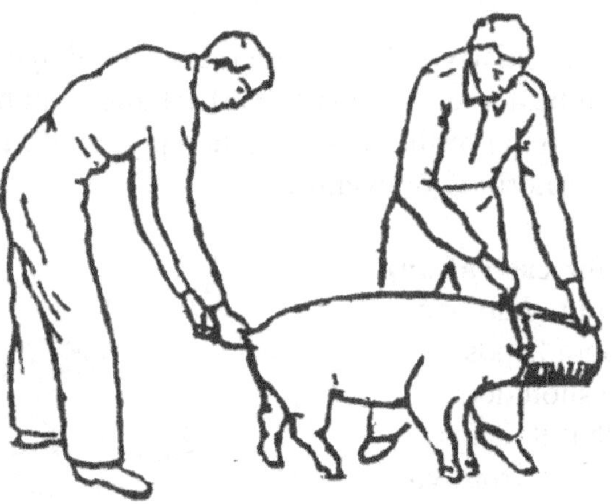

Methods of safely tying pigs so they cannot slip out of a rope or suffocate by strangling.

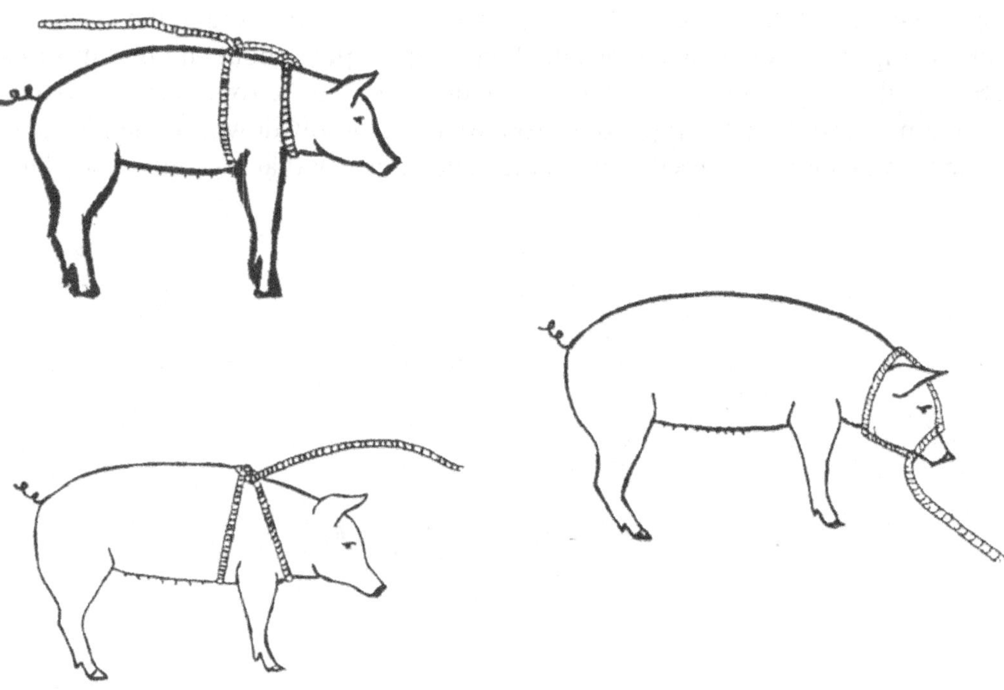

RABBITS

- Grasp the rabbit gently by the loose skin on the back of its neck.

- Lift it up, immediately grab the back legs (to prevent it from scratching you) and support its back end so the rabbit feels secure.

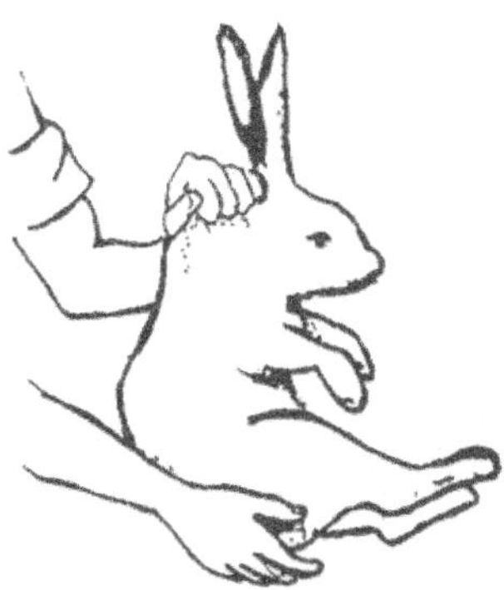

- After catching the rabbit, the rabbit can be tucked gently under your arm in order to restrain it. This is a common method of restraint when determining its sex.

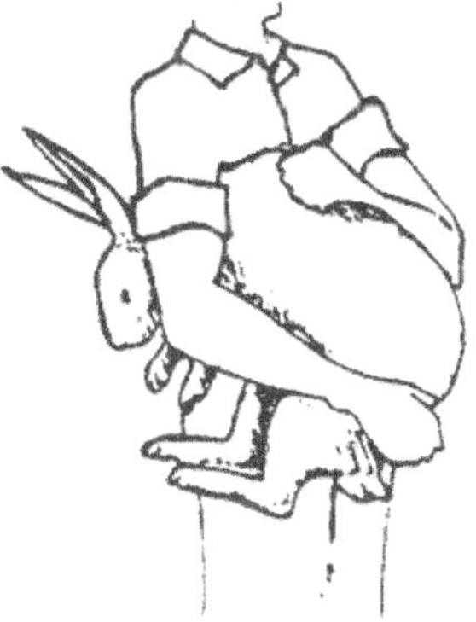

A rabbit must not be picked up by its ears, because it might struggle & break its back.

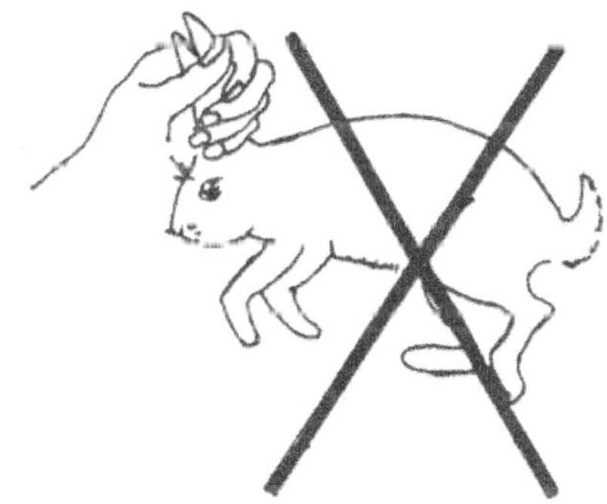

CHICKENS

To handle its head, sit the bird's breast on the palm of your hand and hold the legs between your fingers.

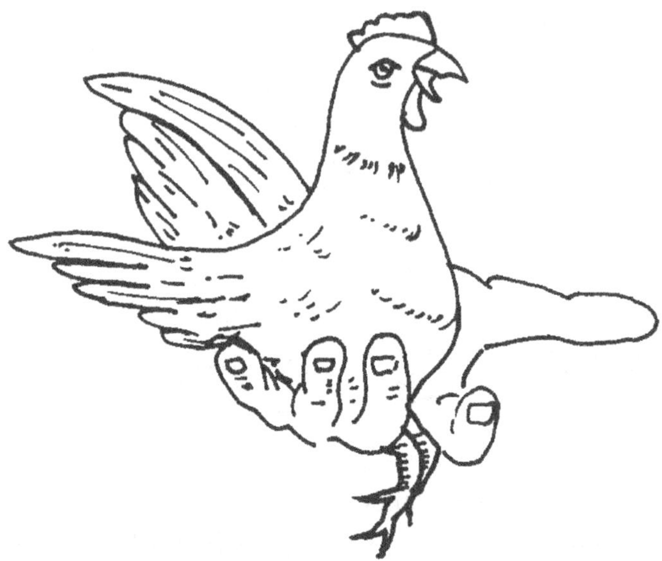

For injections in the breast muscle, turn the bird over and hold its wings between your fingers.

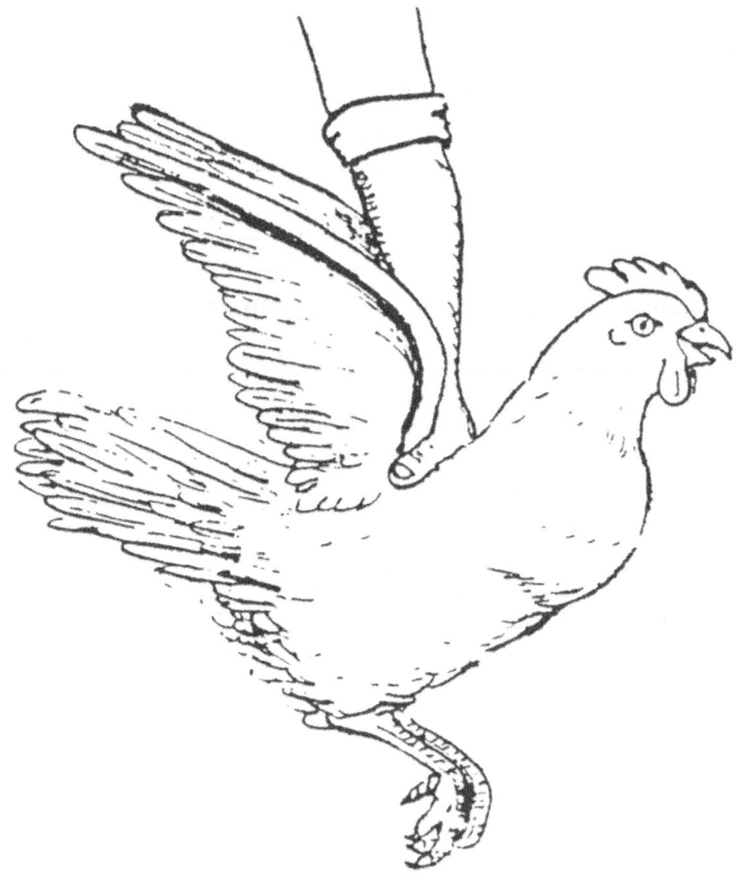

<u>**When is age estimation important?**</u>
When diagnosing a disease: Certain diseases are associated with age.

When purchasing an animal: An animal owner who cannot estimate age may unknowingly purchase an animal that is quite old and unproductive.

When predicting how an animal may respond to treatment: Younger animals recover from injury, especially broken bones, more rapidly than older animals. Older animals are more resistant to certain infectious diseases than younger animals.

Age Estimation of a HORSE, MULE OR BURRO

8 days:	First pair of "milk" lower teeth appear.	
8 weeks:	Second pair of "milk" lower teeth appear.	
8 months:	Third pair of "milk" lower teeth appear.	
2.5 years:	First pair of "adult" lower teeth replace milk teeth.	
3.5 years:	Second pair of "adult" lower teeth replace milk teeth.	
4.5 years:	Third pair of "adult" lower teeth replace milk teeth.	
5 years:	Canine tooth appears. (However, not every horse, mule or burro develops canine teeth.)	

Note: After five years, age estimation is less exact.

6 years: First pair of lower teeth develops a flat surface
- i.e. the hole in the tooth disappears.

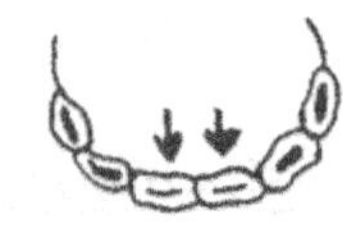

7 years: Second pair of lower teeth develops a flat surface.

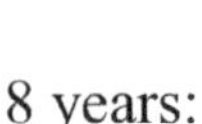

In some horses a "hook" develops on the third pair of upper teeth.

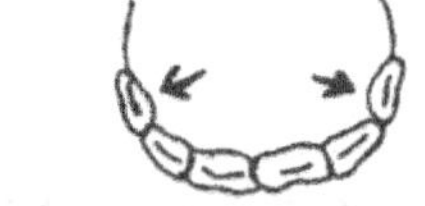

8 years: Third pair of lower teeth develop a flat surface.

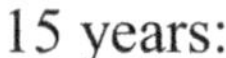

10 years: In some horses, a line begins at the top of the third pair of upper teeth.

15 years: In horses that develop a line in the third pair of upper teeth, the line appears half-way down the tooth.

Also, the teeth start changing from oval-shaped to triangular-shaped.

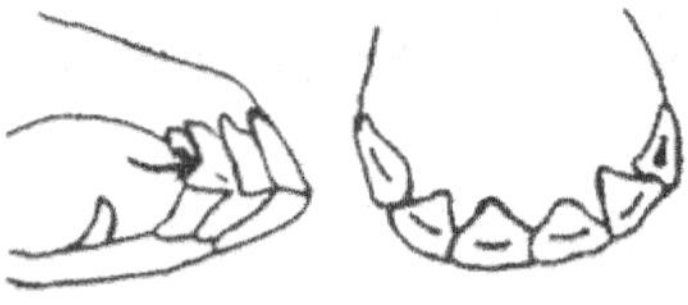

20 years: In horses with a line, the line is complete from the top to the bottom of the tooth.

25 years: In horses with a line, the top-half of the line disappears.

In general:
When <u>young</u>, the teeth are straight up and down and oval-shaped.

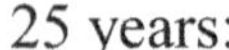

When <u>middle-aged</u>, the teeth begin to slant and change shape.

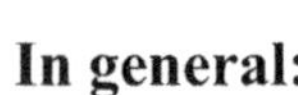

When <u>old</u>, the teeth are quite slanted and triangular-shaped.

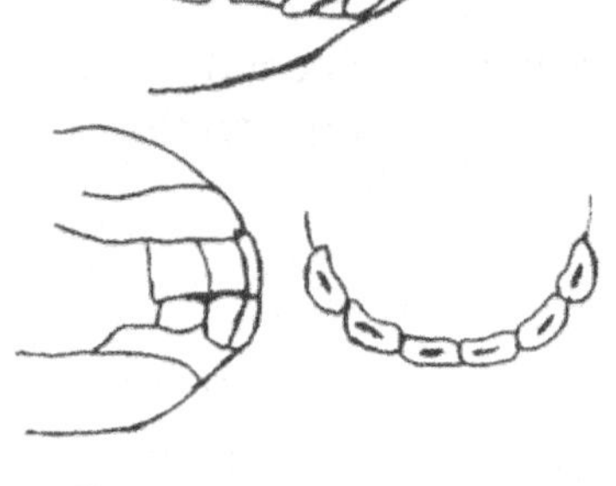

Age Estimation In CATTLE

30 days:	Four pairs of "milk" teeth have erupted.	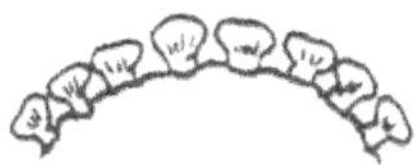

1.5 years:	First pair of "adult" teeth erupt to replace the milk teeth.	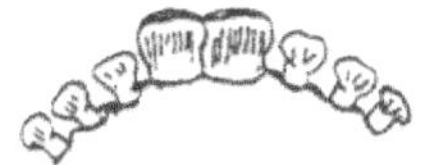
2.0 years:	First pair of adult teeth are full-grown.	

2.5 years:	Second pair of adult teeth erupt to replace the milk teeth.	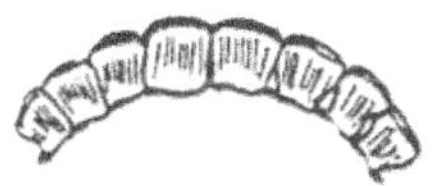
3.0 years:	Second pair of adult teeth are full-grown.	
3.5 years:	Third pair of adult teeth erupt to replace the milk teeth.	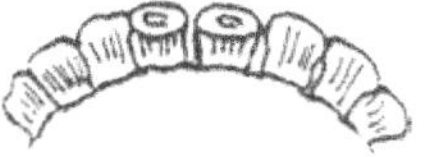
4.0 years:	Third pair of adult teeth are full-grown.	

4.5 years:	Fourth pair of adult teeth erupt to replace the milk teeth.	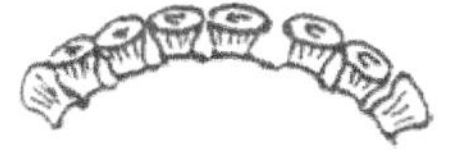
5.0 years:	Fourth pair of adult teeth are full-grown.	

Note: After five years of age, age estimation in cattle is less exact.

Approximately 8 years:	The surface of the first pair of teeth flattens.	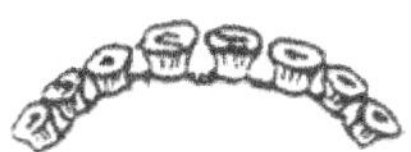

Approximately 9 years:	The surface of the second & third pair of teeth flattens.	

Approximately 10 years:	The surface of the 4th pair of teeth flattens.	

In general:
When young, cattle have oval shaped teeth.

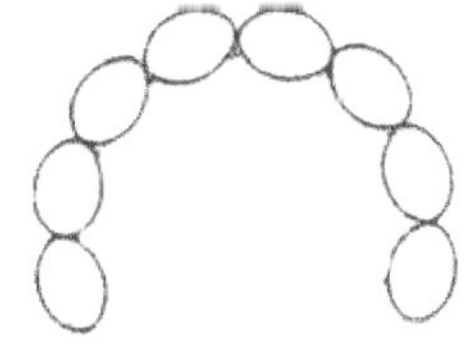

When older, cattle have triangular shaped teeth.

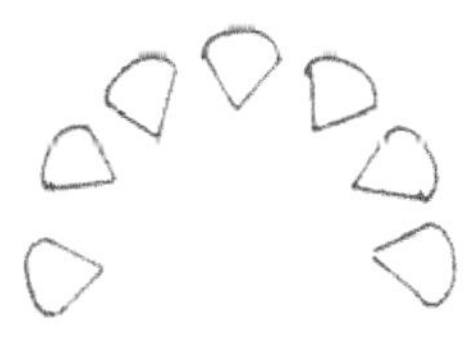

Age Estimation In SHEEP & GOATS

Less than 1 year of age: Four pairs of milk teeth.

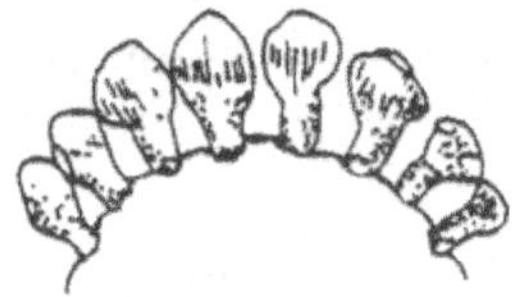

1 year of age: First pair of adult teeth erupt to replace milk teeth.

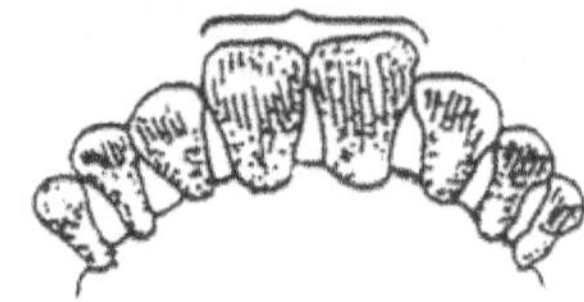

2 years of age: Second pair of adult teeth erupt to replace milk teeth.

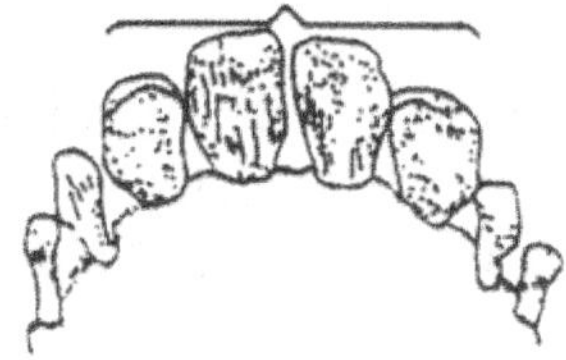

3 years of age: Third pair of adult teeth erupt to replace milk teeth.

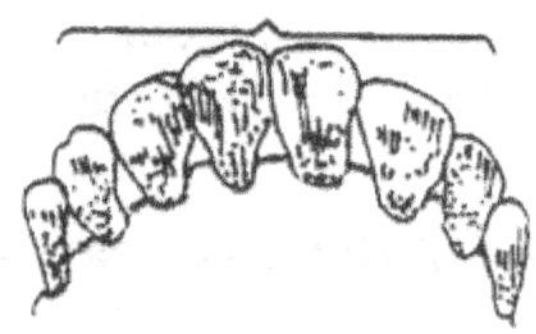

4 years of age: Fourth pair of adult teeth erupt to replace milk teeth.

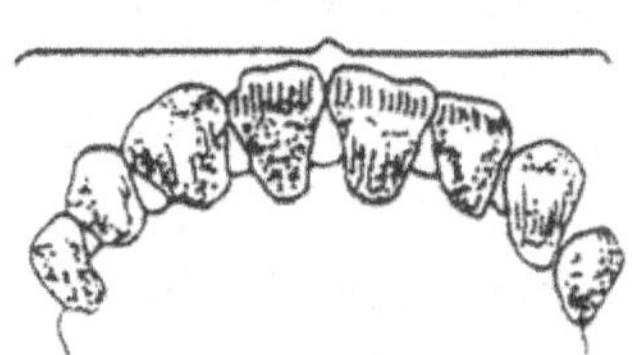

Remember, a goat or sheep with four pairs of adult teeth is four years of age *or greater*.

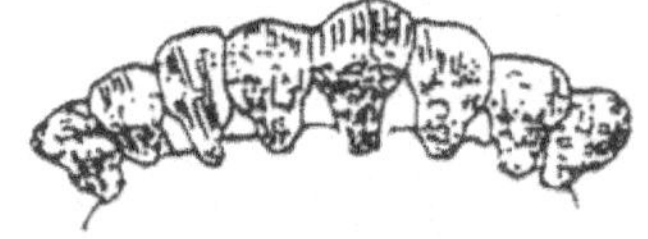

In old sheep or goats, the teeth begin to separate.

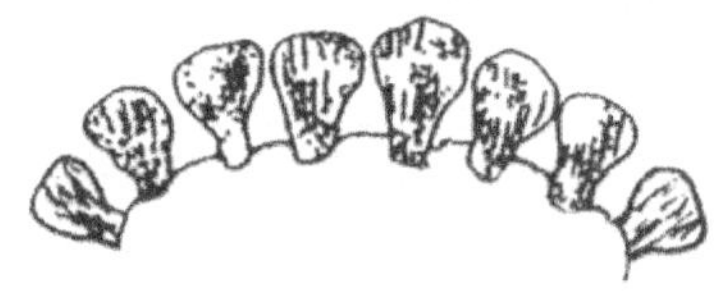

2.3 WEIGHT ESTIMATION

When Is Weight Estimation Important?

When calculating a dose of medication: Doses are often based on the animal's weight.
When selling an animal: In some places, animals are sold by weight.
To monitor weight gain: An owner may want to monitor an animal's weight gain or loss.

Methods of Weighing Animals

Using a Scale: This method is most accurate if the scale is good.
Using a Tape Measure: This method requires only a tape measure and can be used almost anywhere. Once the animal is measured, then one of two methods can be used:

- a **table** is used to look up the weight of the animal, or
- a **calculation** is made based on the measurements.

Centimeters versus Inches
Some tapes measure in inches rather than centimeters. It is sometimes necessary to convert from measurements made in inches to centimeters. This is not difficult to do. Simply use the following equation: _____ inches X 2.54 = centimeters.

For example: 12 inches = ?? centimeters   ----> 12 inches X 2.54 = 30.5 centimeters.

Weight Estimation of Cattle - Method One
To estimate the weight of cattle, wrap a flexible measuring tape (that measures in centimeters) around the thorax (i.e. chest) of the animal. This measurement is called the circumference, or "girth." Use the table on the following page for the corresponding weight.

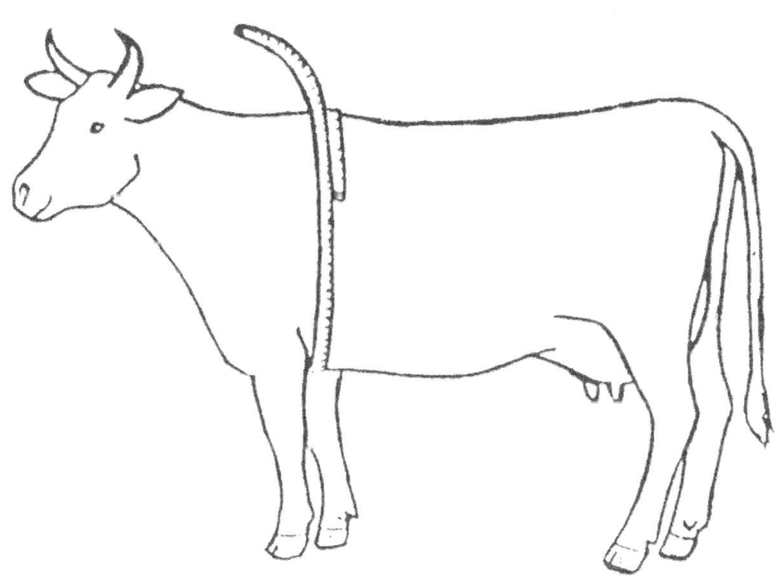

Table for Estimating Weight in Cattle[1]

Thorax Measured in Centimeters (Girth)	Weight in Kilograms (Larger or Imported Cattle)	Weight in Kilograms (Smaller or Local Cattle)	Thorax Measured in Centimeters (Girth)	Weight in Kilograms (Larger or Improved Cattle)	Weight in Kilograms (Smaller or Local Cattle)
66 cm	37 kg	27 kg	130 cm	189 kg	179 kg
69 cm	38 kg	30 kg	132 cm	197 kg	189 kg
71 cm	41 kg	33 kg	135 cm	207 kg	200 kg
74 cm	44 kg	37 kg	137 cm	217 kg	210 kg
76 cm	46 kg	40 kg	140 cm	227 kg	222 kg
79 cm	49 kg	44 kg	142 cm	239 kg	234 kg
81 cm	54 kg	47 kg	145 cm	251 kg	246 kg
84 cm	58 kg	52 kg	147 cm	263 kg	258 kg
86 cm	63 kg	57 kg	150 cm	276 kg	271 kg
89 cm	67 kg	62 kg	152 cm	289 kg	284 kg
91 cm	72 kg	67 kg	155 cm	303 kg	298 kg
94 cm	77 kg	72 kg	157 cm	318 kg	312 kg
96 cm	82 kg	78 kg	160 cm	332 kg	327 kg
99 cm	87 kg	84 kg	163 cm	348 kg	341 kg
102 cm	95 kg	91 kg	165 cm	363 kg	357 kg
104 cm	102 kg	97 kg	168 cm	379 kg	372 kg
107 cm	109 kg	103 kg	170 cm	395 kg	389 kg
109 cm	117 kg	110 kg	173 cm	412 kg	405 kg
112 cm	125 kg	118 kg	175 cm	430 kg	421 kg
114 cm	134 kg	125 kg	180 cm	466 kg	457 kg
117 cm	143 kg	134 kg	183 cm	485 kg	476 kg
119 cm	152 kg	143 kg	185 cm	504 kg	496 kg
122 cm	161 kg	152 kg	191 cm	543 kg	535 kg
124 cm	170 kg	160 kg	193 cm	563 kg	555 kg
127 cm	179 kg	170 kg	196 cm	583 kg	576 kg

---

[1] In many countries the local cattle are smaller, tougher and better adapted to the local conditions. In contrast, imported cattle are often larger and require more feed. Careful studies show that the weights of these two types of cattle are different, even if the tape measurement is the same. Therefore this table contains estimated weights for both types of cattle.

Weight Estimation of Cattle - Method Two

Wrap a flexible tape measure (that measures in inches) around the thorax of the animal to measure the **"circumference"** or **"girth"** of the animal. Wrap the tape around the animal just behind the front legs.

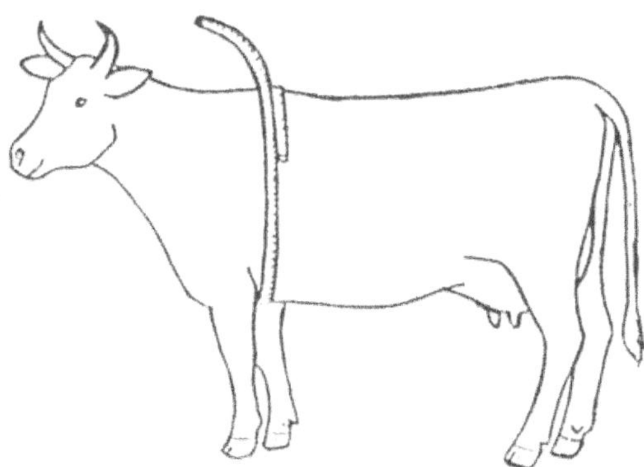

Measure the **"length"** of the animal from the point of the shoulder to the most posterior point of the hip.

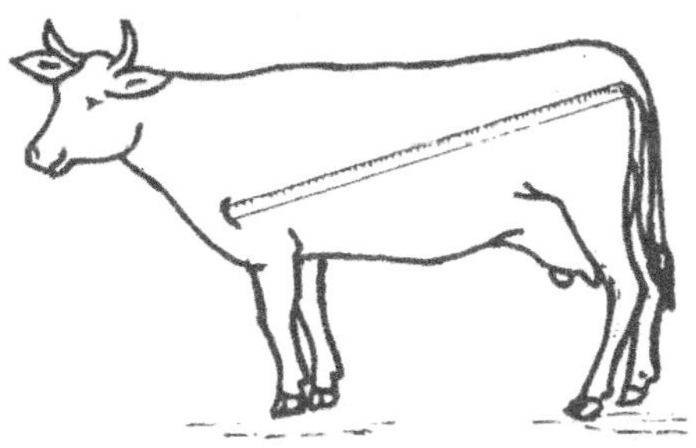

Calculation: (girth x girth x length) / 10,840 = Weight (in kilograms).

Conversion (to pounds): weight in kilograms X 2.2 = weight (in pounds).

For example, a cow has the following measurements
      Girth = 140 cm   Length = 124 cm

      Calculation: (140 x 140 x 124) / 10840 = 224 kilograms

Conversion: 224 x 2.2 = 492 pounds

Weight Estimation of Pigs

To estimate a pig's weight: Measure the "length" and "girth" of the pig. Then refer to the table below.

Measure the "length" from between the pig's ears to the base of its tail.

Measure the girth by wrapping a measuring tape around the pig's thorax just behind the front legs.

Calculation: $\dfrac{\text{girth (cm)} \times \text{girth (cm)}}{120. \text{ g}}$ = weight (in kilograms)

Weight table for pigs

On the **horizontal row** at the top of the table, find the closest number representing the **"length"** and put a finger of your right hand on that number. On the **vertical column** to the left of the table, find the closest number representing the **"girth"**, and put a finger of your left hand on that number. Slide your **right** index finger **down** the table and your **left** finger horizontally **across** the table until your two fingers meet. The number on which your fingers meet is the estimated weight of the pig *in kilograms.*

Length (cm)

Girth (cm)	80	90	100	110	120	130	140	150	160	170
80	36	42	50	58	69	80	93	107	121	137
90	40	47	54	65	74	86	98	111	126	143
100	48	55	63	72	82	94	106	120	135	151
110	60	67	75	84	94	105	118	132	146	162
120	75	82	90	99	109	120	133	147	161	177
130	94	101	108	117	120	139	161	165	180	196
140	118	123	130	139	150	161	173	187	202	218
150	141	148	156	165	175	186	189	212	227	243
160	170	177	184	193	203	215	227	241	256	272

Kilograms

Weight Estimation of Horses

Measure the diameter of the horse by placing a measuring tape around its "girth" (i.e. its chest or thorax) just behind the front leg. Use the table to find the corresponding weight.

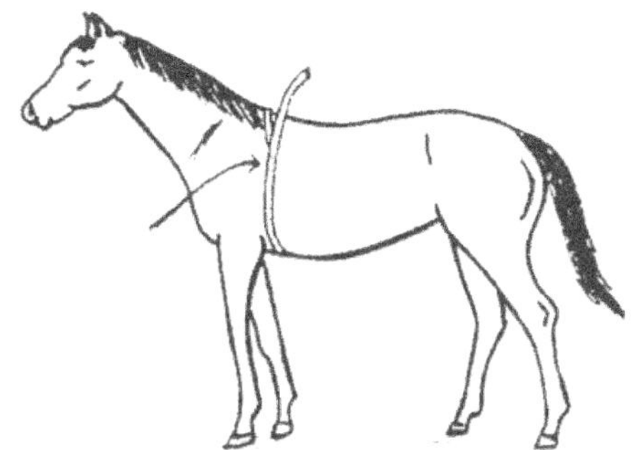

Weight Table For Horses

Measurement in Centimeters	Weight in Kilograms	Measurement in Centimeters	Weight in Kilograms
66 cm	36 kg	129 cm	188 kg
68 cm	38 kg	132 cm	197 kg
71 cm	40 kg	134 cm	207 kg
74 cm	43 kg	137 cm	217 kg
76 cm	46 kg	139 cm	228 kg
79 cm	49 kg	142 cm	239 kg
81 cm	54 kg	145 cm	251 kg
84 cm	58 kg	147 cm	263 kg
86 cm	63 kg	150 cm	276 kg
89 cm	67 kg	152 cm	290 kg
91 cm	72 kg	155 cm	304 kg
94 cm	76 kg	157 cm	318 kg
96 cm	82 kg	160 cm	333 kg
99 cm	87 kg	162 cm	348 kg
101 cm	94 kg	165 cm	364 kg
104 cm	102 kg	167 cm	380 kg
106 cm	109 kg	170 cm	396 kg
109 cm	117 cm	172 cm	413 kg
111 cm	125 cm	175 cm	430 kg
114 cm	134 cm	177 cm	450 kg
116 cm	143 cm	180 cm	470 kg
119 cm	152 cm	182 cm	490 kg
122 cm	161 cm	185 cm	505 kg
124 cm	170 cm	187 cm	525 kg
127 cm	179 cm	190 cm	545 kg

Measure the girth of the goat or sheep by placing a measuring tape around the animal's thorax just behind the front leg. Use the table to find the corresponding weight.

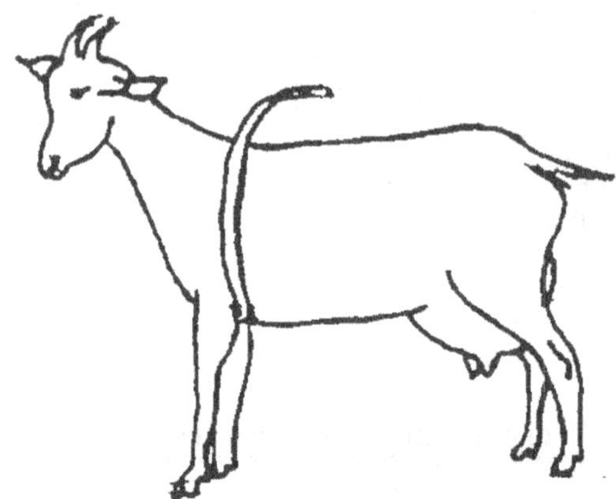

Weight table for goats and sheep.

Measurement in Centimeters	Weight in Kilograms	Measurement in Centimeters	Weight in Kilograms
25 cm	2 kg	68 cm	34.5 kg
28 cm	2.5 kg	71 cm	37.5 kg
30 cm	3 kg	73 cm	40.5 kg
33 cm	4 kg	76 cm	43.5 kg
36 cm	5 kg	79 cm	46.5 kg
38 cm	6 kg	81 cm	50.5 kg
41 cm	7.5 kg	84 cm	55 kg
43 cm	9.5 kg	86 cm	60 kg
46 cm	11.5 kg	89 cm	65 kg
48 cm	13.5 kg	91 cm	70 kg
51 cm	15.5 kg	94 cm	75 kg
53 cm	17.5 kg	96 cm	80 kg
56 cm	19.5 kg	99 cm	85 kg
58 cm	22.5 kg	102 cm	90 kg
61 cm	25 kg	104 cm	95 kg
63 cm	28.5 kg	107 cm	100 kg
66 cm	31.5 kg		

Note: In thin goats and sheep, this table tends to overestimate the weight.

3.0 CLINICAL EXAMINATION and DIAGNOSIS

A fundamental and critical skill of a good AHA is to properly handle and examine an animal.

A proper clinical exam consists of four parts, followed by the diagnosis.

1) HISTORY TAKING (Asking the right questions about the situation)
2) OBSERVATION OF THE ANIMAL
3) EXAMINATION OF THE ANIMAL (PHYSICAL EXAMINATION)
4) EXAMINATION OF THE ENVIRONMENT (Food, water & living area.)
5) DIAGNOSIS

Special Note: HEALTHY, SICK, DYING AND DEAD ANIMALS
Healthy animals should be examined BEFORE sick, dying, or dead ones to avoid possible exposure of healthy animals to disease.

Sick animals should be immediately isolated from healthy animals. Sick animals will also recover better if they are kept separate, given extra care and don't have to compete with healthy animals for food.

The examination of a dead animal is called a "post-mortem," "necropsy," or "autopsy." A necropsy can help determine whether illness was due to a poison, deficiency, or infectious disease. It takes training and practice to recognize some diseases inside a dead animal. Other diseases, such as parasites, may be easy to recognize in a dead animal.

3. 1 HISTORY TAKING

Carefully <u>question and listen</u> to the animal caretaker before looking at the animal. This is critical since the caretaker "knows" the animal and may recognize subtle symptoms. Ask questions that require more explanation than simply a "yes" or "no" response. To verify uncertain responses, ask the same question more than once in different ways.

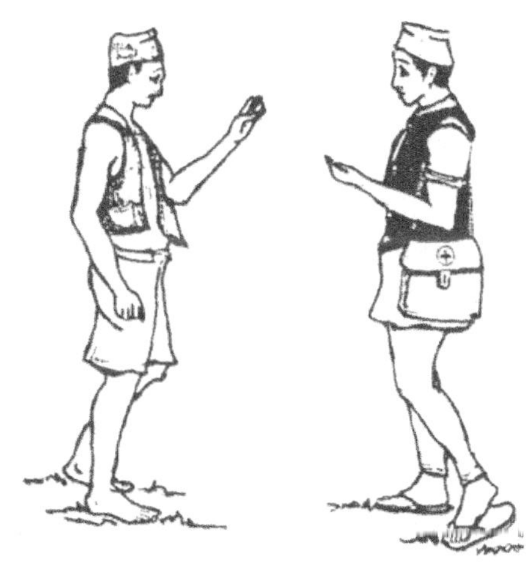

Some important questions include:
"Why did you call me? What do you think is wrong with your animal?"

"How long has your animal been sick? Is it getting better or worse?"

"Describe the symptoms."

"Have you treated the animal? With what? For how long? Did it improve?

"What medicines or injections (vaccines) have your animals received in the past?"

"Is this a milking animal? When was the baby born? Is it giving as much milk as usual?"

"Is it pregnant or was it bred? When?

Is it possible that it was bred without your knowledge? Are there loose animals that may have bred it, or does your animal run loose?"

"Is this a working animal? What work does it do? Is it working now?"

"How old is your sick animal?" If the age is unknown:
- Ask: *"How many years has it plowed? or*
  "How many times has it given birth?
  (Usually each "ring" on the horn represents a calving)
- Or: Examine the animal's teeth.

"Do you have other animals? Are they well? Have some of them been ill like this? Are animals in the community sick? How were they treated? Did they improve?"

"How much did your animal eat today? How much does it usually eat? Is it eating well? When did it stop eating?"

"How much water does your animal drink? Where does it get its drinking water? Is it drinking well? When did it stop drinking?"

"Did you see it urinate today? The usual amount? What color was the urine?"

"How is its manure? Hard? Soft? Liquid? Bloody? Anything unusual about it?"

"Who cares for the animal? Have other people recently cared for the animal?" "Has anything changed recently?"

"Where does the animal stay? In a pen, staked out, loose?"

"How long have you had your animal? Did you just buy it? From where? From an individual? From a market? Were/are other animals at the market also sick?

"Was the animal transported a long distance? Were the animals crowded during transport? How many were on the truck? Was the animal recently exposed to bad weather or some other stress?"

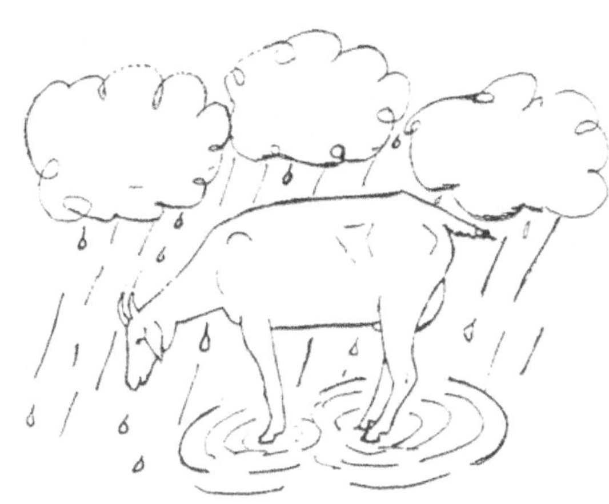

Observe the animal from a distance without disturbing it by going too close or touching it.
If the animal becomes upset or excited, it will breathe more rapidly and act differently.

3.2.1 Condition

In what condition is the animal?
Thin? Weak? Pregnant? Lactating?
Bloated? Is it well grown? Is it stunted?

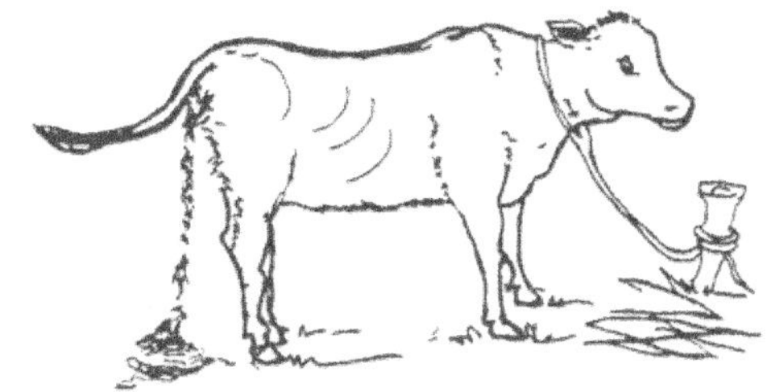

This calf is thin and has a poor hair coat

3.2.2 Behavior

Is the animal behaving
normally? Is it unusually nervous, crazy,
aggressive or excited? Is it unusually slow
or lazy? Does it stay alone? Is it walking
into things? Is it scratching? Is it looking or
kicking at its abdomen, rolling on the
ground, or injuring itself as if in pain? Are
animals (especially piglets or chickens)
huddled together because they are cold?

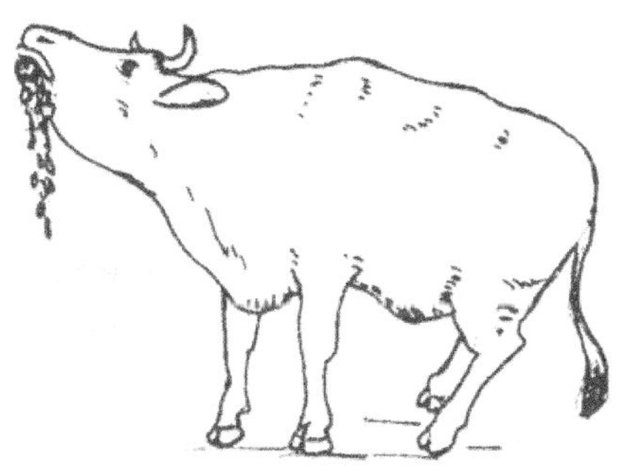

*This cow is nervous, has weak back legs
and cannot swallow. It has rabies.*

3.2.3 Movement

Can the animal walk? Does it stagger or not seem
to know where its legs are?
Do the back legs seem weaker than the front legs?
Does it walk in a circle? Is its head tilted to one
side? Is it limping? Is it weak? Is it making
strange movements or noises? Can it keep up
with the rest of the herd?

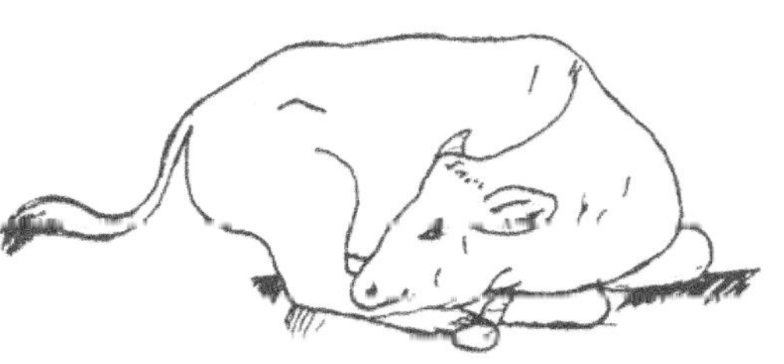

This animal cannot stand.

3.2.4 Discharges

Are there discharges (like blood or pus) from any body openings (the eyes, ears, nose, vulva, rectum or penis)? Does the discharge smell rotten or putrid? Do the animal's manure and urine look normal?

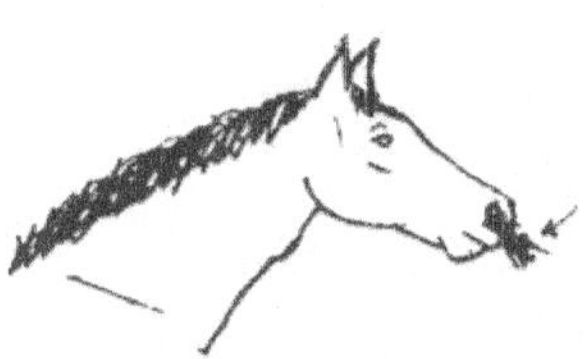

This horse has a nasal discharge.

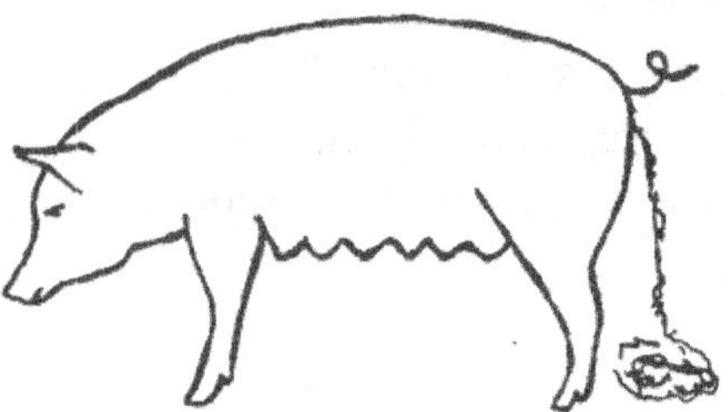

This sow has a discharge from the vulva.

3.2.5 Respiration

Respiration refers to breathing. Normally, an animal breathes with a smooth and effortless movement of the ribs. What is the *respiration rate?* See page 200. The following signs may signal problems in the respiratory system.

- sudden or jerky breathing
- coughing and sneezing
- rapid breathing
- breathing with difficulty or extra effort
- wide-open nostrils in a resting animal (especially horses)
- breathing with the mouth open

Note: Breathing with the mouth open may also be due to overheating.

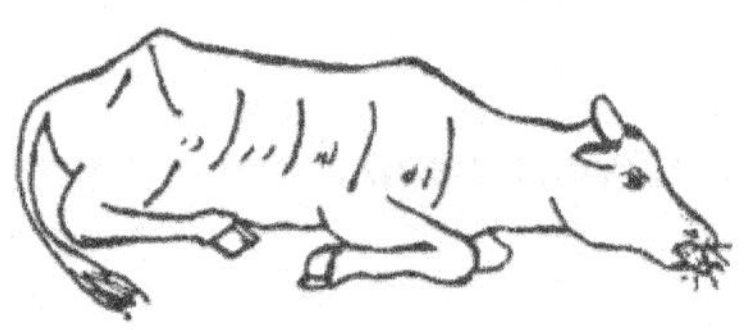

This calf is coughing, has difficulty breathing, and has a nasal discharge

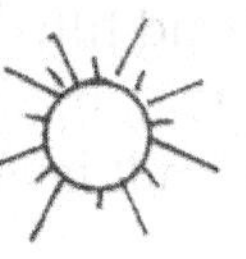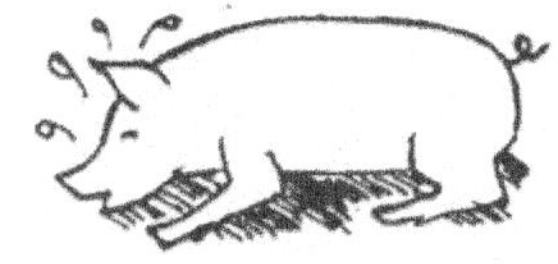

This sow is hot and is breathing with her mouth open.

3.3 PHYSICAL EXAMINATION

The physical exam should be done as **quietly and gently** as possible. Gentle **restraint** may be needed if the animal is not tame. If the animal becomes upset, the temperature, respiration and pulse may increase.

Where to start? If possible, the exam should be done with the animal standing. We prefer to start the exam from the rear for cattle, buffalo, sheep, goats and pigs, and work towards the front of the animal. For horses, we prefer to start the exam from the head of the horse and work towards the rear. Whichever is the <u>least upsetting</u> to the animal is the best place to start.

Be Consistent: Try to follow the same order whenever you examine a sick animal, so you will be less likely to skip a part of the exam.

3.3.1 Body Temperature

"Fever" means an elevated temperature (above normal). One of the most common reasons for fever is **infection** because the body's temperature rises as it fights the infection.

Elevated temperatures also occur:
-        With exercise, fear and direct sunlight (especially in dark colored animals).
-        Mother animals giving birth and newborn animals which cannot control well their body temperature. (e.g. sows during farrowing often overheat in hot climates.)
-        At a young age (i.e. young animals normally have slightly higher temperatures).

Below-normal temperature may occur:
-        In cows with "milk fever."
-        In baby animals that are small, weak, underfed, or have diarrhea.
-        In cases of poisoning.
-        Just before death.

HOW TO TAKE THE TEMPERATURE
-Grasp the thermometer <u>firmly</u> at the end with the highest numbers. Shake the thermometer so that the liquid is forced to the end with the lowest numbers.

-Moisten the thermometer with water, spit, oil or soap. Gently insert the thermometer into the rectum and hold it against the wall of the rectum. Do not force it! Do not leave it in the middle of a mass of feces.

-Either hold the thermometer firmly with your hand while taking the temperature, or tie a string to the end of the thermometer and attach a clip on the free end of the string. When the thermometer is in the rectum, attach the clip to a tuft of hair or wool on the tail. Otherwise, the animal may push the thermometer out and break it. Leave the thermometer in the rectum for 2 to 3 minutes.

-Remove thermometer and wipe it off with a leaf, piece of straw, or rag.

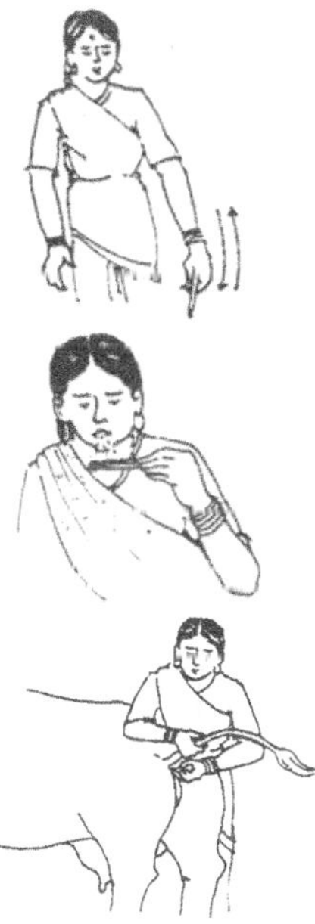

-To read the thermometer, grasp the thermometer at the end with the highest numbers. Then slowly rotate it until a clear liquid line is visible. At the point where the liquid line abruptly ends, read the number marked on the thermometer. This is the temperature of the animal.

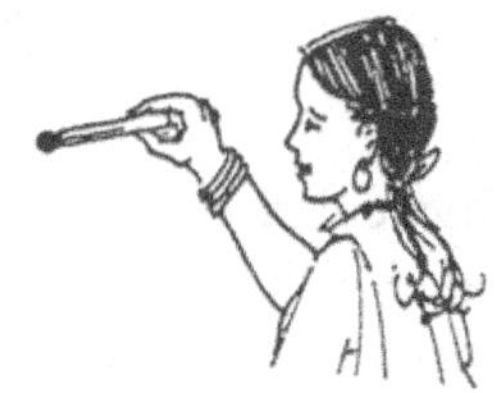

-Clean the thermometer with soap and water; store it in a case to prevent breakage.

Table 1: Normal Body Temperatures Measured by a Thermometer in the Rectum

Animal	Rectal Temperature Fahrenheit (F)	Rectal Temperature Celsius (C)
Man / Woman	98.6	37
Cattle less than 1 year	102.5	39.2
Buffalo less than 1 year	102.0	38.9
Cattle more than 1 year	101.5	38.6
Buffalo more than 1 year	100.5	38.1
Horse	100.5	38.1
Mature Goat (varies with weather)	104	40
Young Sheep / Goat	103.1	39.5
Mature Sheep	103	39.5
Young Pigs	103.6	39.8
Mature Pig	102.2	39
Rabbit	102.7	39.3
Chicken	107.6	42
Dog	102	39
Cat	101.5	38.5

3.3.2 Pulse

"Pulse rate" or "heart rate" is the number of heart beats per minute. "Pulse" also refers to the quality of the heartbeat. Is it strong or weak? Regular or irregular? To measure the pulse rate, place your fingertips against an artery and count the number of pulsations per minute. With practice you can determine whether the pulse is regular and strong. **Try to measure the pulse rate when the animal is calm and resting.**

A rapid pulse may result from fear, exercise, pain, heart problems, overheating, and from an elevated body temperature.

A weak, irregular pulse is a bad sign, indicating that the heart is not effectively moving blood through the body, or the animal is in "shock," or close to death.

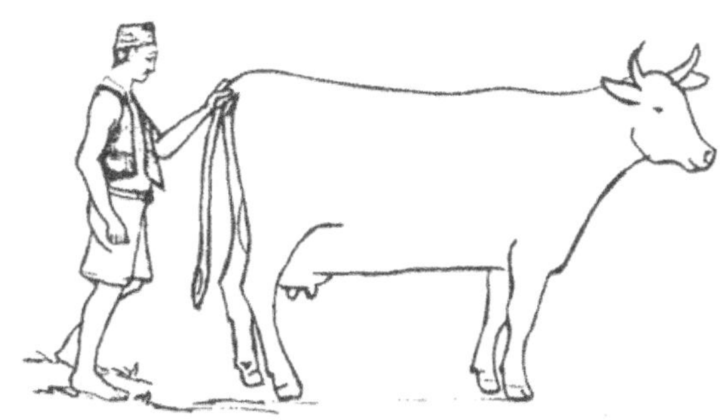

In cattle, buffalo and yak, grasp the tail near the rectum, placing the fingertips in the groove on the underside to feel the pulse.

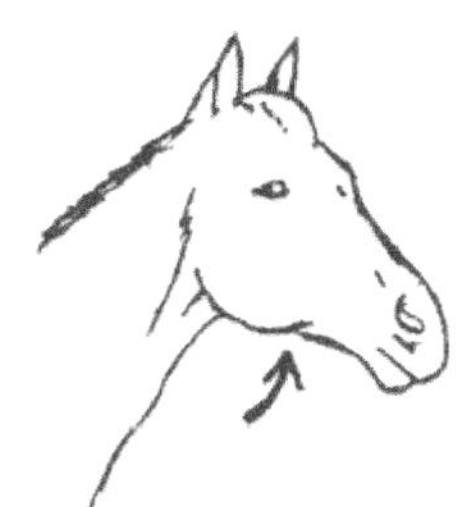

For horses, burros, mules, sheep, and goats, the pulse can be counted by feeling the facial artery on the inside of the lower jaw.

Table 2: Average Pulse and Respiration Rates in Cool Weather

Animal	Respiration Rate	Pulse Rate / Minute
Man / Woman	12	70
Calf (few days old)	56	125
Calf (6 months old)	30	96
Cattle (up to 1 year)	27	91
Cattle (adult)	16	50
Buffalo (calf 6 months)	28	-
Buffalo (adult)	12	45
Horse	10-12	44
Goat / Sheep (adult)	15	75
Goat / Sheep (young)	20	110
Piglet (2 weeks)	25	138
Pig (12-14 weeks)	18	112
Pig (Adult)	15	65-85
Rabbit	55	130
Bird (varies considerably)	12-40	100-200

3.3.3 Skin

If the animal's hair coat is not smooth, shiny and lying flat, something is wrong....

Is the animal constantly scratching?
Does it have skin that is dry, injured,
scaly or red? Does it have sores, hair
loss or wool loss? If yes, consider
parasites as a diagnosis.

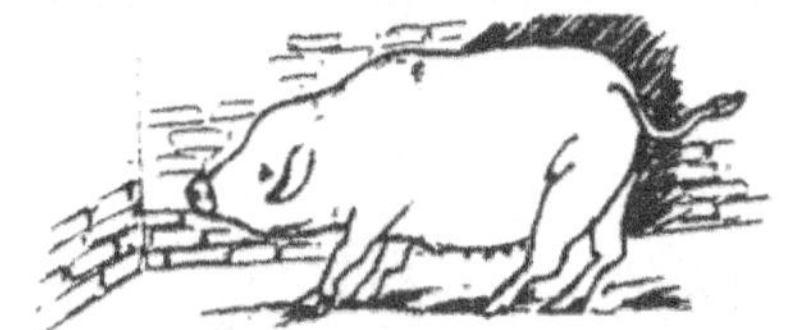

This pig is constantly scratching

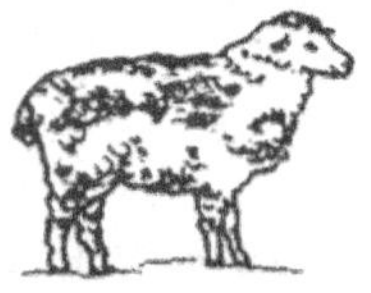

This sheep has
areas of wool
loss to due mange

Are there parasites on the skin
such as ticks, lice or fleas?

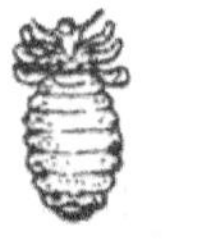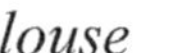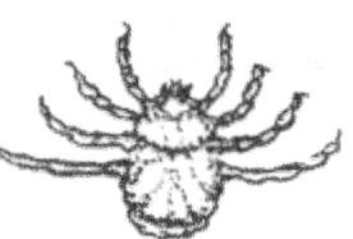

louse   tick

Is the skin or hair dry, and the hair rough, dull in color
and standing up? Consider internal parasites and/or
malnutrition.

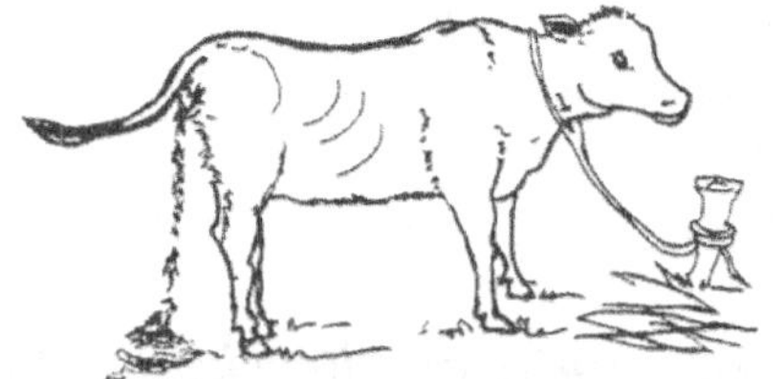

This calf has rough, dull hair.

Are there blisters (vesicles) on the udder, near
the mouth or near the hooves? This may be
Foot and Mouth Disease (FMD). In sheep this
may be contagious ecthyma.

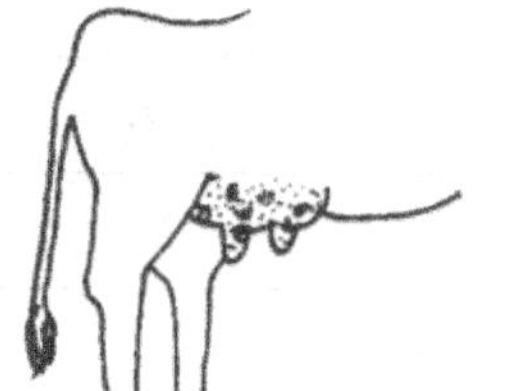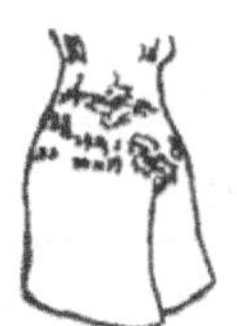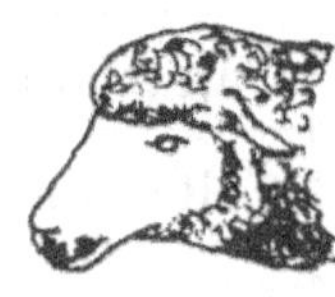

When you pull a fold of skin, does it snap back when you let go or
does the fold remain standing? If it remains standing, the animal
doesn't have enough liquid in its body. This is called
"dehydration."

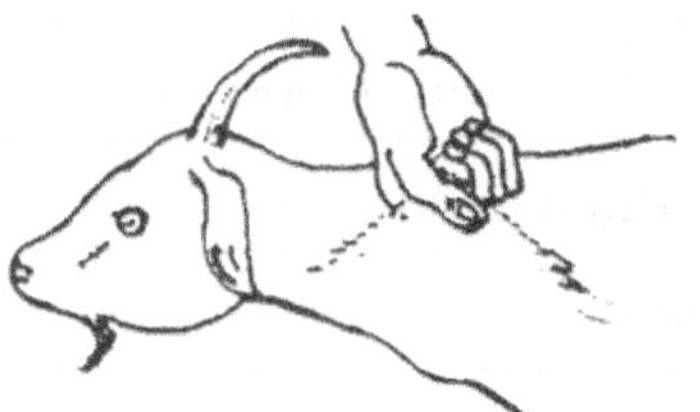

Are small holes burrowed in the skin or wounds? Are there white, ugly worms wiggling in the
 holes? These are screw worms or maggots.

Are there warts, lumps, bumps or swollen areas? Are there signs of injuries to the skin?
Is the skin sunburned? (Especially on white pigs or white areas of cattle and horses).

3.3.4 Eyes

Is there pus or excess tears from the
eyes?

Are there stains down the side of the
face?

Is the animal blinking excessively like it
has pain in the eye or is bothered by
light?

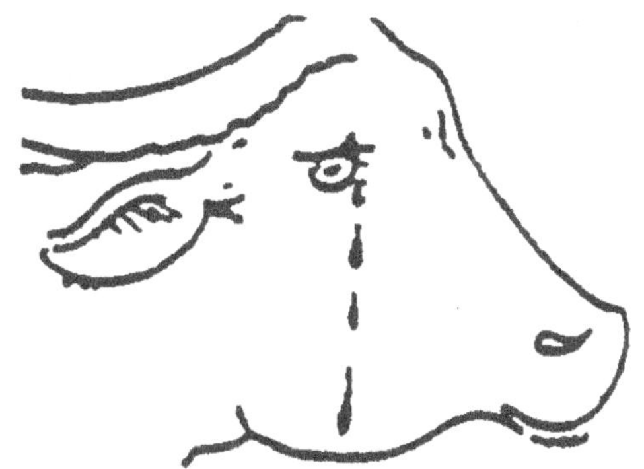

Are there cloudy areas on the surface of
the eyes (due to infection or injury)? Are
the eyes sunken in the sockets? This
may be due to serious dehydration.
What color is the tissue surrounding the
eyeball (called "conjunctiva")?
Normally, it should be pink:

-       *Reddened* conjunctiva indicates
        inflammation due to irritation or
        infection. It may also indicate
        fever.
-       *Dark red, purple or brown*
        conjunctiva indicates severe
        toxemia (blood poisoning) and is
        a very bad sign.
-       *Pale or white* conjunctiva
        indicates shock, or anemia
        usually due to parasites.
        See page 125.
-       *Yellow* conjunctiva indicates a
        liver problem (i.e. liver flukes) or
        that blood cells are being
        destroyed (i.e. anaplasma or
        Babesia), and is called
        "jaundice." The yellow color can
        be seen best in the white part of
        the eye called the "sclera."

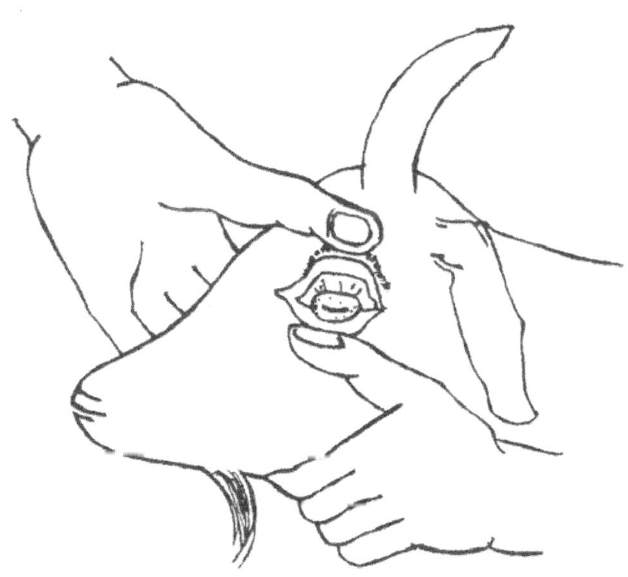

3.3.5 Ears

Are there signs that the animal has been scratching its ears because of parasites? For example, is there redness <u>behind</u> the ears? Are there crusty areas, sores or discharges from the ears? Is the animal shaking its head frequently? Are there ticks inside the ears?

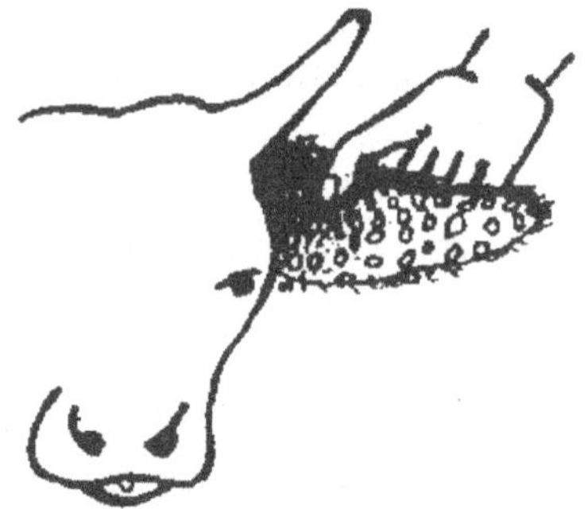

This ear has many ticks in it.

3.3.6 Nose

A healthy animal's nose is moist and cool.
- Is there discharge of pus that might be a sign of infection in the nose, throat or lungs?

- Is there a foul odor from the animal's mouth indicating infection in the nose or mouth?

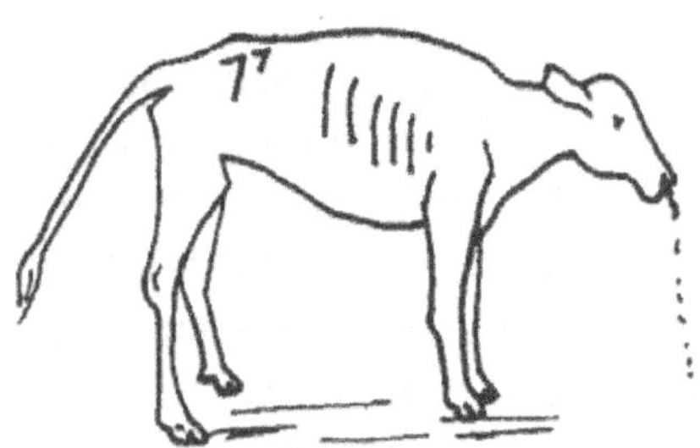

This calf has a discharge of pus from its nose.

3.3.7 Mouth and Throat

Do the teeth appear normal and able to chew food?   An animal with missing or deformed teeth or with a mal-aligned jaw may have trouble eating and therefore appear very thin. Is there extra fluid accumulated under the jaw? (This is a sign of internal parasites).

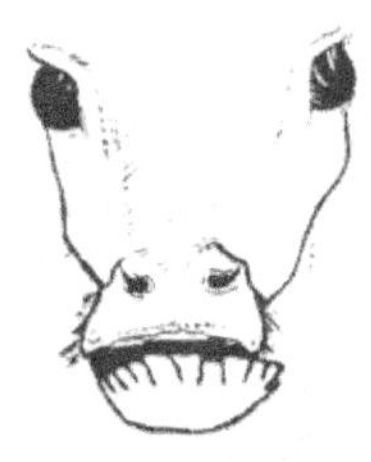
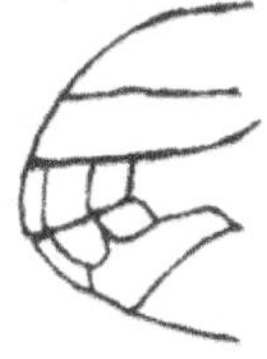
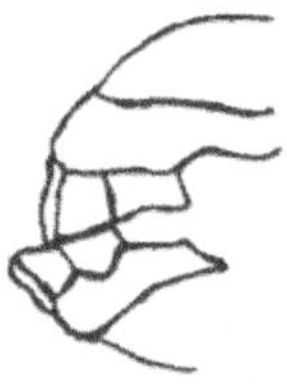
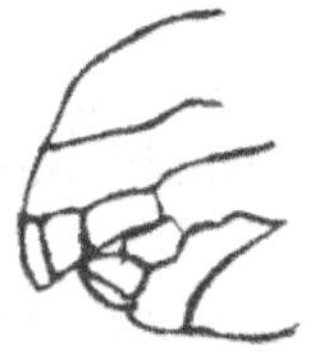

Cow with crooked mouth   *Horse with normal teeth*   *Horse with underbite called "monkey mouth"*   *Horse with overbite called "parrot mouth"*

Can the age be estimated? See pages 32-35 on age estimation? What color are the gums? Gum color may provide a clue for certain types of toxicities. Are there any sores or blisters on the gums or tongue? Several diseases cause sores or blisters, such as FMD.

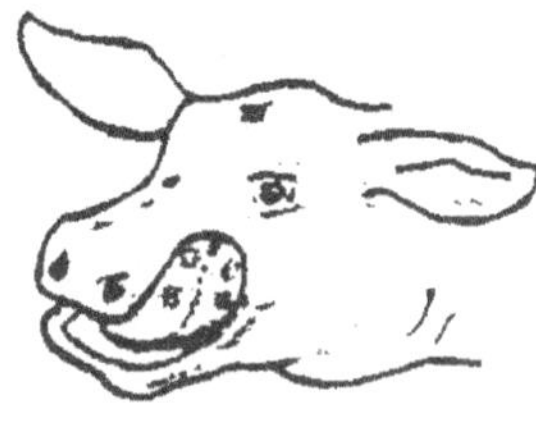

Is the animal able to swallow? An animal that can't swallow often drools excessively.

WARNING!!! An animal that can't swallow may have something caught in its throat or it may have **RABIES**.

IF THERE IS ANY POSSIBILITY OF RABIES, DO NOT EXAMINE THE MOUTH WITHOUT WEARING GLOVES. Any contact with the saliva of a rabid animal may give a person rabies. See pages 251-253, 281.

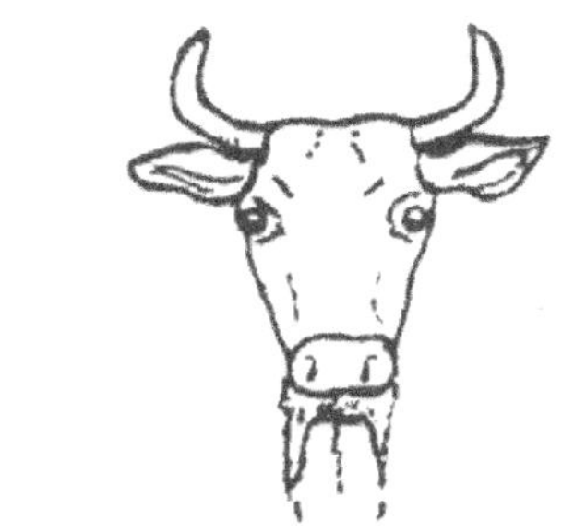

This animal is drooling because it cannot swallow

Next examine the area under the lower jaw. This becomes filled with fluid when an animal has thin blood (i.e. anemia) due to worms and other internal parasites. The owner may call it "big head" or "bottle jaw."

The throat can become swollen if there are problems with the windpipe or food pipe, such as an abscess developing (especially in horses and pigs) or anthrax (especially pigs).

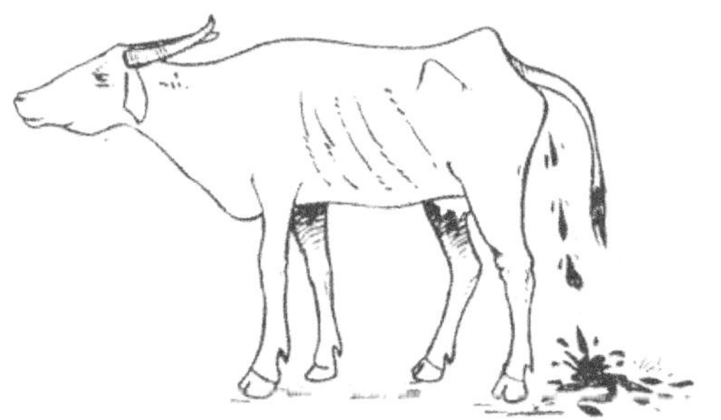

Buffalo with extra fluid under its throat

3.3.8 Hooves / Feet

Does the animal limp or have sores, wounds or swellings at the top of the hoof or between the toes (i.e. FMD or foot rot)?

Are the hooves long and deformed due to footrot, birth defects, or improper feeding?

Do the hooves have horizontal lines (ripples), due to a past fever, a change in feed, or a lactation period?

Are there cracks in the hooves? These can often be resolved by trimming and filing.

Are there sores or drainage (like blood or pus) from any part? Are the feet unusually hot indicating inflammation, injury, or infection such as an abscess?

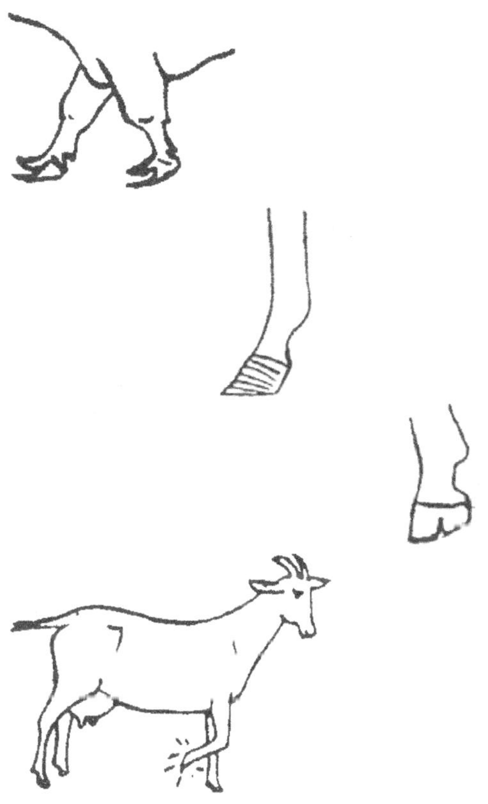

3.3.9 Legs

Are there deformities? This could be due to
a birth defect, an injury, or improper feeding.
Are there injuries or scars which indicate past
injuries? Are there swollen areas, lumps, or
areas that seem unusually hot? This could be
inflammation due to injury or infection.

3.3.10 Navel

In young animals, is the navel hot, swollen
or having a discharge? This often occurs along
with swollen joints and is due to an infection
of the navel in young animals, particularly
those that did not receive colostrum. See pages
56, 238.

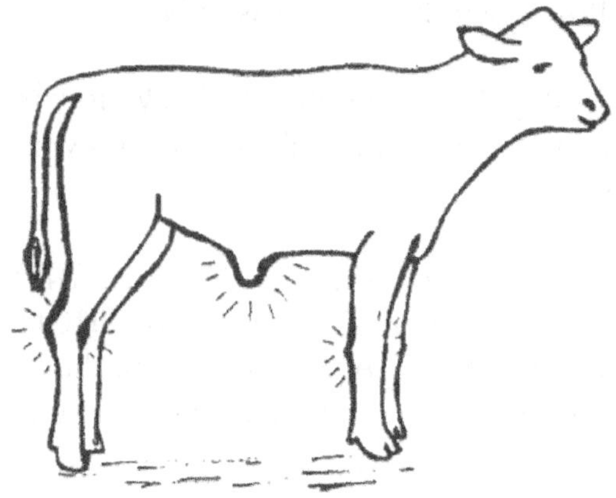

Calf with joint and naval infection

3.3.11 Abdomen

Animals that chew cud are called "ruminants" and
include cattle, buffalo, yaks, sheep, goats, llamas
and alpacas. One of their "stomachs" is called the
"rumen." Place your ear against the left flank of a
gentle, healthy ruminant and hear the rumen
rumble one to three times per minute to mix food.
**Rumen movement is a sign of health and
absence of it is a sign of illness.** In a "non-
ruminant" animal, such as a horse, put your ear
close to either flank (if it is tame enough) to hear
gurgling sounds of the intestines. A healthy
animal at rest has constant sounds like this.

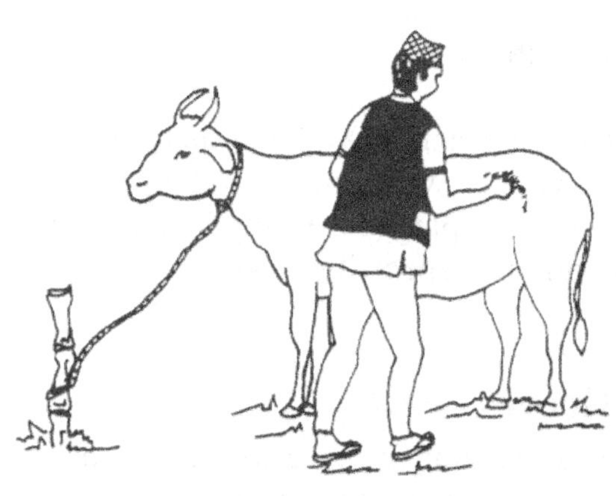

3.3.12 Teats / Udder

The teats and udder should be soft, normally
shaped, and evenly placed. A hard, hot, painful or
swollen udder or milk that is bloody, watery, or
lumpy are sign of "mastitis."

3.3.13 Vulva

Is the vulva normal in size and shape? Is there
discharge that looks abnormal and/or smells bad?
A discharge indicates infection in the uterus
called "metritis." Remember, some animals
normally have a discharge during heat, or during
the week after giving birth. Normal cows have
some bloody discharge 1 to 3 days after they are
in heat.

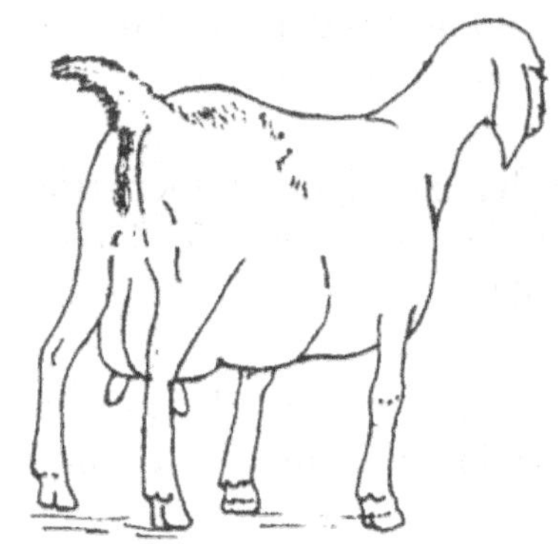

Goat with normal udder, teats and vulva

3.3.14 Testicles

Are there <u>two</u> testicles of <u>normal</u> and <u>equal size</u>? Animals with unusually small testicles or only one testicle (called a "cryptorchid") should not breed. Are there swellings or strange shape of the testicles indicating current infection such as "brucellosis?" Are there injuries or sores?

3.3.15 Penis

Is the penis normal in size and shape? Is there any sign of injury? Is there abnormal discharge? Sometimes an animal may have a birth defect which makes it impossible to extend its penis.

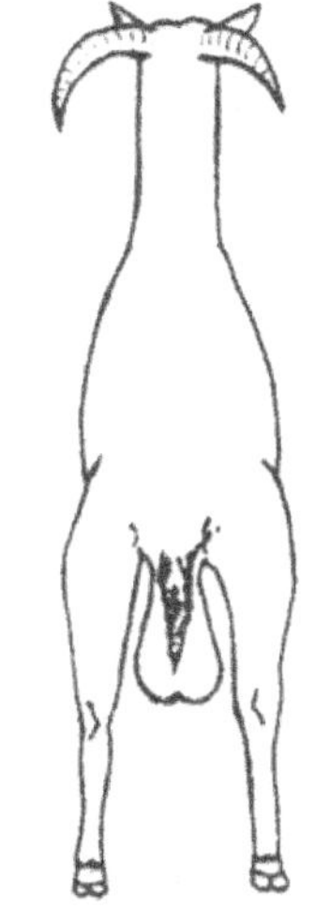

Goat with normal testicles

3.3.16 Rectal Examination

A rectal exam consists of inserting an arm (often covered with a plastic sleeve and glove) in the rectum of the animal. This is done to push urine from the bladder, check for pregnancy, detect a uterine infection or check for loops of intestine that are blocked or distended with too much gas. Technicians use this same procedure for artificial insemination of an animal. Rectal examination takes supervised practice to learn well.

WARNING: If done improperly, a rectal examination can lead to a punctured rectum and death, especially in horses. Therefore, this procedure is usually done only by a veterinarian or a trained technician.

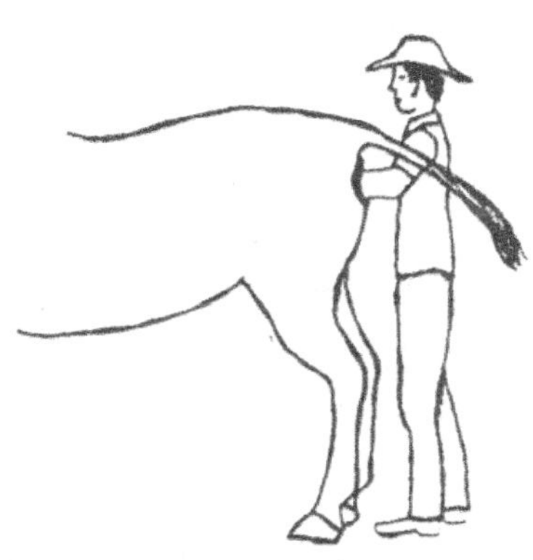

Rectal examination

3.4 EXAMINING THE ENVIRONMENT

A good AHA always verifies how the animals are managed, as well as the type of shelter, food, water and soil. This becomes especially important when <u>many</u> animals are sick.

Minerals

Soils in tropical countries often lack adequate minerals such as phosphorous. Animals eating forages from these soils may also become deficient in these minerals. This happens especially if animals' diets are not supplemented with minerals using a "mineral-salt block" or a special "feeder" or "tank" of minerals. See page 101. Information on the soil in your area can usually be obtained at the Ministry of Agriculture.

Check carefully:
- Food & water sources
- Pastures
- Shelter & pens
- Birthing areas
- Number of animals
- Space available

Vitamins

Animals can also lack certain vitamins in their diet. Sometimes, feed stored for months in a hot place may lose its vitamins, particularly vitamins A and E. Wet feed can also spoil and lose its vitamins and/or make animals sick.

Poisons

If one suspects poisoning, one should check all feed and water sources as well as pastures, pens and shelters where the animals stay. Animals running loose may have easy access to poisons such as rat poison.

- *Molds*. Moist feed can become moldy. The mold may produce a toxin or poison which can cause illness and death. Molds also make the food less tasty so that the animals do not want to eat it.
- *Poisonous plants* may also cause problems. During drought periods, some plants concentrate nitrates and become poisonous. Often poisonous plants do not taste good to animals. However, when feed is scarce, hungry animals are more likely to eat poisonous plants.
- *Garbage*. Some garbage like old car batteries, antifreeze or used motor-oil are poisonous and should not be left where animals can find them.
- *Animal feeds.*
    - Feed can be accidentally contaminated with toxic chemicals.
    - Animals may be fed the wrong feed. For example, pig feed may contain enough copper to poison sheep. Horses die if fed *Monensin or Rumensin* - a common feed additive for livestock.

Water

<u>Always</u> check the water source.

- *Contamination:* If water is contaminated, stagnant, has a dead animal floating in it, or is too warm or cold, animals may not drink it. <u>Thirsty</u> animals may drink from a contaminated water source and become sick.
- *Salt poisoning:* Pigs receiving salt in their diet and inadequate quantities of water may die due to brain swelling. This is commonly called "salt poisoning" or "salt toxicity", but is actually due to lack of water. See pages 254, 269, 313.
- *Electric currents:* If the drinking water source has an electrical current in it, animals may not drink it.

Pasture

Animals that are overcrowded or kept continuously in the same pasture will have more problems with internal parasites. If a pasture is overgrazed, it will no longer meet the nutritional needs of the animals.

Shelter

Animals need protection from the sun (in hot climates) and wind. Baby pigs need to be kept at about 91 F (33 C), otherwise, they will get diarrhea or pneumonia. Animals closed inside a shelter without fresh air may develop pneumonia. Animals kept in a wet pen frequently develop infected feet and diarrhea.

Crowding

Crowding too many animals together in a pen is asking for trouble! They are more prone to many diseases and injuries. Pigs and chickens that are crowded may cannibalize (eat) their pen mates.

Birthing Areas

Animals giving birth in dirty conditions often develop uterus infections, and their babies get navel and joint infections as well as diarrhea. Animals should give birth in clean, dry, and "fresh" areas where other animals have not been.

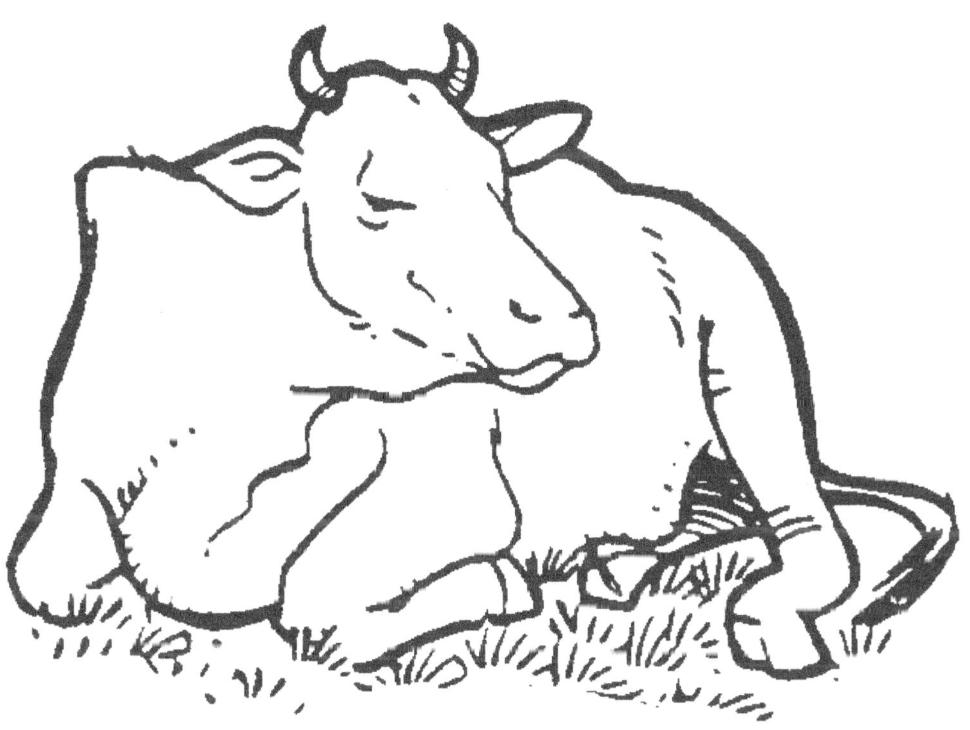

3.5   THE DIAGNOSIS
Which System & What Disease?

Which system of the body? Information from the history, observations, and examination must be used to *decide what body system is affected.* The following table might help.

Table 3: Systems of the Body

Body System	Organs within the System	System Function
Reproductive System	Female: ovaries, oviducts, uterus, vagina, mammary gland Male: testes, vas deferens, glands, penis	Reproduce offspring and provide milk for the young offspring.
Digestive System	Mouth (teeth, tongue, gums), throat, esophagus, stomach, intestines, liver, pancreas	Obtains, chews and digests food.
Respiratory System	Nose, larynx, epiglottis, trachea, lungs, bronchi	Allows air to move in and out of the body; takes oxygen from the air; filters and warms air; cools the body.
Muscular System	Muscles, tendons	Enables movement of the body and organs.
The Skin	Skin, sweat glands, hair, nails and hooves	Protects the body and regulates body temperature.
Skeletal System	Bones, cartilage	Cartilage protects joints; bones support and protect the body.
Urinary System	Kidneys, ureters, bladder, urethra	Cleans the blood (makes urine); removes waste; balances water and salts.
Nervous System	Brain, spinal cord, nerves	Responsible for sensing, moving, coordination of the body and thinking.
Circulatory System	Heart, blood vessels (arteries, veins, capillaries)	Supplies and regulates blood flow to all parts of the body.
Blood & Lymphatic System	Blood cells (red, white, platelet), plasma, lymph vessels and nodes, spleen	Carries oxygen and nutrients; removes wastes; contains cells and proteins that fight infection.
Endocrine System	Hormones and all glands in the body which make hormones (pituitary, thyroid, parathyroid, adrenal, pancreas and reproductive glands)	Hormones act as chemical messengers which travel in the blood and regulate most functions of the body.
Special Systems	Eyes, ears, nose, tongue	Detect stimuli to allow interaction with the environment outside the body.

What disease?

After deciding which body system is affected, the next step is to determine what disease the animal has. *But how?*

1. ***First, know the most common diseases in your area***. Discuss with other experienced Animal Health Agents, visit slaughter houses, observe or perform autopsies whenever possible, attend meetings where AHAs, extension agents and veterinarians gather to discuss technical issues.

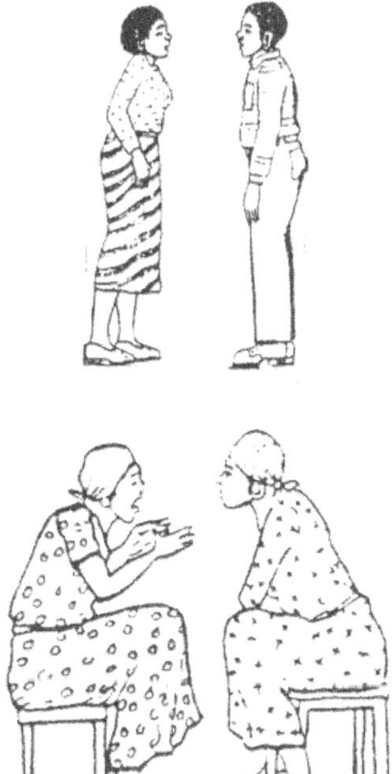

2. ***Learn from local people and AHAs more experienced than you***. Learn from local farmers about the diseases of their animals and how they treat and prevent them. Working and discussing technical issues with a competent and experienced AHA is often an effective way to learn how to diagnose and treat the most common problems in your area.

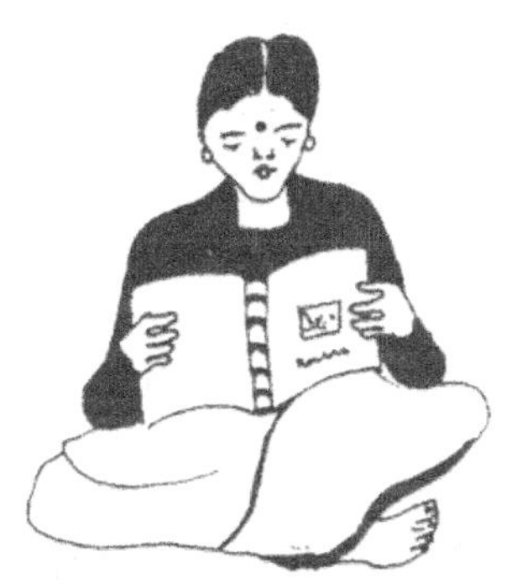

3. ***Study and have an open mind to new ideas.*** Use this book and any other available books to learn more. Keep an open mind about new treatments and techniques. This book is organized by body systems. Once you identify the body system affected, turn to the chapter on that body system and learn about the most common diseases affecting that system.

What if I am unable to diagnose or treat a problem??

Do not panic or get discouraged!! Even the best AHAs are sometimes unable to diagnosis or treat a problem! Diagnosis is especially difficult when an AHA is working alone in a remote area.

If unable to make a diagnosis, all information (history, observations, examination) should be recorded and sent to the nearest veterinary officer, or to a veterinarian in the Ministry of Agriculture. This specialist may then help you diagnose the problem. Even if the animal dies, a diagnosis will be important for other animals in the future with the same problem. The veterinary specialist will be more likely to help AHAs who provide good information. Sometimes, a diagnosis may require specimens from the sick or dead animal. If this is the case, be sure to ask exactly what and how specimens should be taken and preserved.

Sending For Help

Include the following information when sending a report to a district or regional veterinary / animal health officer, or to a veterinarian in the Ministry of Agriculture.

Information from the History

- Species, sex and age of animal.

- When the problem began.

- How the problem began; how it progressed.

- Whether it is getting better or worse.

- Whether there are other animals in the area with similar symptoms.

Information from Observation and Examination

- Important findings after examining the animal and the environment, including the animal's temperature and any observed abnormalities.

- A list of possible diseases based on the history and examination findings. (This list is called a "differential diagnosis.")

- Presumed diagnosis based on findings.

Information Regarding Treatment

- How the animal was treated, including the name and dose of medicine given, method of administration, and length of treatment.

- How the animal responded after treatment.

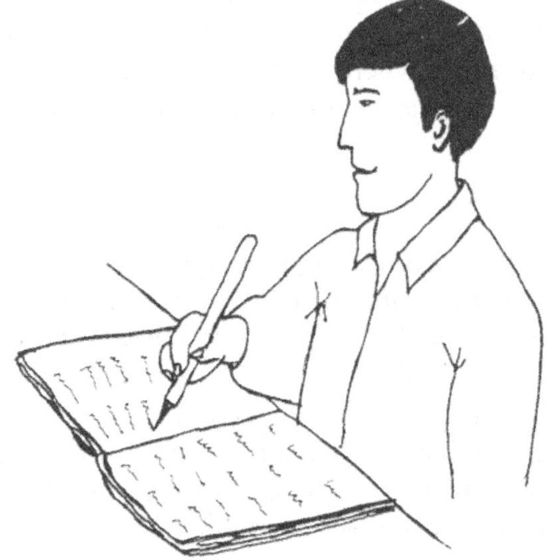

Include the proper information in your requests for help.

4.0   PRINCIPLES OF TREATMENT

4.1   IMPORTANT!!   TREAT AN EMERGENCY QUICKLY
(Also see First Aid, Page 80)

4.2 WHAT TO DO IN THE CASE OF A DISEASE OUTBREAK??

The occurrence of an unusually large number sick animals is called a disease "outbreak."
Large outbreaks of disease are often called "epizootics" or "epidemics." When outbreaks
occur, "control measures" should be taken prevent further spread.

Isolate Sick Animals

First, separate sick animals as well as their urine, manure and bedding from healthy animals.
Do not let people or animals contact sick animals and then go to healthy ones. This is called
"isolation." See page 95.

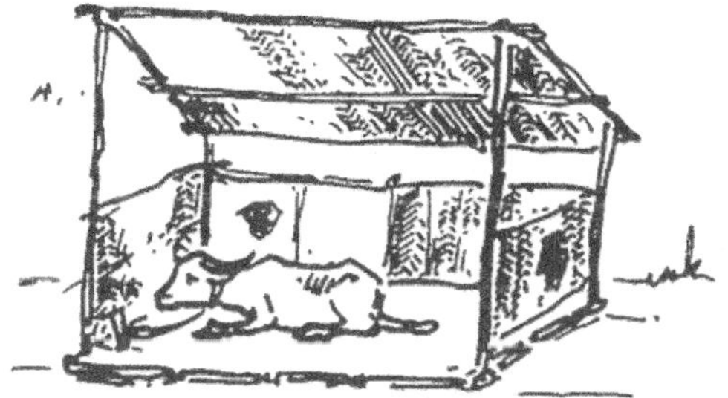 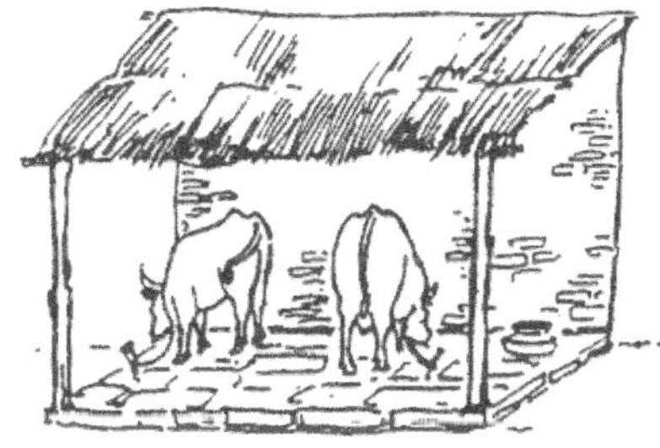

Visit Area Affected and Examine Animals

Investigate the epidemic. Where and when did it start? Were new animals brought into the
area? Where did they come from? What are the initial symptoms, age, sex, species and breed of
animals affected? How many animals are affected? If possible, do physical exams on several sick
animals. Make careful notes.

Notify The Ministry of Agriculture

Inform the Department of Veterinary Services of your findings. Depending upon the situation,
they may want to take over the investigation. If so, the animal health agent should co-operate
fully with the Ministry's actions. If the disease threatens peoples' health, the Ministry of Health
must be informed.

Confirm The Diagnosis

If possible, confirm the diagnosis This may require laboratory specimens and special supplies.
If the laboratory or Ministry request specimens, ask exactly <u>which</u> specimens and <u>how</u> they
should be taken. Someone with special training may need to do this.

Properly Manage Sick and Healthy Animals

Decide how sick and healthy animals in the area should be managed. If there is a large epizootic,
these decisions should be made at the central or intermediate level of the Ministry of Agriculture.
In the case of a small epizootic, if the central or intermediate level does not act, authorities from the
local level should decide what to do. The animal health agent may have to meet with local leaders to
enlist their support in controlling the epidemic. Decisions about treatment should be based on the
ease of use and price of available medicines, as well as the value and number of affected animals.
If there is not enough medicine, difficult decisions must be made regarding <u>which</u> animals to treat.

4.3   CHOOSING A TREATMENT

The treatment chosen depends on several things:
- diagnosis
- number of animals involved
- medicines available
- price of treatment
- value of the animals
- probability that animals will survive and become productive again
- ability of the owner or AHA to use the medicines properly
- ability of the owner to pay
- preferences of the owner

The AHA must explain to the owner the treatment options, price, work involved, and likelihood for recovery. Only then can the owner make the best decision, taking into account the situation and the value of the animal.

It is often impossible to give the best or most complete treatment. For example, the best treatment may require daily injections and be impossible for an owner living far away (unless someone nearby can give the injections). Perhaps another medicine must be chosen. Or, the owner may not have enough money for full treatment. The AHA must use her/his best judgment with each situation.

There may also be certain pressures placed on the AHA. Some farmers <u>expect</u> an AHA to give injections, even if unnecessary! **However, some medicines, such as antibiotics, lose their effectiveness when overused or used needlessly!** Moreover, medicines cost money and are often in limited supply.

On the other hand, if an injection is not given, the owner may think an AHA is incompetent and destroy her credibility in the community. In these situations, an AHA may try to explain and persuade the owner, and use her best judgment in these situations. Sometimes there is no easy solution.

AHAs should try to attend community meetings and spend time in the community learning the knowledge, attitudes and practices of local livestock owners. By establishing a good relationship with the community, as well as asking, observing and listening, an AHA can learn about the most common diseases and the way these diseases are perceived and treated. Meetings and time spent in the community are worthwhile to establish credibility and community participation in addressing local problems. Once credibility is established, an AHA can teach livestock owners some critical concepts about treating, controlling and preventing animal diseases (including the issue of injections!!).

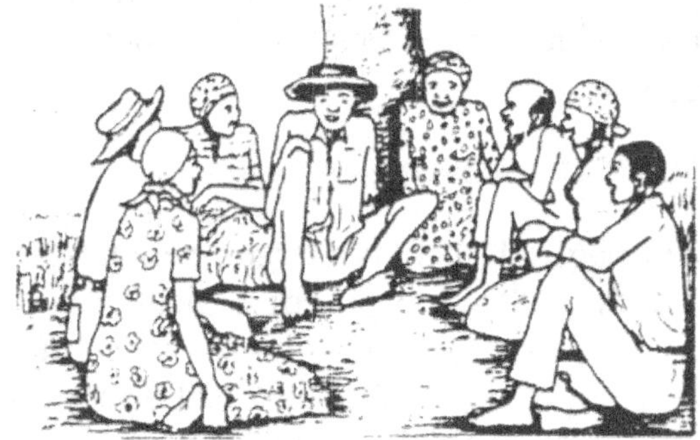

To be effective, an AHA should develop a good relationship with the community.

4.4 SUPPORTIVE CARE FOR A SICK ANIMAL

Regardless of the diagnosis and treatment chosen, certain things should be done for any animal that is sick. This is called "**supportive care.**" Most animals will recover more quickly and completely when good supportive care is provided along with treatment.

Provide high quality food and water for a sick animal to encourage it to eat and drink. A sick animal should always be in a clean, dry, shady and protected environment. It should never be left in the sun, wind, or mud. Protect sick animals from other animals that may attack or injure them.

Supportive care includes:

- *Good food*
- *Plenty of clean water*
- *Good shelter*
- *Protection*

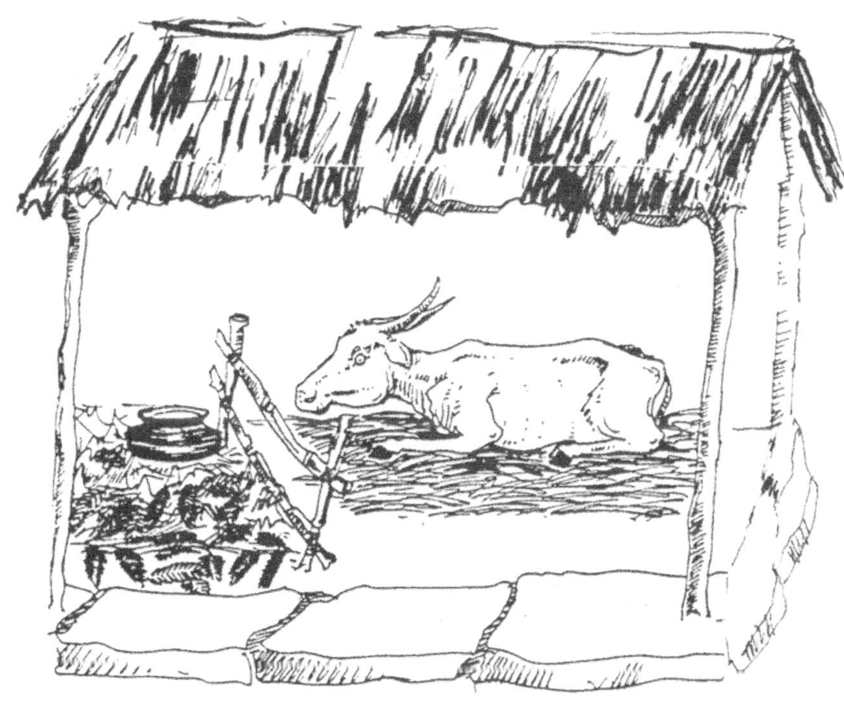

A sick animal needs supportive care: good food, clean water, and a good shelter

4.5 GENERAL TREATMENT FOR A HIGH FEVER

When an animal has a high fever or is overheating, it is should be treated immediately. Otherwise, the fever may rise too high and kill the animal or cause it to abort.

Thoroughly examine the animal and try to determine the cause of the high temperature. Then treat the animal for the specific cause, if possible.

- To bring the temperature down, pour cool water over the animal.
- Keep the animal in the shade.
- Offer the animal cool water to drink. Encourage it to drink by putting the water near its mouth or pouring some water into its mouth. In some cultures, people believe that a drink of water will kill an animal with a fever. This is not true!

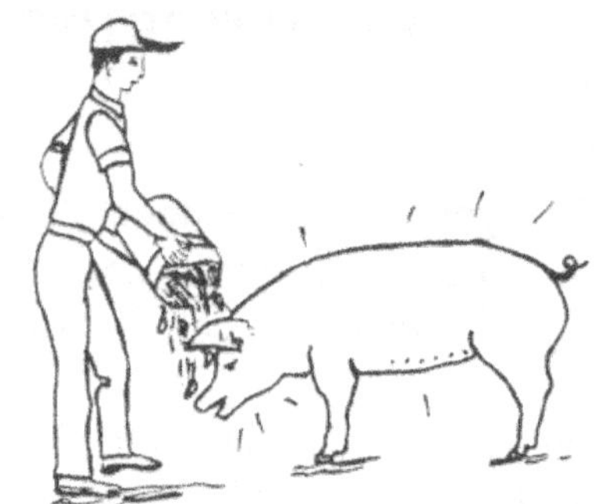

Pouring cool water over the animal can help to cool down an overheated animal.

A sow (mother pig) often cannot regulate her temperature during farrowing (giving birth) and may overheat in hot weather. In this case, pour cool water over her. If this does not work, give her an ice-water enema. It may save her life. Pass a <u>smooth-ended</u> tube <u>gently</u> into the sow's rectum and pour ice water down the tube. If ice water is not available, use the coldest water you can find, for example from a spring or deep well.

The following drugs may also reduce a high temperature:

ASPIRIN: If you can find aspirin for animals, use it according to the instructions. If not, use aspirin for people. Crush the pills, mix the powder with water and put this mixture down the animal's throat. For ruminants or horses, a syringe <u>without the needle</u> works well to squirt the mixture into the back

 of the animal's mouth. Or put the aspirin-water mixture in a narrow-necked bottle, put the opening

of the bottle into the corner of the animal's mouth (in the space where there are no teeth), raise the animal's head and tip the bottle to deliver the medicine. Don't try this with pigs because they will probably bite the syringe, bottle or you. Do not use aspirin for cats since it will poison them. Information on dosage is listed in the back of the book.

DYPYRONE 50%: This is sometimes also called *"Novin."* It can be injected IV, IM or subcutaneous. Give 1 ml / 50 kg bodyweight every eight hours until the fever is gone.

FLUNIXIN MEGLUMINE: A brand name for this is *Banamine*. It can be administered IV or IM. Give 1 ml / 50 kg once daily until the fever is down. It is also available in oral paste and powder. This drug is expensive but very effective.

4.6 DIFFERENT ROUTES FOR GIVING MEDICATIONS

4.6.1 How to Calculate the Amount of Medicine to Give
See Chapter 28 on Medicines.

4.6.2 Where And How, To Give The Medication
There are six common ways to administer a medication.
1. "per os", "PO" or "orally." (Other names for "in the mouth"). See pages 64, 67.
2. By injection under the skin ("sub-cutaneous" or "SQ" or "SC.)" See page 72.
3. By injection in the muscle ("intra-muscular" or "IM.)" See page 73.
4. By injection in the vein ("intra-venous" or "IV.)" See page 74.
5. By local application ("topically)" (i.e. on the surface of a wound, the skin or hoof).
6. By special application to the organ involved. For example:
    - intra-mammary (into the teat), See page 158.
    - intra-uterine (into the uterus), See page 86.
    - intra-ocular (into and around the eye), See page 86.

4.7 HOW TO GIVE MEDICINE IN THE MOUTH (ORAL MEDICATIONS)

> *When giving medicines, an animal should be properly*
> *restrained to avoid injury to the animal or people.*

There are special instruments (tools) for
giving pills or boluses in the mouth of
animals.

balling gun to give pills or boluses

Many species, (i.e., cattle, buffalo, goats, sheep, llamas, alpacas, horses, BUT NOT PIGS!)
have a space <u>without teeth</u> on the side (or corner) of their mouth where a medicine applicator
can be inserted. This will prevent crushing the applicator in the animal's teeth.

4.7.1 For Pills

For large pills, called "boluses", a "balling gun" can be inserted GENTLY into the "corner"
of the animal's mouth <u>where there are no teeth</u>. Gently maneuver the balling gun over the
gums and tongue. **Never jam the balling gun into the mouth or force it deep into the throat**
because this may cause serious injury and infection. Once the balling gun is inserted, push
the plunger gently to place the bolus onto the back of the tongue.

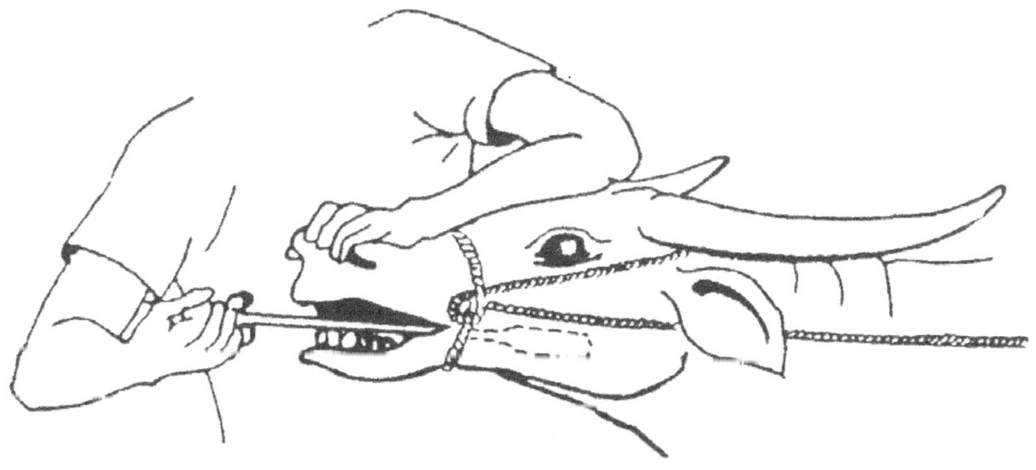

Note: If there is no balling gun, a smooth-edged stiff tube may be inserted as described for the
balling gun. Then slide the pills through the tube onto the back of the animal's tongue. This tube
must be long enough for the pills to fall into the back of the mouth.

4.7.2 For Liquids

For animals other than pigs, feeding liquid medicines, called "drenching", can be done by using a narrow-mouthed bottle <u>with smooth edges</u> or a large syringe (WITHOUT THE NEEDLE!).

Enter the bottle or syringe in the corner of the animal's mouth where there are no teeth, lift the animal's head slightly, and tip the bottle or push the plunger of the syringe.

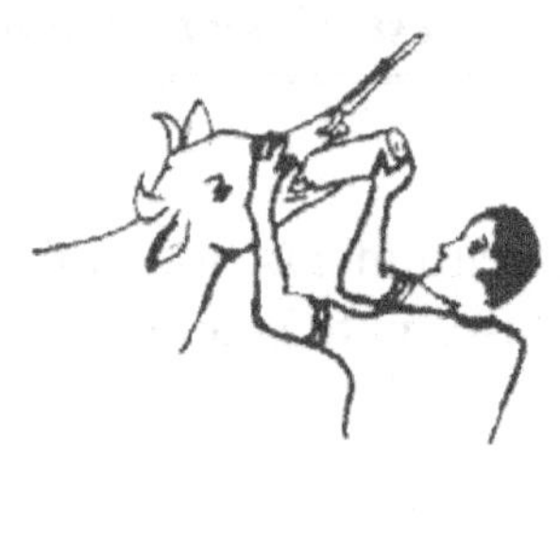

If there is no balling gun, boluses can be dissolved in water and given <u>as a liquid</u> in this manner. Wrap the neck of the bottle with heavy tape or other protective material in case the animal breaks the bottle by biting it.

A special "drenching gun", available in some countries, is useful to treat many animals rapidly and accurately. It is like an automatic syringe that delivers a set amount of medicine each time the trigger is pulled.

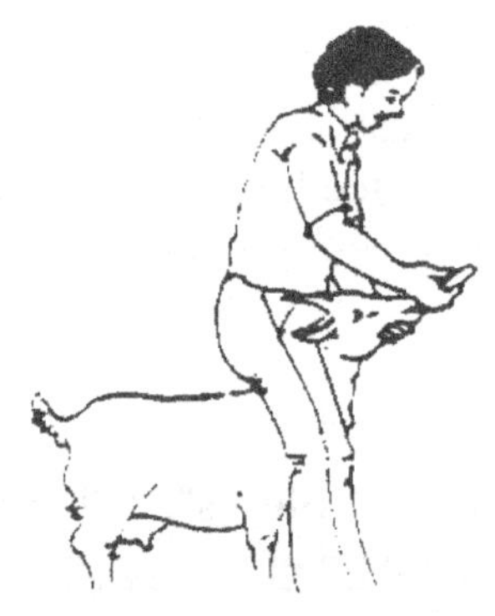

The smooth end of the drenching gun is placed in the corner of the animal's mouth and over the tongue. The trigger is then pulled to deliver the medicine as the animal swallows. The gun refills automatically from a tube that is attached to a plastic bottle.

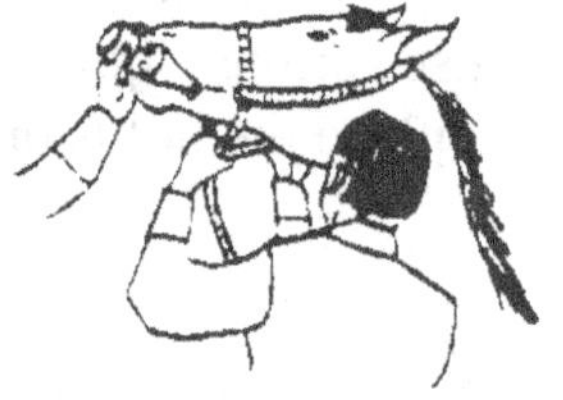

WARNING!!! When lifting an animal's head to give liquid medicine, be careful not to lift it too high. Also be careful not to give the medicine too rapidly. Otherwise, the medicine may enter the windpipe (trachea) and lungs (causing suffocation or pneumonia) instead of the food pipe (esophagus). This is especially true with baby animals.

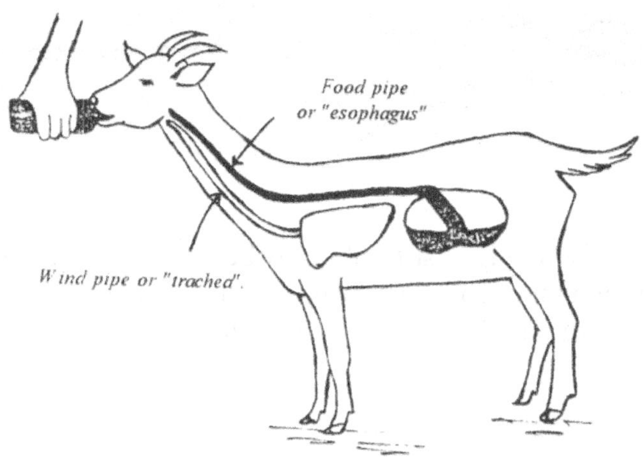

4.7.3 Passing a Stomach Tube in Ruminants
(to Give Fluids or to Relieve Bloat)

To pass a stomach tube in ruminants, a long, flexible (rubber or plastic) tube and a short, hard pipe (called a "speculum") made of metal or bamboo are needed. Both the tube and the speculum should have smooth edges to avoid injuring the animal's mouth or throat. To prevent the animal from biting the tube, first gently insert the speculum into the animal's mouth <u>and hold it firmly so that the animal does not swallow it!</u> Pass the tube through the speculum until it touches the back of the throat and stimulates swallowing. As the animal swallows, gently push the tube down the animal's throat and into its rumen. You can often observe the tube pass down the left side of the animal's neck.

Check to make sure the tube is not in the windpipe! If while passing the tube, the animal starts struggling and coughing, withdraw the tube and start again (the tube may have entered the wind pipe instead of the food pipe). In ruminants, once the tube is in the rumen, check to see if the smell f rumen gas comes out of the tube. If the animal is bloated, gas may rush out. It may be necessary to move and twist the stomach tube or press on the animal's side until the tube is in a pocket of gas. Before putting medicine down the tube, blow air down it and have someone listen on the left flank for gurgling sounds in the rumen (in ruminants). **If there is any doubt about whether the tube is in the rumen, withdraw the tube, let the animal rest, and start again.** When the tube is in the rumen, attach a funnel to the free end of the tube and pour the liquid medicine down the tube.

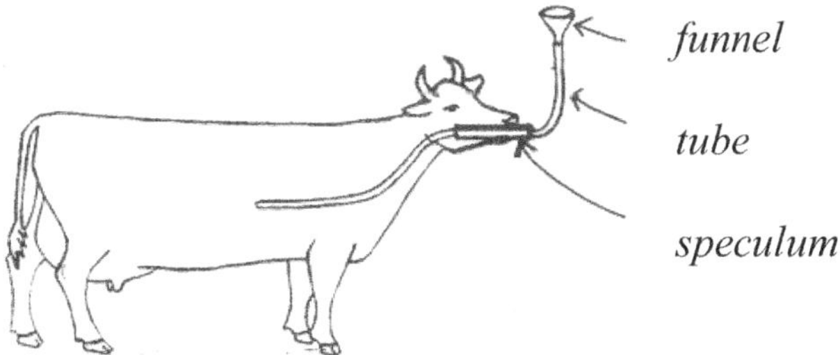

To remove the tube, first blow in the tube to empty it. Then, cover the end of the tube with your thumb and pull the tube out rapidly. Finally, remove the speculum.

Size of tubes and speculums: In cattle, the speculum should be about 25 centimeters in length and a diameter that comfortably fits in the mouth. The flexible tube should be approximately two meters in length and a diameter that can fit through the pipe. In sheep and goats, the hard tube should be about 12 centimeters in length and a diameter that fits comfortably in the mouth. The flexible tube should be at least one meter in length and a diameter that fits through the speculum.

Caution about passing stomach tubes in horses: In horses, the procedure is similar except a speculum is not needed and the tube is passed along the <u>bottom</u> surface of the **nose** (not the top surface, otherwise the nose will bleed!), down the throat and into the stomach. <u>Be extremely careful in horses because it is much easier to accidentally pass the stomach tube down the wind pipe and into the lungs.</u>

4.7.4 Giving Oral Medicines To Pigs

Warning! Adult pigs have sharp teeth on the side of their mouths and powerful jaws. When giving oral medications, they may try to bite you or the applicator.

Pigs can be fed oral liquid medicines by holding them with a snare, (See page 28) and squirting the medicine into one nostril using a syringe (without the needle!). Begin by giving the medicine slowly until the pig starts to swallow. Then rapidly give the rest of the medicine.

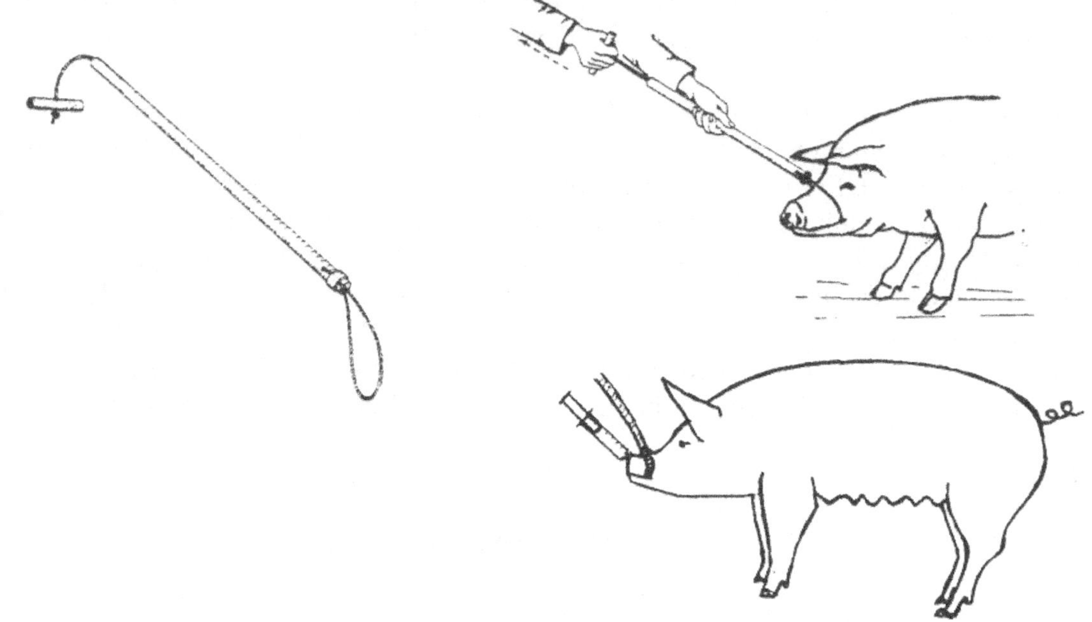

4.7.5 Special mouth speculums

Although there are special mouth speculums for each species to help give oral medicines, <u>local materials</u> can usually be used and are less expensive.

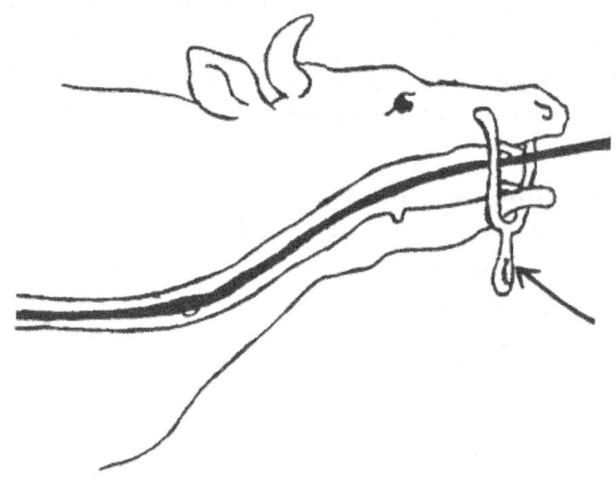

A SPECIAL SPECULUM CAN BE USED TO KEEP THE MOUTH OPEN.

4.8.1 Syringes

Syringes come in many sizes indicated by the number of milliliters (ml's) or cubic centimeters (cc's) they contain. (Note: 1 ml = 1 cc) Syringes are made of durable plastic, metal or glass. Glass and metal syringes usually last longer and are easier to clean and re-sterilize. However, they are expensive and glass parts are easily broken.

Some syringes come in the form of a "pistol" or "dosing syringe." They are designed to inject several animals consecutively with the same product before it is necessary to refill the syringe.

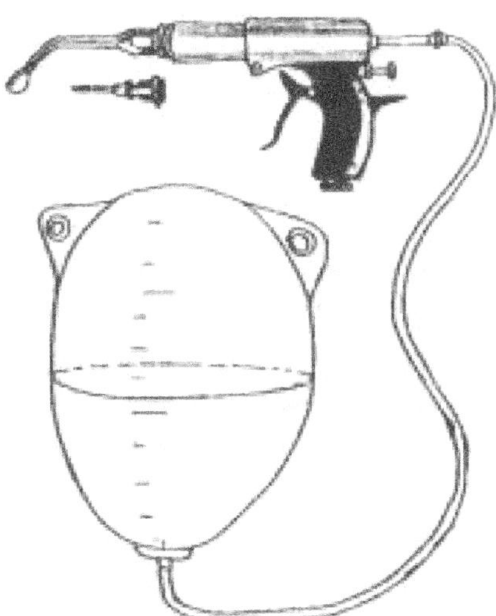

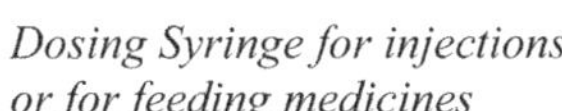

*Dosing Syringe for injections
or for feeding medicines*

The dosing syringe can be adjusted to automatically deliver a set amount of vaccine or oral medicine at each injection. Dosing syringes can be connected by a plastic tube to a "backpack" that contains a large quantity of medicine or vaccine. This avoids having to refill the syringe repeatedly. It is especially useful if many animals will be injected consecutively and rapidly with the same product. However, if the needle is not changed between animals, certain diseases can be spread from animal to animal.

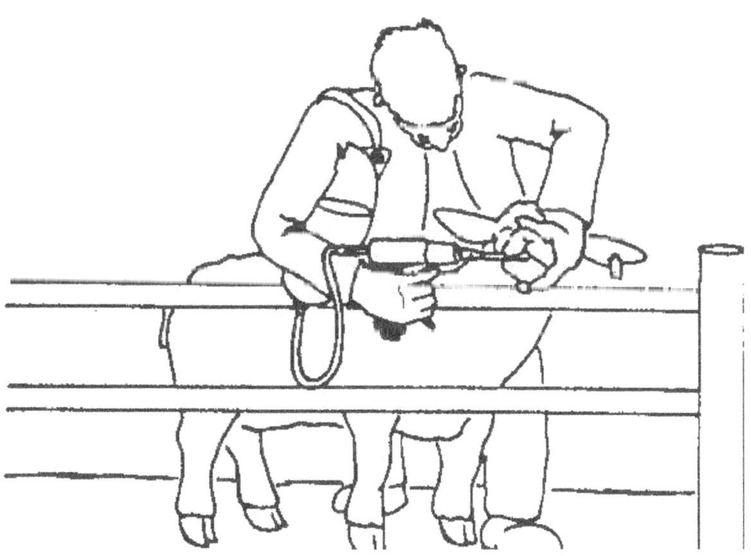

4.8.2 Needles

Needles come in different lengths and bore sizes (i.e. diameters). On the base of the needle or
needle package, the length is indicated in inches or centimeters, and the bore size is indicated as a
"gauge." It is usually written like this:

"16G x 1"   This means a 16 gauge needle that is one inch in length.

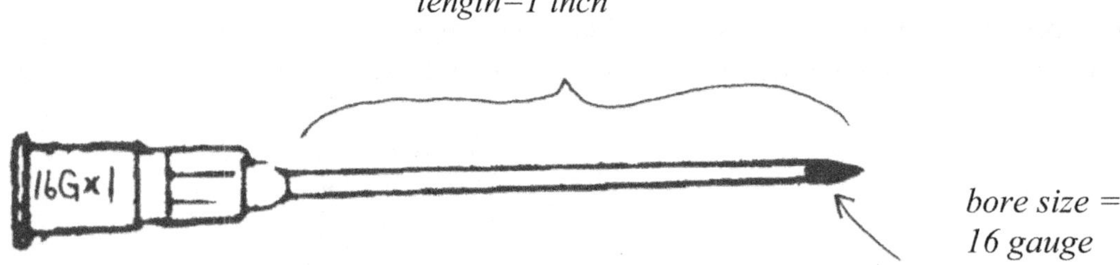

LENGTH
Most medicines for livestock require a needle 1 to 1.5 inches in length. For subcutaneous
injections, 1.0 inch needles are sufficient, although 1.5 inch needles can be used. For deep
intramuscular injections, choose 1.5 inch needles if you have them, except in baby livestock
where 1 inch needles are sufficient.

DIAMETER OR BORE SIZE
Most medicines for livestock require 16 to 22 gauge needles; the larger the gauge, the smaller
the bore size. The choice of bore size depends on the animal species and size as well as the
"viscosity" (thickness) of the medicine.

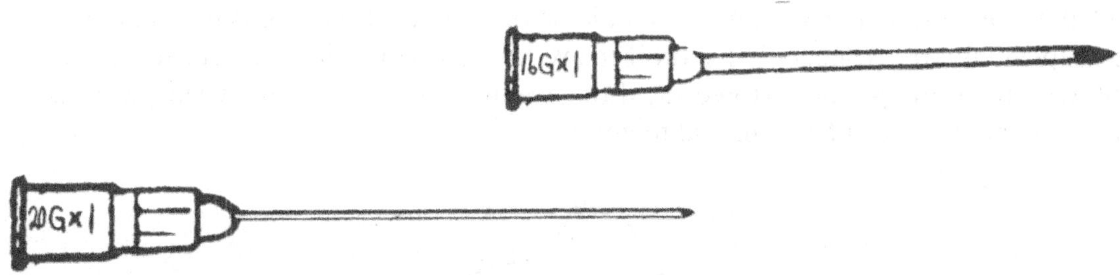

For baby livestock, 20 or 22 gauge needles are appropriate, unless the thickness of the medicine
requires a larger bore. For example, most penicillin cannot be given through a needle smaller
than 19 gauge. In adult livestock, 16 to 19 gauge needles are used depending on the thickness
of their skin. Large bore (small gauge) needles make it easier to inject medications and don't
bend as easy as small bore needles. But more medicine can leak back from a large bore injection
site and be wasted.

4.8.3 Preparing A Syringe and Needle for Injection

Carefully calculate the amount of medicine
needed, based on the animal's weight and
concentration of the drug as specified on
the label.

Wash hands with soap and water.

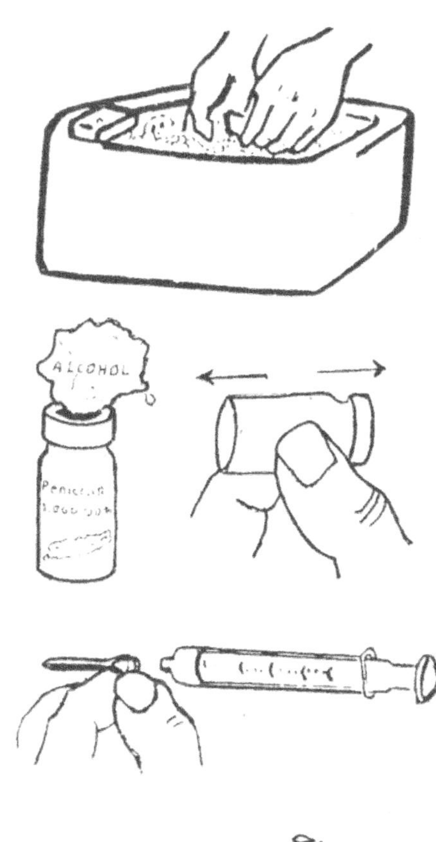

Clean the rubber top of the medicine vial
with disinfectant and shake the vial to mix
the medicine.

Attach a <u>sterile</u>, <u>capped</u> needle securely to a
syringe.

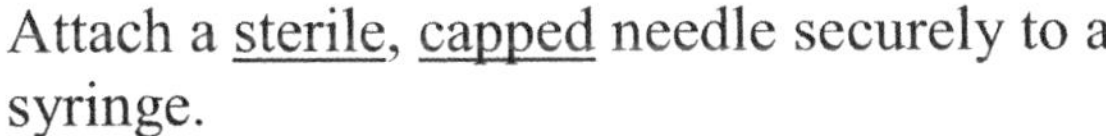

Remove the needle cap and introduce the
needle into the vial. Making sure the tip of
the needle is submersed in the medicine,
pull on the plunger to fill the syringe with
the necessary quantity of medicine.

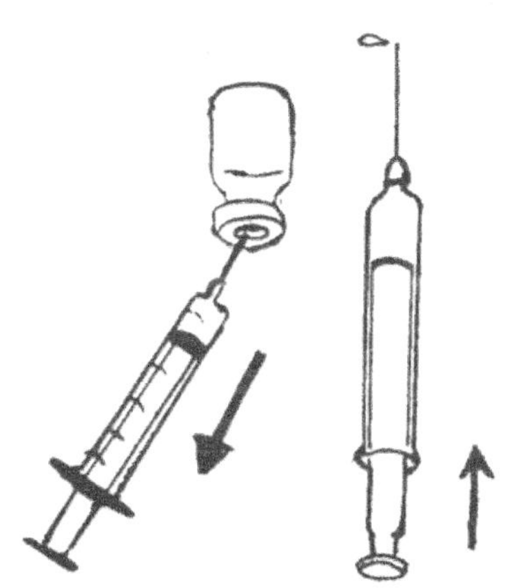

Remove the needle. With the needle
pointed up, push the plunger slightly to
remove any excess air in the syringe. After
removing the air, make sure enough
medicine still remains in the syringe.

Give the injection immediately or replace
the needle cap to avoid contamination.

**Whenever the needle cap Is removed, avoid touching the needle (except at the base)
or allowing it to touch other things that may contaminate it.**

USE STERILE, SHARP NEEDLES

Needles and syringes should be discarded, or they should be
rinsed and re-sterilized before their next use.

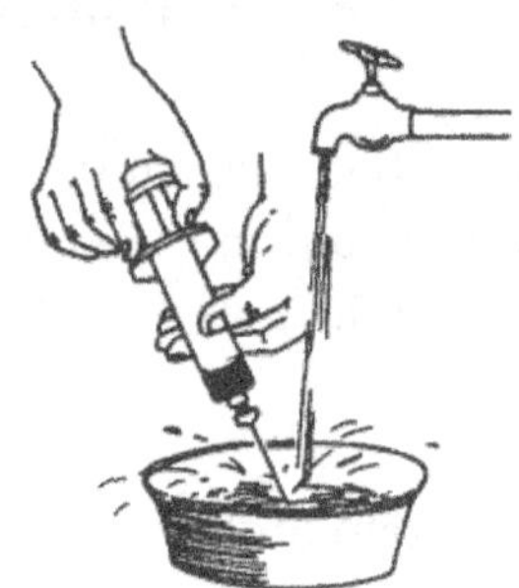

Dull needles should be re-sharpened or discarded
since they may cause abscesses.

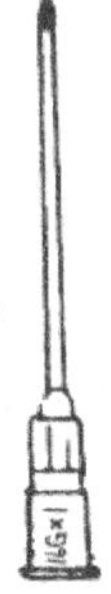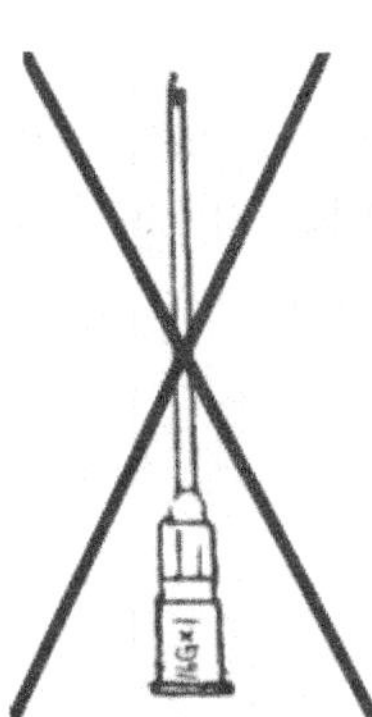

DISCARD PROPERLY AND SAFELY!

Needles should be discarded in a narrow-mouthed container with a secure
lid. When the container becomes full, it should be discarded by burning or
burying.

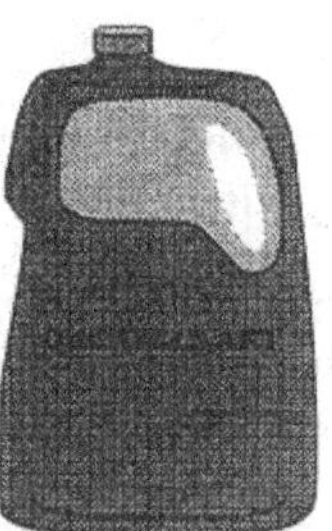

Needles should NEVER be discarded by tossing them on the
ground or in the general (municipal) garbage. This may result in
needle stick injuries to people or animals.

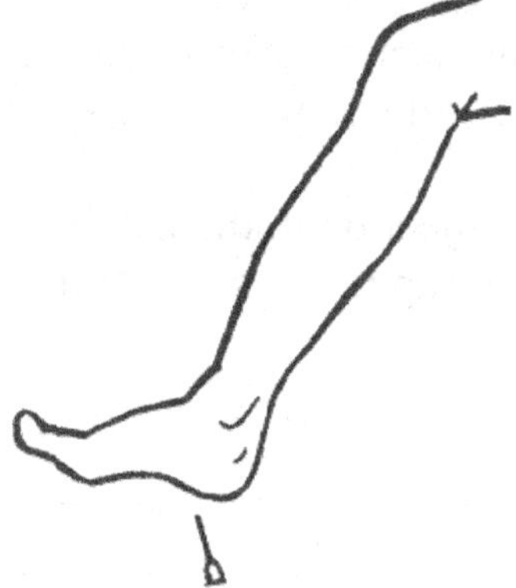

NEVER insert a <u>used</u> needle into a bottle of medicine or vaccine. Always use a sterile needle.
Otherwise the entire bottle of medicine can be contaminated.

4.8.4 Subcutaneous & Intramuscular Injections

Sub-cutaneous injections: A sub-cutaneous (or SQ or SC) injection is given under the skin.
The preferred sites to give SQ injections are where:
-     there is loose skin.
-     it is easy to give an injection without getting kicked, hit by horns, or otherwise hurt.
-     there will be good drainage if an abscess develops.

Intra-muscular injections: An intra-muscular (or IM) injection is given in the muscle.

The black circles marked on each animal below are the preferred sites for SQ and IM
injections.

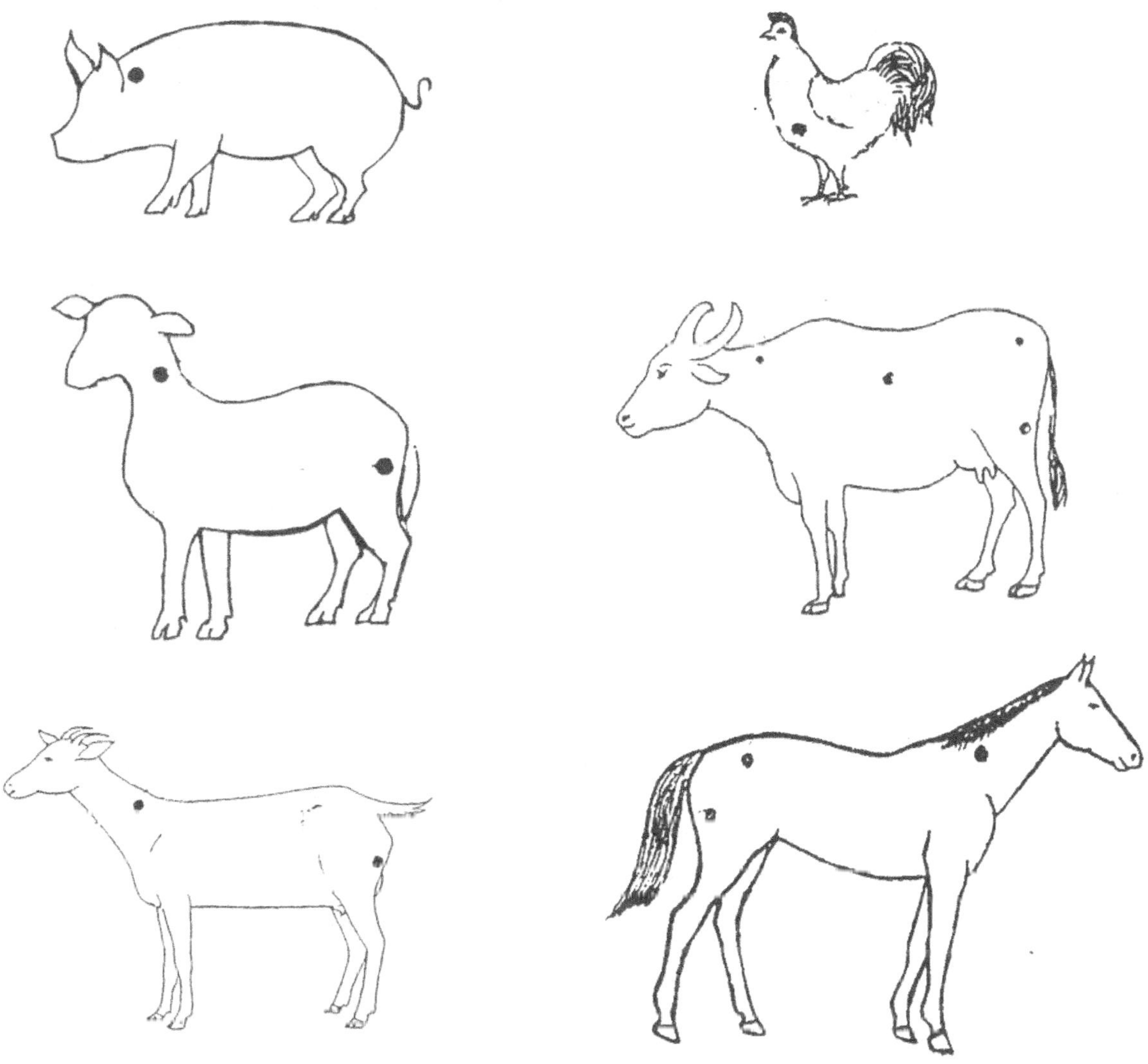

NOTE: Injections into the large muscles of the rump or back leg can cause extensive damage to
the tissue and the loss of a large amount of meat. Injections in the neck area are preferred.

HOW TO GIVE A SUBCUTANEOUS OR INTRAMUSCULAR INJECTION

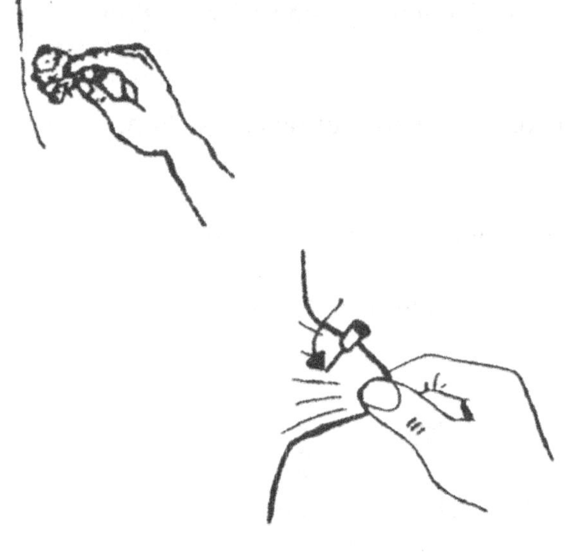

Prepare the syringe and needle. Restrain the animal properly and choose the site for injection. If the site is dirty, wash it or choose another site. If the site is clean, remove the needle from the syringe. Hold the base of the needle firmly with your thumb and forefinger.

Warn everyone around you to stand back or to be ready in case the animal reacts.

For SQ injections: Pull (tent) the skin with one hand and insert the needle so that point lies between skin and the underlying muscle.

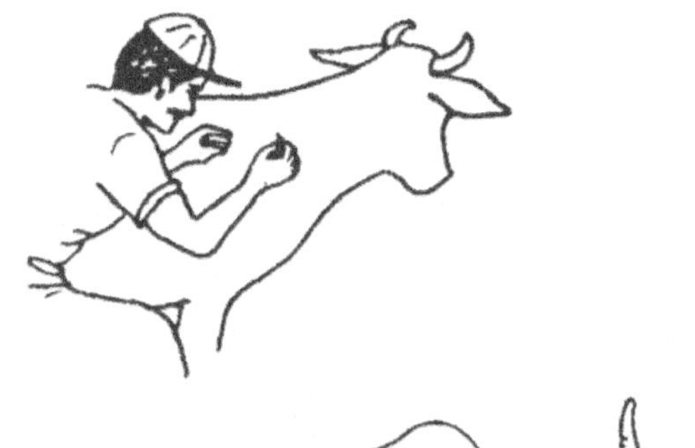

For IM injections: Place the needle boldly and quickly through the skin and into the animal's muscle by directing the needle at a right angle to the skin as it enters the animal.

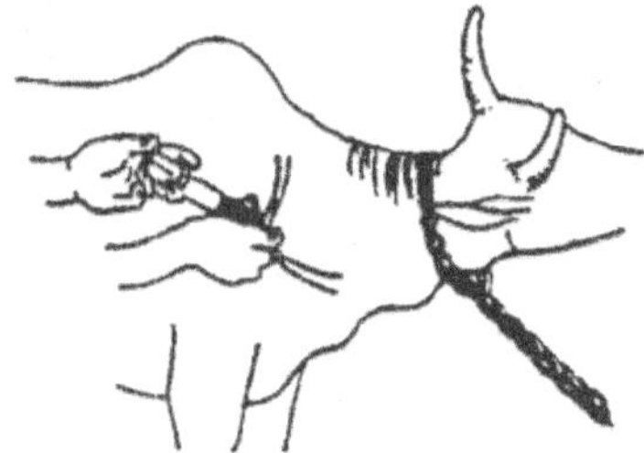

Attach the syringe securely to the needle.

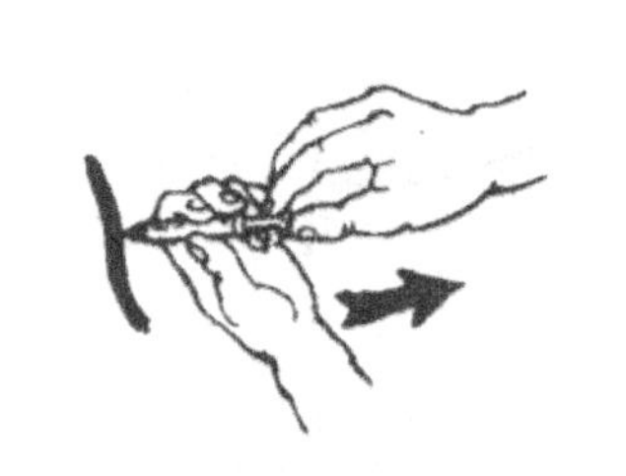

Pull back on the plunger slightly and see if blood enters the hub of the needle or the syringe. If so, this means the needle accidentally entered a vein. Partially withdraw the needle and reposition it.

If there is no sign of blood, push the plunger to administer the injection. Then withdraw the syringe & needle.

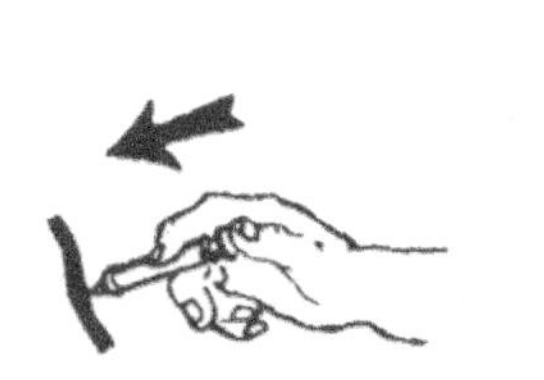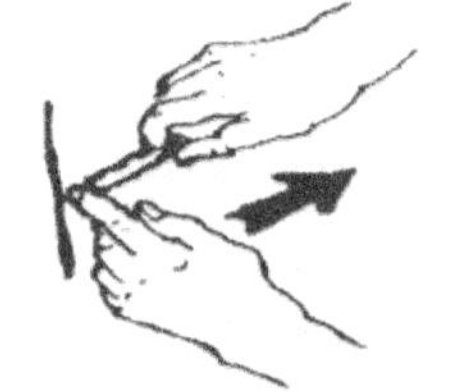

4.8.5 Giving Intravenous Injections In Ruminants & Horses

In general, the most commonly used medicines can be given in the mouth, SQ or IM. Occasionally, an AHA may have to give an intravenous injection (or IV) injection, although generally this is done by experienced technicians or veterinarians.   The preferred site for IV injections is the jugular vein. This vein is quite large and easy to find in adult cattle, horses, goats and sheep.

Prepare the syringe.

Restrain the animal properly with the animal's head slightly lifted and away from you. Cattle that cannot stand up can be restrained by placing a halter or nose tongs on its head or nose and tying the free end of the rope to the back leg. Clean the site.

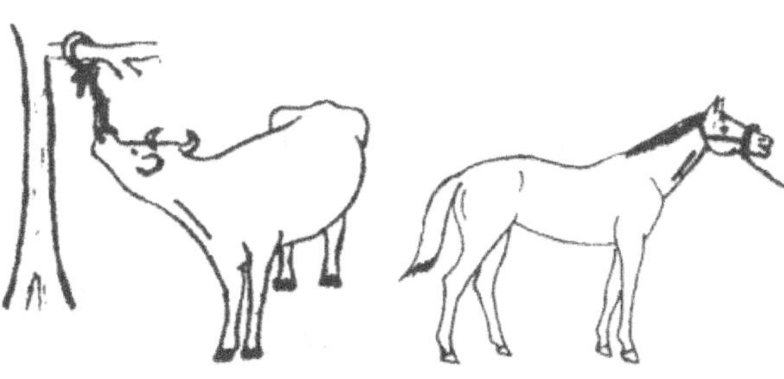

Remove the needle from the syringe and grasp the needle firmly with your thumb and forefinger.

Find the jugular vein by lifting and slightly turning the animal's head away from you and finding a groove in the animal's neck. Press your thumb into this groove. This will cause the jugular vein to bulge above your thumb and is called "holding off" the jugular vein.

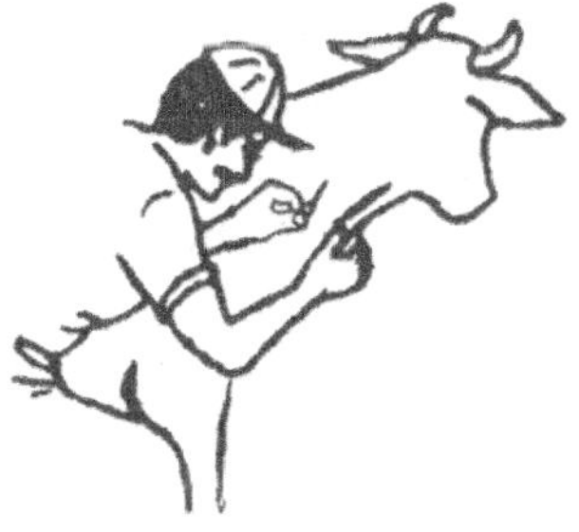

Warn everyone around that you are going to place the needle and to stand back or be ready in case the animal reacts.

While still holding off the vein, quickly and boldly insert the needle through the skin and into the vein by directing the needle at an angle as it enters. You will feel the needle enter the vein and blood will trickle out the needle hub. Before administering any medicine, the needle should be "threaded" into the vein until the hub is touching the skin. Blood should drip from the properly threaded needle.

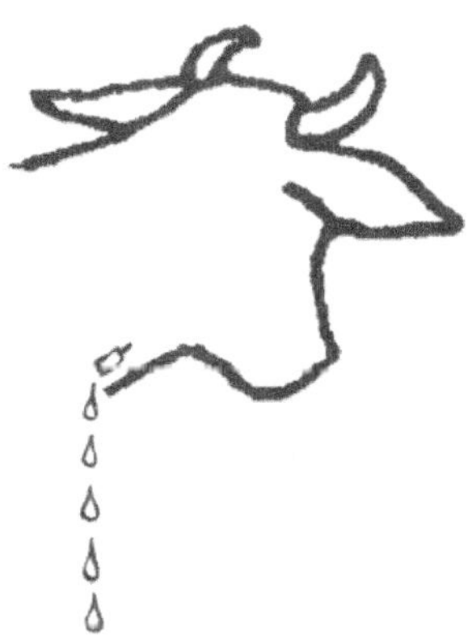

Use a 19 gauge needle or larger bore when giving IV injections. Otherwise, it may not be possible to detect if the needle entered the artery because blood is usually too thick to pulsate out of a smaller bore needle.

When you are sure that the needle is in the vein, attach the syringe securely to the needle. Withdraw the plunger slightly to see that blood enters the syringe. This is to assure that the needle is still in the vein. If not, re-position the needle. If blood flows easily into the syringe, push the plunger to administer the injection.

Never give an injection in the artery!

WARNING: Blood PULSATING or spurting out of the needle is a sign that the needle accidentally entered an artery instead of the vein. This is a rare event that happens most commonly in horses, llamas and alpacas. <u>NEVER give an injection in the artery!</u> If you are not sure where the needle is, withdraw it and try again.

WARNING: Some IV injections should be given slowly or the animal may collapse. Check the label or ask an experienced person.

WARNING: Some IV injections are quite caustic and can severely damage the surrounding tissue if accidentally given outside the vein. This is true for a drug called "phenylbutazone" often given to horses. Check the label or ask an experienced person.

4.8.6 Intravenous Injections in Pigs

An intravenous injection is usually given to pigs in an ear vein. Carefully restrain the pig with a snare and place an elastic band or rope around the base of the pig's ear. Clean off the ear and wait for the ear veins to fill up with blood. The largest vein is usually a vein that runs along the back edge of the ear flap.

Choose a vein that is full of blood and easy to see. Insert a 19-gauge needle and thread it into the vein as far as possible. This minimizes the possibility that the needle will slip out of the vein if the pig shakes its head or resists. Attach the syringe and withdraw slightly on the plunger to verify that the needle is still in the vein. If it is, blood will enter into the syringe. <u>Release the elastic band before injecting</u>. Then push the plunger to give the injection.

CAUTION: The ear veins of pigs are fragile. IV injections must be administered slowly to avoid rupturing the vein. Excellent restraint is essential!

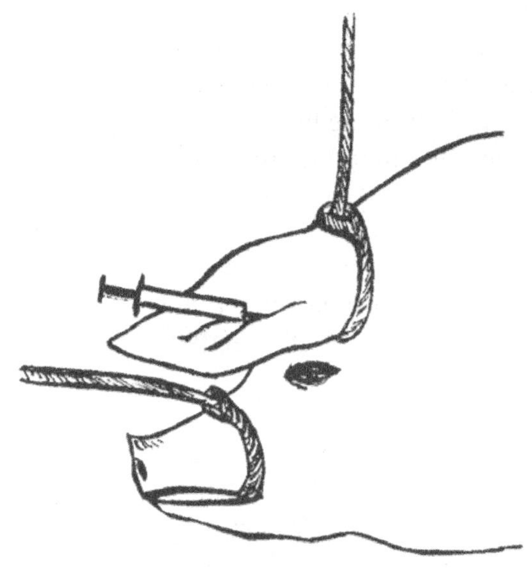

4.9 CLEANING AND STERILIZING EQUIPMENT

Cleaning and/or sterilizing instruments reduces the risk of spreading disease by these instruments. The following methods may be used on glass, metal and plastic equipment, but will eventually damage plastic equipment. Note: For some organisms like anthrax spores, the following methods may not be sufficient.

Step 1: Clean

Equipment should be cleaned immediately after use. It may be necessary to scrub with a brush to clean blood from joints and the inner surfaces of the instruments.

Step 2: Disinfect &/or Sterilize

DISINFECTION

***Savlon* Method:** Use 10 ml *Savlon* for every liter of water. (1:100 solution). Soak instruments and suture for 20 minutes before using.

Chlorine Bleach Method: Use 1-part chlorine to 7 parts of water and soak for 20 minutes.

Alcohol/Spirit Method: Soak instruments, suture and cotton wool for about 20 minutes in concentrated (70%) ethyl alcohol or drinking alcohol.

STERILIZATION

Flaming: Pour alcohol over <u>metal</u> instruments and ignite the alcohol.

Steam Method: Metal instruments, nylon suture and cotton wool are placed in a steam sterilizer for 15 minutes. If no steam sterilizer is available, the surgery tray can be placed into a pressure cooker for 15 minutes.

Boiling Method: Boil metal or glass instruments for 20 minutes.

Step 3. Rinse

<u>After disinfecting</u>, all syringes and other instruments should be rinsed with sterile (boiled) water. <u>Do not rinse instruments after sterilizing them.</u>

Step 4. Dry

After cleaning and disinfecting, sterilized instruments should be covered with a sterilized cloth and allowed to air dry. They should be kept wrapped until just before use. Equipment should be stored in a dry, dust-free place.

Do not <u>store</u> equipment in disinfectant. Storing instruments in disinfectant solutions will destroy the equipment.

Note: Sometimes equipment such as needles, syringes, scalpel blades, syringes, scissors, or forceps are needed frequently on a busy day. In this case, the equipment can be stored <u>temporarily</u> in a covered glass or metal tray and filled with disinfectant. After the clinic, remove the instruments from the disinfectant, clean them, dry them, and store them properly.

Prepare fresh disinfectant daily and replace solution that becomes dirty or contaminated during use. If equipment is kept in disinfectant often, add sodium-nitrate at a rate of 4 grams per liter to the solution to help protect the instruments.

5.0   First Aid

5.1   SYMPTOMS OF AN EMERGENCY   -   QUICK REFERENCE LIST

> *A good AHA knows which symptoms need treatment immediately!*

MAJOR First Aid: Accidents, Poisons, Sudden Illness, Allergic Reactions, Shock

-Injuries or accidents	Page 78
-Broken bones (fractures)	Page 232
-Toxicity (poisonings)	Pages 80-83, 254-255
-Bloat (tympany)	Pages 185-188
-Snake or insect bites	Pages 82, 255
-Shock	Page 85
-Bleeding, heavy or continuous	Page 78
-Bleeding from nose	Pages 186, 202
-Difficulty breathing	Pages 199-200
-Inability to stand up or move (paralysis)	Page 259
-Has not urinated for two or more days	Page 247
-Has not drunk anything for two days or more	Page 267
-Dark colored or black manure (intestinal bleeding ulcer)	Page 194
-Painful abdomen (colic)	Page 190
-Watery discharge from the teat of a lactating cow	Page 155
-Sudden stiffness (tetanus)	Page 258
-High fever	Pages 62-63
-Accumulation of fluid under the jaw.	Page 52
-Strange, aggressive or crazy behavior	Page 250
-An animal having tremors or convulsions	Page 257
-Wound that suddenly becomes more inflamed and hot	Page 219
-Birthing problem	Pages 139-147
-Prolapsed rectum or uterus	Page 149
-Severe dehydration with sunken eyes & weakness	Pages 50, 267
-Any wound that may need suturing	Page 213
-Exposure to a large number of dead or dying animals	Page 60

MINOR First Aid   Eye Injuries, Wounds, Broken Horns, Burns

-Eye Injuries	Page 85
-Wounds	Page 212
-Broken Horns	Page 225
-Burns	Page 220

5.2   FIRST AID: DEFINITION

First Aid is the immediate treatment of injuries or sudden illness with whatever facilities and materials are available to save the animal's life or prevent permanent damage.

5.3   MAJOR FIRST AID

5.3.1 Injuries/Accidents

In the case of most serious injuries and accidents, first aid should consist of the following:

Check if the animal is breathing.

Pull the animals head up or back to "straighten" the wind pipe and open the airways as wide as possible. If there is fluid or blood in the airways, small animals can be held upside down to allow the fluid to drain. If the animal is not breathing, give artificial respiration by pushing on the chest 10-20 times per minute. For small animals and newborn babies, artificial respiration can be given by covering the nose and breathing into the mouth about 10 times per minute.

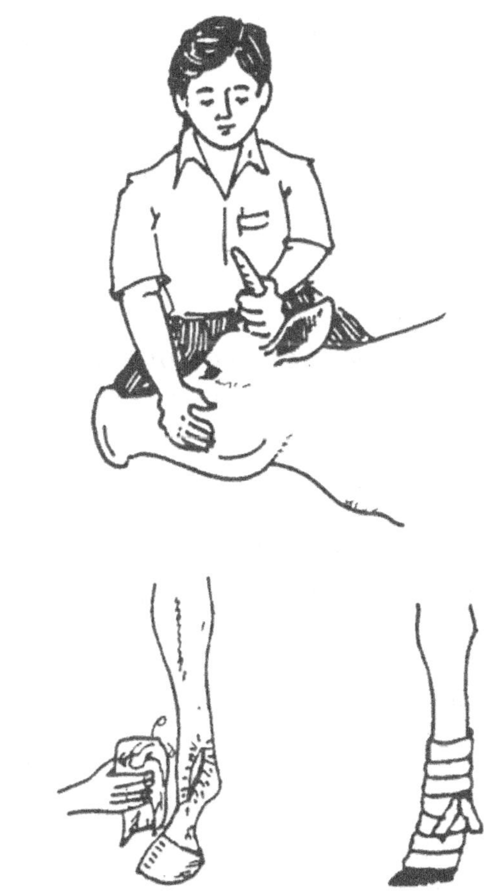

Stop serious bleeding.

Use any of the following measures:

Apply pressure directly to the wound itself with a clean piece of cloth or a tight bandage; or apply pressure to the major blood vessel which supplies blood to the injured area. When the serious bleeding has stopped, thoroughly clean and care for the wound, and give antibiotics.

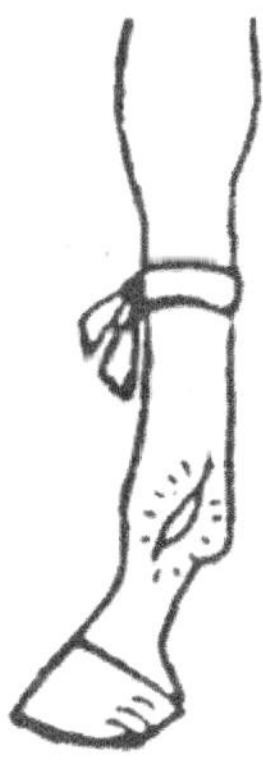

Apply a tourniquet. If blood is spurting or pulsating with great force from a wound, it is likely that an artery is cut. If the wound is on a limb, a tourniquet, which is simply a rope or thin strip of cloth, can be tied tightly around a limb ab<u>ove</u> the wound (i.e. somewhere between the wound and the heart). It stops blood flow to the area and allows a clot to form. A tourniquet should be released every 20 minutes to check for bleeding and to allow some blood to flow into the area.

For hard tissue like horns and hooves, apply potassium permanganate crystals (if available) with a damp piece of cloth.

For bleeding horns, one can tie (temporarily) a tight band around the base of the horn to block some of the blood vessels going into the horn. Likewise, for castration wounds in calves, sheep, and goats that continue to bleed hours after the castration is done, one can tie a tight band temporarily around the base of the scrotum (the sac of skin that held the testicles).

A red hot piece of iron or metal can also be used to cauterize bleeding arteries on horns, hooves and castration wounds, although care should be taken to avoid burning surrounding tissue.

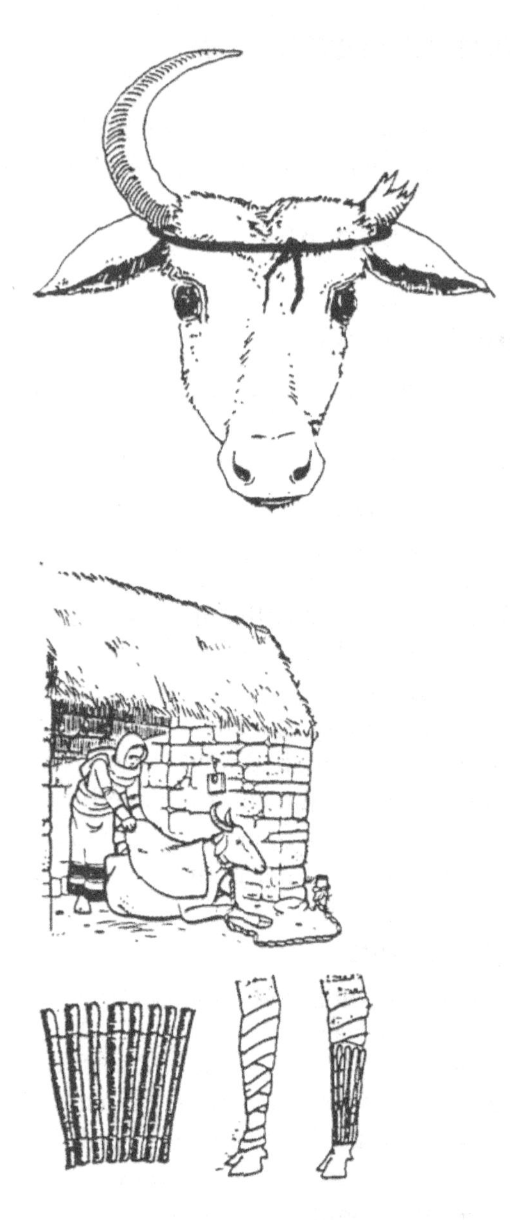

Keep the animal warm, dry and comfortable.
Protect the animal from extreme heat, cold, sun and wind.

Do not move the animal until it is stable.
Check for fractures. If a lower leg fracture is present, apply a splint before moving the animal. See page 233. It may also be necessary to relieve pain with aspirin or another pain killer. The animal can be moved when its condition is stable.

Transport an animal as comfortably and quietly as possible to prevent it from struggling and injuring itself more. For example, do not carry the animal upside-down or on its back! A large animal can be carried by placing strong pieces of wood underneath the animal's belly and having several people lift the end of the boards.

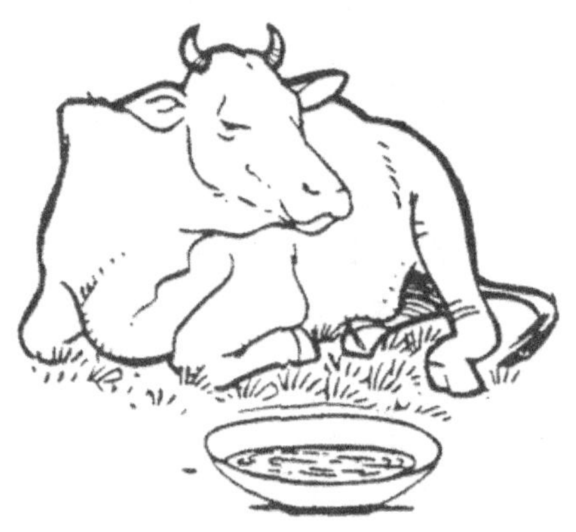

Offer water to the animal.
As soon as it can drink, offer water to the animal. However, **do not force it to drink** if it cannot swallow.

5.3.2 Poisons and Toxicity

When poisonous plants or other toxic feeds may have been eaten:

a. Take a thorough history. Determine whether the owner or caretaker is sure that the animal(s) ate something poisonous and the amount of time elapsed since the poison was eaten.

b. Examine the environment to try to identify the source of the poison. Be sure to check all feed and water sources, pastures, and any shelters where the affected animals stay. Collect samples of suspect plants or other substances.

If animals with symptoms were grazing in an area with poisonous substances, assume the animal ate the poison and treat it. Most poisonous plants do not taste good. However, when animals are hungry, such as during the dry season, they may eat poisonous plants.

c. Examine both sick and healthy animals. Verify how many are sick with the same or similar symptoms and compare these animals to the healthy ones. Try to determine what the sick animals were exposed to that the healthy ones were not.

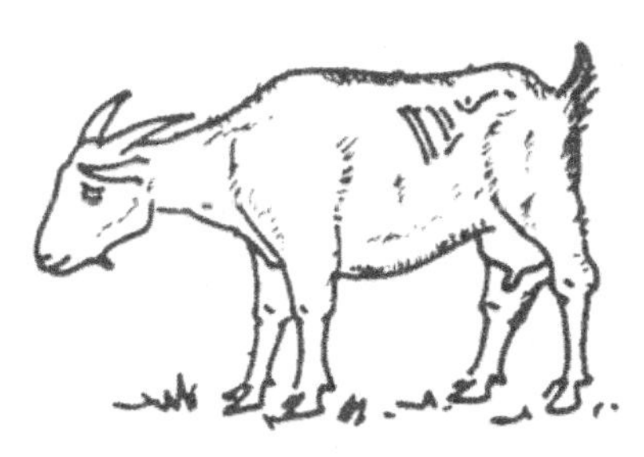

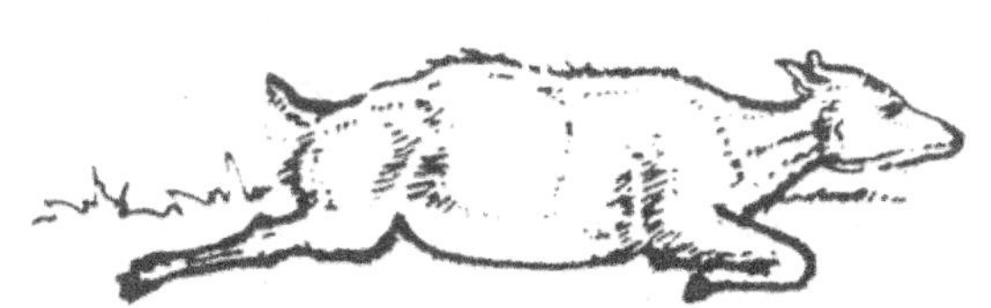

General symptoms of poisoning:
Although the symptoms usually depend on the type of poisonous plant that was eaten, many poisonous plants cause the following symptoms.
- Suddenly dull or with odd behavior.
   - No appetite.
   - Bloating. This may also be accompanied by difficult breathing.
   - Diarrhea & excess salivation (i.e drooling or frothing at the mout
   - Off-colored gums or conjunctiva (the tissue around the eyes). If the gums o conjunctiva are brownish, suspect nitra toxicity. If they are bright red, suspec cyanide toxicity.
   - Sudden death.

Note: A high temperature is usually NO a sign of plant poisoning.

General Treatment of Toxicity

Empty the stomach. Since it is difficult to make ruminants vomit and since horses cannot vomit, empty the stomach and intestines by feeding one of the following medicines that cause diarrhea. Mix these medicines in water and give it orally.
-    **Magnesium sulfate:** This is most commonly available (dose: 250 mg/kg or one teaspoon per five kg of bodyweight). 200-300 gm for large animals; 20-40 gm for small animals.
-    **Sodium sulfate (Glauber's salt):** If available, this is preferred over magnesium sulfate. The dose is the same as magnesium sulfate.
-    **Sorbital:** The dose is two grams/kg of body weight.

Give activated charcoal: If available, activated charcoal can be given with the medicines above. Activated charcoal helps to absorb the poison. A dose of two gm/kg body weight diluted 1:10 in water can be given by mouth. Do not confuse activated charcoal with ordinary charcoal!
Note: In general, activated charcoal should not be mixed with mineral oil or other oils.

Note: In small animals (dogs and cats), the stomach may be emptied by making them vomit. This is usually only effective if no more than two hours have passed since the poison was eaten. Soapy water and certain local plants (those recognized as traditional medicines) often work to make a small animal vomit.

Treat for bloat: If the animal is bloated and cannot breathe properly, pass a stomach tube or use a trochar, cannula, or knife. Once the bloat is relieved, give magnesium sulfate. See section on *bloat*. See pages 186-187.

Some common plant poisonings

Cyanide or Prussic Acid Poisoning
Cyanide is found in the seeds or leaves of certain plants. Young, rapidly growing plants or those wilting due to frost or drought are more likely to have cyanide. Toxic levels of cyanide are also found in some rat poisons.

Symptoms: The symptoms occur rapidly and include bright red gums and rapid, difficult breathing. Sometimes animals are simply found dead.

Treatment:
1. Give **magnesium sulfate** in the mouth to cause diarrhea and get rid of the toxin.

2. In mild cases, give oral **sodium thiosulfate:** 30 gm for large animals; and five gm for small animals. Repeat it every hour until the animal is better.

3. In serious cases, mix 66 grams of **sodium thiosulfate** in 500 ml of sterile water and give in the vein at a dose of 500 ml per 100 kg body weight.

Plants that can produce cyanide:

Hoecius lunatus	velvet grass
Hydrangea spp.	hydrangea
Linium spp.	flax
Lotus corniculatus	birdsfoot trefoil
Phaseolus lunatus	lima bean
Prunus spp.	cherry
	apricot
	peach
Pyrus malus	apple
Sambucus canadensis	elderberry
Sorghum spp.	sudan & johnson grass
Suckleya suckleyena	poison suckleya
Trifolium repens	white clover
Triglochin maritima	arrow grass
Vicia sativa	vetch seed
Zea mays	maize

Prevention of Cyanide Poisoning:
Avoid grazing pastures where cyanide-producing plants are known to grow. Especially avoid these pastures when the plants are growing rapidly and when they have been recently wilted by frost or drought.

Nitrate Poisoning

Nitrate poisoning can occur when animals eat plants following a period of drought, or when they drink water contaminated with nitrates. Soils high in nitrates or ammonia, particularly acid soils, are more likely to cause nitrate toxicity. Similarly, soils low in the minerals molybdenum, sulfur, or phosphorous are more likely to cause nitrate poisoning. Finally, low temperatures also increase the risk of toxicity.

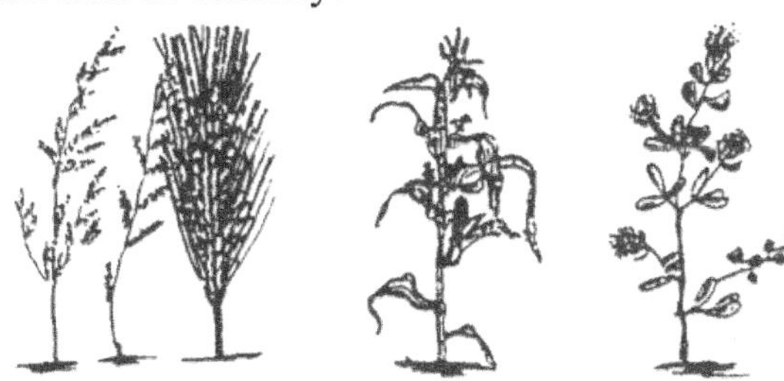

Symptoms: The symptoms occur rapidly and include rapid, difficult breathing, rapid pulse, and sometimes sudden collapse when forced to move. In addition, the animal has brown-colored gums, conjunctiva, and blood.

Treatment: Mix ten grams of **new methylene blue** with 500 ml (1/2 liter) of boiled, cooled water. This is given IV at a rate of two ml per five kg body weight. It may be repeated at 6-8 hour intervals if a large amount of toxic material was ingested.

Poisoning from Snake & Insect Bites:

Symptoms: Sharp pain and local swelling at site of the bite wound, difficult breathing, shock (weak pulse), and salivation. Horses and cattle often experience snake bites on the muzzle. See page 255. This can lead to swelling of head and nose.

Treatment:
1. Try to stop the poison from spreading by:
- cleaning the wound with soapy water.
- keeping the animal quiet.
- applying suction to the wound (useful only if done within 15 minutes).
- applying a tourniquet to reduce the spread of venom.
2. Give steroids to reduce swelling and epinephrine to counteract shock.
3. Give painkillers if needed to control pain.
4. Administer antibiotics to prevent infection.

Plants most commonly known to cause nitrate poisoning:	
Weeds	
Amaranthus spp.	pigweed
Chenopodium spp.	lamb's quarters
Cirsium arvense	Canada thistle
Datura spp.	jimsonweed
Helianthus anuus	wild sunflower
Kochia scoparia	fireweed
Malva parviflora	cheeseweed
Melilotus officinalis	sweet clover
Polygonum spp.	smartweed
Rumex spp.	dock
Salsola pestifer	Russian thistle
Solanum spp.	nightshades
Sorghum halepense	Johnson grass
Crop plants	
Avena sativa	oats
Beta vulgaris	beet
Brassica napus	rape
Glycine max	soybean
Linum usitatissimum	flax
Medicago sativa	alfalfa
Secale cereale	rye
Sorghum vulgare	sudan grass
Triticum aestivum	wheat
Zea mays	maize

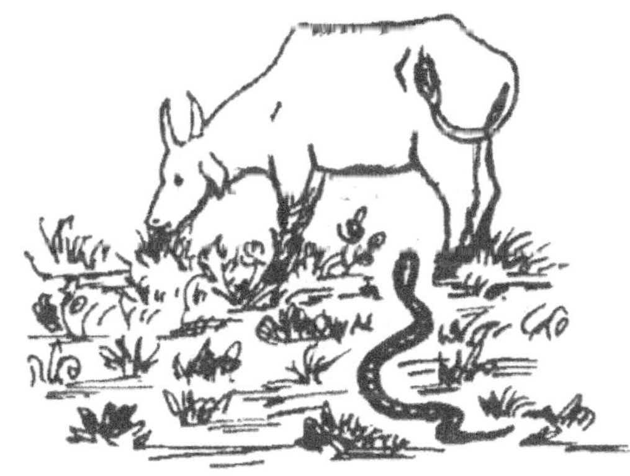

Pesticide Poisoning or Toxicity

Livestock may be accidentally exposed to
toxic amounts of pesticides in their feed or by
improper mixing of sprays or dips for
external parasites. Cats and most baby
animals are more sensitive to pesticides.
Symptoms vary with different pesticides. **If
the pesticide container is available, read
the label for signs and treatment of
toxicity.**

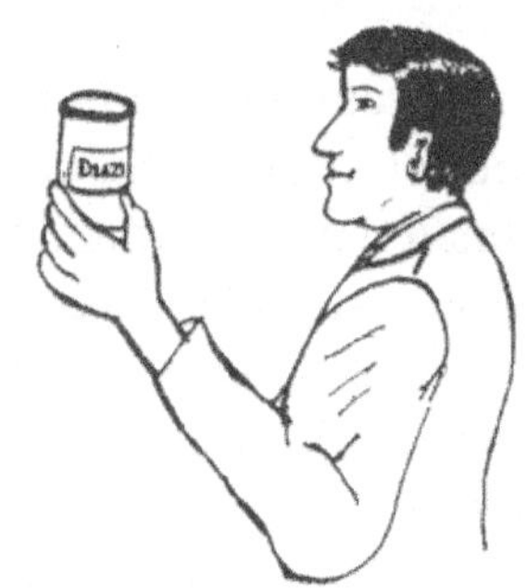

Chlorinated Hydrocarbon toxicity
(i.e. BHC, Chlordane, Lindane, Aldrin, Dieldrin)
Symptoms:
1.   First the animal acts overly nervous, crazy or excited. This can resemble rabies.
2.   Then the animal shivers, trembles and convulses until it dies.

Treatment: There is no good treatment. If the exposure was to the skin, try to rinse off the
pesticide with soap and water. If exposure was by mouth, give magnesium sulfate and <u>activated</u>
charcoal by mouth. Continue to feed activated charcoal daily in the feed for two weeks to
absorb any remaining toxin from the gut.

Organophosphate (OP) toxicity:
(i.e. Dichlorvos, Fenthion, Malathion, Parathion, Ronnel, Ruelene, Levamisole)

Symptoms:
1. Difficult breathing.
2. The signs of: "**SLUD**": <u>s</u>alivation,
   <u>l</u>acrimation (tears coming from eyes),
   <u>u</u>rination, and <u>d</u>iarrhea.
3. Possible convulsions.

Treatment of OP toxicity:

1.   Animals that were overdosed by skin exposure (during dipping or spraying) should be bathed
   with mild, soapy water.
2.   Give **atropine sulfate** (IM) at the following
   doses:

Cattle:	30 mg/45 kg BW
Sheep:	50 mg/45 kg BW
Horses:	6.5 mg/45 kg BW
Dogs:	2-4 mg total BW

(These injections may have to be repeated every 4 or 5 hours if symptoms return.)

Rat Poison
Sometimes livestock accidentally eat seed grains treated with rat poison. The treatment or antidote
will vary depending on the type of rat poison. **Therefore, read the container of the rat poison for
information on toxicity and treatment**. Sometimes livestock do not eat enough of the poison to
have serious symptoms. Nevertheless, remove the source of poison and provide **supportive care**
until the animal recovers.

5.3.3 Sudden Infection

Livestock with acute, severe diseases such as anthrax, hemorrhagic septicemia, or *Clostridia* can have symptoms that resemble poisoning. Usually these diseases also cause a fever. In this situation, the best treatment is penicillin or tetracycline. If the animal has black blood from the anus or mouth/nostrils, assume it has anthrax and be very careful to avoid exposing yourself or others. <u>If the animal dies of anthrax, do not cut it open</u> since this will contaminate the ground with anthrax spores. See page 196.

In a case of sudden illness, always perform a thorough clinical exam to determine which system is affected. Remember that an animal that is suddenly and severely ill may have a deadly organism (such as clostridia, anthrax, or the cause of hemorrhagic septicemia) in its blood spreading throughout the body. This is called "septicemia." If an organism produces a poison that circulates in the blood, it is called "toxemia."

5.3.4 Allergy

An allergy occurs when the body reacts to a substance inside, or in contact with the skin. This substance may be something that does not cause problems in other animals. Allergies can be divided into two types:
1. Severe allergic reactions can cause shock, difficult breathing, and sometimes death; and
2. Mild allergic reactions can cause itching, swelling or redness of the skin, urticaria (hives), blisters in the mouth, sneezing, eye irritation, or excessive tears from the eyes.

Major Allergic Reactions Affecting Breathing (Anaphylaxis)

These may be caused by insect bites, food, or medicines.

Symptoms: The symptoms often start soon after exposure and may include difficult breathing, a rapid, weak pulse and collapse. The throat may also be swollen inside.

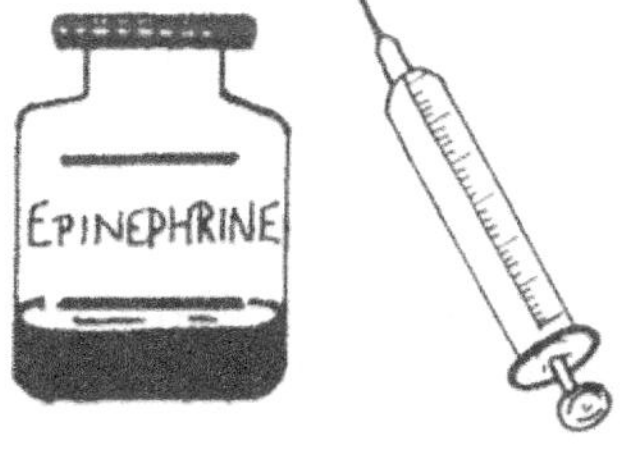

Treatment: Immediately remove the source of the allergy; give **adrenalin** (also called **epinephrine**), **antihistamines,** and **steroids** (see dosages in pharmacy section) immediately or as soon as possible if these medicines are available.

Mild Allergic Reactions

These most often result from insect bites, food, medicines, plants, insects (like caterpillars) or chemicals. These are not usually serious conditions that will kill an animal quickly.

Symptoms: Mild allergies often occur soon after exposure. They are usually seen as skin allergies (red spots, itching and/or swelling of the skin), blisters in the mouth, red teary eyes and sneezing.

Treatment: Try to identify the substance causing the allergy and prevent exposure to that substance. Treat with **antihistamines** or **steroids**.

5.3.5 Shock

Shock occurs when the circulatory system cannot deliver enough
blood to the tissues with the appropriate force (or pressure).
Shock may be due to an allergy or occur following massive
hemorrhage (blood loss), infection, poisoning, brain damage,
or injury with severe tissue damage and pain.

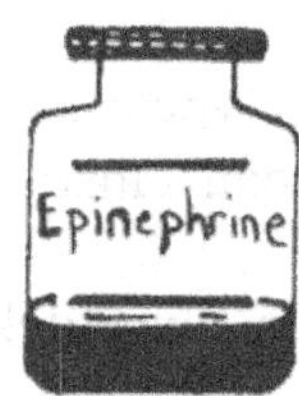
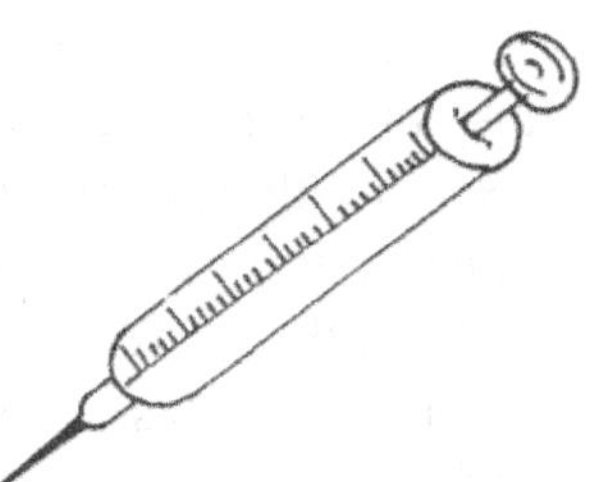

Symptoms:
1. Weakness or loss of consciousness.
2. Pale, cold, clammy skin.
3. Rapid breathing.
4. Weak pulse, either fast or slow.
5. Low temperature.

Treatment:
1. Check the animal's airway to make sure it is straight and open.
2. Stop any serious hemorrhage.
3. If available, give **adrenaline** (also called **epinephrine**), and **steroids.**
4. Give fluids, preferably in the vein. Give the animal oral rehydration fluids by mouth when it is strong enough to swallow.
5. Keep the animal warm (not hot).
6. Do not disturb or frighten the animal.

Prevention of Shock: Prompt and effective treatment of excessive pain, injuries, infections and
poisonings is the best way to prevent shock. In these situations, ensure adequate breathing, stop
excessive bleeding, keep the animal warm, provide pain relief and avoid excitement or exercise.
Once an animal is known to be allergic to a substance, avoid exposure to that substance.

5.4   MINOR FIRST AID

5.4.1 Eye Injuries, infections and conjunctivitis

Note: Conjunctivitis is inflammation of the
pink membrane surrounding the eye.

Symptoms: An injured or infected eye is
unusually red, the animal squints, and the
eye may have excessive tears or pus coming
from it.

Treating the eye -   Remember:
- The eye is very **sensitive**. Injuries to it are very painful.
- Always **wash hands** before examining an eye.
- Use only **medicines made for use in the eyes**.
- Acute injuries should be treated immediately.
- Chronic problems in the eye are difficult to treat successfully.

Treatment:

If the problem is chronic (i.e. has been there for a long time), warn the owner that the eye will probably not improve much with treatment.

If the problem is acute:

- Restrain the animal properly and wash hands well.
- Look in the eye for a foreign body; and remove it, if possible.
- Look for cloudiness in the colored part of the eye. Cloudiness is a sign of infection or injury in the eye. Red and/or swollen conjunctiva (pink membrane around the eye) is a sign of conjunctivitis.
- Wash eye well with boiled, cooled water. If available, add boric acid at a ratio of one-part boric acid to 100 ml water.
- Put antibiotic ointment in the eye at least twice daily for seven to ten days. Be sure to use only ointment that is made for use in the eye. Often eye ointment for people can be found in the local market and is safe to use in animals.

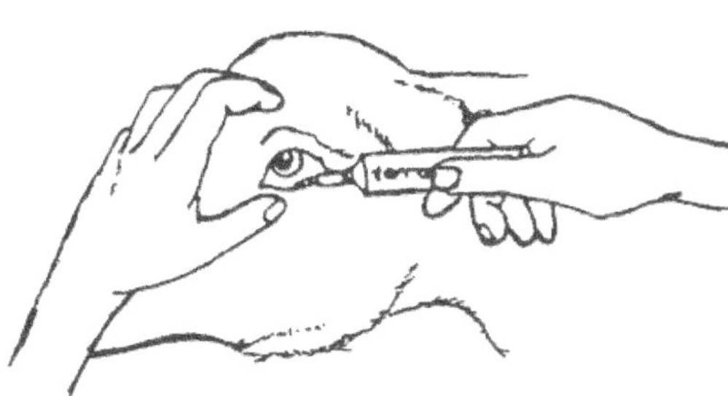

- Keep the eye clean. Regularly rinse the excess discharge from the eye and protect it from flies.

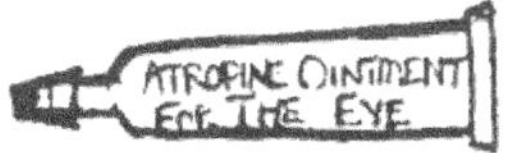

- If the eye is injured, put **atropine** drops or atropine ointment in the eye (if available). This will help relieve much of the pain and may prevent permanent damage.

    Caution: Avoid getting the atropine drops or ointment in your own eyes or your eyesight will be blurry for a while.

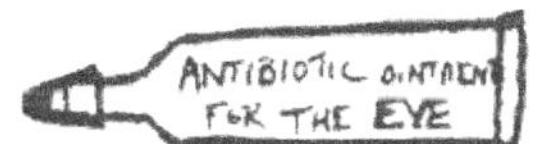

5.4.2 Removing worms from the eye

Dilute sterile **local anesthetic** with distilled water to make a 0.5% solution and squirt several ml into the eye. Wait several minutes, then flush the eye with distilled water. The worms should be flushed out with the distilled water.

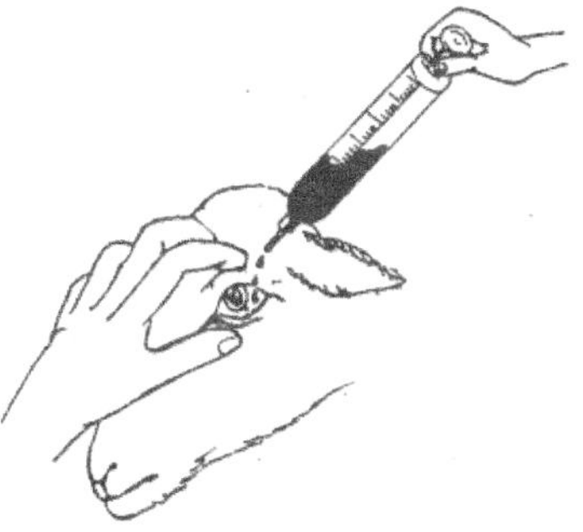

Minor first aid also includes smaller wounds like wild animal bites, lameness, broken horns and burns. For these problems, see Chapter 14, the Skin System.

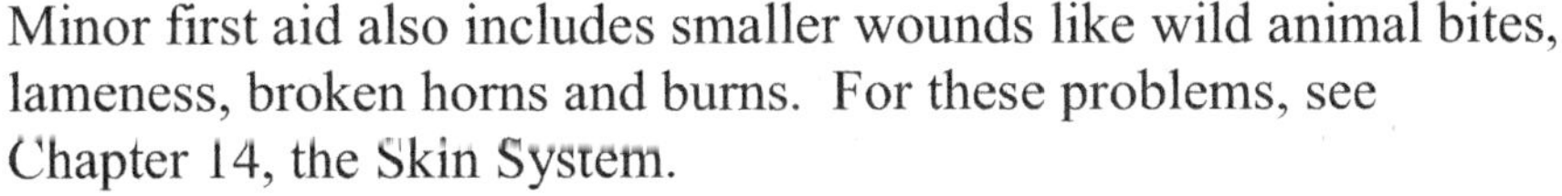

5.4.3 Minor Wounds

The first step in the treatment of wounds is to stop the bleeding. See page 78. After the bleeding is stopped the wound must be treated so that it heals as quickly as possible.

5.4.4 Broken Horns

Broken horns require immediate first aid to prevent maggot infestation. See page 225.

5.4.5 Burns

See page 220

6.0   Infectious Diseases: Prevention & Control

6.1   DEFINITIONS

Infectious disease: *A disease caused by living organisms such as bacteria, fungi, parasites, protozoa, and viruses.*

Infection: *Occurs when living organisms enter the body, reproduce, and cause damage.*

Contagious: *When disease is spread directly between animals.*

Non-contagious: *Does not spread directly.*

Micro-organisms: *Living organisms too small to be seen without a special instrument called a "microscope." Micro-organisms may or may not cause disease.*

Germs: *Another word for micro-organisms that cause disease.*

Microscope: *An instrument that makes tiny things look larger.*

Bacteria: *Tiny, one-celled organisms that can usually be killed by antibiotics. Examples of bacterial infections include anthrax, hemorrhagic septicemia, erysipelas, and most cases of mastitis and metritis.*

Viruses: *Micro-organisms smaller than bacteria. There are no safe, effective, readily available medicines to kill viruses once they enter the body and multiply within cells. Antibiotics do not kill viruses! The body's own defenses must fight the virus. Examples of serious viral infections are equine infectious anemia, foot & mouth disease, hog cholera, Newcastle disease, and rinderpest. Correct treatment for viral diseases includes treating severe symptoms and providing good supportive care. Some viruses (like EIA) survive in infected animals for long periods of time. It is often best to destroy animals carrying chronic virus infections so they are not a source of infection for healthy animals.*

Fungi: *Micro-organisms that most commonly infect the skin. Antibiotics do not kill fungi and may even make the fungal infection worse. Anti-fungal drugs are needed to treat severe fungal infections.*

Protozoa: *One-celled micro-organisms often classified as internal parasites. Ticks and biting flies may carry certain protozoa and spread these protozoa while feeding on other animals. Treatment of infections caused by protozoa requires special drugs. Examples of protozoal infections include anaplasmosis, Babesiosis, coccidiosis, theileriosis ("East Coast Fever") and trypanosomiasis.*

Internal & external parasites: *Organisms that live in or on an animal and cause harm to it. Parasites can be large and easy to see like roundworms or ticks; or they can be small and difficult, or impossible to see, like mites and protozoa.*

6.2   EXAMPLES OF INFECTIOUS DISEASES

Disease Causing Organism	Name of the disease	How it enters the body or is spread	Principle treatment
Bacteria	Diarrhea	Through food, water, or containers contaminated with manure	Antibiotics
	Infected wounds	Entry of filth into the wound	
	Pneumonia	Through the air or contact with saliva (coughing), nasal discharge, contaminated food or water	
	Metritis	Contact with filth during or following delivery or abortion	
	Mastitis	Damage to udder or teat, dirty milking practices, unsanitary housing	
	Swollen joints	Germs from manure entering through mouth, wounds, or umbilical cord	
Virus	Foot and Mouth, Rinderpest	From another sick animal (through the air or saliva)	Painkillers like aspirin. (These medicines do not fight the virus directly. They just help the body to heal itself.)
	Rabies	From a bite (saliva)	
Fungi	Ringworm	Contact between animals or contaminated stalls	Iodine
Protozoa	Trypano-somes	From blood (of an infected animal), carried by a biting insect	Specific parasite medicine
	Coccidia	From manure of an infected animal	Specific parasite medicine
Internal Parasites	Liver fluke	From an intermediate host (snail)	Specific parasite medicine
	Roundworm	Directly from the manure of another animal or contaminated pasture	Specific parasite medicine
External Parasites	Lice	From touching infested animals or infested stalls	Specific parasite medicine
	Maggots in wounds	Flies lay eggs in open wounds	Specific parasite medicine

6.3 RESISTANCE & IMMUNITY

6.3.1 Definition of Resistance:

The ability to avoid sickness or death when exposed to an organism.

6.3.2 Resistance depends on:

1. The overall health of the animal: If an animal is strong and healthy, it will be better able to resist a disease. The overall health of an animal depends on:

- **Nutrition**. See page 97.
- **Presence of other diseases**. Other diseases may weaken the animal making it less able to resist the disease.

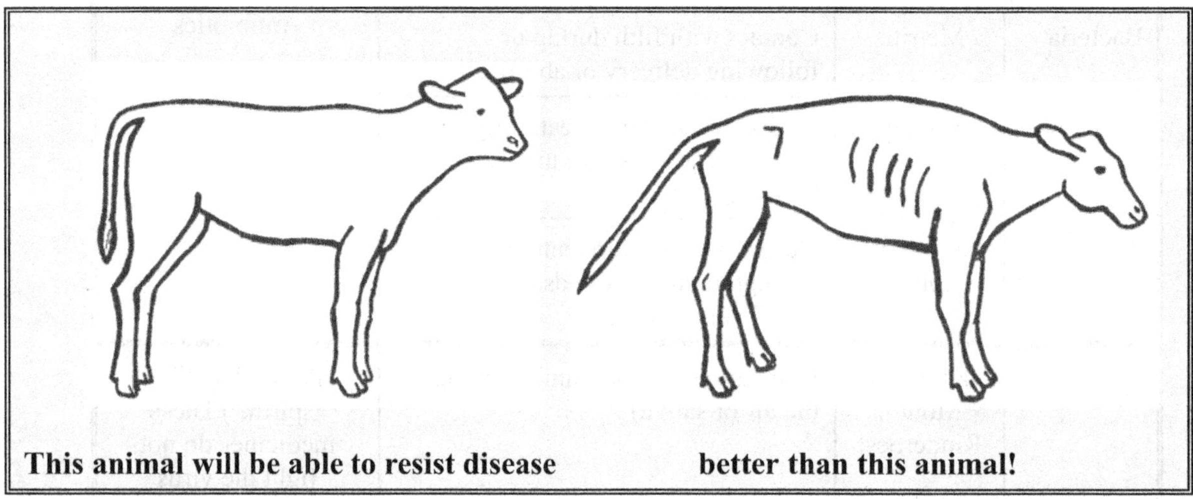

- **Tolerance.** Resistance is acquired by certain breeds of animals over a long period of time. For instance, African cattle have thick skin which allows them to resist certain diseases spread by biting insects.

2. The number of infectious organisms: If only a few infectious organisms enter an animal, then the animal may develop a mild disease or none at all.

3. Immunity: Immunity is when an animal develops its own protection against a specific organism. The animal is then said to be "immune" to the organism and will resist the disease. White blood cells protect the body against invading organisms or foreign bodies called **"antigens."** White blood cells directly attack and kill infectious organisms or make substances called **"antibodies"** to do this.

If an animal has antibodies against the organisms causing a specific disease, then it has "immunity" or "resistance" to that disease.

If an animal has no immunity or other resistance to a disease, then it is "susceptible."

Susceptible animals usually become sick when exposed to infectious organisms.

6.4.1 Passive Immunity

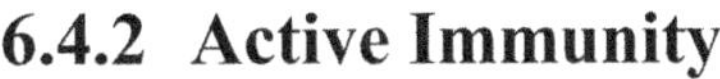

> **To receive this protection, the newborn must drink the colostrum during its first day of life.**

This immunity occurs when an animal receives antibodies made by another animal. This type of immunity provides immediate protection but does not last long. Newborn animals receive antibodies (passive immunity) from their mother by drinking colostrum, the mother's first milk. Without the colostrum, the animal has no protection against common diseases in the area and may die.

6.4.2 Active Immunity

This immunity may result from contact with an infectious organism. When that organism enters the body again, white blood cells or antibodies recognize and destroy it immediately.

6.5   USING VACCINES TO INCREASE IMMUNITY

A vaccine is given to animals or humans to expose them to a specific micro-organism (or a piece of micro- organism) so that active immunity develops against that particular germ. The micro-organisms in the vaccine are killed or altered so they won't cause serious illness in the animal. Most vaccines are given by injection. Some are given orally.

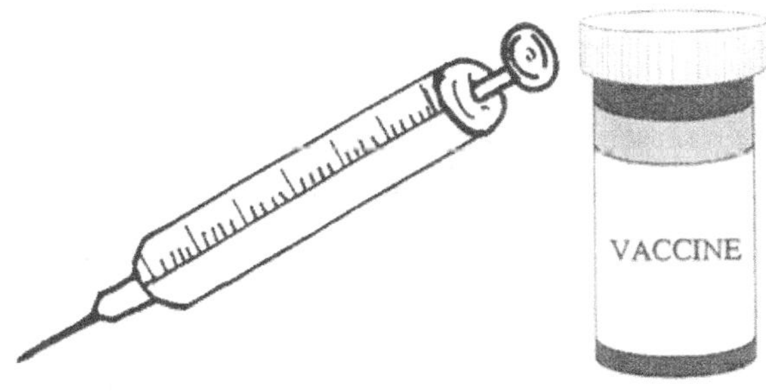

6.5.1 Basic Principles of Vaccine Use

Many types of vaccines provide immunity of varying duration against different diseases. Always follow the instructions and heed the precautions provided with the vaccine. Remember the following general principles:

1   Vaccines should be obtained from a reputable source. Poor quality vaccines can kill and mishandled vaccines can lose their effectiveness. When vaccines cause damage or are not effective, farmers lose confidence in both the AHA and the vaccine.

2.   A vaccine is used to **prevent** disease, not to treat it. Once the animal is sick, it is too late to vaccinate it against that disease. Vaccinating sick animals seldom produces immunity and may make the disease worse.

3.   In general, do not vaccinate sick animals.

4.   Follow the manufacturer's instructions about vaccinating pregnant animals since some vaccines can cause abortion.

5.	Most vaccines provide protection one to two weeks after the vaccine is given. If the animal already has the organism in its body when the vaccine is given, or if the animal is exposed to the organism within one or two weeks after vaccination, it may still become ill. Some vaccines require two injections given three to four weeks apart to provide good protection. The animal is therefore not protected until a few weeks <u>after the second vaccination</u>. The AHA must carefully explain this to livestock owners to avoid being blamed if the animal becomes ill before it is protected by the vaccine.

6.5.2   Cold Storage of Vaccines (*Cold-chain*)

Most vaccines should be kept at 0 to 8°C. Some vaccines, when stored for longer periods of time (i.e. more than one month), should be frozen. Other vaccines become ineffective if frozen even once. Some vaccines are not sensitive to freezing, but lose their effectiveness if they become warm.

> **Always follow label instructions on how to store and care for vaccines.**

The process of keeping the vaccine at the correct temperature from the moment it is manufactured, to the moment it is administered, is called the "COLD CHAIN."

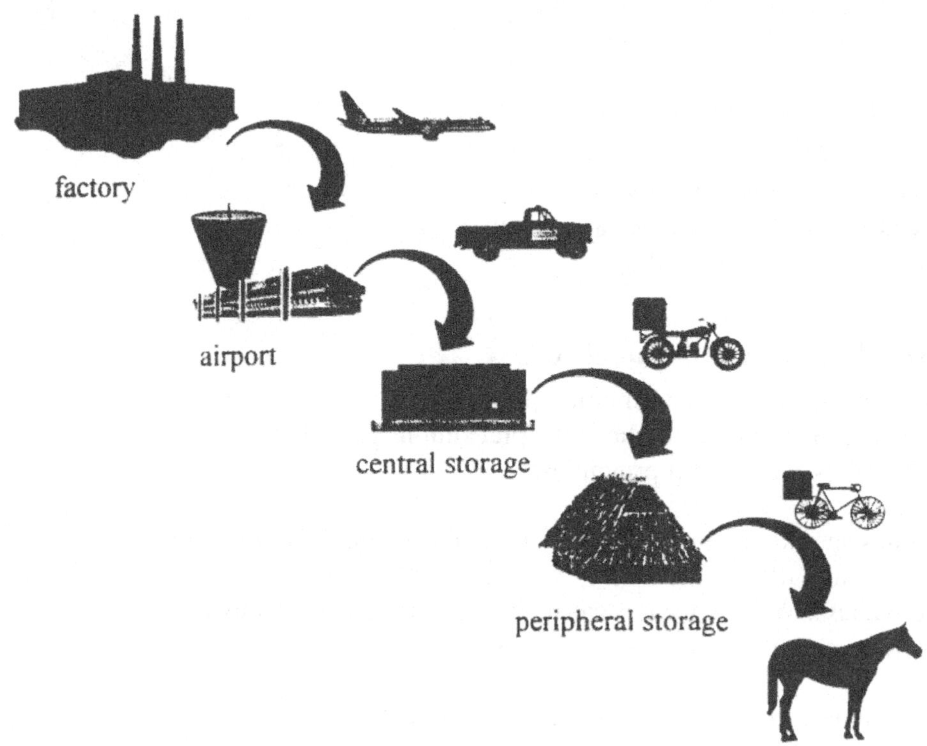

For many vaccines, if the cold chain is broken just once, the vaccine is ruined or at least less effective. There are a few vaccines that don't need refrigeration. These vaccines are called "heat stable" vaccines. For example, a new rinderpest vaccine is heat stable for 30 days.

6.5.3 Five factors that can damage vaccines

1. *HEAT*

Most vaccines are "heat-sensitive" and must be maintained in
a cold chain. They must be stored in a refrigerator at 0 to 8°C,
transported in a thermos with ice or cold packs and used
immediately once drawn up in a syringe. If the syringe full of
vaccine is not used quickly, it should be placed on a cold pack
until it's time to inject the vaccine.

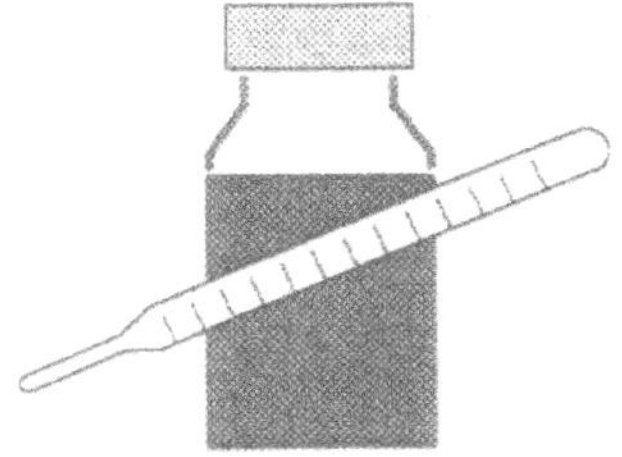

2. *FREEZING*

Vaccines sensitive to freezing will lose their effectiveness if
frozen. Many doses of vaccine have been wasted due to
accidental freezing. Keep a thermometer INSIDE the freezer
and check it daily. Other vaccines should be frozen if they
will be stored for a long period of time. Be sure to follow
carefully the manufacturer's instructions.

3. *SUN*

Never leave vials or syringes containing vaccine in direct
sunlight. When working in the field, open the thermos of
vaccine and fill syringes in the shade.

4. *CONTAMINATION*

Always use sterile needles and syringes when preparing or
mixing vaccine or drawing it out of a vial. Never place a used
needle in a vaccine vial because this can contaminate the
vaccine and cause illness or an abscess at the injection site.

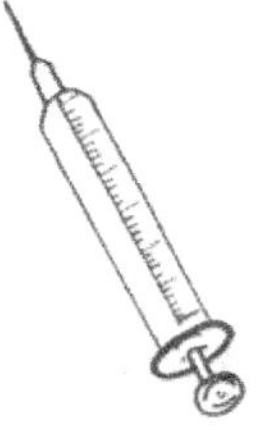

> **If you suspect that a vaccine vial is contaminated, discard it.**

5. *DISINFECTANT & DETERGENT*

Disinfectant or detergent may make vaccine
ineffective. Therefore, avoid contaminating
vaccine with disinfectant or detergent. For
example, do not use syringes or needles for
vaccination that have residues of disinfectant
or detergent left in them from cleaning. Do
not use disinfectant when re-sterilizing
needles and syringes. For sterilization, rinse
thoroughly with <u>water only</u> and then boil in
clean water for at least 15 minutes.

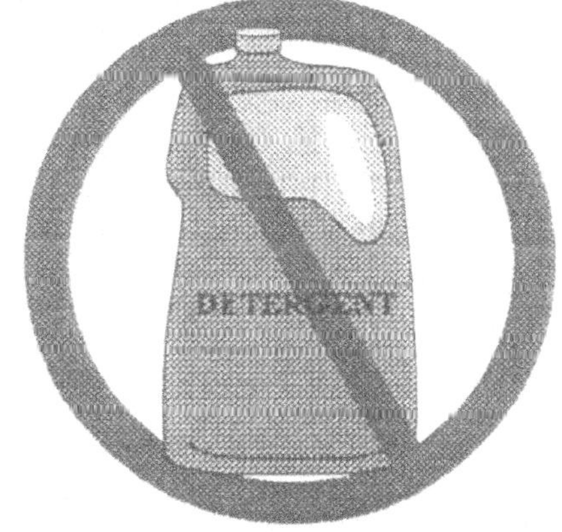

6.6   IMPORTANT PRINCIPLES FOR THE PREVENTION OF INFECTIOUS DISEASES

1. Nutritious food, clean water, adequate shelter

These will help keep an animal strong and more able to resist infections.

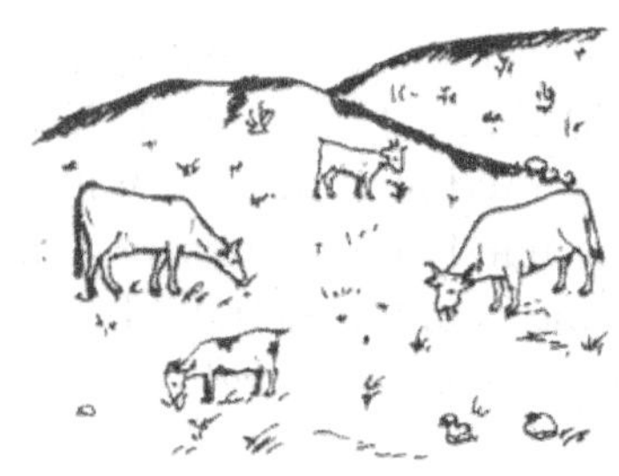

2. Sanitation & Pasture Rotation

This is as important as nutrition. Germs and parasite eggs can survive for long periods of time in old, moist manure and other dark, damp, dirty places. Many health problems can be prevented by providing a **clean**, **dry** environment with **adequate sunlight**. The following measures can also help prevent disease by improving sanitation:

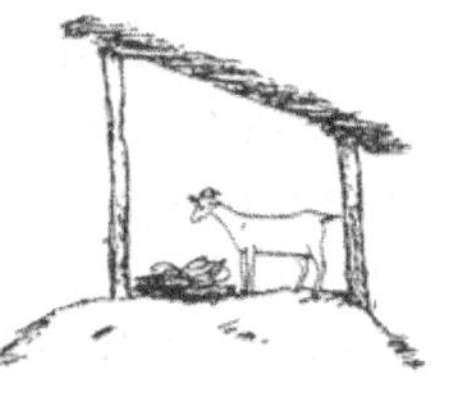

- **Locate pens** and pastures on high **well-drained land**.

- **Rotate the pens and pastures often** and leave them unused for at least one month; or plant crops on them. When the land is left empty, particularly with exposure to sunlight, the immature parasites in the soil dry-out and die.

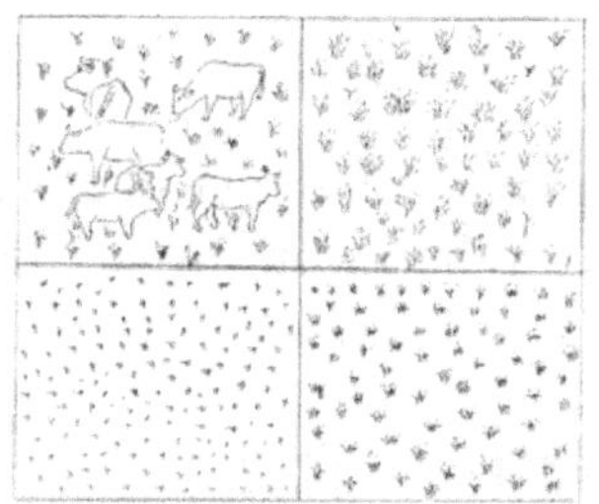

- **Place nursing mothers and babies in "fresh" areas** where other animals have not been for several months, as babies are most susceptible to disease.

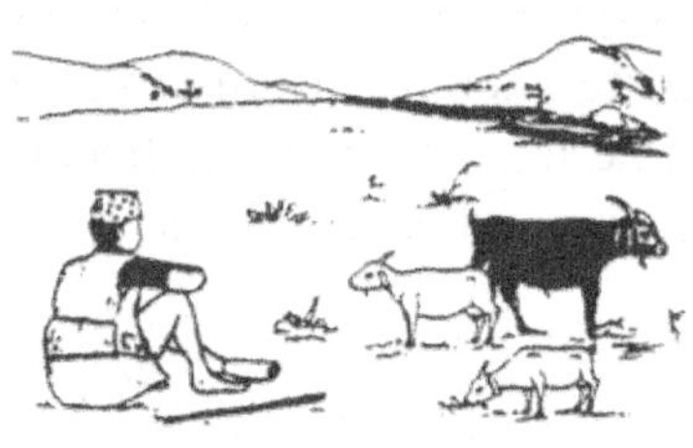

- **Keep food and water clean**. If feeding areas are dirty, the animals will take in germs and parasite eggs when they eat and drink. Therefore, avoid putting food on the ground or using troughs in which the animals can step or lie. Use feed and water troughs that keep the food and water clean and prevent the animal from laying or climbing in the trough.

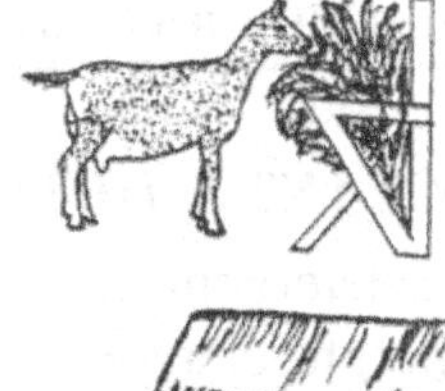

- **Clean permanent buildings often** with soap and water and let the surface dry. Bedding material should also be removed and replaced with clean bedding often. Whenever animals leave a farm, the buildings should be cleaned and left empty for one to three months before housing new animals.

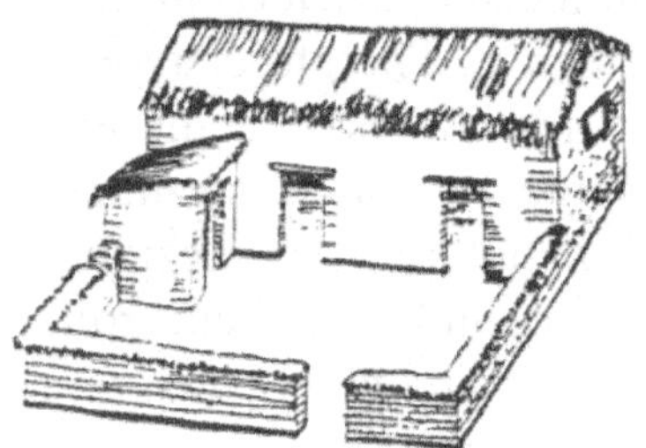

- **Move temporary buildings often.** This is the great advantage of temporary buildings or pens. Simply move the building or pen to a fresh area and expose the previous area to sunlight and drying, so that germs and parasite eggs are killed.

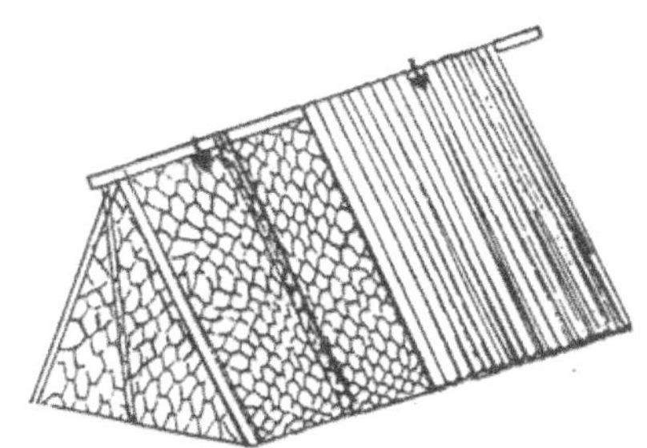

Mobile Poultry Pen

- **Use disinfectants correctly.** Some people use disinfectants, like phenol or chlorine, as a part of their sanitation program to kill germs in buildings, pens, and troughs. Disinfectants are most effective when the place is cleaned beforehand of all organic matter and then rinsed with disinfectant. Some disinfectants can be poisonous, however, and must be used properly to avoid harming people and livestock. Disinfected food and water troughs should be rinsed before re-use.

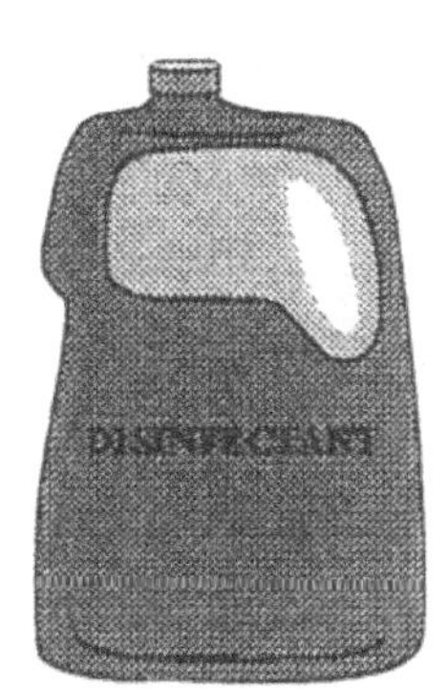

3. Use good vaccines that are known to be effective against important diseases in the area.

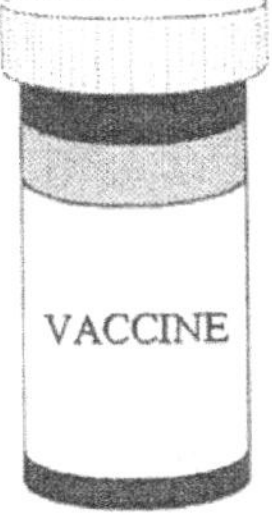

4. Treat regularly for parasites. A good parasite prevention, control and treatment program is critical for good livestock health and production.

5. Use proper chemicals and medicines to control intermediate hosts like insects, ticks, mites and snails. Use them in a manner that does not harm the environment.

6.7 CONTROLLING OUTBREAKS OF CONTAGIOUS DISEASES

"Control" refers to the situation where a disease outbreak has already started but must be contained to **prevent its spread**.   Highly contagious diseases spread rapidly, making control more difficult. Most countries have **laws** to control animal diseases, if the laws are enforced. The following actions are usually taken to control an outbreak:

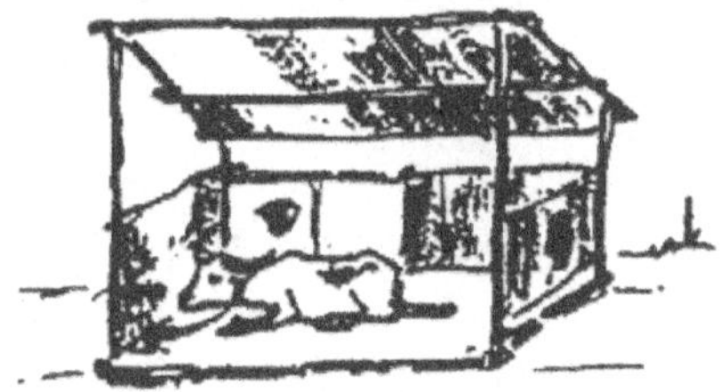

Sick animal isolated from......

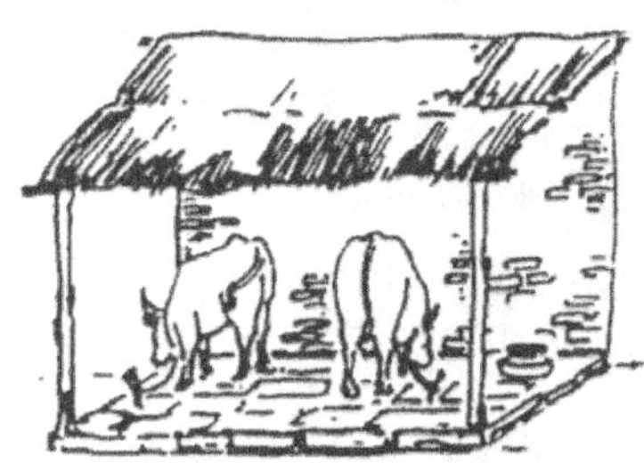

......healthy ones

Isolate Sick Animals.

- **Separate sick animals from healthy ones** to prevent spread of infectious disease. This is called **isolation**.

- **Avoid as much as possible contact with sick livestock.** Do not allow people who have been working with sick livestock to have contact with your healthy livestock, as this may spread disease. When buying new animals, try to isolate them for at least two weeks to verify that they are healthy before mixing them with your healthy livestock.

Determine how the disease is transmitted.

It is often necessary to determine how the disease is spread in order to implement effective control measures. For example, is the cause a contaminated water source or poisonous plant? Is it exposure to an animal with a contagious disease? Is it transmitted by flies or insects called "vectors"? Sometimes a person trained in "epidemiology" is needed to properly investigate the outbreak and identify the cause of the problem.

Quarantine the affected area.

During outbreaks of certain contagious diseases, the government may declare an area "under quarantine," meaning that no animals can be moved in or out of that area.

Vaccinate.

Use an effective vaccine for healthy, susceptible livestock. The vaccine should be available and affordable.

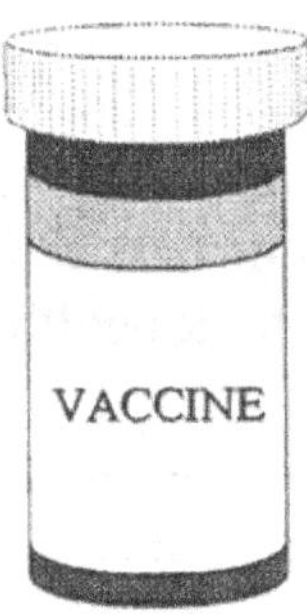

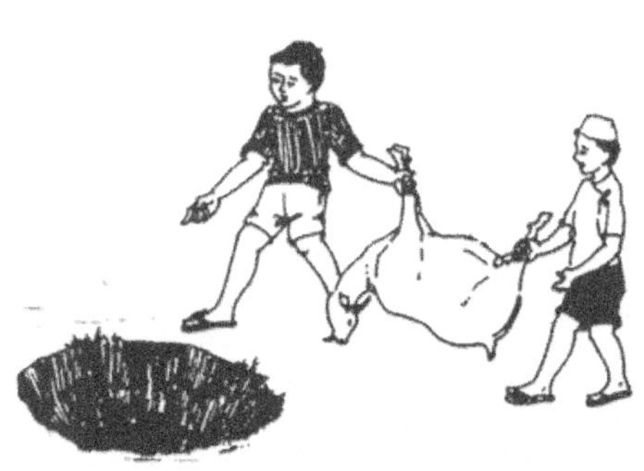

Properly dispose of dead animals

All dead animals should be buried or burned.

Disinfect buildings, pens and troughs.

If the outbreak is due to an infectious disease, buildings, pens, and troughs for the sick animals should be thoroughly cleaned, disinfected, and allowed to stand empty for one to three months.

Slaughter exposed or positive animals.

Some governments require that all animals exposed to a particular disease must be killed and their bodies burned or buried; or all animals are tested and those found positive are slaughtered. In some countries, this method of disease control is not possible due to cultural or religious beliefs.

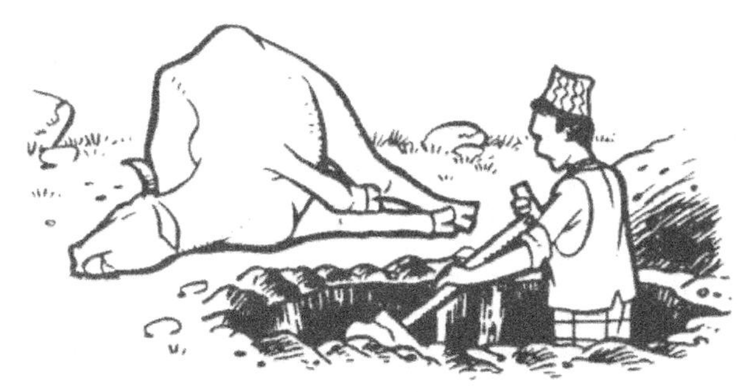

Require health certificates.

Many governments require inspection of all animals before they are transported across borders or to certain destinations. The veterinary doctor or a trained technician inspects the animals and signs a certificate stating that they are healthy. Without this certificate, the animals may not be moved.

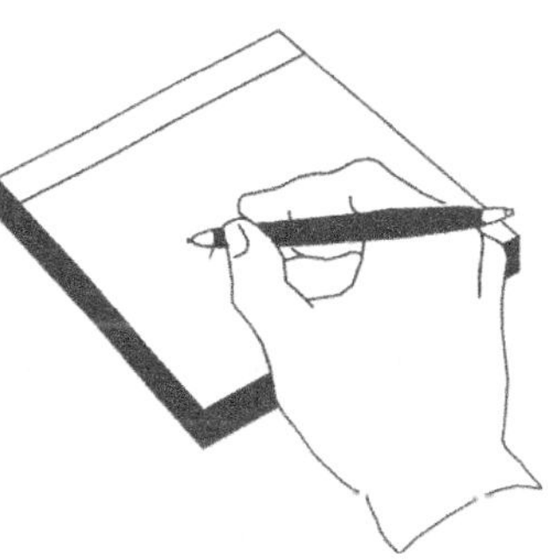

Enforce obligatory reporting of dangerous diseases.

Most governments require that certain diseases be reported to the district veterinary officer so that immediate actions can be taken. These are usually contagious, deadly and economically important diseases such as Hemorrhagic Septicemia, Foot and Mouth Disease, Rinderpest, African Swine Fever, Swine Erysipelas, and Newcastle Disease.

Track the epidemic -
"DISEASE SURVEILLANCE"

For serious diseases, the government may establish a disease reporting system, called "disease surveillance" to answer the following questions:

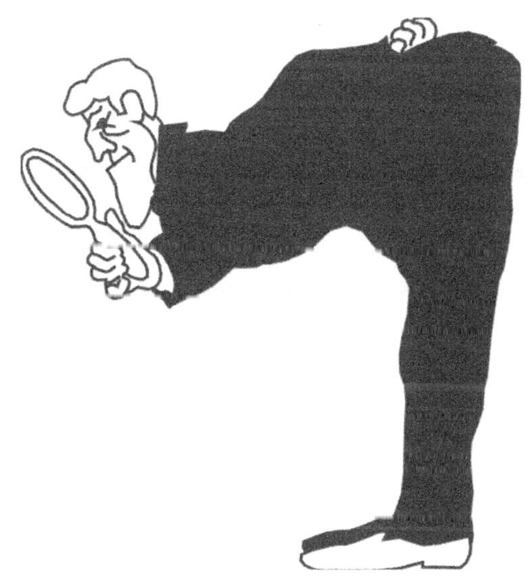

1.   Which animals are affected and how many?

2.   Where are the areas at highest risk?

3.   How many are dying?

4.   Is the amount of disease increasing or decreasing? Is it seasonal or periodic?

5.   With this information, veterinary health authorities can determine the magnitude of the problem and target resources and disease control efforts to areas and animals at highest risk.

7.0   NUTRITION

7.1 THREE KEYS TO UNDERSTANDING NUTRITION

1.   **Different animals require different nutrients; and the same animal will require different nutrients at different times in its life.**
For example: a growing calf, a cow giving milk, and an adult bull require different nutrients.

2.   **Different foods provide different nutrients.** Foods are divided into different groups according to the key nutrients they provide.

3.   **Livestock need a <u>balance</u> of <u>different foods</u> from the different food groups to remain healthy and productive.**
No single food, by itself, provides all the nutrients a body requires.
Exception: A newborn baby receives all the nutrients it needs from its mother's milk.

Review: a **nutrient** is a substance provided by food. A **diet** is the overall mixture of foods that an animal eats.

More About Nutrients:

There are five different groups of nutrients, each having its own role in an animal's body. If the body does not have enough of a certain nutrient, then we say that it has a nutrient **deficiency**.

7.2 FIVE GROUPS OF NUTRIENTS
1. Proteins: Body-Building Foods

Protein is used by the body for **growth** and **milk production**.

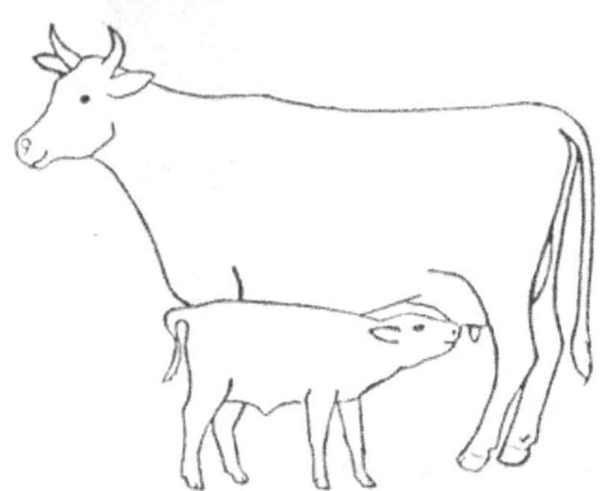

Animals needing extra protein in their diets:
-mothers giving milk
-female animals during late pregnancy
-young, growing animals, especially after weaning

Foods <u>high</u> in protein:
-milk and milk products
-beans, lentils and their products
  (e.g. soy bean meal)
-oil seed cakes (e.g. mustard or rape seed cake)
-special "leguminous" forages (e.g. clover,
  leucaena, and alfalfa / lucerne)
-meat/fish by-products (e.g. blood meal, fish
meal)

Foods with some protein:
-grass when it is still young and
tender (before it becomes mature
and makes seeds)
-hay and silage made from grass
that is cut when green
-grain and grain by-products (e.g.
high-quality rice bran)
-by-products left from alcohol
production

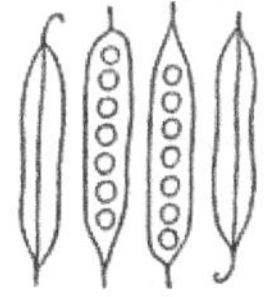
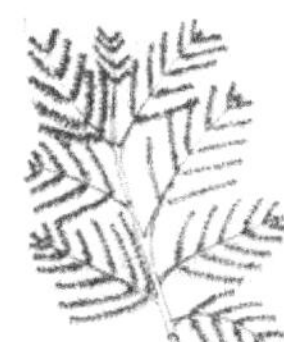
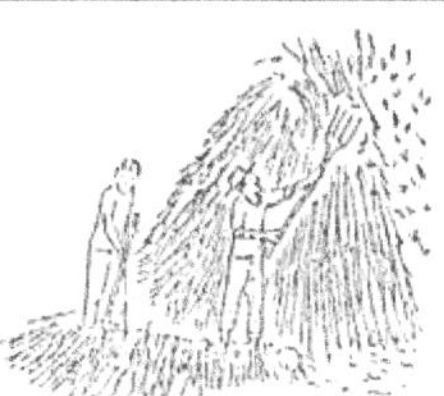
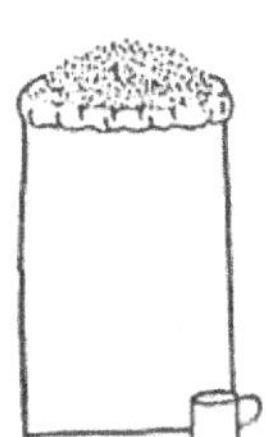
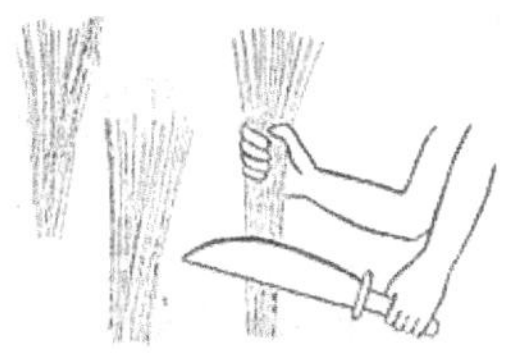

Protein deficiency:
(Most common among young animals)

<u>Young animals</u> will be thin and sickly, often have a
big belly, big head, and thin legs. They will
grow slowly, and have rough hair coats.

<u>Adult animals</u> will give less milk than they should, or
give birth to smaller, weaker babies.

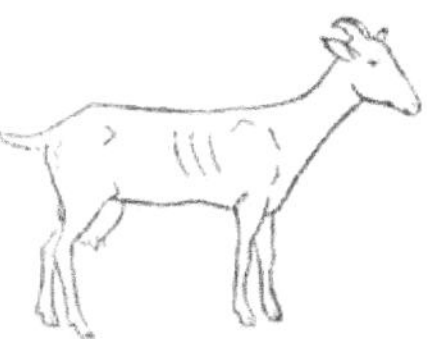

Treatment of Protein Deficiency:
Feed protein-rich food!

Prevention of protein deficiency:
<u>Before</u> protein deficiency develops, feed protein-rich feeds to **young animals, lactating
animals (nursing mothers)**, and **animals during late pregnancy**.

Note: <u>Prioritize</u> your more expensive food! Protein-rich foods are more expensive.
Reserve this food for animals needing it most - (e.g. young, pregnant and lactating animals).

2. Carbohydrates & Fats: Energy-giving foods

Energy is used for daily processes like walking and chewing; as well as for working, growing, making milk and staying warm. When an animal eats more energy than it needs, it stores the extra energy as fat.

Carbohydrates make up the largest part of the diet for most livestock - around 75-80 percent of the total.

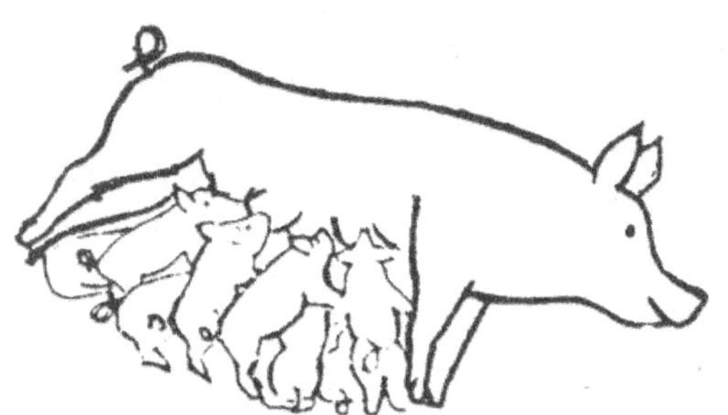

Animals especially needing energy:
-Milking animals
-Growing animals
-Animals exposed to cold weather
-Working animals

"**Energy**" is found mainly in:
- grains (wheat, wheat bran, maize, and barley)
-rice & rice bran
-dried & fresh fruit
-yams, potatoes & other roots
-molasses and other by-products of sugar production
-animal fat by-products
-by-products from alcohol production
-vegetables & garbage
-tender, green grass
-hay which is cut when the grass is green

Important: Old, dry grass, and straw contain only a small amount of energy that the body can use. The energy in most tough feeds, like grass and straw, can be digested only by grass-eating animals.

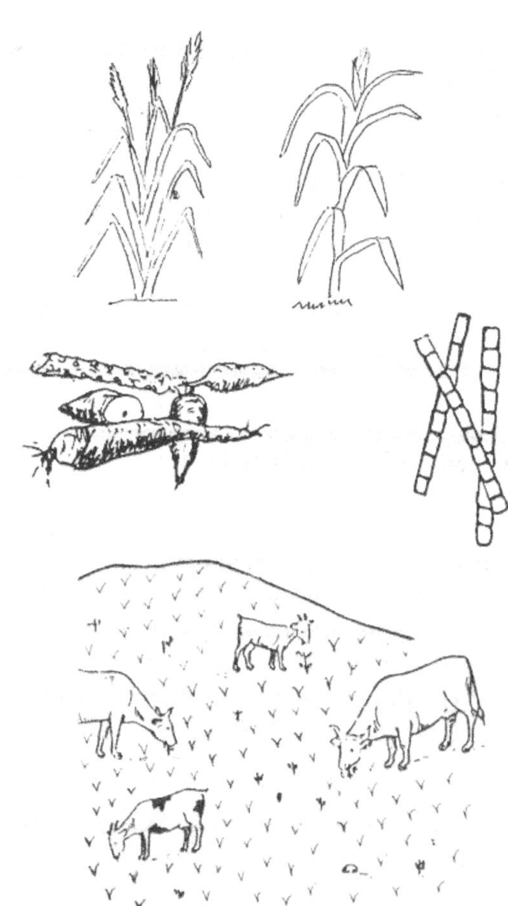

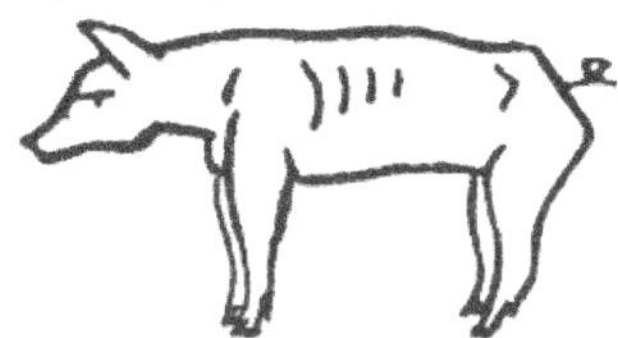

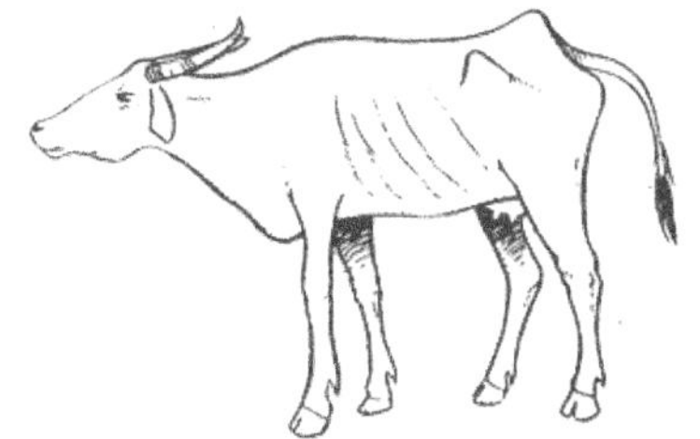

Treatment of Energy Deficiency
Feed more food rich in energy.

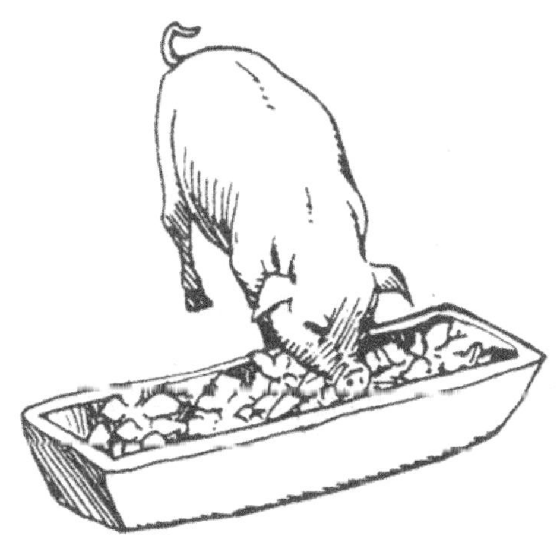

Prevention: Feed more energy foods to young, pregnant and lactating animals, as well as animals exposed to cold weather <u>before</u> they become thin.

Note: Sows not receiving extra energy while nursing <u>will</u> become <u>very</u> thin by the time the babies are weaned. These sows may be infertile for several months after weaning their piglets.

3. Minerals

Minerals are necessary for healthy bones and teeth, for normal body functions, and for milk production. All animals need small amounts of ordinary salt for normal body functions.

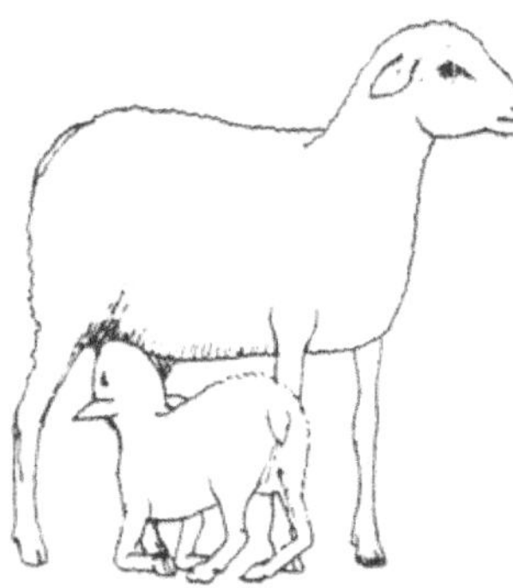 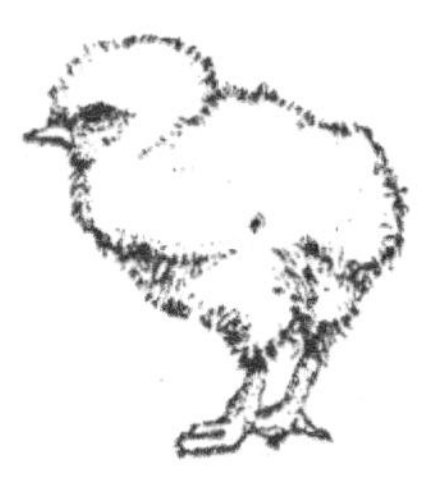

Animals that especially need minerals:
-young, growing, and nursing animals
-mothers giving milk

Mineral Sources:

-milk
-salt
-ground-up bones, egg shells, sea shells
-molasses
-forages, soil, & limestone
-special mineral mixes for livestock

Animals eating forages from soils lacking certain minerals will become deficient in those same minerals, unless they are supplied from another source.

Deficiencies occur most when animals receive a <u>single type</u> of food from a <u>single source</u> or <u>graze only in one area</u>.

For example, a lactating sow receiving only grain by-products will often become deficient in calcium. She will become weak, often starting in her hind legs, until she cannot stand up at all.

Signs of Mineral Deficiencies

- animals lick & chew on anything salty

- animals chew on old bones

- young animals may have bumps on their ribs or deformed legs

- young, nursing pigs may die without an obvious cause (iodine deficiency)

- sows may sit like a dog and not be able to stand up (calcium deficiency)

- nursing cows, especially heavy milk producers, suddenly cannot stand up (calcium deficiency)

- infertility

Caution: Although all animals need some salt, too much salt can be harmful. Never force salt down an animal's throat. Always provide plenty of fresh drinking water to prevent salt poisoning.

Treatment & Prevention of Mineral Deficiencies

Find out what minerals are lacking in the local soils. Phosphorous is often lacking in tropical soils.

Use easily available sources of minerals such as ground bones, shells, and ash. These are often found locally at reasonable prices.

Feed a variety of food or graze in more than one area.

Feed the animals salt, but make sure they have access to adequate water (especially pigs). Generally, animals will eat only the amount of salt they need. If iodine deficiency is a problem, then mix small amounts of iodine with the salt.

Do not spend money on expensive mineral mixes unless advised by someone trustworthy. Many shopkeepers sell mineral mixes even when it is not necessary.

4. Vitamins: Protective Foods

Vitamins are needed in small amounts for growth, reproduction and normal body functions. Vitamins are necessary to protect from diseases and for wound-healing.

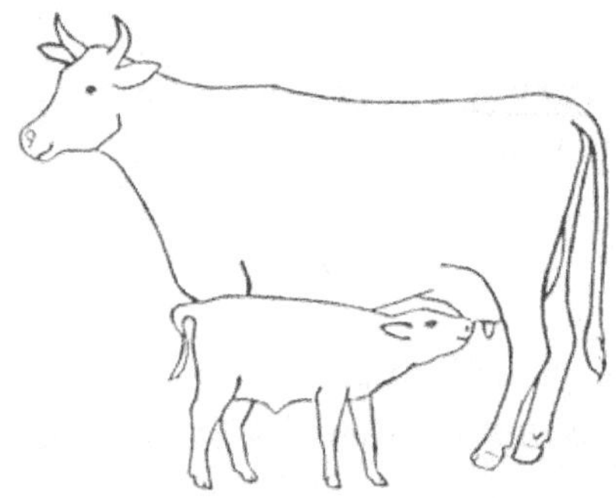

Animals that especially need vitamins:

- Young, pregnant and lactating animals

Sources of Vitamins

-Fresh, green forage
-Fresh fruits & vegetables
-Protein sources provide small
   amounts.

Signs of Vitamin Deficiencies
The signs depend on which vitamin is lacking and which kind of animal is affected. (See Page 311, which lists the most common deficiencies.)

Treatment of Vitamin Deficiencies

Unless the animal is unable to eat, it is least expensive to **give the animal fresh, green forage to eat**.

Inexperienced AHAs tend to give unnecessary vitamin injections to sick animals. This is sometimes due to pressure by the owner for "an injection."

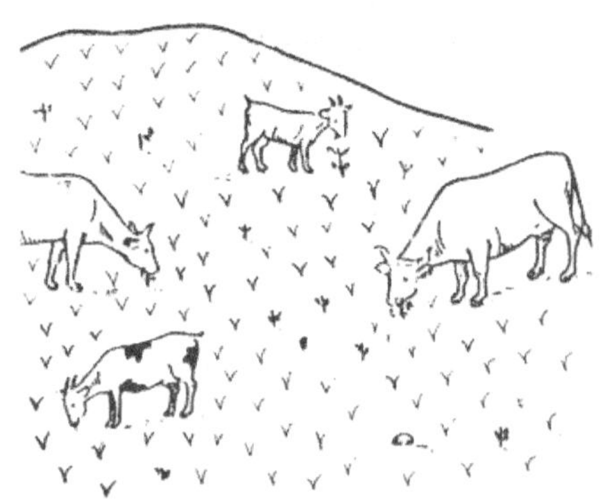

5. Water: The Most Important Nutrient

A fresh, plentiful, constant source of water is essential for all functions of the body.

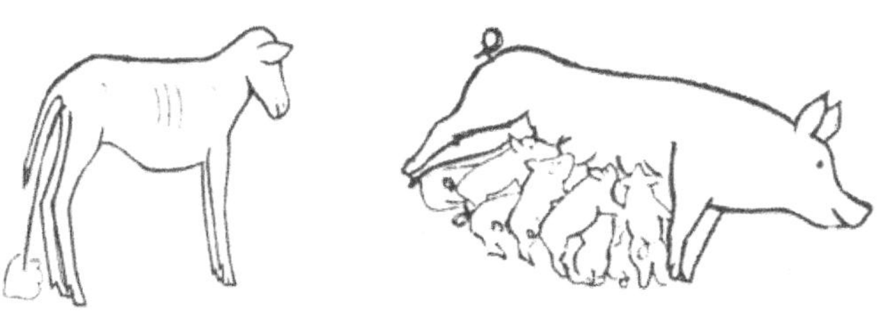

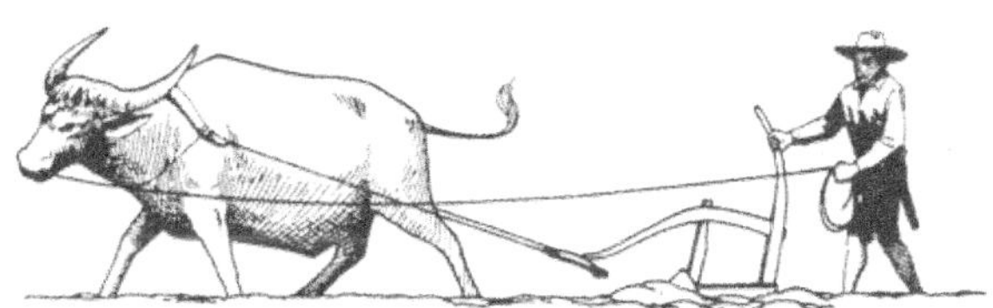

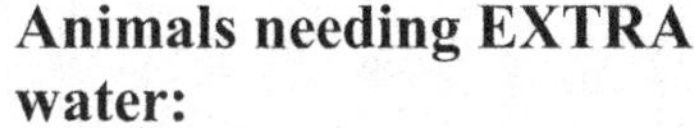

Animals needing EXTRA water:

-Sick animals, especially those with diarrhea or vomiting.

-Lactating animals

-Working animals

-Animals living in **hot and/or dry climates**.

Sources of Water

All foods, contain <u>some</u> water, especially fresh, green forage. Although <u>some</u> animals can survive on this amount of water, <u>it is not enough for good health, and production.</u>

All animals should be given clean, fresh water to drink at least four times daily. When water is given, the animal should be given time to drink as much as it wants. If it drinks all the water, it should be offered more.

The best way to give water is to have fresh water available all the time for the animal.

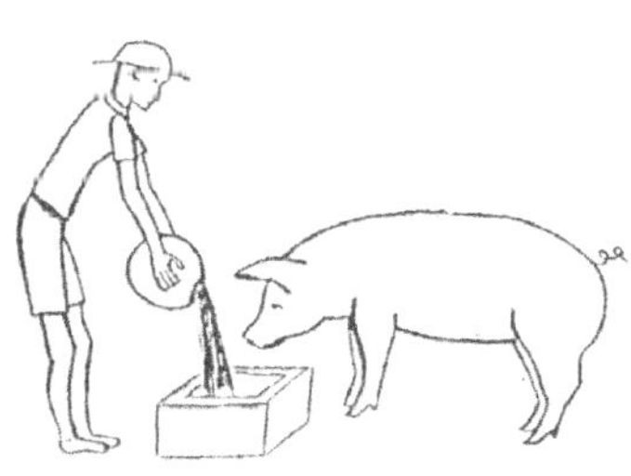

Signs of Water Deficiencies

For mild deficiencies, the animal may have dark or very little urine.

Animals, especially pigs, that receive salt in their diet but no water may show signs of salt toxicity (neurologic symptoms) and even die.

See Page 49,191,267 regarding dehydration, a severe deficiency of fluid in the body.

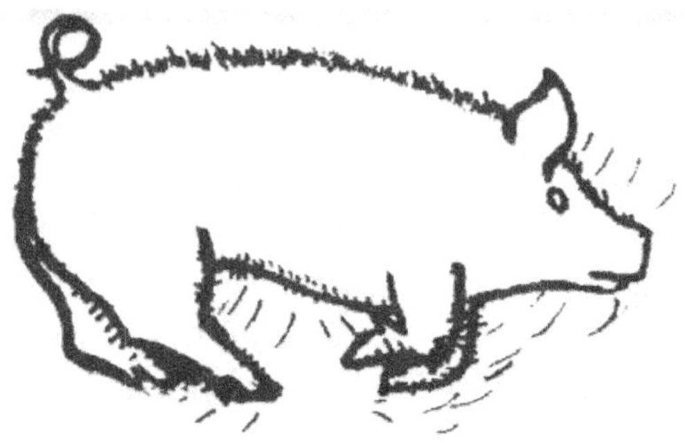

Pig trembling and convulsing due to salt toxicity (lack of water)

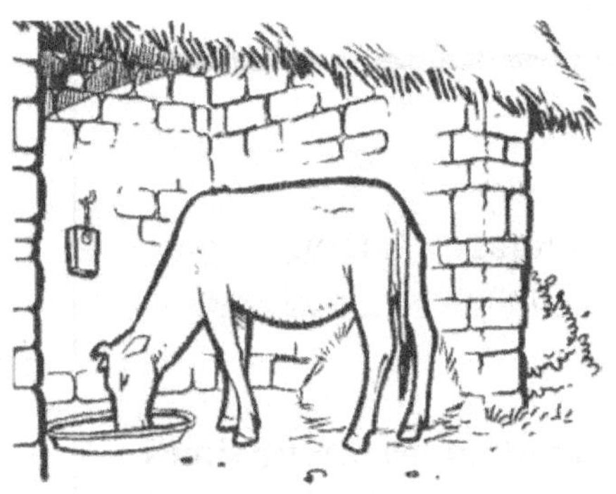

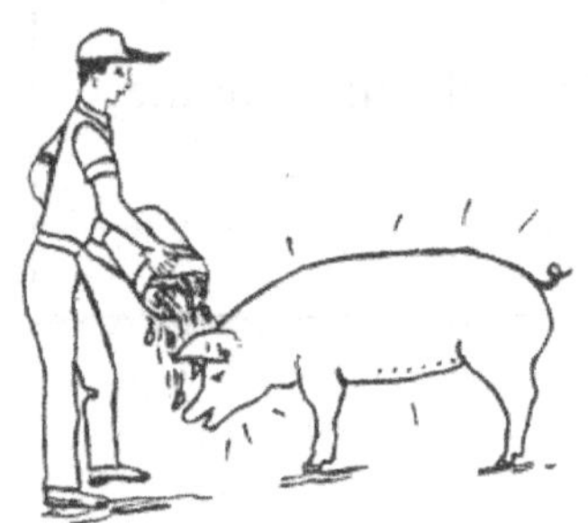

Treatment of Water Deficiencies (Dehydration)

For mild dehydration, provide clean, fresh water throughout the day and night.

See Page 268-269, for treatment of dehydration if the water deficiency is severe.

Note: An overheated animal may not drink until it has cooled down. Allow the animal to rest quietly in the shade, and, if possible, pour some cool water over it, particularly its head. Then, offer it water again.

7.3 SOME GUIDELINES AND HINTS FOR FEEDING LIVESTOCK

1. A balanced diet contains food from both protein and carbohydrate sources.

2. Higher quality feed should be reserved for pregnant and nursing mothers, as well as for growing animals. These animals especially need more protein in their diet.

3. Poorer quality feed can be fed, with less problems, to adult animals that are being kept for meat, adult oxen and buffalo that are not working, and adult females that are not in late pregnancy or giving milk.

4. Avoid sudden changes in the diet of animals. For instance, an animal eating straw or hay that is suddenly changed to green grass will often get diarrhea or bloat.

5. All animals, even grazing animals, need fresh, clean water. Offering water before other foods can help prevent bloating.

6. **Minerals and vitamins have their best effect <u>when livestock are already getting enough water, energy and protein</u>**. Antibiotics, as well as vitamin or mineral injections, will not make your livestock healthy and productive <u>if they are not being fed well</u>. It is more effective and less expensive to feed a proper combination of energy and protein, and to seek <u>local</u> sources of vitamins (green forage) and minerals to feed <u>by mouth</u>.

7. Young animals, particularly at the time of weaning, need extra protein in their diet. They should be fed some protein-containing foods like soya beans or protein-rich forages.

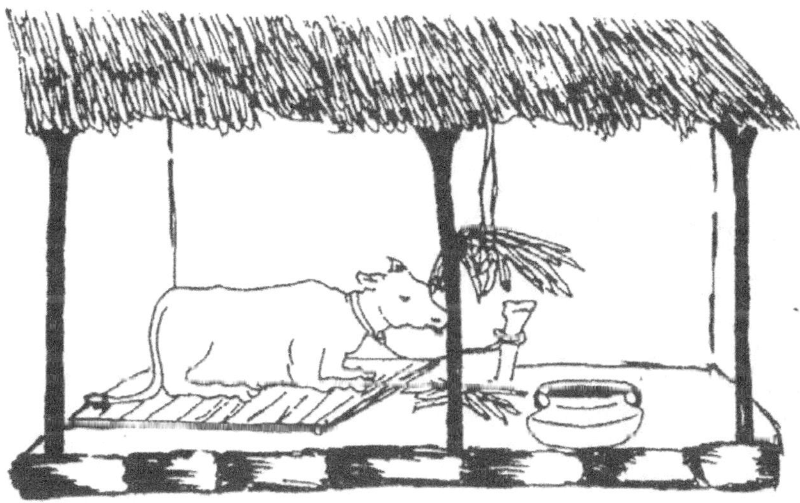

8.0   PARASITES FOUND ON THE SKIN

Parasites which are found **on** or **in** the skin are commonly called "ectoparasites" or "external parasites." Flies, fly larvae, and lice are called **insects**, and have six legs in their adult stage. Ticks and mange mites are called **arachnids** and have eight legs in the adult stage. The ectoparasite that causes ringworm is a tiny plant-like organism called **fungi**. Most ectoparasites can be seen with the eye. However, some of them, like fungi and some small mange mites, can only be seen with the help of a microscope.

Important parasites found <u>on</u> the skin include ticks, lice, flies, and fleas. Important parasites found <u>in</u> the skin include fungi, mites, maggots, screw worm, and warbles (or grubs).

Many important livestock diseases are spread by ticks. Therefore, the section on ticks is covered first. This section covers principles regarding the use of chemicals to kill ticks. The principles used to control ticks can be applied to the control of other parasites as well.

8.1   GENERAL SYMPTOMS OF EXTERNAL PARASITES IN LIVESTOCK

- itching
- scratching
- hair or wool loss
- wounds on the skin
- dry, scaly, and/or thickened skin
- parasites or their eggs

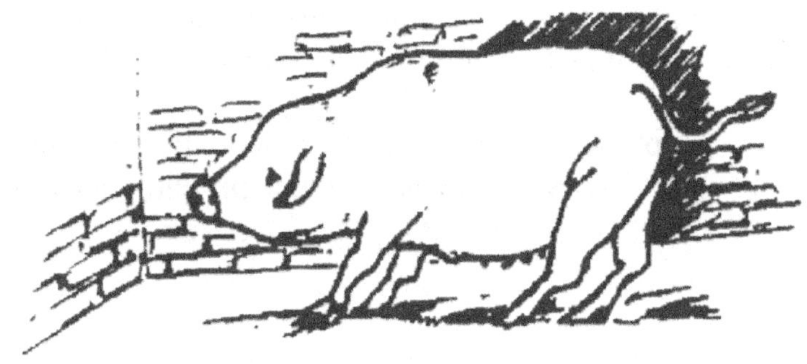

Pig constantly scratching due to manage or lice

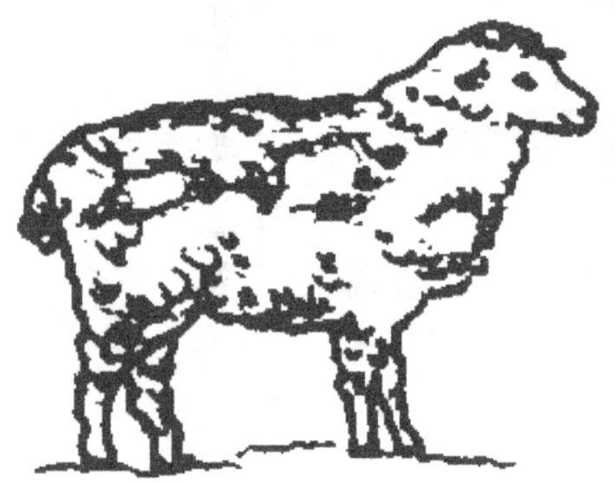

Wool loss and dry, scaly skin due to mites or lice

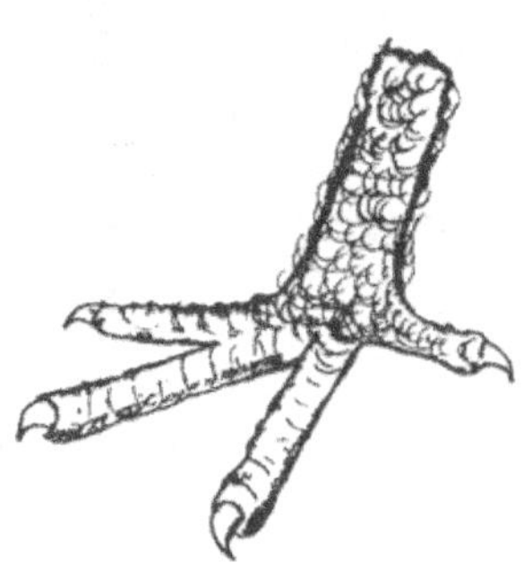

Scaly leg due to leg mites in poultry

8.2　GENERAL CONTROL OF EXTERNAL PARASITES

Many external parasites can be controlled by new medicines (pesticides or insecticides) that are available. Some pesticides come in a liquid form, and others come in the form of a dust. A number of traditional treatments for external parasites also work quite well. For instance, see page 120, to make a pesticide from tobacco leaves.

There are several major methods of applying pesticides:
- **Sprays:** Some pesticides are mixed with a water solution and sprayed onto the animals.
- **Dusts / dust bags:** Some pesticides are applied directly as dusts or put into bags that the animals rub against.
- **Backrubbers:** Some dusts are mixed with oils and placed in backrubbers that the animals rub against.
- **Ear Tags:** Some ear tags have pesticide in them, and slowly release the chemicals into the animal's body.
- **Direct Applications:** Using a cloth, sponge, or brush, some pesticides are directly applied to the area of skin where the parasites are present.
- **Pour-Ons:** These insecticides can be poured on the back of the animal in small amounts. They are absorbed into the blood, and then kill external parasites located almost anywhere on, or feeding on, the body.
- **Dips:** Some medicines are put into a water solution and the animals are bathed or dipped into the solution.
- **Injections:** Some injections, like "Ivermectin," kill most internal and external parasites.

Speak with a local expert about the products available in your area to treat external parasites.

CAUTIONS: Medicines for external parasites are poisons. Successful treatment involves poisoning the parasites without harming the livestock. Parasite treatments work properly only when the correct product in the right amount is used at the appropriate time. Wildlife, fish and beneficial insects may be poisoned by some products if careless use allows the medicine to contaminate food or water.

8.3　TICKS

Tick can be seen attached to the animal's skin, or sometimes inside the ear flap, or around the udder, scrotum, tail, anus, and vulva.

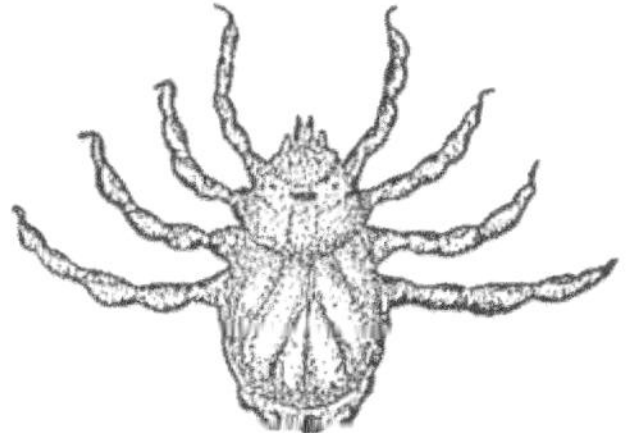

Symptoms and Diagnosis / Lifecycle

Direct Damage: Ticks directly damage an animal by sucking blood, causing:
- reduced growth and/or weight
- anemia (thin blood) and weakness
- damage to hide or teats
- licking and scratching, instead of contented grazing
- sores or breaks in the skin that become infected or attract screw worm flies
- reduced fertility and/or milk production
- reduced immunity to other diseases
- paralysis

Indirect Damage: Ticks also carry and infect animals with serious diseases such as anaplasmosis, Babesiosis, heartwater disease, and theileriosis. These are called **"tick-borne diseases,"** since they are transmitted by ticks.

Life cycle of ticks

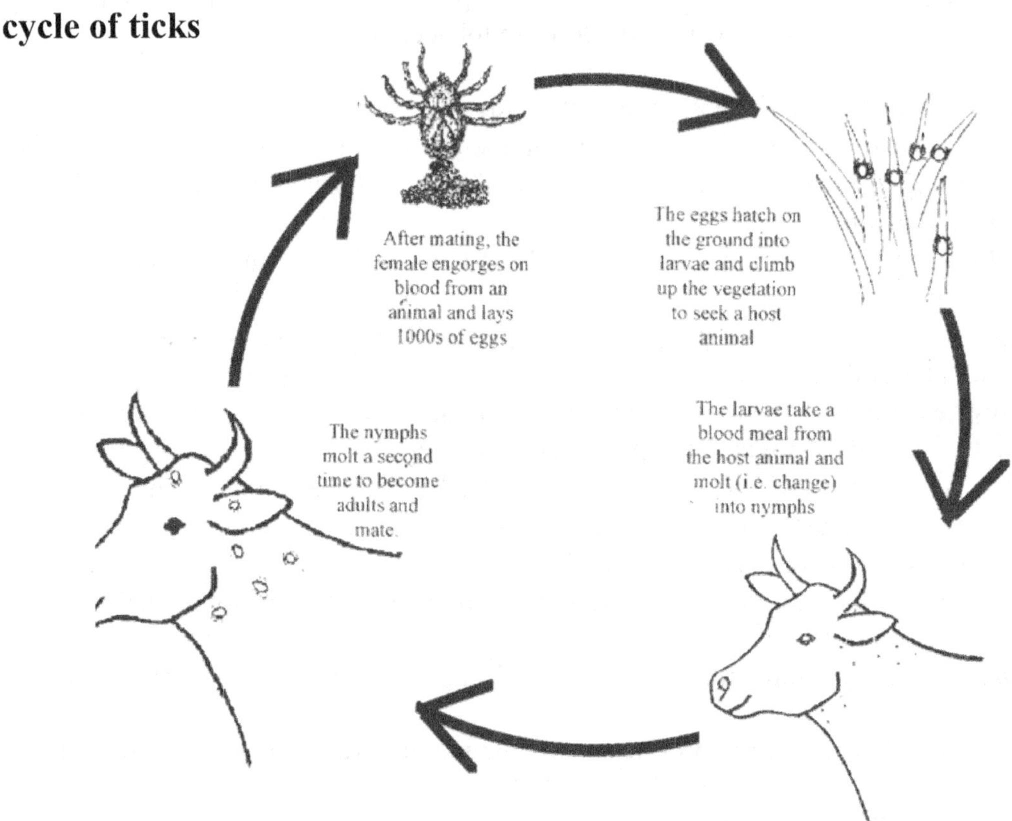

Ticks spend part of their lives on the ground, and part on the host-animal. The amount of time spent on the host-animal varies with the species of tick. The process when the tick matures from one stage to another stage is called a "molt." In general, eggs are laid on the ground and hatch into six-legged larvae. After sucking blood from an animal, the larvae molt (mature) into eight-legged nymphs. The nymphs attach themselves to a host-animal, fill with blood, and drop off. On the ground they molt into adult ticks. The adult ticks crawl up on grass or bushes, attach to a passing host-animal, mate, and feed on blood. The female adult tick then drops off the host-animal, lays its eggs on the ground, and the cycle begins again. The entire cycle may take up to one, two, or three years, depending on the species of tick and the weather conditions.

Types of ticks

Ticks are described as 'hard-bodied' or 'soft-bodied,' based on their body form. They are further described as 'one-host,' 'two-host,' or 'three-host,' based on the number of host-animal species they feed-on during their life cycle. A 'one-host' tick feeds on the same host-animal as a larva, a nymph and an adult. It drops off only to lay eggs. 'Two-host' and 'three-host' ticks change host-animals between stages of development.

- Control measures against ticks vary, depending on the type of tick involved. Australia and Latin America have one-host ticks. Africa and North America have a mixture of one-host, two-host, and three-host ticks.

Natural or acquired resistance to ticks or tick-borne diseases

Animals imported from an area without ticks, and European breeds, tend to be less resistant to ticks and tick-borne diseases. Some animals, such as the "zebu type" of cattle, are more naturally resistant to ticks and the diseases they cause. Animals that are born and raised in a tick-infested area are usually more resistant than imported animals. Even 'resistant animals' may lose their resistance if they have no exposure to ticks for long periods of time.

> **Warning!** Importing less resistant animals into tick infested areas can be disastrous. Many animals may become sick and/or heavily infested with ticks. Imported cattle usually require more intensive tick control measures than native cattle.

Diagnosis: Finding the ticks on the animal provides a definitive diagnosis. However, a diagnosis can also be made by observing the symptoms and knowing that ticks are common in the area.

Treatment / Control and Prevention: Chemicals used to kill ticks are called "acaricides," "pesticides," or "ixodicides." The following information is needed for good tick control:
- What are the main types of ticks in the area? One-host, two-host, or three-host ticks?
- Are tick-borne diseases killing or making many animals sick in your area?
- What specific areas, seasons, and type of animals develop problems?
- What acaricides are available, in what form, and at what cost?
- Are the ticks in your area known to be resistant to certain acaricides?

These questions can usually be answered by an agricultural extension agent or agricultural college in your country.

> **DANGER!!! (The following holds true for most pesticides - not just those used for ticks.)**
>
> - All pesticides are poisonous if mixed improperly.
>
> - Pesticides must be stored safely away from children and animals.
>
> - Always <u>read</u> and <u>carefully follow</u> the instructions which should <u>always</u> be issued with the pesticide. Do not use pesticides which are unlabeled or have no instructions. If you are not sure how to mix them, seek advice from someone who knows how to use them - or do not use them.
>
> - Use pesticides only from reputable chemical companies.
>
> - Make sure antidote (or treatment) is available to treat accidental overdose of the pesticide you are using. Know how to use the antidote. Quick access to an antidote is important, particularly, if you are treating a large number of animals.

WARNING!!
- Avoid splashing pesticides on your skin or in your eyes.
- Wear rubber gloves when mixing or applying pesticides.
- Avoid contaminating drinking water or feeds with pesticides.
- Do not mix different pesticides together unless the manufacturer specifies that the chemicals may be mixed.

For the details regarding these different methods, See Chapter 26, "Insecticide Use for Control of External Parasites."

Controlling ticks through pasture management

This method might work in Australia and parts of South America where only one-host ticks exist, and where there are few wild animals to maintain the tick population. Tick-infested areas should be fenced off, and no livestock allowed to enter for three to six months. During this time, the ticks die because they have no host-animals on which to feed. The amount of time required depends on the temperature and humidity. Hot, dry weather kills ticks more quickly (i.e. within three months), than cold, wet weather. Tick control through pasture management may fail in windy areas, since strong winds can carry tick larvae for considerable distances and re-infest pastures.

In areas where there are many wild animals, and where two-host and three-host ticks exist, good tick control through pasture management is not possible.

Ineffective methods of tick control

FIRES: In some areas, fires are used in an effort to control ticks. This does not work well because the tick eggs and larvae buried in the soil are protected from the fire. This practice is also harmful to the environment as it burns the organic matter in the soil and the soil becomes less fertile.

PASTURE SPRAYING: Pasture spraying is largely ineffective and very expensive. It may also harm the environment by contaminating drinking water and killing useful insects.

Controlling ticks by spraying or burning pastures is INEFFECTIVE and degrades the environment.

8.4   FLEAS

Fleas are jumping insects that bite and suck blood. Although livestock owners often complain about them, fleas are seldom a serious problem for livestock. They may become a problem if large numbers build up in animal housing. Large numbers of fleas may seriously weaken animals by sucking their blood and causing intense irritation at the site of the bite.

Fleas from livestock can also bite people who live nearby, causing intense itching and irritation. In areas where people and animals live in the same building, fleas can create human health problems.

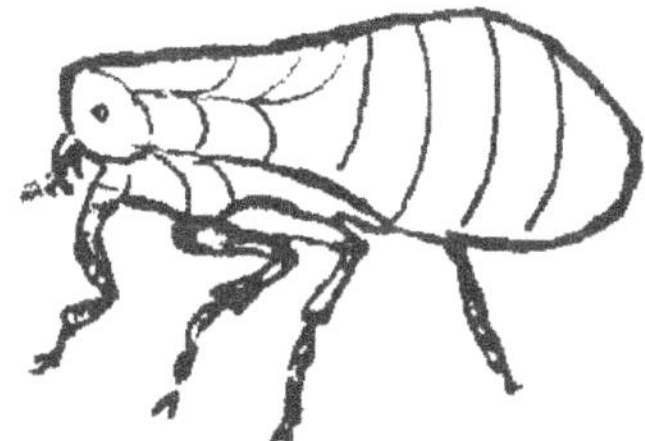

Lifecycle: Fleas are hard to control because there are four stages of development (egg, larvae, pupa, and adult) and only the adult stage lives primarily on the animal. The other stages hide in bedding, clothes, rugs, furniture, and cracks and corners where dust and dirt collect.

Symptoms / Diagnosis: The main symptom is itching and scratching. Some people and animals get an allergic reaction from flea bites. Fleas may be diagnosed by finding the adults jumping around. Or, small black specks that look like dirt may be seen. These black specks are really the feces from fleas. To test, put the black specks on white paper, and place a few drops of water on the specks. A red stain will appear on the paper if it is flea feces because they contain the red color of the blood that the fleas have eaten.

Treatment: Insecticide dust, and many types of sprays applied to animals help to reduce the flea problem but kill only those fleas which happen to be on the animal. Fleas that are living off the animal can later re-infest the animal. Check the labels for specific instructions. Note: Injectables and pour-ons which get into the blood of animals are also often effective for control of fleas and other insects. However, they are expensive.

Prevention / Control: Before any type of spraying or dusting is done, the housing should also be thoroughly cleaned. Especially clean in the corners of buildings where dust and dirt accumulate, and any hides or fabric that provide hiding places. This area should then be sprayed or dusted.

8.5   LICE

Lice are described as biting or sucking types, depending on their mouth parts and method of feeding. Both types can cause problems in livestock   They seem to affect animals that are malnourished, and young animals. In general, lice that infest one species of animal do not infest other species of animals.

Lice live amongst the hair. They bite the skin or suck blood when feeding. This irritates the animal. Animals with lice spend much time rubbing and scratching. This damages the hair and wool. The white eggs of the lice, called nits, may be seen by parting the hair / wool and looking carefully near where the hair enters the skin.
- In pigs, sucking lice are usually seen around the head, neck, and legs. They cause the pig to be restless and spend much time scratching. The pigs spend less time eating, and become thin and unhealthy.
- In buffalo, the eggs of lice are seen stuck in the hair of the animal. However they do not seem to cause many problems except for young or malnourished buffalo.

- In sheep with thick wool, heavy infestation with lice damages the wool.
- In chickens, biting lice cause lowered weight gain or egg production.
- In camels, llamas, and alpacas, lice cause itching and excessive dandruff.

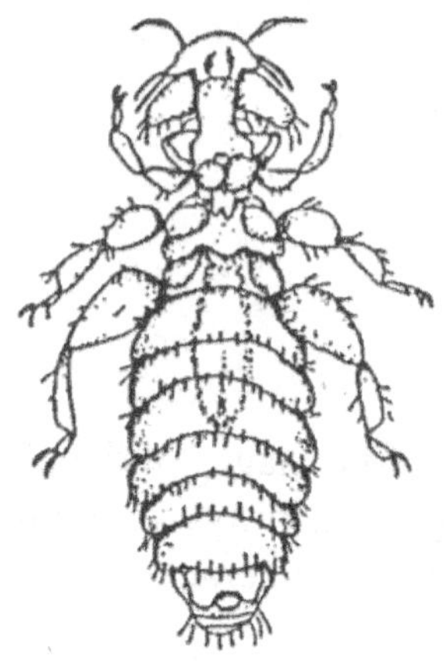

Biting Louse

Lifecycle: Adult lice live mostly on the animal. They spread from one animal to another by direct contact or through infested equipment. In general, adult lice cannot survive for more than one week off the animal.

Symptoms / Diagnosis: Itching, scratching and damage to skin, wool and hair are seen.

Treatment / Control: Many dips, sprays, or pour-on products may be effective against lice. Ivermectin injection works well against sucking lice, but not against biting lice. Severe infestations may require re-treatment in 10-21 days to kill lice that hatch from eggs laid before the first treatment.

When treating for lice, it is important to treat all animals in the group at one time. Otherwise the lice will spread from untreated animals back to the treated ones.

8.6   MITES

Adult mites are very small and have eight legs. It is hard to see a mite clearly without the use of either a microscope or a magnifying glass. In livestock, mites cause a disease called, "mange." Mange is a common skin problem of sheep, goats, buffalo, cattle, pigs, rabbits, camels, llamas, and alpacas.

People also have their own kind of mites that cause a disease called "scabies," that is common in young children. Occasionally people who handle animals with mange become infested with the mites from animals. This causes only temporary itching and discomfort because livestock mites live on people for only a short time.

Mites burrow into the skin and cause severe irritation and itching. One particular type of mite in sheep causes bad itching and scab formation. The infested animals become very thin and weak. This disease is commonly called "scab." It is very infectious and dangerous, and can spread to cattle and other animals. If an AHA suspects "scab," they should report it to the local veterinary authorities.

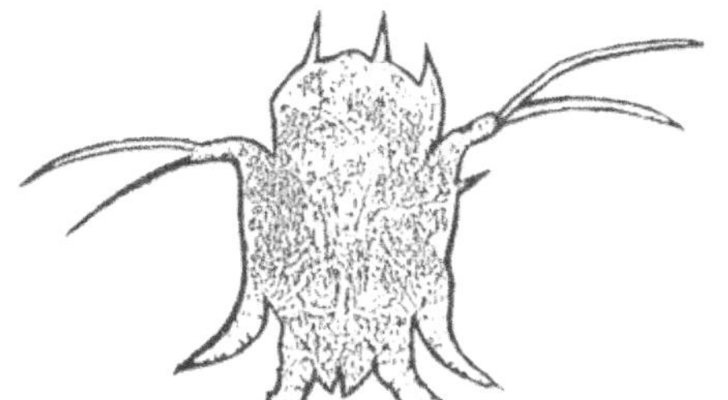

Common Mange Mite

Lifecycle of Mites: Adult mites live on the skin, and in the skin. They burrow into the skin and reproduce there. Mites often spread from one animal to another when the animals touch each other. They may also be spread through grooming equipment or harnesses used by both mangy and non-infested animals.

Symptoms / Diagnosis:

Type One Mange: Itching, scratching, and damage to skin, wool, and hair are seen. If an animal does not respond to treatment for mange, a trained technician should scrape the skin and examine the scrapings using a microscope. If the animal has mange, mites should be visible in the scrapings.

Type Two Mange: There is also a type of mange that is not as itchy. It is called "demodectic mange." It often starts on the head, shoulders and neck. Small bumps develop and they contain thick, greasy material, and sometimes pus. The skin becomes thick and forms heavy folds. The animals may get better on their own. This type of mange is almost impossible to treat successfully. Microscopic examination of the material from the bumps should show the demodectic mites.

Treatment / Control: As mentioned above, demodectic mange is very difficult to treat. Any animal with any type of mange should be washed well with soap and water. If the wounds are already infected, the animal may also need an antibiotic injection. Long-acting penicillin (benzathine penicillin) or amoxacillin are often effective against skin infections. Several methods can be used to kill the mites causing the mange.
>   **Sulfur ointment** can be made from one part sulfur powder mixed with ten parts of cooking oil or giu. This mixture must be rubbed into the wounds at least once a week for four or five weeks. This is very safe and easy to use.
>   **Motor oil** is quite effective for pigs and buffalo/calves. Used motor oil can be applied in small amounts and rubbed into the affected areas at the beginning of an infestation. Do not apply used motor oil to large, infected wounds because it may contain harmful chemicals that could poison the animal. As with sulfur ointment, it should be used weekly for four or five weeks.
>   **Benzyl Benzoate** is very good for ear mites in rabbits. After cleaning with disinfectant water, several drops of medicine can be put into the ear; and the ear should be massaged. This should be repeated at least once a week for four or five weeks. Some people treat all their rabbits regularly to prevent this problem.

Cythion, Malathion or other pesticides. Follow the label carefully.

Ivermectin can also be used for some types of mange, but it is quite expensive.

8.7   FLIES

Flies are harmful to the health of livestock for several reasons:
- Flies irritate animals and prevent them from eating and resting.
- When many flies bite an animal, it can become weak.
- Flies carry infection to wounds and to the eyes.
- Some flies lay eggs which hatch as maggots on the animal. The maggots feed on the flesh of the animal, causing extensive tissue damage.
- Biting flies can spread blood-borne diseases, such as the tsetse fly which carries trypanosomiasis in Africa.

Life Cycle of Flies

All flies go through a cycle where the adult female mates and then lays eggs. The eggs hatch and become larvae (sometimes called maggots). The larvae develop into pupae, and then adult flies. This whole life cycle can be as short as one week in some species, or it may be as long as one year.

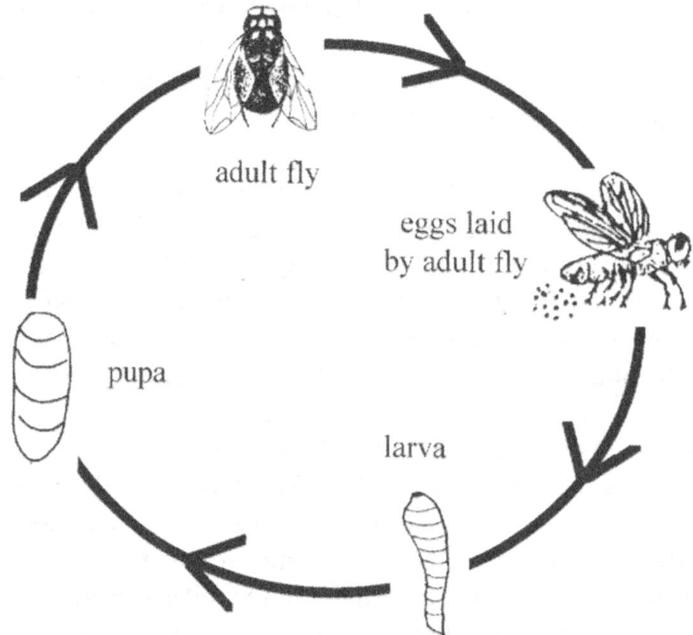

Symptoms / Diagnosis: Adult flies themselves are easily seen. In addition, livestock bothered by adult flies often move nervously, and may run in groups as they try to escape the biting, buzzing, and irritation. For other flies, the larvae (maggots) are the form of the insect that cause animal health problems. Diagnosis of larvae infestation often requires close observation.

Treatment / Control: Flies are difficult to completely control. However different methods may help reduce the number of flies and the level of aggravation.
- Eliminate the places where fly larvae may develop.
- Spread manure thinly over the pasture so it dries out. Fly eggs cannot hatch and develop properly in dry manure.
- Some ducks eat insects, and chickens eat ticks. Keeping ducks and chickens with animals like cattle helps to control flies and ticks.
- Cover or remove rotting material, manure and compost where larvae develop.

As with medicines for tick control, **insecticides** for fly control must be used carefully. See page 108 and Chapter 26, Insecticide Appendix.

- **Direct Application:** Insecticides may be directly applied to the animal through sprays, pour-ons, or ear tags that have the insecticide in them. Pyrethrins are often quite effective against flies.

- **Self-applicators or back rubbers** can be made from a sack containing insecticide dust, or soaked in insecticide oil. Coumaphos can be used in oil or as a powder. (Mix 300 ml of 11.6% EC in 4 liters of diesel fuel.)
    - Put the powder in a burlap sack, or soak the burlap sack in the oil mixture. Then tie the sack around a tree or post, or wrap it round a wire between two posts. Animals learn to rub against it to control their own flies. It may need replacing after several weeks.

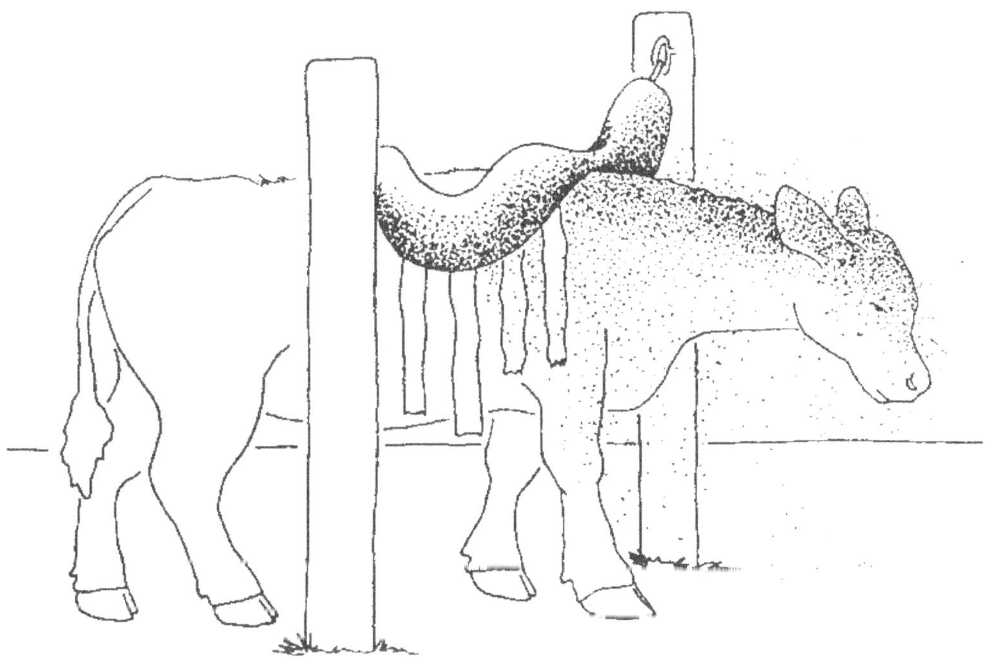

Cow Walking Under Back Rubber That Has Insecticide On It

8.7.1 Some Specific Examples of Fly Problems

8.7.1.1 *Midges (Culicoides), blackflies (Simulium species), and mosquitoes (Culex species)*

- Midges transmit diseases, including Bluetongue in sheep.
- Midges are found where it is wet. They breed in swampy places and are found more often in cool climates.
- Midges are tiny (one to three mm long).
- Blackflies (five mm long) breed in running water.
- Mosquitoes breed in still water. Control is difficult. Drain wet areas where flies breed.
- Keep animals away from swampy areas, especially during insect-feeding times in the early morning and late afternoon.
- Insect repellents are often used on a daily basis during certain times of the year.
- Other insecticides may be used with the advice of a local expert.

8.7.1.2 *Horn flies and buffalo flies*

- Horn flies are found in the Americas and North Africa; buffalo flies are found in Asia and Australia.
- Their bites irritate livestock.
- They breed in manure, but live mostly on the animal. Thousands may live on a single animal.
- Back rubbers for applying insecticide provide good control.

8.7.1.3 *House flies and bush flies*

- House flies are found worldwide and bush flies are found in Australia.
- They cause annoyance and spread diseases.
- Control measures include proper handling of manure and use of fly baits. If manure is spread out and dries quickly, the housefly population decreases.

8.7.1.4 *Stable flies (Stomoxys)*

- They look like house flies, but they bite the skin and blood oozes out at the site of the bite. Stable flies are very irritating.
- Control measures include removing dung and rotting material. Insecticides are not necessary if sanitation is good.

8.7.1.5 *Horse flies (Tabanids)*

- They bite like stable flies, causing pain, and leaving open wounds in the skin.
- If present in high numbers, they may make animals weak from blood loss.
- They may transmit trypanosomiasis.
- Control is very difficult because they are on the animal for only a short time. Repellents may work, but must be applied frequently.

8.7.1.6 *Sheep Keds (Sheep ticks)*

- These are really flies without wings. They resemble big lice in the wool of sheep. They bite and suck blood, and the infested sheep scratch and damage their wool.
- Dips and sprays provide effective control.

8.7.1.7 *Tsetse flies (Africa)*

- Tsetse flies bite and feed on blood. During the feeding process they transmit trypanosomiasis. See page 275.
- Control is not easy. Where the flies live, most breeds of cattle cannot be kept without expensive control measures. To avoid trypanosomiasis in the presence of the flies, check with the nearest extension agent the possibility of making and using tsetse fly traps. New kinds of traps use small amounts of insecticide and are simple to make.

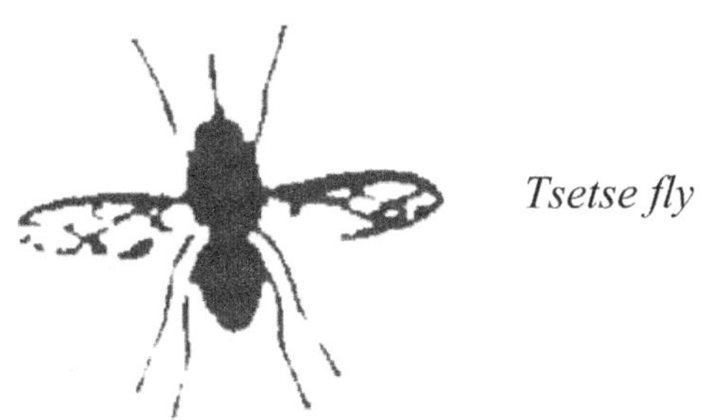

Tsetse fly

8.7.1.8 *Maggot Infestation (Myiasis)*

Maggots are the larvae stage of flies. When maggots develop and feed in, or on, living animals, this is called **myiasis**. Maggots can cause serious problems in wounds or where wet manure sticks to the skin of livestock. During fly season, maggot infestations occur in castration wounds, injuries, sore feet from foot and mouth disease, cuts, broken horns, umbilical cords on newborns, under the tail of sheep, and around the anus of animals with diarrhea.

Symptoms and Diagnosis: Adult flies mate and lay their eggs which hatch into larvae (maggots). The larvae crawl further into wounds. Some maggots damage the tissue; others prevent the wound from healing. Some flies lay eggs on, and around, the nose of sheep and goats. These eggs hatch into larvae which then crawl up the nose and into the sinuses or horns. Animals with these larvae may shake their heads, rub their horns against things, sneeze, and move restlessly.

Treatment and Prevention / Control of Myiasis:
This is truly one condition where **prevention is better than cure!**

Methods of **prevention** include:
- Clip wool short around the tail so that manure does not collect in the wool.
- Treat diseases, for example worms, which cause diarrhea and soiling of the wool.
- Insecticides with a long-lasting effect can be used to prevent maggots on woolly sheep.
- During fly season, all wounds must be watched carefully. Maggot infestations can be prevented by putting insecticide powder around the wounds, and putting insecticide creams, ointments, or home remedies in the wound itself. (Note: Insecticides and home remedies may cause irritation to the tissue, and slow-down the healing process. It is best to keep wounds clean and covered, and to apply repellents around the wound and on the dressing. If this is not possible, then go ahead and apply medicines directly into the wound itself to prevent the development of myiasis.)

Treatment includes:

- Clip wool or hair away to expose the maggots.
- Clean the wound with soap or antiseptic (e.g. *Savlon*).
- Use a locally available method to kill the maggots or to get them to leave the wound.
  - Crush mothballs - dissolve them in water and squirt the solution into the wound.
  - Liquid insecticides - spray, brush or sponge on the places where maggots are seen. Organophosphates like diazinon or chorfenvinphos (*Supona*) kill the maggots in about half a day.
  - Turpentine oil, creoline or kerosene can be used. Put on cotton wool or a clean cloth, and put this over the maggot infested wound. Hold in place with a bandage made of a strip of cloth.
  - Use other locally-made solutions like tobacco solutions or certain crushed leaves.
- Remove after two or three hours, pick out dead maggots, clean the wound, and rinse it thoroughly.
- Apply a locally available insect repellent around the wound to prevent flies from laying eggs again.

8.7.1.9 *Screw worm*

Symptoms / Diagnosis: Screw worm infestations occur in Latin America and Africa when the larvae of screw worm fly hatch from eggs laid on the edge of a wound. The larvae look a bit like a wood screw, and the pointed head goes deep into the flesh. Groups of maggots feed together, burrow deep into the flesh, prevent the wound from healing, and provide a site for infection by bacteria or fungi. Screw worms cause great irritation to an animal.

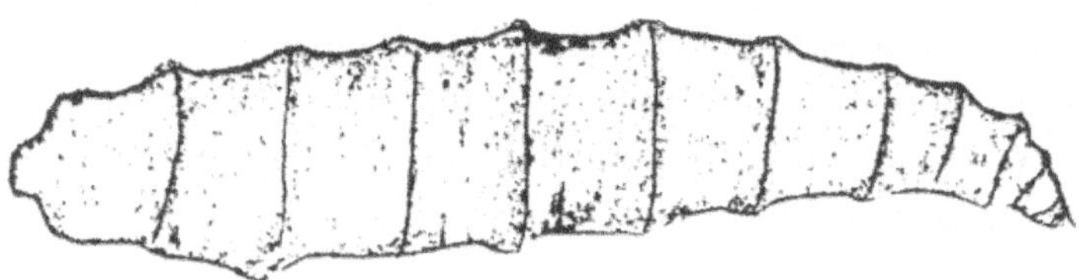

Screw worm larva that burrows into wounds

Treatment: The earlier the treatment begins, the less damage will be done. Check other animals in the group to see if there is an early infection.

- Clean the wound (use soap or antiseptic).
- Apply insecticide powder or creoline deep into the wound, for example Coumaphos wettable powder.
- Remove the dead larvae, clean the wound, and apply insecticide grease to prevent re-infestation.
- Since most wounds are already infected, also give an antibiotic injection like penicillin or oxytetracycline.

Prevention: In areas with screw worm, use insecticide grease or spray on wounds caused by simple surgical procedures (like castration or dehorning). Make the grease with one part *Coumaphos* 5% powder to 30 parts *Vaseline* (or new car oil). Or, use one part *lindane* to 20 parts *Vaseline* (or new car oil).

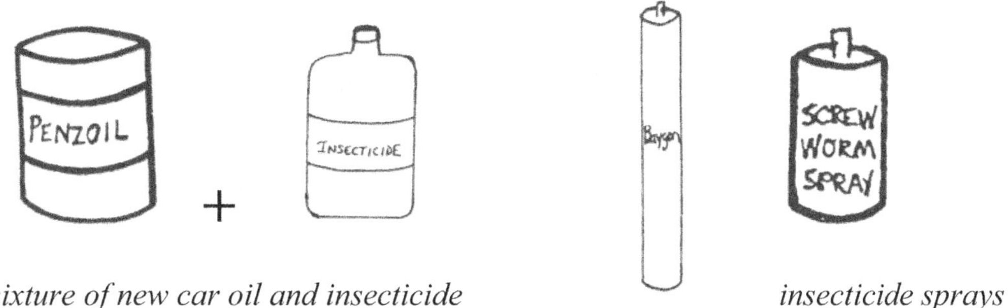

mixture of new car oil and insecticide   *insecticide sprays*

Note: Ivermectin kills young larvae but is not as effective against the older ones. Direct treatment of infested wounds is the best method to ensure all larvae are killed and removed.

Insecticide made from Tobacco

It is possible to make your own solution of tobacco insecticide using the following instructions:
- Soak 300 grams of dried tobacco leaves in one liter of water.
- Add one tablespoon of salt.
- After three hours, use the tobacco leaf as a sponge and rub the liquid over infested areas of the animal's body. (Ethno veterinary Medicine in Asia, Volume 2: Ruminants. Page 50.)

8.7.1.10 Bots

Symptoms / Diagnosis: Bots are maggots (fly larvae) which live inside the body. Some live attached inside the noses of sheep, others live attached to the stomach of horses. The bot eggs can often be seen as yellow specks on the hair of a horse, particularly its legs.

Sheep nose bots cause sneezing, a thick discharge from the nose, and shaking of the head. The sheep may become thin because they cannot graze normally. Horse bots live attached to the stomach or intestine, and cause few problems.

Treatment / Control
Sheep nose bots:
- Treat the sheep with ivermectin, or
- Spray inside the nose with a solution such as chloroform spirit, *Dettol*, tobacco, or insecticides such as trichlorphon.
    - Use a syringe without a needle, or a hand-held spray pump. Place the sheep upside down, on its back, and hold the sheep's head level Spray the solution into one nostril so that it runs back, deep into the nasal area. Hold the sheep on its back for about one minute, then quickly turn it over, and allow it to get up on its feet. After a minute or two of rest, repeat the treatment in the other nostril.

Horse bots:
- Regularly treating horses with trichlorphon, dichlorvos or ivermectin will control bots.

8.7.1.11 Warbles (Cattle Grubs)

This condition occurs mainly in the Northern Hemisphere. Heel flies lay eggs on the hair of the lower legs, and larvae hatch from the eggs, penetrate the skin, and migrate through the body to sites under the skin.

Symptoms / Diagnosis: These larvae are seen as bumps under the skin along the back, and are called "warbles" or "grubs." Each bump contains a grub about three centimeters long. Many types of animals can be affected, but warbles are most common in cattle and dogs. Warbles stress cattle and damage the hides.

Treatment and Prevention of Warbles: Migrating larvae can be killed with insecticide spray or pour-on, or ivermectin. However, if big larvae die inside the animal, they can damage the animal's nerves. It is best to treat larvae before they become big. Treatment at the end of the fly season, after adult flies stop laying eggs, kills larvae before they get big and migrate.

- Squeezing the bumps to remove the grubs is effective (and feasible if the number of grubs and animals is small.)
- Use famphur (*Warbex*), fenthion (*Tiguvon*), or (*Ivomec*) pour-on or injection. On milk cows, do not use insecticides that enter the milk. Rotenone is effective when brushed on the animal's back, and does not get into the milk of cows.

8.7.1.12 Torsalo or nuche maggots

Symptoms / Lifecycle: The scientific name for this maggot is "Dermatobia hominis." Nuche maggots are larvae that hatch from fly eggs. The fly deposits eggs on mosquitoes, which then deposit the eggs on cattle. The eggs hatch into larvae (or maggots) that burrow into the hide and damage it.

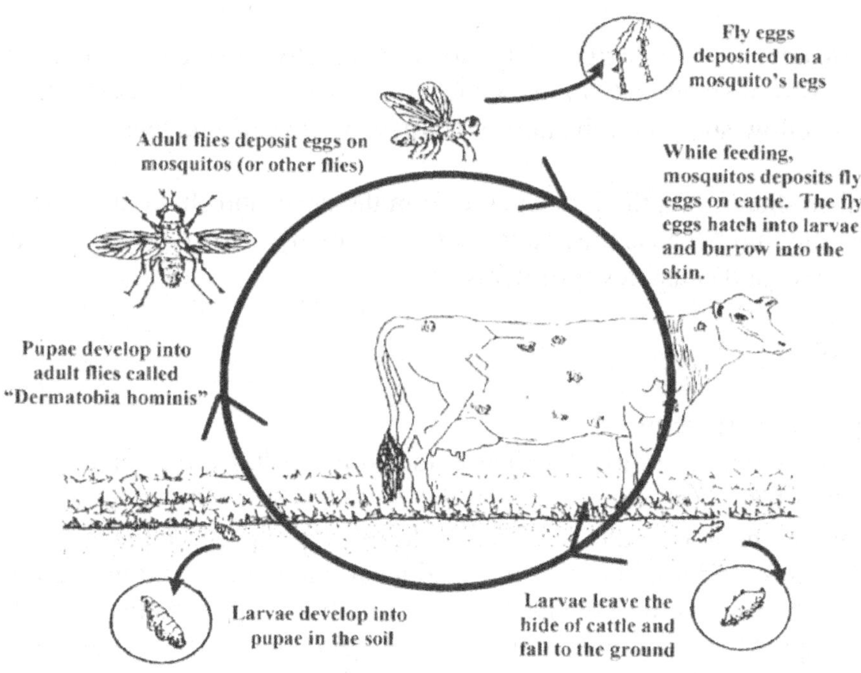

Diagnosis: Affected cattle develop bumps (with little air holes) on their backs, joints and any other area where maggots have burrowed.

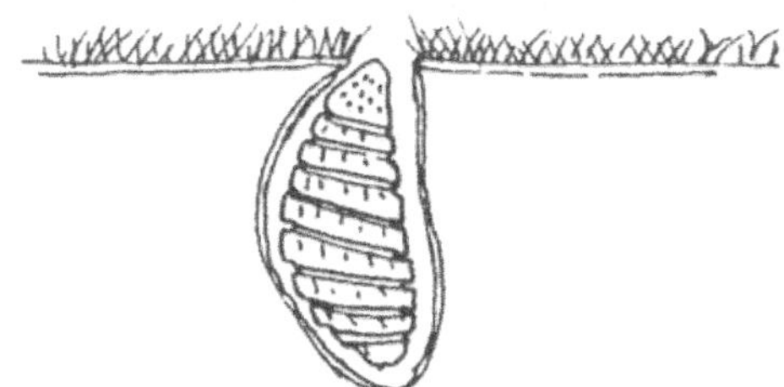

Treatment / Control / Prevention: There are several options for treating nuche maggots. Ask a local agricultural agent about the most effective and affordable product in your area. Options include:

1. Apply insecticide using back-rubbers or dust bags to help prevent nuche maggots.

2. Pour oil (cooking or new car oil) or grease into the air hole to suffocate the maggot. This oil or grease can be mixed with insecticide to make it more effective. For example, mix one part *Coumaphos* 5% powder to thirty parts grease or oil.

3. Administer ivermectin as an injection or oral paste, according to instructions.

8.8   LEECHES

Leeches are different from other parasites. There are two major types of leeches affecting livestock:
- leeches that live and feed in the nose and throat.
- leeches that attach to the skin of an animal, suck blood, and then drop off.

Symptoms / Diagnosis: Nasal leeches cause serious problems in some areas. (They can also affect people sometimes). When the animal is drinking water, baby leeches enter the mouth with the water. These leeches attach to the lining inside the nose, and begin to suck blood and grow. They cause blood loss and irritation. As a result, the animal eats less, and growth and production are decreased.

Treatment of Nasal Leeches: Treatment depends on what is available. Local remedies can work well.
- Some farmers prevent the affected animal from drinking for about one day. Then they offer water, and when the animal starts to drink, the leech also sticks its head out to drink. Then the farmer grabs the leech and pulls it out. Because leeches are slippery, they must grab the leech with a piece of cloth, or a pair of pinchers.

- Another treatment is to use a solution applied in the nose of the affected animal. A nicotine solution prepared from tobacco, a chloroform / spirit solution, or other solutions may be used.
  1. Restrain the animal properly (preferably in a crate).
  2. Hold the animal's head level so that the fluid put into its nose will remain there. (If the nose is pointed down, then the solution runs out of the nose; and if the nose is pointed up, then the solution runs down the throat and the animal swallows it.)

3.   Using a syringe with the needle removed, squirt 20-30 ml of the solution into the nostril where the leech is. (5 ml for small animals).
4.   Hold the animal's head level for one to two minutes.
5.   If there is a leech in the other nostril also, then repeat the process for the other side. Sometimes the leech falls out and is seen immediately. However, often the leech is not seen again. Apparently the solution kills the leech, it slides down to the throat, and the animal swallows it.

8.9   FUNGI (RINGWORM)

Ringworm is a disease that affects the hair and skin. This disease is found all over the world. It is caused by a single-celled organism called a fungus. In particular, young animals kept in damp, dark conditions seem to suffer from it. When the animals are moved to a dry, clean, sunny place, the fungus infection often clears up on its own. People can also get ringworm, so technicians should also be careful when handling animals with ringworm.

Symptoms: Round shaped areas of hair loss develop mostly on the head and neck. These areas become dry and crusty, and turn a gray color. Sometimes the animal spends time scratching these spots.

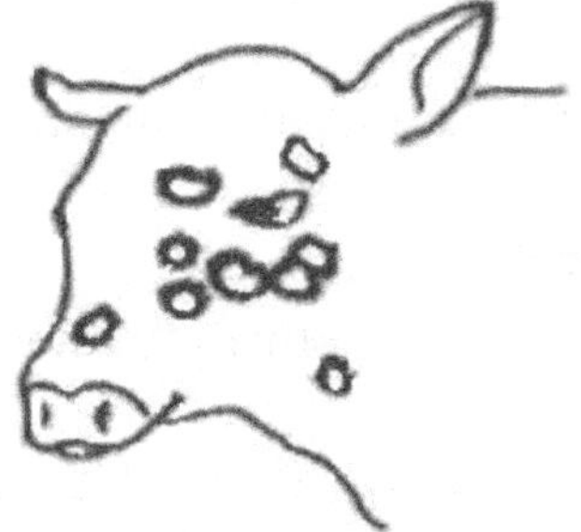

Classic round, crusty ringworm lesions on the head of this steer

Diagnosis: Based on the observed symptoms. One can also remove some of the hairs and crust from the edge of the area of hair loss. Place these hairs on a microscope slide with dilute potassium hydroxide solution for examination. The hairs and crust can also be placed in a clean bottle and sent to a laboratory for fungus identification.

Treatment: The infection spreads easily from animal to animal. It may also spread from feed racks and water troughs where animals scratch themselves.

Treatments applied directly (locally) to infected areas include:
- Tincture of Iodine every other day for seven to fourteen days. Don't get this into eyes or on sensitive tissue.
- Copper Sulfate powder mixed with petroleum jelly (*Vaseline*). Apply once and remove completely after 24 hours to avoid burning sensitive skin.
- *Thiabendazole* paste: one or two applications several days apart.
- Anti-fungal salves or creams that may be available in the market. (e.g. human preparations, *Tinactin*, etc.)

Systemic treatments include:
- Sodium Iodide given IV   or   Fulvicin (griseofulvin) boluses

Prevention / Control: Clean and dry pens, sunshine, and good diet, all help to prevent ringworm.

9.0 Parasites Inside The Body - "Internal Parasites"

The problem of internal parasites can devastate a farmer through lost production or dying animals. It is one of the most important and common problems seen by AHA's. The following section provides a simple, practical approach to treating and controlling internal parasites. Chapter 27 provides a more detailed approach. See pages 325-351.

THE GENERAL LIFE CYCLE OF INTERNAL PARASITES

Although the life cycle of each type of internal parasite varies, most have a life cycle with two stages: an adult, reproductive stage; and an immature, infective stage.

Adult, reproductive phase

The adult stage usually occurs inside the body. The adult parasite lays eggs that are then passed out of the body in the feces, urine, or saliva and can infect other animals. These adult parasites can be killed (i.e. treated) with medicines *before* they lay eggs.

Immature, infective stage

The infective stage usually occurs outside the animal's body in the soil, on pastures, or in water. The eggs either change to become "infective eggs" or immature parasites. An animal becomes infected when it takes in food or water contaminated with immature parasites or infective eggs. Some parasites also pass through an "intermediate host" while in the environment. The large roundworm may also infect unborn animals through the mother's bloodstream.

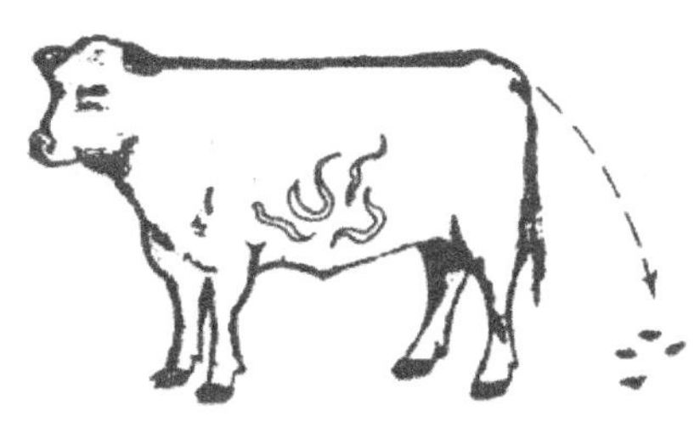

Adult parasites inside the animal lay eggs which are passed in the feces.

The eggs mature and become "infective eggs" or immature parasites.

Another animal eats the infective eggs or immature parasites while grazing, which then become adult parasites in the animal's intestines.

9.1   RECOGNIZE THE SYMPTOMS OF INTERNAL PARASITES

Parasites interfere with nutrition and may suck the blood of an animal. Then the animal does not have enough nutrients for itself and will suffer from malnutrition.

Four Keys to Treating and Controlling Internal Parasites

1.   Recognize the symptoms of internal parasites.

2.   Know which internal parasites are common in your area.

3.   Know which medicines treat internal parasites common in your area.

4.   Know which management practices control internal parasites.

Animals with internal parasites and / or malnutrition may have the following symptoms:

- have diarrhea
- are thin and often sickly
- have dull, dry hair that does not lay flat
- have heads that appear too big
- are pale due to anemia (check under the eyelids)
- have extra fluid under the jaw due to *severe* anemia (bottle jaw)
- have big abdomens
- produce little milk
- do not grow well

Pale under the eyelids
due to anemia

Extra fluid under the jaw
due to *severe* anemia

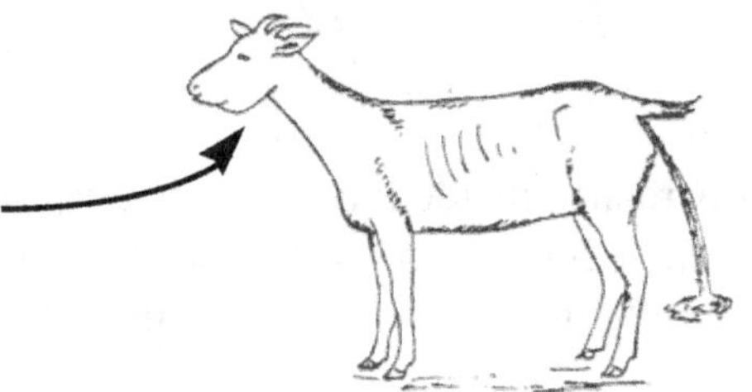

9.2   KNOW INTERNAL PARASITES COMMON IN YOUR AREA

The following three procedures can identify the most common parasites in an area:

1. **Parasite survey:** Manure samples from several animals are examined using a microscope to identify the most common parasites in an area. Information from parasite surveys is often available from government veterinary workers.

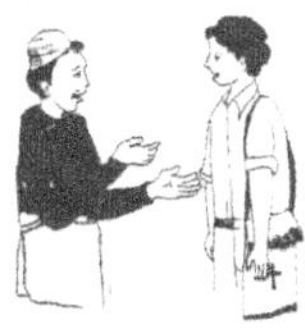

2. **Autopsy:** The bodies of dead or slaughtered animals are examined, particularly the digestive systems and livers. This is an easy way to learn whether liver flukes are a problem because they can be seen in the liver ducts without a microscope.

3. **Ask:** Other local veterinarians or AHA's may already know which parasites are common in your area. In addition, the Ministry of Agriculture may have useful information.

9.3   KNOW WHICH MEDICINES ARE COMMON IN YOUR AREA

Once the common parasites are identified, the most appropriate and inexpensive medicine can usually be found in the local market. Every medicine should be from a reputable source and have a label indicating for which parasites it is effective. Sometimes only the scientific names are listed on a label. Therefore, you may need the assistance of a veterinary doctor or someone else who knows these scientific names.

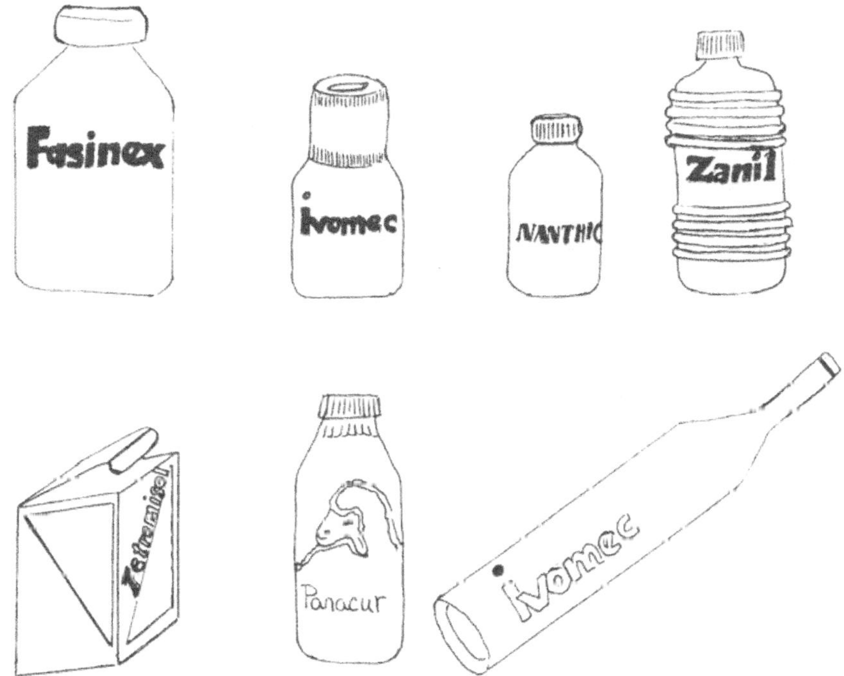

Examples of various worm medicines

Note: Animals that have had a chronic or severe load of parasites can remain sickly even after treatment if the parasites have already caused permanent damage to the animal's internal organs. **Therefore livestock owners should give parasite medicine routinely to avoid the permanent damage.**

Note: Parasites can become resistant to medicines that have been used for a long period of time in an area. When a certain medicine that once worked no longer works, the parasite may have become resistant and a change in medicine is necessary.

9.4   KNOW MANAGEMENT PRACTICES TO CONTROL PARASITES.

Immature parasites and eggs can often survive for long periods in the environment. This is especially true if the environment is moist, dark, and dirty. However, immature parasites and eggs can usually be killed by sunlight, heating or drying.

The following management practices help control internal parasites
- Keeping pens clean, dry, and exposed to sunlight
- Keeping babies and mothers separate from other animals and on the cleanest, least used (by animals) land.
- Putting water and food in troughs or mangers where animals cannot defecate.
- Giving parasite medicine regularly to all animals as well as to mothers before giving birth and during lactation.
- Keeping animals away from wet, swampy areas.
- Moving the animals to different pens or pastures every 1-2 months (called "pasture or pen rotation").

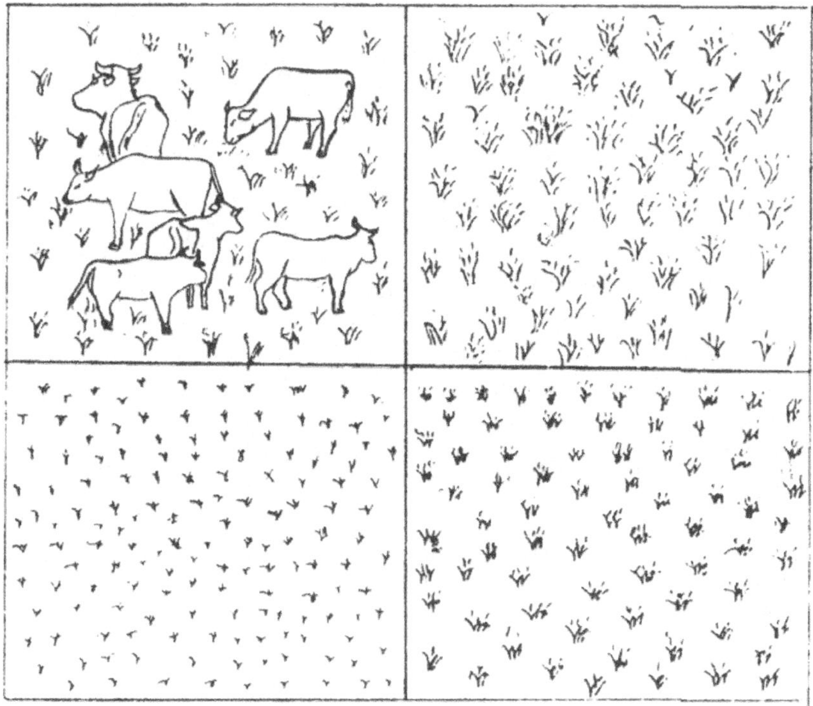

Example of pasture rotation: Animals graze on 1 pasture for 1-2 months and then are moved or "rotated" to a new one. The other 3 pastures remain empty for 3-6 months. During this time, parasites die from exposure to sunlight and drying, and the grass is able to grow properly.

9.5 THE PRACTICAL STEPS

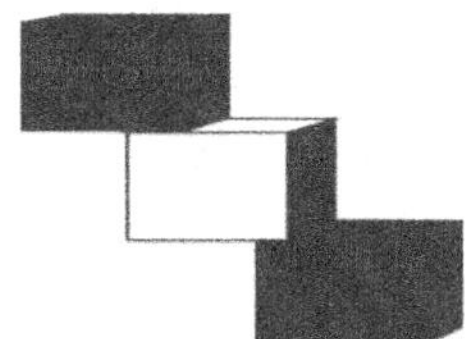

1. Take a complete history and examine the animals. Be sure to ask the owner about the animal's nutrition and whether it has been treated for any parasites in the last 1-3 months. Be sure to also examine the animal for external parasites.

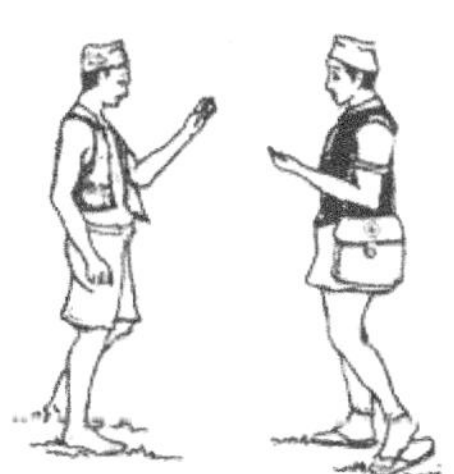

2. If the animal has not been treated for internal parasites in the past 1-3 months, treat it. Based on the most common parasites in your area, choose the most appropriate and least expensive medicine available.

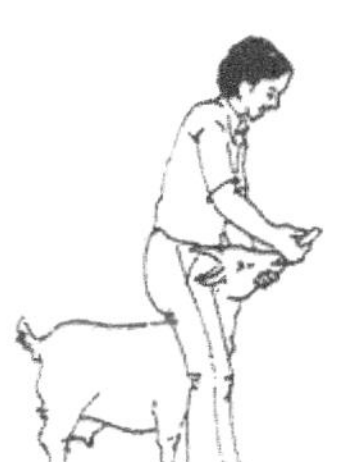

3. Treat the animals for any other problems found during the history or examination.

Caution: Always follow label instructions. Remember to use the proper medicines on pregnant animals as some medicines may cause abortions.

Important note: Imported animals may have less resistance to the local parasites and diseases, and may require parasite treatment more often as well as extra efforts in controlling parasites.

Another important note: Animals suffering from internal parasites often have external parasites as well. Be sure to check and, if necessary, treat for both.

A True Story

In Nepal, a veterinarian conducted parasite surveys, talked with farmers and examined dead animals. He learned that liver flukes are a problem in grazing animals and large roundworms a problem in calves. He developed simple rules about treating animals in the hilly areas of Nepal for internal parasites that cost little, worked well, and required no microscope.

Simple Rules for Treating Internal Parasites in the Hilly Areas of Nepal

1. **For adult sheep, goats, cattle, and buffalo that graze regularly:** First treat for liver fluke. If the animals are still doing poorly after several weeks, treat for small roundworms also. The best method, if affordable, is to treat for both liver fluke and small roundworms at the same time. Treat the animals every 6-12 months depending on the severity of the parasite problem.

2. **For adult sheep, goats, cattle, and buffalo that are kept mainly in a pen:** First treat for small **roundworms**. If the animals are still doing poorly after several weeks, treat for liver flukes also. The best method, if affordable, is to treat for both liver fluke and small roundworms at the same time. Treat the animals every 6-12 months depending on the severity of the parasite problem.

3. **For baby buffalo and baby cattle (calves):** Treat for large roundworms sometime during their first four months and repeat the treatment four weeks later. As they get older and begin to eat grass, they can be treated the same as adults (i.e. according to rules 1 and 2).

4. **For young sheep and goats:** Treat for small roundworms and tapeworms every 6 months or even more **frequently** depending upon the severity of the parasite problem. At one year of age, they can be treated the same as adults (according to rules 1 and 2).

5. **For pigs:** Treat for roundworms every 6 months. In addition, treat pregnant sows 5-10 days before giving birth (e.g. before putting her in a farrowing crate) and baby pigs at weaning and 4 weeks after weaning.

6. **For horses:** Treat for small and large roundworms every 6 months or more frequently depending upon the severity of the parasite problem. Begin treating young horses by one month of age and every 3 months until they are 1-year-old.

7. **For chickens:** Treat for large and small roundworms as well as tapeworms, depending upon what you see in the intestines when killing chickens for meat. The most common worm is usually the large roundworm.

8. **For all animals** with **bloody diarrhea:** Treat for coccidia.

Note: If a reliable laboratory technician is available, it is best to do a fecal exam when an animal does not respond to treatment the first time.

When the Simple Approach Does Not Work:

If an animal suffering from internal parasites is treated correctly, at least some improvement in its condition should be apparent within a month of treatment. If there is no improvement, the AHA should consider the following possibilities:

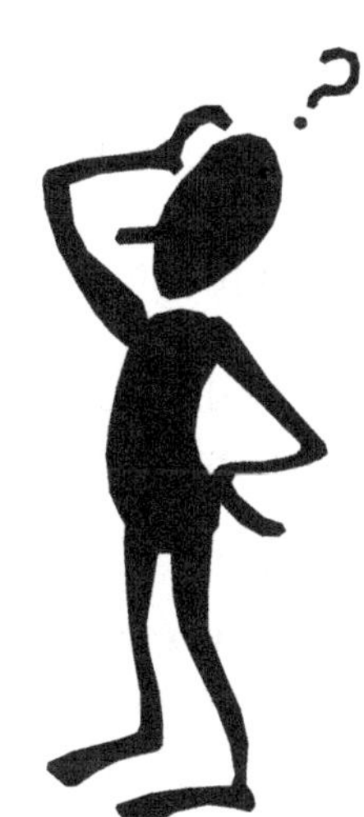

- Was the medicine spilled?
- Did the animal spit the medicine out before swallowing?
- Was the medicine mixed improperly?
- Was the medicine out-of-date?
- Were the animal's internal organs already permanently damaged by the parasite before the medicine was fed (i.e. how long had it been sick before it was treated?)?
- Does the medicine label indicate that it is effective against the parasite involved?
- Has the medicine been used for a long period of time in the area, making the parasite resistant to it?
- Is the animal getting enough food to eat?
- Does the animal have bad teeth, an infection or some other problem in its mouth?
- Is the animal suffering from some other condition besides internal parasites?

If there is no obvious reason why the medicine failed, then try one of the following approaches:

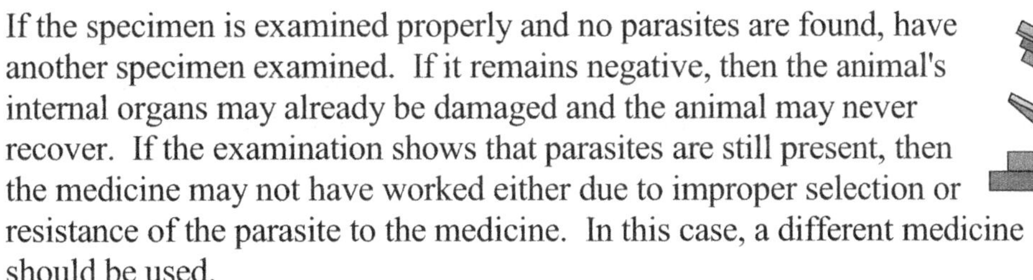

1. Take a specimen of fresh manure to the nearest laboratory to have it examined by a knowledgeable person using a microscope to identify any parasites or eggs.

    If the specimen is examined properly and no parasites are found, have another specimen examined. If it remains negative, then the animal's internal organs may already be damaged and the animal may never recover. If the examination shows that parasites are still present, then the medicine may not have worked either due to improper selection or resistance of the parasite to the medicine. In this case, a different medicine should be used.

2. If it is not possible to have a fecal specimen examined, then try using a different medicine and see if the animal responds. Be sure to follow the label instructions carefully. If the animal still does not respond, then its internal organs may be damaged.

10.0   Reproduction

10.1 INTRODUCTION

Reproduction is the process by which animals have babies (i.e. reproduce). The body system responsible for this process is called the **reproductive system**. AHAs need to understand the reproductive system for the following reasons:

1. Most livestock producers cannot afford to keep animals that do not reproduce or give milk.

2. Many different medicines and treatments affect the reproductive system. If used improperly, these medicines may endanger the livestock or their owners.

3. Offspring have the combined qualities, both the good and bad, of their parents. **Genetic improvement** involves careful selection of breeding animals to improve their offspring, and is dependent on understanding the reproductive system.

10.2 THE START OF A NEW LIFE

A variety of *hormones* control the process of reproduction. A hormone is a chemical substance produced naturally by the body. Hormones travel in the blood to parts of the body where they cause a certain action. In male animals, the testicles produce these hormones. In female animals, the uterus and ovaries produce these hormones.

10.2.1 Hormones in Females

Estrogen
This is the female hormone associated with heat or "estrus" (the period when the female can become pregnant, if bred).   Estrogen causes the female animal to stand for the male so that mating can take place. Some medicines contain estrogen, and cause female animals to come into heat. These medicines can cause abortions (death of the baby before it is born) and they may also damage the ovaries.

Progesterone
The ovary produces this female hormone after the animal comes into heat. Progesterone helps maintain pregnancy.

Prostaglandin
This hormone can cause a female animal to come into heat about three days after injection. It is safer than estrogen, but usually more expensive. It causes pregnant animals to abort.

10.2.2 Hormones in Males

Testosterone

The testicles produce this hormone. It is responsible for the changes that occur in a male's body at maturity. For example, testosterone causes the following: the penis enlarges, male goats develop an 'odor', oxen develop their 'humps' and their muscles, male animals develop a desire to breed female animals, and sperm begin to mature in the testes. If a male animal is castrated, then the source of testosterone is removed and these changes do not occur.

Reproductive System of a Male Animal (Bull)

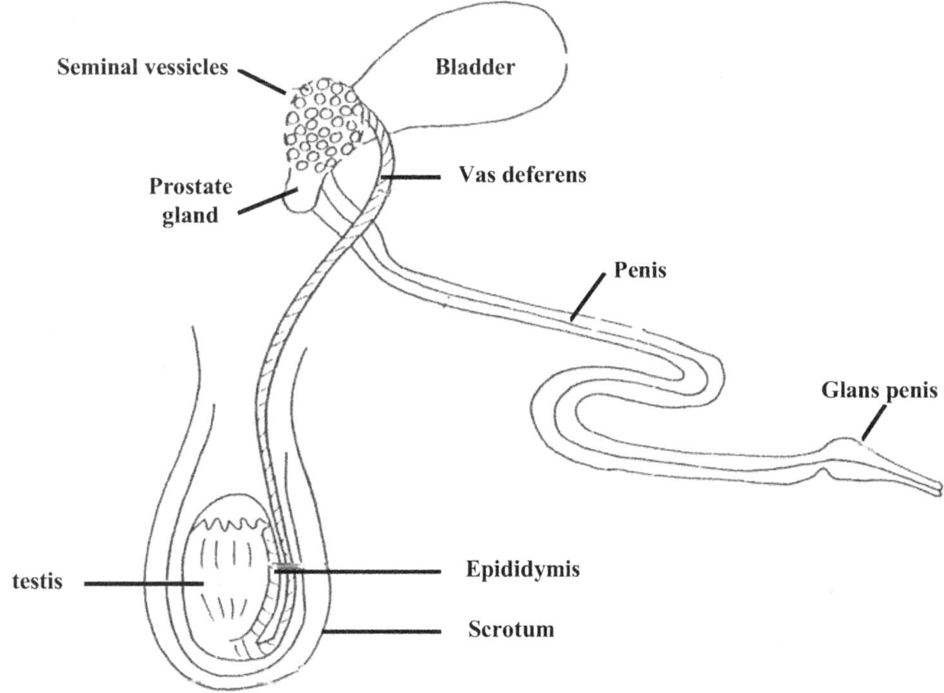

Reproductive System of a Female Animal (Cow)

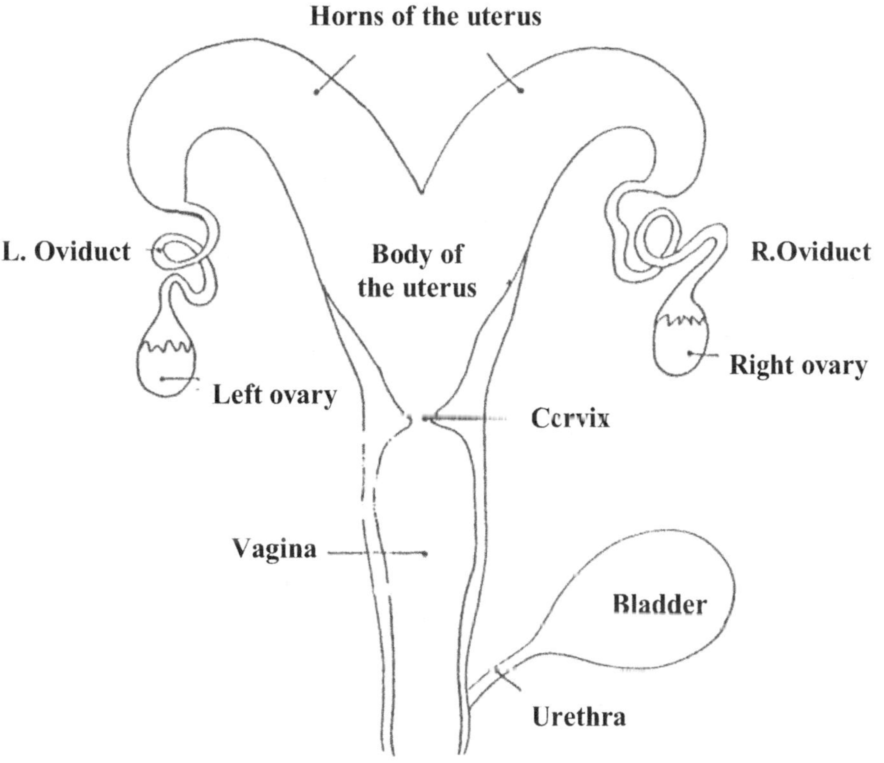

10.2.3 Terms of Reproduction

Sperm

Sperm are tiny cells present in the male's testicles at birth, which mature when the animal reaches puberty. The sperm move from the testicles into the epididymis, where they become mature. When a male animal sees or smells a female animal in heat, he usually wants to mate (or breed) with her. His penis becomes rigid and is inserted into the vagina of the female. At the moment of breeding, many sperm travel from the epididymis, through the vas deferens, and into the urethra. Certain glands (e.g. prostate and seminal vesicles) secrete fluid into the urethra to combine with the sperm, and form semen. The semen flows from the penis into the vagina of the female near the cervix. The sperm then move through the cervix, into the uterus, and up the oviduct.

'Heat' or 'Estrus'

From birth, females have many **eggs (ova)** in their ovaries. Following puberty, an egg (ovum) matures inside a fluid-filled bubble called a "follicle" on the surface of the ovary. The ovum produces the hormone "estrogen" which enters the bloodstream and reaches the brain, causing the female to come into **'heat'** or **'estrus'**, and to stand still while mating. Estrogen also causes ova to mature inside a follicle and prepares the uterus for pregnancy. In animals that usually have only one baby at a time, only one ovum develops during each estrus. In animals that have litters, such as dogs, many ova develop during each estrus.

Ovulation

Ovulation is when the follicle ruptures and releases the ovum. Ovulation usually occurs at the end of estrus. After ovulation, the ovum enters the oviduct.

Fertilization

If sperm are present in the oviduct at the time of ovulation, the egg might combine with a sperm cell. This process is called **"fertilization."** If the egg is fertilized, the mother becomes **"pregnant."** The new cell formed by fertilization contains everything needed to form a baby, which will have characteristics of both the mother and father. The new cell divides and multiplies millions of times throughout pregnancy to form a baby.

10.3 THE HEAT CYCLE (OR ESTRUS CYCLE)

After ovulation, the empty follicle on the ovary then develops some new tissue, called the **corpus luteum**, or **"CL."** The CL produces progesterone, which is used to maintain the pregnancy if fertilization occurs. If fertilization does not occur, the ovum in the oviduct and the CL on the ovary dissolve, and a new ovum forms on the ovary, to continue the cycle. The following table reviews this process using a cow's heat cycle as an example.

HEAT (ESTRUS) CYCLE OF A COW

The average heat cycle length of a cow is 21 days, consisting of the following four stages:

Stage I: 3-days in length
- Follicle develops.
- Ovum matures.
- Estrogen prepares the uterus for pregnancy.

Stage II: 1-day in length
- Female comes into "heat" (stands for the male).
- Follicle ruptures at the end of heat and the egg is released (ovulation).

Stage III: 3 - 5 days in length
- Corpus luteum or "CL" develops on the ovary.
- CL begins producing progesterone
- Sperm and egg meet in the oviduct (fertilization).

Stage IV: 13 days in length
- Uterus is ready to receive fertilized egg.
- If uterus does not receive the fertilized egg (if cow is not pregnant) then the CL dissolves and a new follicle develops to repeat the cycle.

If the animal becomes pregnant, the CL continues producing progesterone to maintain the pregnancy, and the cycle stops. If the animal does not become pregnant, the cycle continues.

Animals may vary in regards to their breeding cycles. For example, horses, sheep and goats come into heat during certain seasons of the year. They are called "**seasonal breeders.**" The rabbit, llama, and camel only ovulate after mating. That is, the act of mating makes ovulation occur. This is called "**induced ovulation.**" See Breeding Table for more information.

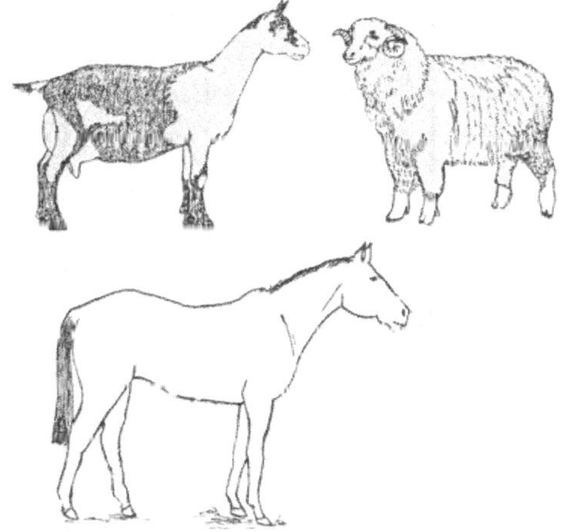

Seasonal breeders

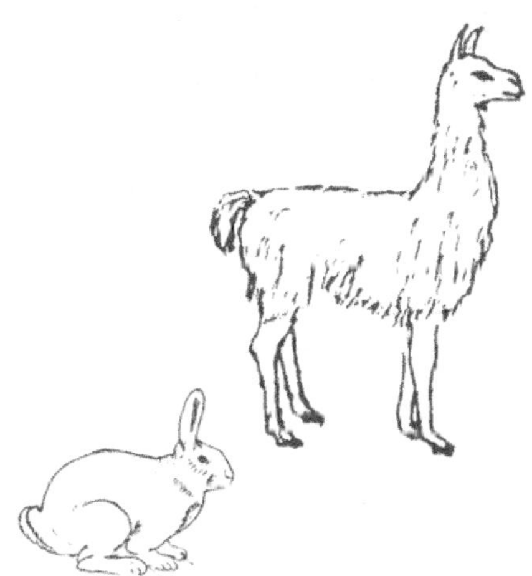

Induced ovulators

Breeding Table for Common Animals

Animal	Minimum Age to Breed - Puberty (Months)	Type of Heat Cycle / Length of Heat Cycle	Signs of Heat	Length of Heat Period	Best breeding time	Gestation Time (length of pregnancy)	First Heat After Giving Birth
Buffalo	18 - 24 months (20 average).	Somewhat Seasonal 18-24 days (22 average).	Swollen vulva. Crying out. Clear discharge.	1-2 days (1 day average).	----	300-325 days (310 ave.).	Varies. Seasonal breeders.
Cow	10-24 months (18 average).	All year 18-24 days (21 average).	Mounting by other females, Clear discharge.	4-24 hrs. (18 hrs. average).	From mid heat until 6 hrs. after end of heat.	280 days.	Varies Breed after 60 days.
Sheep	7 - 12 months (9 average).	Somewhat Seasonal 14-20 days (17 average).	Change in behavior.	1-2 days.	Not too important.	145-150 days.	Next season.
Goat	4 - 8 months (6 average).	Somewhat Seasonal 18-21 days (20 average).	Change in behavior.	2-3 days.	Daily when in heat.	145-155 days.	Next season.
Horse	10 - 24 months (18 average).	Seasonal Length of cycle varies (21 days average).	Frequent urination. Vulva opens and shuts.	3-8 days.	Last 2 days of heat. Or, breed every 2 days.	330-345 days.	4 - 14 days after giving birth.
Pig	4 - 9 months (7 average).	All year 16-24 days (21 average).	Swollen vulva. Stands with pressure on back.	2-3 days.	After first day of heat.	114 days.	4 - 10 days after weaning.
Rabbit	4 - 12 months (7 average).	All year.	No real heat period.	No real heat period.	Breed when vulva is pink and swollen.	30 days.	Almost immediately.
Dog	5 - 24 months.	2 times / year average.	Change in behavior.	1 week.	After day 2 of heat.	58-70 days.	A few months.
Cat	4 - 12 months (10 average).	Somewhat Seasonal 14 – 21 days.	Change in behavior.	4 days (if mated).	After day 2.	58-70 days.	4-6 weeks.
Llama	24-36 months.	All year 18-21 days induced ovulators.	Female is receptive to male during certain days of heat cycle, but no outward signs of heat.	Can be receptive to male during 10-12 days of heat cycle.	1-2 times daily when receptive.	330-360 (342 ave.).	-----

Note: The minimum age at breeding varies, depending on the breed and quality of nutrition. The length of pregnancy may also vary according to breed.

10.4 NORMAL PREGNANCY

The process of pregnancy is similar in most animals. The following details are true for most types of livestock - except poultry.

The fertilized egg in the oviduct moves to the uterus where it continues to grow. The fertilized egg is called an "embryo" and, as it begins to take shape, a "fetus." The length of time from fertilization until the baby is born is called the "**gestation period.**" The length of the gestation period varies by animals. (See Breeding Table on previous page).

Throughout pregnancy, the cervix is closed tightly with a plug of thick mucus that prevents germs from entering the uterus and infecting the baby. The baby is also surrounded by a fluid (called "amniotic fluid") that forms a cushion and protects the baby from injury. The baby is fed by the nutrients that pass from the mother's blood, through the placenta and umbilicus, and into the baby's blood.

10.4.1 Care of the Pregnant Mother

Protection

The pregnant mother should not be stressed during pregnancy. Therefore, she may need a shelter or pen to protect her from excessive heat, sun, wind, cold, or fighting with other animals. Try to make the mother gentle and accustomed to humans, so she will not be stressed during delivery and milking, when humans may need to assist her. Do not let a mother become too thin or too fat.

Fresh feed and water

A pregnant mother should have clean drinking water available at all times. She should also have a "complete feed" (See the nutrition chapter regarding the special needs of pregnant mothers). Use local feeds and give the mother as much **variety** as possible, especially green feed. This will minimize the risk that the diet is missing some essential vitamin or mineral.

Never depend on only one type of feed! In some places it is common practice to give a pregnant mother only one type of feed and nothing else. This practice should be avoided as it often leads to nutrient deficiencies.

10.5 NORMAL DELIVERY OF THE BABY (OR BABIES)

The weeks before delivery

During the last few weeks before delivery, the udder enlarges. During the last few days before delivery, the level of progesterone in the blood decreases and the estrogen level increases. This causes the muscles around the vulva to relax. Just before delivery, the mother may act differently. She may be nervous, lie down and get up many times, or look at her side as if it hurts. Her udder may become very large and may even appear swollen. Horses may have a bead of waxy substance at the tip of their teats during the last 24 hours before delivery.

Preparing for the delivery

When these signs are seen, the delivery place should be prepared. The delivery place should be quiet, clean, dry, and warm - but not hot. There should be enough space for the mother to lie down comfortably. The delivery place should be nearby the animal keeper so that the mother can be monitored. The mother's hair and udder should be clean, and she should be untied so that she can lie down comfortably.

When labor begins

When labor begins, the hormone called **oxytocin**[2] begins contracting the uterus and usually the mother begins pushing. Both activities help to open (dilate) the cervix so that the baby (or babies) can be born. During labor, the fluid-filled sack around the baby breaks and fluid rushes out, making the birth canal slippery.

Time Required: The cervix should open within an hour of the time the mother begins pushing. The baby cannot come out until *after* the cervix opens. Labor usually lasts 2 to 3 hours from the time the mother begins to push until the baby is born. If labor lasts more than 8 hours and someone does not intervene, the baby (or babies) may die. If labor lasts more than 24 hours, the mother may die also. If labor continues beyond 48 hours and the mother does not die, the dead baby (or babies) will begin to bloat. At this point, delivery will be very difficult and the uterus may tear, in which case, the mother will probably die.

Position:

In animals that have only one baby at a time (such as cows, buffalo, sheep, goats, horses, yaks, llamas, and camels), the mother can normally deliver a baby only if it is in one of following two positions:

1. With the 2 front feet and the head coming out at the same time; or

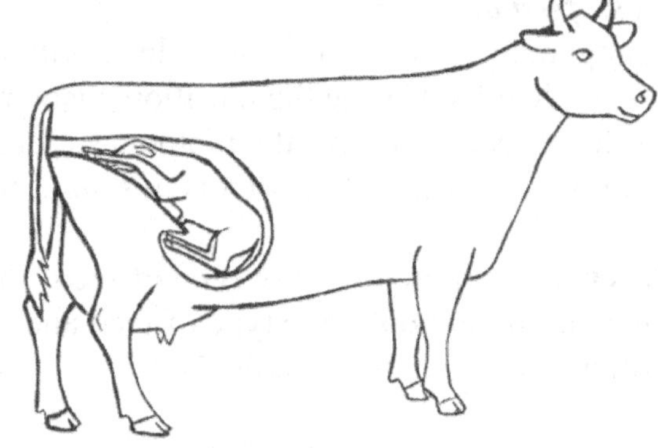

2. With the 2 hind feet and the tail coming out at the same time.

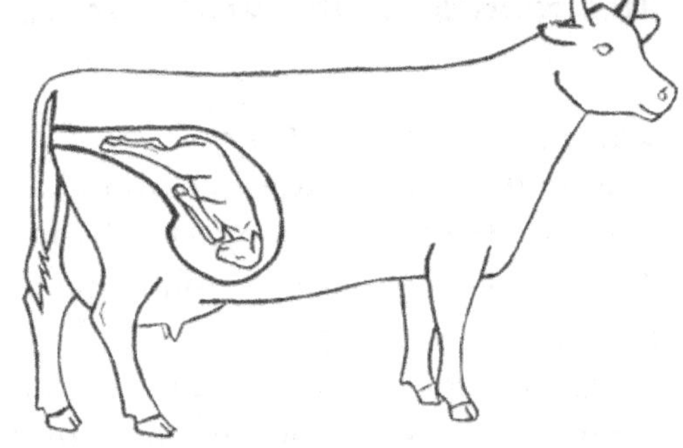

---

2 Oxytocin has two functions. Firstly it helps the uterus to contract. Secondly it also helps in the process of "milk letdown". See page 263.

If the baby is not in one of these two positions, the AHA must reposition it.
In animals that have a number of babies at one time (such as pigs, rabbits, dogs and cats),
the position of the baby's head, legs and tail is not as critical. However, if the baby is turned
sideways in the uterus, the AHA must reposition it. In addition, the uterus must squeeze
(contract) to push the babies towards the cervix. If the uterus does not contract properly, the
birth of the babies may be delayed and oxytocin may be needed to make the uterus contract.
In pigs, if there is a delay between births of more than 30-60 minutes, the AHA should rub the
mother's teats (causing a natural release of oxytocin into the mother pig's body), or give her
an injection of oxytocin. See page 213.

10.6 CARE OF THE NEWBORN

Observe that the baby breathes, is warm and dry and, within the first 6 hours, drinks colostrum.
However, do not interfere with the mother or baby unless necessary. If you need to interfere,
be very careful of the mother who may aggressively protect her baby.

1. **Breathing:** Make sure that the baby is breathing properly. It may be necessary to clean the
    fluid out of its nose and mouth with your hand, or to hold the baby upside down for several
    seconds so that the fluid can drip out. It may also be necessary to push on or squeeze the
    baby's chest to stimulate breathing.

2. **Warm and dry:** If the mother does not lick the baby clean and dry, the AHA can dry the
    baby with some clean grass or a clean cloth. If possible, do not move the baby, unless it is
    in a cold or wet place.

Colostrum - the first milk

It is critical that all babies receive colostrum within six hours of birth. Colostrum is critical
for the baby because:
- it provides antibodies to protect the baby from disease
- its laxative effect helps the baby pass its first feces called "meconium"
- it is very nutritious

An important note: Colostrum must be fed *within 6 hours of birth* to absorb the antibodies.
If the baby receives colostrum late, it cannot properly absorb the antibodies.

Allowing the baby to suck at once also helps the mother because the sucking stimulates a
release of oxytocin in the mother's body which:
- contracts the uterus and pushes out the placenta and birth fluids
- stimulates milk let down

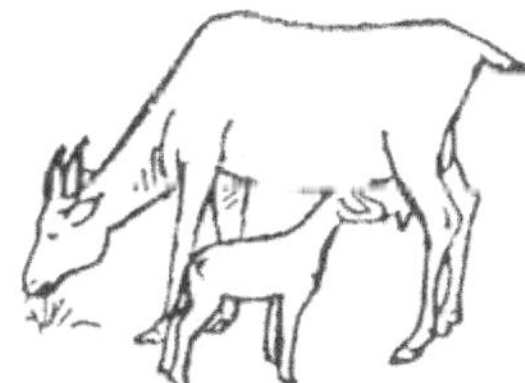 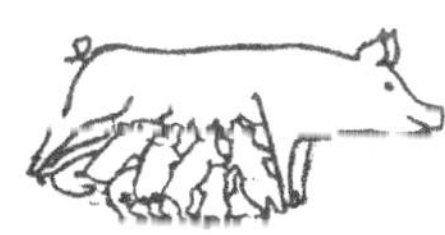 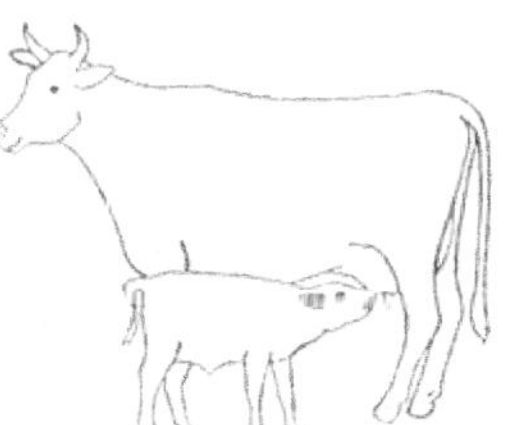 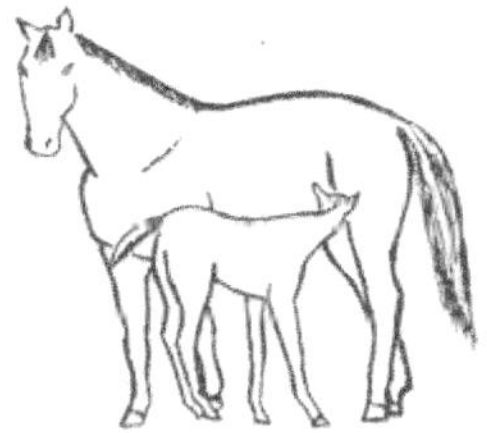

Colostrum must be fed within 6 hours of birth. If not, the baby may get sick.

10.7 DISEASE CONDITIONS ASSOCIATED WITH REPRODUCTIVE SYSTEM

10.7.1 Difficult Births (Dystocias)

A difficult birth is called a "dystocia." There are many causes of a dystocia:

- the mother may be weak and unable to push
- the cervix may not open
- the baby may not be in the correct position
- the baby may be dead and possibly bloated
- the baby may be deformed
- the baby may be too big for the mother (sometimes a problem when a small cow is bred to a big bull)

Equipment Needed for Delivery of Babies

1. Clean water and soap. Disinfectant soap is best, but regular soap also works.
2. Three small ropes about 1.3 meters in length. Nylon ropes are easiest to clean.
3. Plastic sleeves, if possible.

    Note: Women often make excellent birth assistants, especially for smaller animals like pigs, sheep and goats. Their hands are smaller to assist the delivery when necessary, and they tend to take good care of newborn babies.

How to Handle a Dystocia

Step 1. Take a history: Take a history and be sure to ask the following questions:

1. When (what date) is the mother supposed to have her baby? Is it early or late?
2. For how many hours has the mother been trying to deliver the baby?
3. Has someone already put their hand inside the mother to help her?

If the mother has already been trying to have her baby for several days, then the baby is probably already dead and the mother may also die. You must warn the owner before you begin to work or you may be blamed for the death. Also, if someone has already tried to pull the baby out, they may have already injured the uterus inside.

Step 2. Conduct an external examination:
Examine the animal. In particular, note whether she is thin and weak (and so may not be able to push the baby out), and whether there is placenta or smelly fluid coming out of the vulva.

How to handle a dystocia
1. Take a history
2. Conduct an external exam
3. Conduct an internal exam

4. Correct the problem & deliver the baby
    -open cervix, correct position
    -open cervix, incorrect position
    -closed cervix
    -twisted uterus
    -dead and bloated baby

5. Treat for any other conditions found in the baby or mother

Step 3. Conduct an internal examination:
If the animal can move, put her in a clean, dry place. If it is a cow, buffalo, or horse, have someone hold the tail out of the way (or tie it up). Wash around the mother's vulva thoroughly with soap and water. Wash your arm up to the shoulder with soap and water. **If you have sores on your arm, or if the calf is already dead, wear a plastic glove to protect yourself from infections like Brucellosis.** After washing, apply soap again to your arm (or the plastic sleeve) to make your arm slippery. Then gently insert your hand and arm into the vulva and on into the vagina (birth canal).

Have someone hold the animal's tail
or tie it to the side

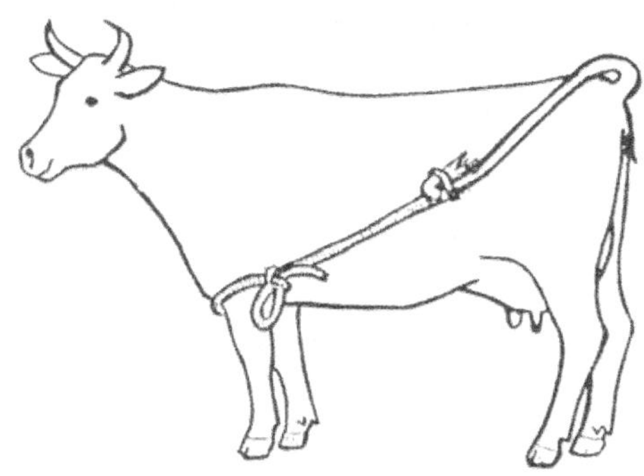

How to tie a tail

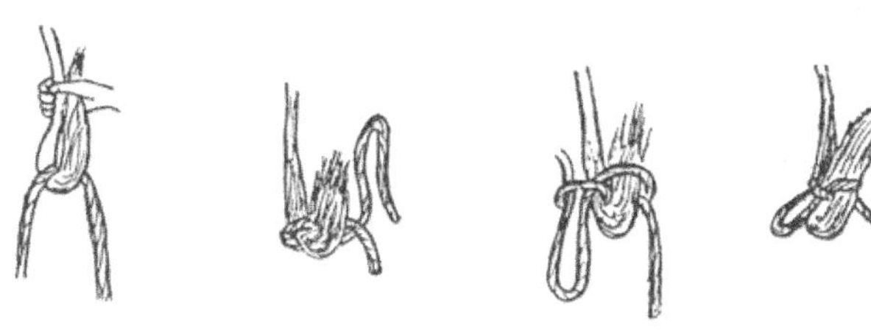

Wash the animal's vulva
and surrounding area

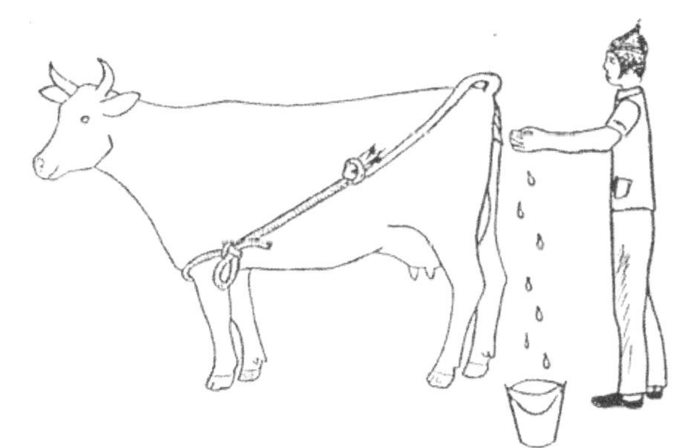

Wash your own hands and arm.
Put on a plastic sleeve if available

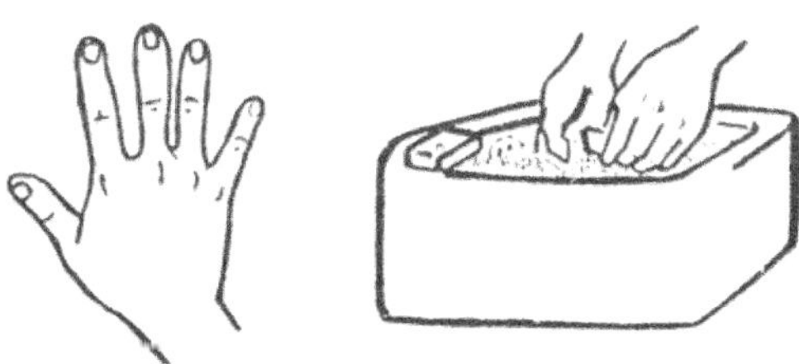

Insert your hand and arm
gently into the animal

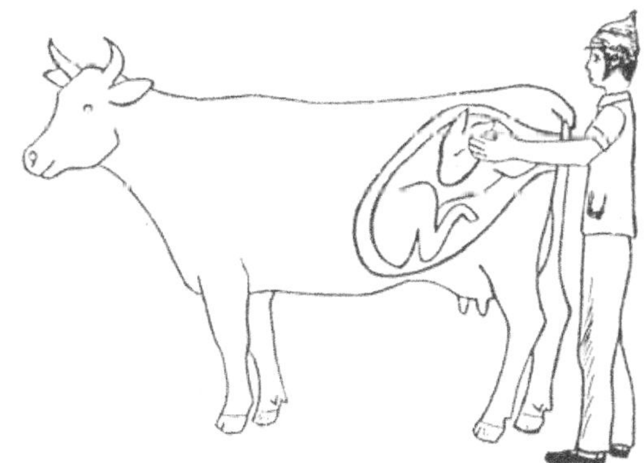

Once your hand is inside the vagina, determine the following:

- Is the cervix closed?
- Is the baby in a bad position?
- Is the baby too large to pass easily through the birth canal?

How to determine whether the cervix is open

Once your hand is in the vagina, if you can touch the baby with your hands, then the cervix is open. If you cannot touch the baby, then the cervix is still closed.

How to determine whether the position is correct

If you can feel the legs, determine whether they are front or back legs. To do this, first find the hoof and then feel up the leg. If the first 2 joints on the leg bend the same way, then it is a front leg. If the first 2 joints on the leg bend the opposite way, then it is a back leg. If you have identified two front legs, then the head should be positioned between them, otherwise the baby is not correctly positioned. Similarly, if you have identified two back legs, and you cannot find a tail, then the baby is incorrectly positioned.

Correct / Normal Positions for Delivery

Most babies are born with the head and two front legs coming first. However, a baby can also be born if both back legs and the tail come at the same time.

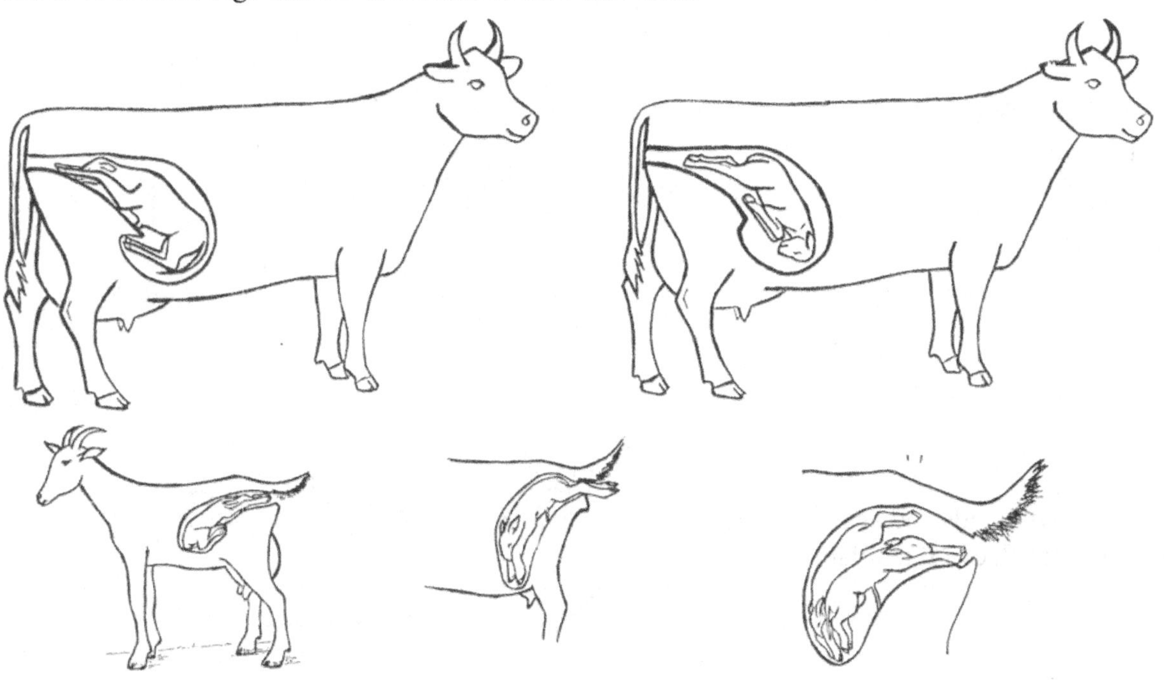

If the baby is not in one of these positions, it is the job of the AHA to move the baby into one of these positions so that it can be delivered.

Problem 1. The cervix is open and the position is correct, but the mother cannot deliver

This problem may occur when the baby is too big for the mother's birth canal, the mother is unable to push properly, the slippery fluids have dried out or a combination of these factors.

Treatment:

- Make sure that the baby is slippery (apply soap if necessary).
- Attach ropes to the legs (with a slip knot).
- Pull on the ropes (particularly as the mother pushes) until the baby is born.

Problem 2. The cervix is open but position is incorrect
The following diagrams show the most common positions that are incorrect.

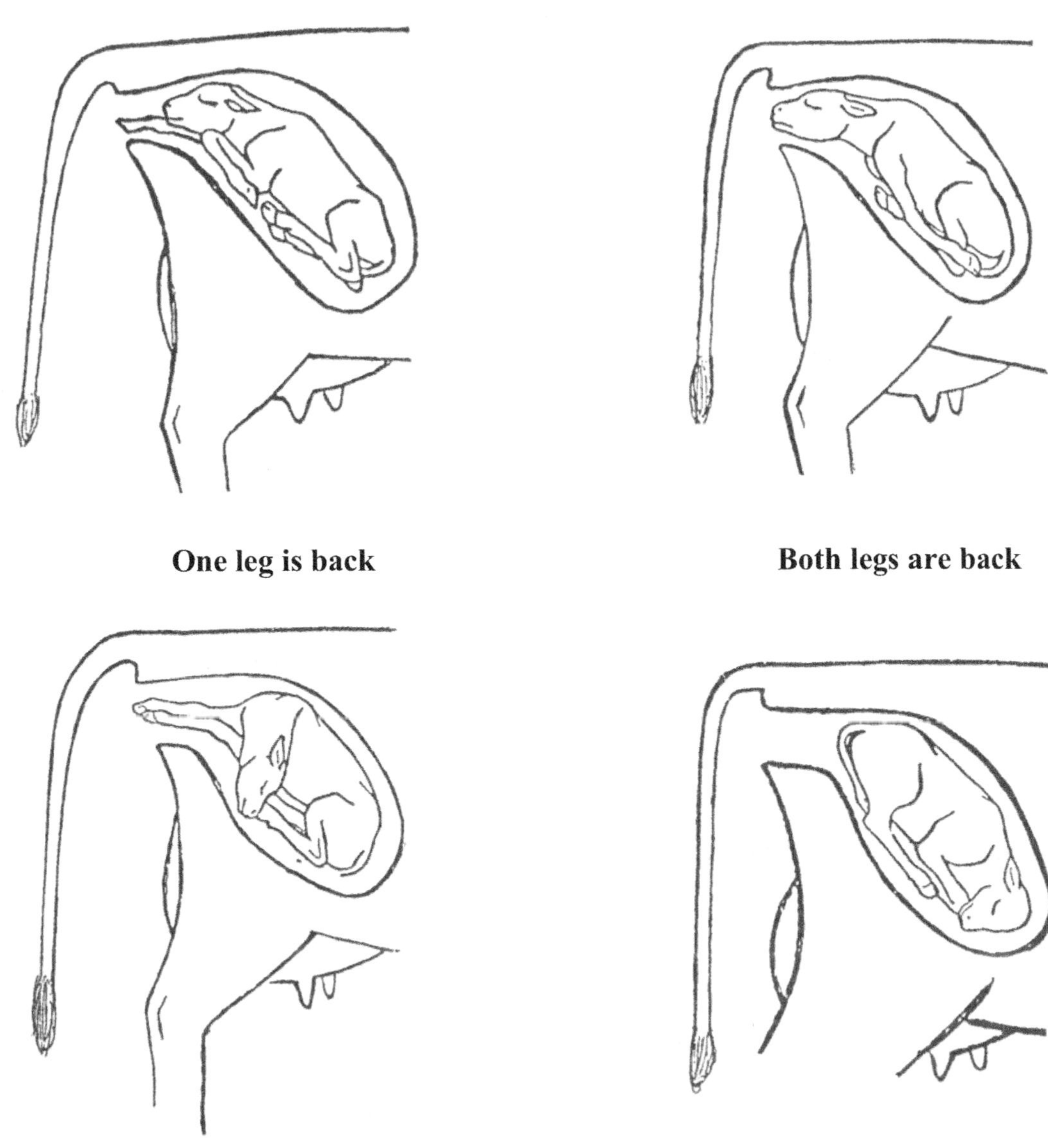

<table>
<tr><td align="center">One leg is back</td><td align="center">Both legs are back</td></tr>
<tr><td align="center">The head is back</td><td align="center">Breech position</td></tr>
</table>

Treatment: Before correcting the problem in the following examples, you must first gently push the baby farther into the uterus to gain more space for maneuvering. **Caution:** To avoid tearing the uterus when maneuvering the baby, only push the baby back into the uterus when the mother is *not* pushing, and cup your hand around the edge of the hoof when repositioning a leg. Once the baby is delivered, antibiotics should be given to the mother to prevent uterine infection.

Caution: Never try to pull baby out of its mother before the baby is correctly positioned. Otherwise, you may kill both the baby and mother! Even if the baby is in the correct position, do not pull too hard. If two strong men cannot pull a baby cow or buffalo out, then stop and re-check that the baby is in the correct position.

Example 1. The head and only one front leg are forward

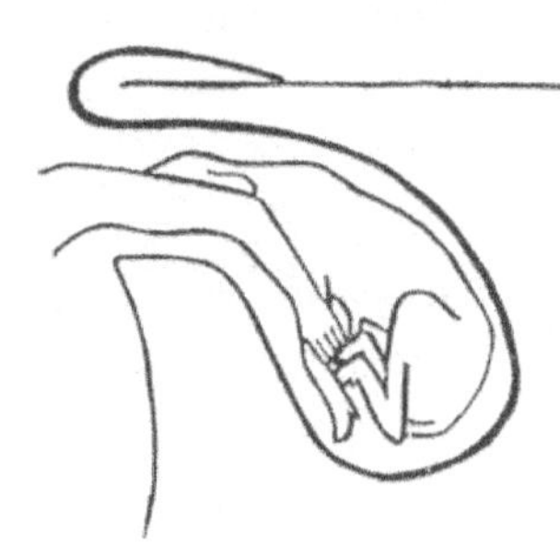

- Attach a rope to the front leg that is forward, but do not pull on it.
- Slide your hand down the opposite side of the animal and find the leg that is back.
- Cupping your hands around the hoof edges to avoid tearing the uterus, carefully move the leg into the correct position.
- Once in the correct position, pull the baby out.

Example 2. The head only is forward, and both front legs are back

- Slide your hand down each side of the baby and grab the legs.
- Cupping your hands around the hoof edges to avoid tearing the uterus, carefully move each leg into the correct position.
- Once in the correct position, pull the baby out. Attach ropes to the front legs if necessary.

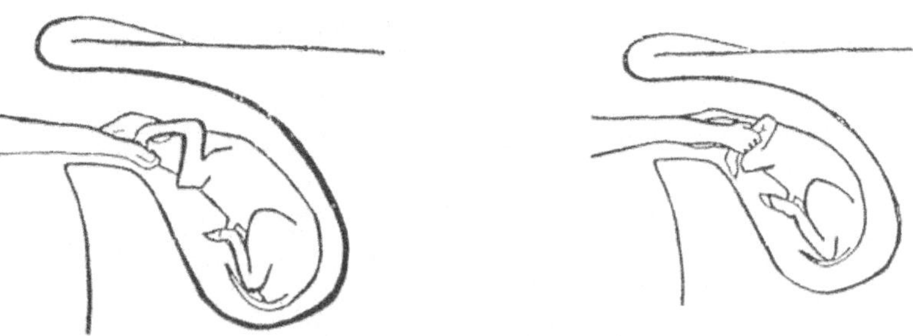

Similar example in sheep and goats

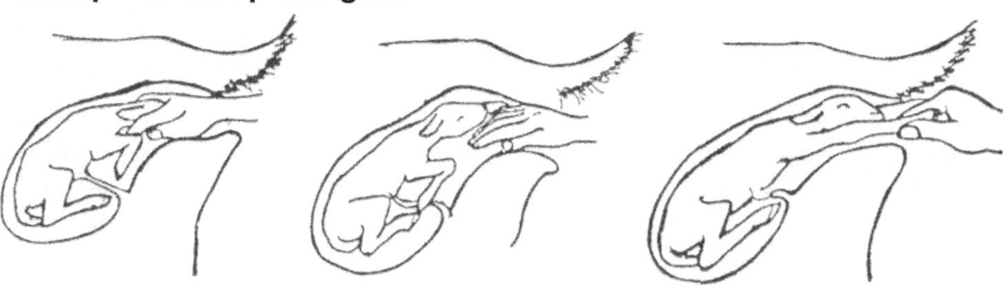

Example 3. Front legs only are forward and the head is turned back.

This position is one of the most difficult to correct. Sometimes, the neck may even be twisted so that the head may be turned up, down, or to the side.

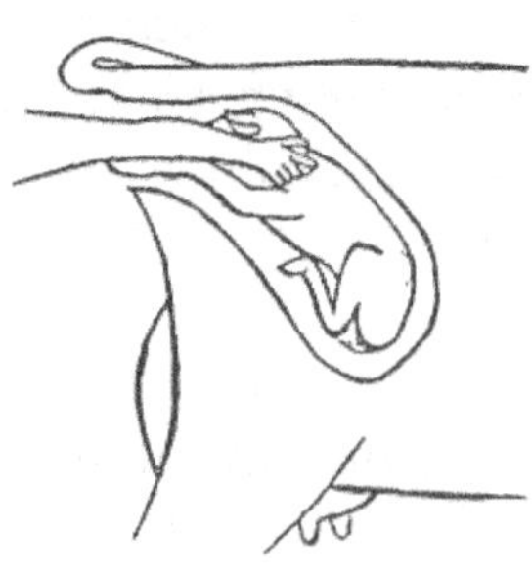

- Check that the legs you feel are truly front legs.
- Attach ropes to the front legs but do not pull on the ropes.
- Search for the head
- After finding the head, grab the mouth, eyes sockets or ears and gently pull into the correct position. It may be necessary to untwist the neck first. **Caution:** Cup your hands around the baby's teeth when pulling the head forward to avoid tearing the uterus with the baby's teeth.
- Once in the correct position, pull on the ropes to pull the baby out

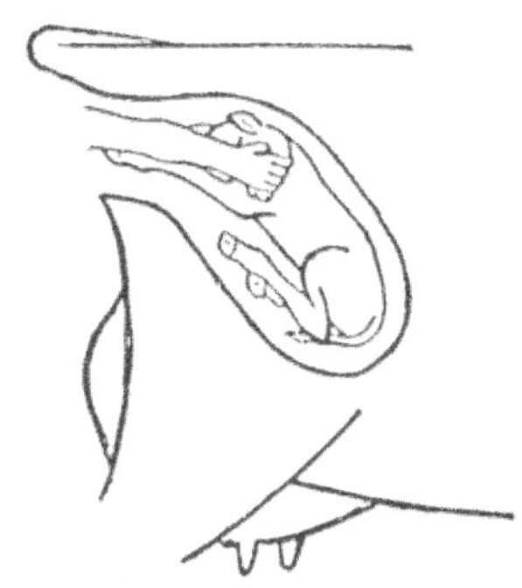

Note: Sometimes the head returns to its original position when you begin to pull. If this occurs, attach a rope to the head and apply tension to the rope to keep the head forward while pulling the baby out. There are two ways to do this that will not injure the baby:
- Tie the rope, in a slip knot, to the bottom jaw only
- Tie the rope in a slip knot under the chin so that, as the baby's head comes out, the knot can be loosened to allow the baby to breathe.

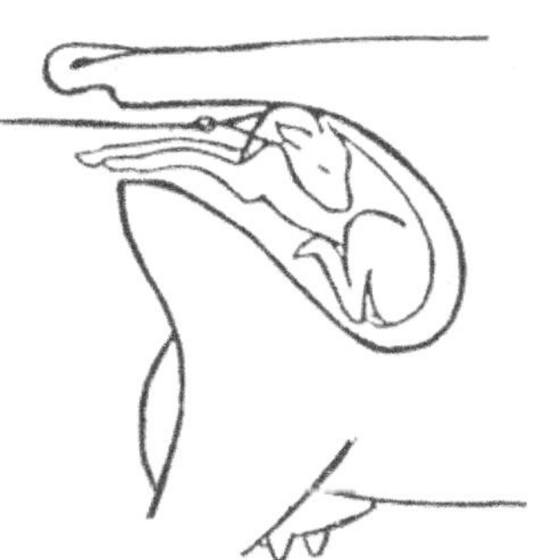

Example 4. The tail only is present without the back legs (Breech position)

Sometimes only the tail is found and both legs are tucked up under the body. This position can be difficult because the baby can be stuck tightly in the birth canal.
- Put your hand on the rump of the baby and gently push it back in the birth canal so that you have room to correct the position of the back legs. Do this carefully, when the mother is not pushing.
- Reach inside and find the hock joint (or knee) on one back leg.
- Pull this knee up into a bent position.
- Put your hand between the legs and push the knee to the outside. Pull the hoof toward the middle (or inside) and toward yourself at the same time. **Caution:** If you pull the hoof to the outside, you may tear the uterus or break the leg - or both!
- Do the same for the other leg until both back legs and tail are in the birth canal.
- Pull on the legs until the baby comes out. It may be necessary to attach ropes to the legs.

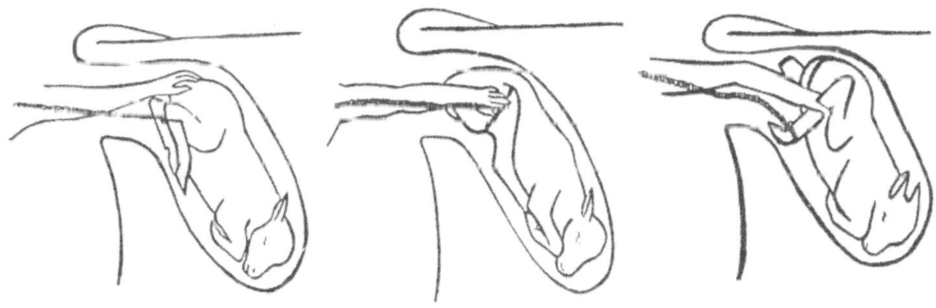

Problem 3. The cervix is closed

The cervix may be closed for the following reasons:
- It is too soon to give birth.
- The cervix was already opened, the mother was unable to deliver the baby, and the cervix then closed (in which case, there is usually a bad odor and discharge from the mother's vulva).
- The mother is too weak to push properly (i.e. pushing helps open the cervix).

Treatment: Re-examine in 1-2 hours to determine whether the mother is beginning to dilate

If the cervix begins to open (dilate):
- Insert your hand into the cervix and apply steady pressure by opening your hand to dilate the cervix completely. This may also stimulate the mother to push.
- If the cervix opens by this technique, then apply soap around the baby to make it slippery and pull the baby out. You may need to reposition the baby or attach ropes to pull the baby out.
- Give oxytocin to stimulate contractions.

If the cervix does not begin to open:
- Insert antibiotics through the cervix (if possible),
- Give an injection of antibiotics.
- Give estrogen (as an injection or tablets).
- Wait for the cervix to open over the following week.
- Re-examine the mother every 2 days to see if she has dilated, at which time remove dead baby, and treat the mother for a retained placenta.

Problem 4. The uterus is twisted so that it is difficult to put your hand in.

When the uterus itself is twisted, the birth canal cannot open properly. This is called a "uterine torsion" (twisted uterus) and happens most commonly in buffalo and cows, and less commonly in smaller animals.

Signs
- The animal is restless, uncomfortable and straining.

- As always, wash your hands and arms with soap. 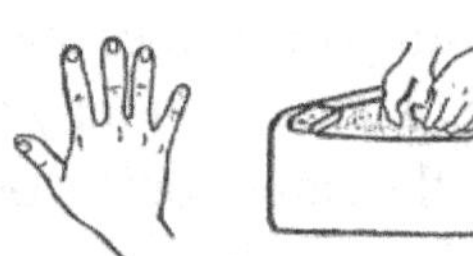

- When you insert your hand into the vagina, it seems narrow and twisted. You may or may not be able to feel the baby.

Treatment

- If the cervix is open enough to put your arm in, try to untwist the uterus by grasping the baby and turning it over inside the uterus. This is often difficult to do unless you are very strong. If this does not work, then do the following:

    - Ask 4-5 strong men to help you.

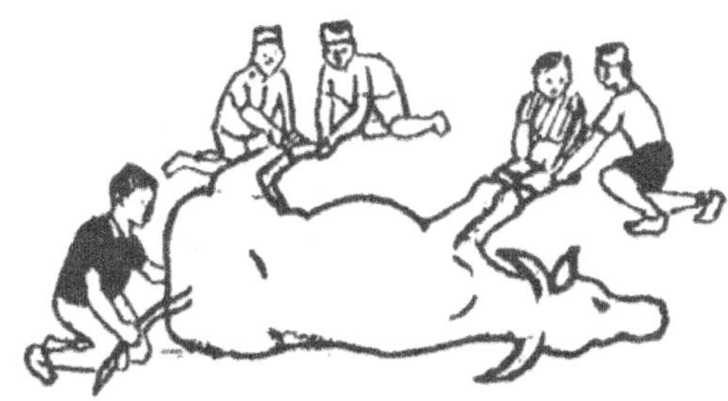

    - Find a clean, dry, level place to make the mother lie down. If the uterus seems twisted to the right (i.e. clockwise), then gently cast the mother onto her right side. If the uterus seems twisted to the left (i.e. counter-clockwise), then gently cast the mother onto her left side.

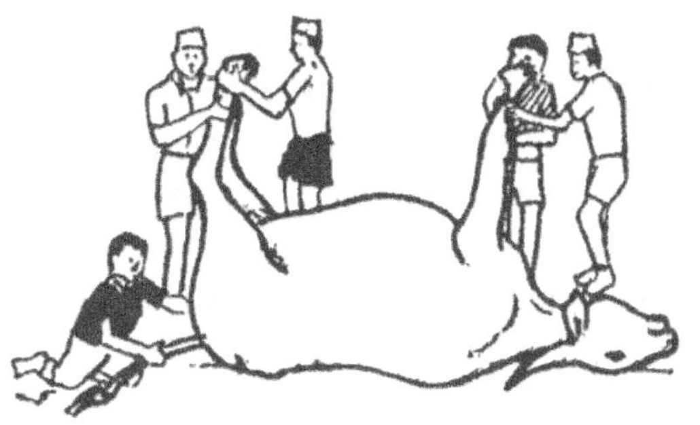

    - Try to insert your hands gently through the twisted part of the birth canal and grip some part of the baby. While gripping the baby, roll the mother onto her back and then to her other side.

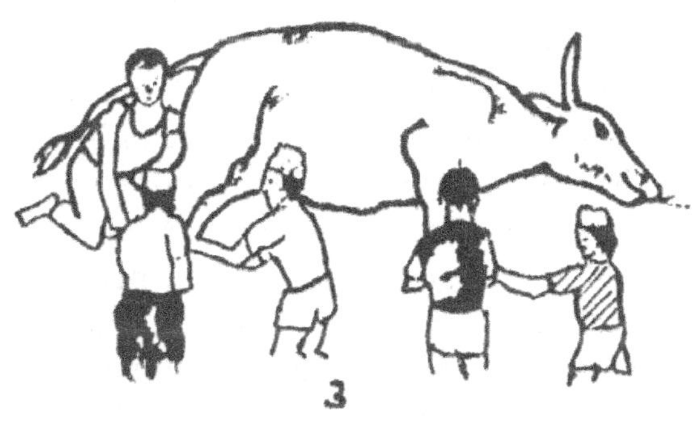

    - If it is impossible to grip the baby, then place a plank across the mother's abdomen (with one end of the plank on the ground) and roll the mother to her other side while applying pressure to the abdomen with the plank. The plank holds the baby in place while turning the mother, thereby untwisting the uterus.

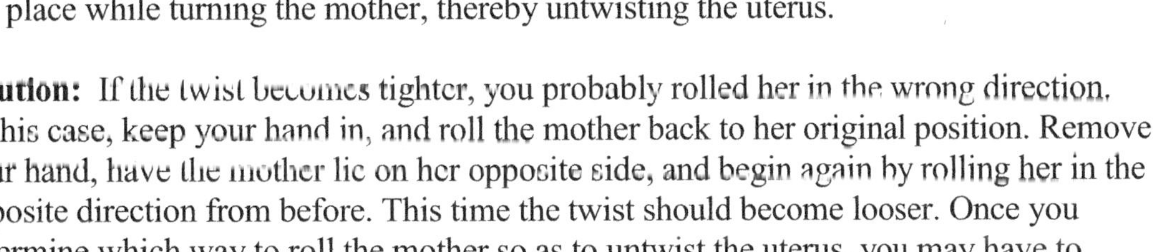

Caution: If the twist becomes tighter, you probably rolled her in the wrong direction. In this case, keep your hand in, and roll the mother back to her original position. Remove your hand, have the mother lie on her opposite side, and begin again by rolling her in the opposite direction from before. This time the twist should become looser. Once you determine which way to roll the mother so as to untwist the uterus, you may have to repeat the procedure 4 or 5 times until the uterus is completely untwisted.

- After the uterus is untwisted and the vagina is straight, the cervix may be somewhat closed. In this case, try to open it with your fingers or wait 1-2 hours for it to open naturally.
- Once the cervix is open, make sure the baby is in the right position, or reposition it.
- Gently pull the baby out.

Problem 5. The baby is dead and bloated inside the mother

This problem causes the uterus to be very weak so that it may easily tear.

Treatment:

- Wash your hand and arm and put on a plastic sleeve. Apply soap to make the sleeve slippery.
- Check to see if the uterus is already torn. If so, inform the owner, so that you are not blamed for a pre-existing condition. You may want to advise the owner to forego treatment (and slaughter the animal). If the owner wants to try saving the mother, warn the owner before you begin to work of the high risk that the uterus may tear during treatment.
- Check the position of the baby. If incorrectly positioned, try to correct it and pull the baby out without tearing the uterus.
- If the baby is bloated, carefully try to split the skin of the baby with a sharp knife so that the air comes out. Then try to pull out the intestines, heart, lungs, bones, etc. Sometimes it all comes out in pieces. **Caution:** Insert the knife cupped in your hand to avoid cutting uterus.
- If you still cannot deliver the baby, you may need to do a fetotomy (see next section) which is a technique of cutting up the dead baby while it is still inside the mother and removing the pieces.
- Once the baby is removed, flush out the uterus and treat the mother for a retained placenta.

Embryotomy (Fetotomy)

Sometimes you cannot remove a dead baby without first cutting it into pieces. There is a special instrument for this purpose called an embryotome or fetotome. Its purpose is to cut the dead baby into pieces without injuring the mother. It looks like a metal pipe, (or two metal pipes welded together). Fetotomes are not easy to use nor is there one method that works in all situations.

A special wire (embryotomy wire or horn cutting wire) is put through the pipes of the fetotome. The pipes protect the uterus from the wire. The exposed loop wire that comes out of the other end of the fetotome is then looped around the part you want to cut off (e.g. the head). A handle is placed on each end of the wire. As one person holds the fetotome so that pipe ends are tightly against the calf, another person pulls back and forth on the handles, in a sawing action, so that the exposed loop of wire cuts through the calf without damaging the mother's uterus. If you do not have a fetotome, use a single pipe with smooth edges and put the two ends of the wire next to each other in the pipe to accomplish the same thing.

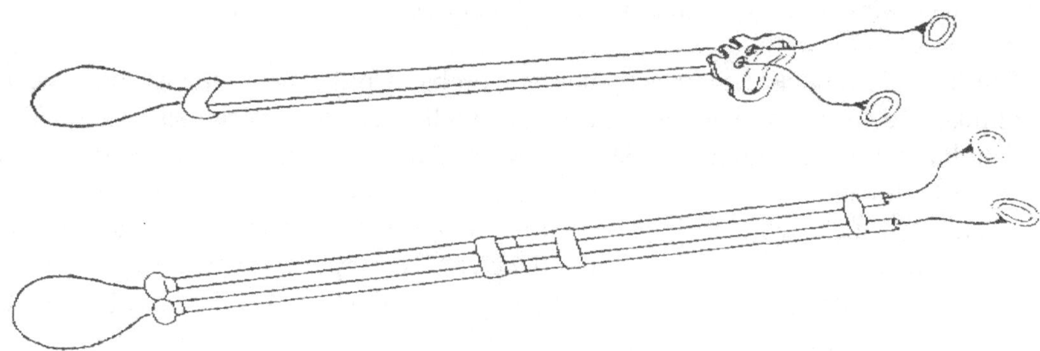

Fetotome Used for Cutting Up Dead Babies Inside the Uterus

10.7.2 Animals That Cannot Stand Up (Downer Animal)

Sometimes an animal cannot stand up, particularly after a long difficult delivery. This can happen due to fatigue, damaged muscles or nerves, or lack of calcium, called "milk fever." See page 270.

Treatment: If the animal has "milk fever," treat it accordingly. If the down animal becomes alert and able to eat, then there is a good chance it will recover. If the animal cannot lift its head or eat (even after treating it for milk fever), it probably will not recover; and the owner should consider killing it for meat.

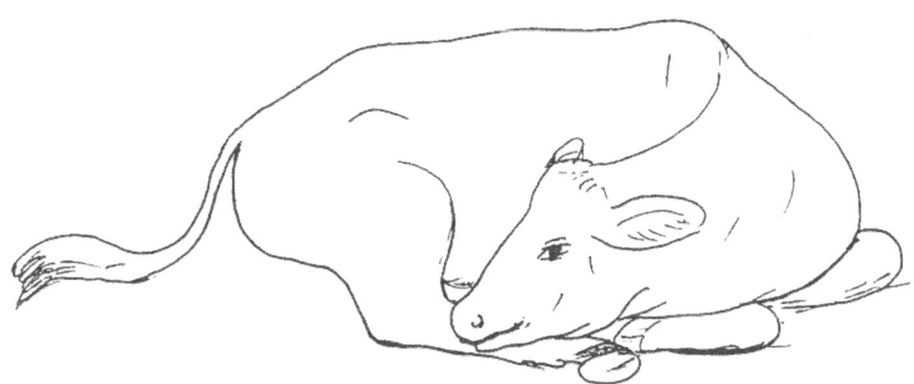

The general treatment for any down animal is the following:
1. Protect the animal from harsh weather (e.g. heat, sun, cold, wind, rain) and other animals
2. Put the animal on soft, clean, dry bedding on level ground. Soft bedding is particularly important for a large animal to avoid serious muscle damage and skin sores from the weight of its own body.
3. Reposition the animal to its other side at least four times daily to avoid muscle damage and skin sores.
4. Give the animal fresh food and water at least four times daily.
5. Use fly powder, if necessary, to keep the animal from being bothered by flies, maggots and screw worm. See page 316.
6. If possible, gather several people together to help lift the animal at least once daily. Do not let the animal try to walk unless the area is level, safe and not slippery; otherwise the animal may fall and injure itself.

If after two weeks there is no sign of improvement, the owner should consider killing it for meat.

10.7.3 Problems of the Uterus & Birth Canal

(Prolapsed Vagina, Prolapsed Uterus, Discharge from the Vulva, Retained Placenta, Metritis)

10.7.3.1 Prolapsed Vagina

This is the term used when the vagina comes outside of the vulva. It is seen as a red ball of tissue that is pushed out of the vulva, and the mother is often pushing and straining, like she is trying to deliver. It usually happens during the last few months of gestation when the baby is big; as the mother lies down, the pressure of the large baby causes the vagina to prolapse.

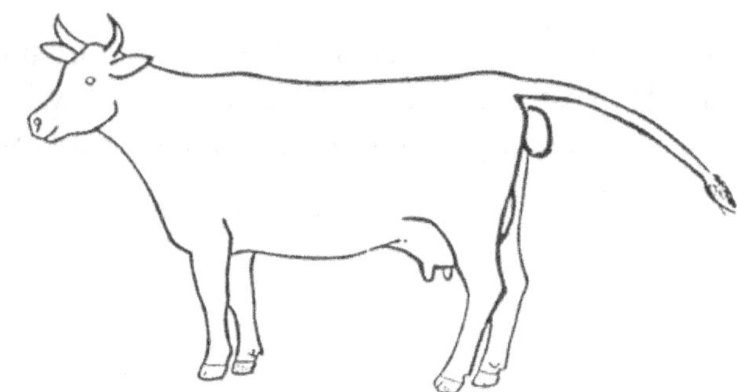

Treatment

- Position the mother so that her head is slightly downhill. If necessary, dig a shallow hole (about 1-foot-deep) where her front feet are.
- With the animal standing up and her head downhill, the red ball of tissue should be thoroughly washed and made slippery with soap. (If there are any wounds or maggots, they must be treated.)
- Slowly push the prolapsed vagina back inside the vulva.
- After the vagina is pushed back inside, gently hold it in place for at least 5-10 minutes or the mother will push it out again. It can be held inside by holding the vulva shut with your hand from the outside.
- After the mother stops straining, release your hand and observe the animal closely for a half hour or so. Prevent her from laying down for the next few hours or she will push it out again.
- Advise the farmer to feed the mother in small amounts many times each day. This will make her rumen take up less space in the belly.
- If the mother starts straining again, watch her and do not let her lay down for several hours.
- If the mother keeps straining and pushing the vagina out, you may have to hold it in with ropes, or with sutures. (See diagrams for prolapsed uterus). However, this is dangerous because you will need to remove the ropes immediately when the mother starts to deliver her baby.

10.7.3.2 Prolapsed Uterus

This is the term used when the uterus turns inside-out and comes out of the vagina. This usually occurs within hours after giving birth. In high producing dairy cows it is often associated with milk fever (lack of calcium). It is also seen fairly frequently in buffalo.

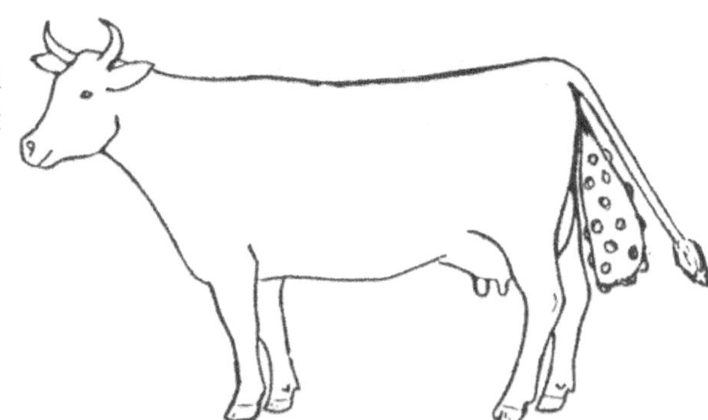

Treatment:

- Respond to the call quickly. If the uterus has been out for more than 8 hours, the mother usually dies. However, 80% of animals which are treated quickly will live.
- Thoroughly clean the uterus and push it back into the mother. This is often difficult to do because the mother usually tries to push it back again! The uterus can be pushed back into the mother animal if she is either lying down or standing up.
- **Laying Down Position:** Position the mother so that her front end is tilted downhill (if possible) to prevent her from pushing hard, and so that the forces of gravity will work with you. Do this by digging a shallow hole and putting her front end in it, or put some straw under her back end, or pull her hind legs out behind her. (See diagram.)

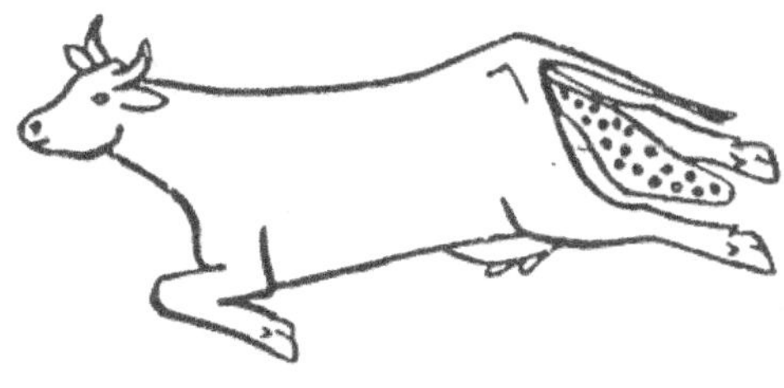

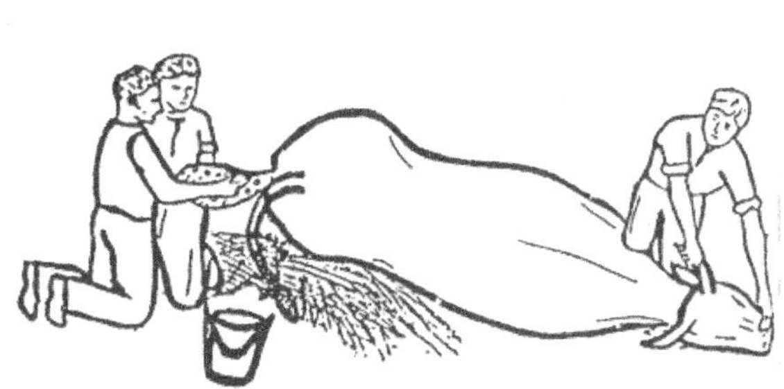

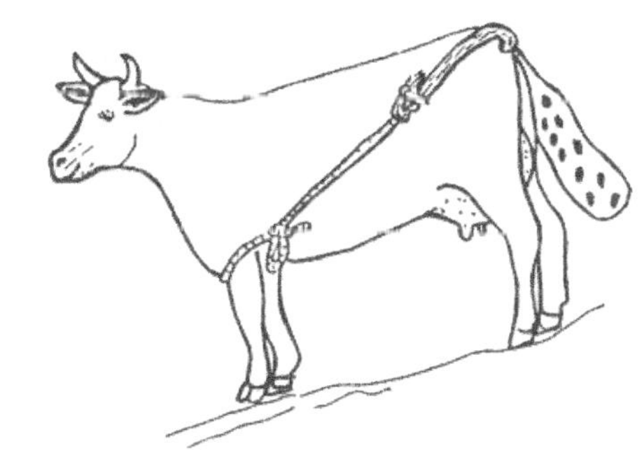

- **Standing Position:** In this position also, try to position the mother so that her front end is tilted downhill.

Step-by-Step Procedure for Treatment of Uterine Prolapse

- Clean the uterus well. It is easiest to put the whole uterus into a bucket of clean water and wash it with soap.

- Remove the placenta, if possible.

- Squat (or stand, if the mother is standing) behind the mother and gently lift the uterus.

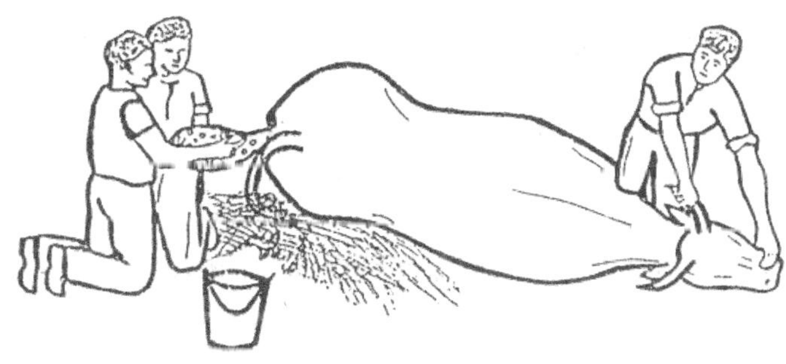

- Apply soap to make the uterus slippery.

- Slowly push the uterus back into the vulva and vagina. It may be necessary to apply more soap to make the uterus more slippery.

    - When pushing, be careful not to poke holes in the uterus with your fingers.
    - The process may take a long time, even an hour or more.

- Ensure that the uterus is pushed into the proper position inside the mother; otherwise, she may push it out again.

- If the uterus is so swollen that it will not go back inside the mother, apply cold water (and possibly sugar) to reduce the swelling. Most importantly, remember to make the uterus slippery and keep the mother's front end tilted slightly downhill.
- Place antibiotic boluses such as those containing sulfa, tetracycline, or furazolidone inside the uterus. If boluses are not available, use 6 capsules that contain 500 milligrams each of tetracycline (for humans).
- Give an injection of antibiotic such as penicillin, ampicillin or tetra-cycline.
- Examine and, if necessary, treat the animal for milk fever.
- Prevent the animal from pushing the uterus back out again by one of the following methods:
    - tie a "ring" around the vulva so that the uterus cannot come back out.
    - place 3 or 4 sutures, using thick suture material in the vulva to close it. The sutures must then be removed in about 3 days.

- Allow the baby to nurse so that oxytocin is released to contract the uterus and prevent it from coming out again. If the baby cannot nurse, then give the animal an injection of oxytocin.
- If the mother was lying down, try to get her onto her feet again. You may have to lift her, using 5 or 6 people. If she is still trying to push her uterus out, then keep her front end tilted downhill.

10.7.3.3 Discharge from the Vulva

The following describes the different types of discharges from the vulva and their significance:

Clear, slippery fluid at the time of heat: a normal sign of heat

Slight, bloody discharge: a normal sign shortly after a heat period (i.e. it's too late to breed her)

Red-colored discharge during the first week following delivery: a normal symptom as long as the cow is eating and does not have a fever

Bad-smelling discharge from the vulva: a sign of metritis (i.e. infection of the uterus).
- Shortly after delivery, this discharge may often be a mixture of blood and pus and can cause severe illness or even death.
- Chronic discharge is often comprised of pus and does not usually cause severe illness, but can lead to infertility.
- For treatment, see metritis. See page 154.

10.7.3.4 Retained Placenta

A retained placenta occurs when all of the afterbirth (placenta) does not come out within a few hours following delivery. This problem may be due to nutritional deficiencies, infectious diseases, a difficult delivery or other factors. A retained placenta may lead to a uterine infection, called "metritis." See page 154. Metritis can make an animal very sick.

Treatment
During the first 6-12 hours following delivery, try tying a rock to the part of the placenta hanging outside of the mother. The weight of the rock may help remove the placenta. Alternatively, fill the placenta that is hanging out of the animal with water.

If, after 12 hours the placenta has not come out, the best treatment is to put antibiotics into the uterus, plus give an injection of antibiotics to prevent metritis. However, in remote areas, where medicines and emergency help are difficult to obtain, remove the placenta by hand. Although removal by hand is less preferable because it can damage the uterus, it may also prevent the development of severe metritis, toxemia or even death.

Exception for Mares: A retained placenta in a mare is more serious than in most other animals, since mares are more susceptible to serious metritis. If the placenta has not come out within three hours after delivery, give 10 IU of oxytocin in the muscle every hour until the placenta comes out. If the placenta still does not come out after 6 hours, give an injection of antibiotics (e.g. penicillin) and continue the antibiotics for 5 days. Do not remove the placenta by hand as this may cause hemorrhaging.

Exception for Pigs: If a sow has a retained placenta, give her 10 IU of oxytocin every two hours during the first day. If by the second day the placenta has not come out, stop the oxytocin injections and give the sow injections of antibiotic to prevent serious illness due to metritis. Continue the antibiotics for 3-5 days.

To manually remove the placenta from cattle, buffalo, goats and sheep
1. Have the owner hold the tail, or tie it to one side
2. Wash the vulva and the area around it very well with soapy water.
3. Put a plastic sleeve on your arm (if available), and wash the sleeve until it is slippery with soap. **Caution:** Never treat an animal that has just aborted without wearing a plastic glove and sleeve. Always wash your hands and arms afterwards. See page 139.

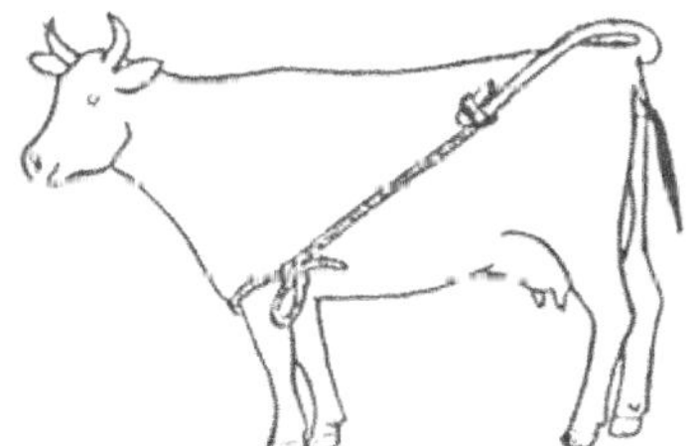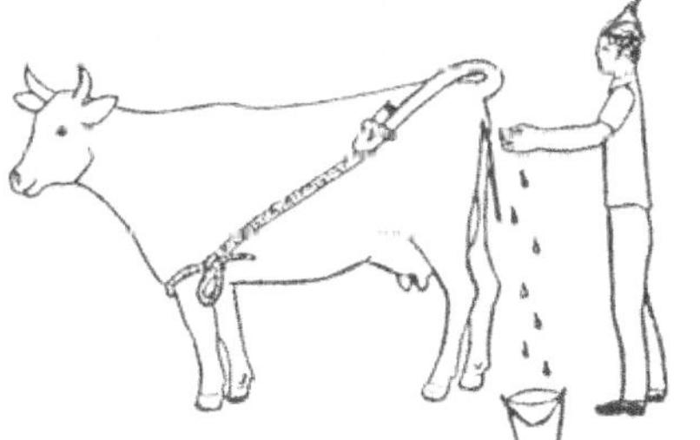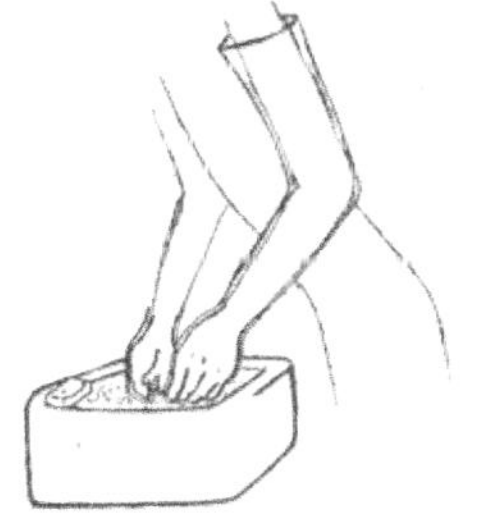

4. Insert your arm as far as possible into the uterus.
    If the cervix is already closed, then your arm
    will not go beyond the vagina.

5. Gently detach and remove as much of the
    placenta as possible. Since the placenta may be
    slippery, try wrapping it around your finger
    several times to hold on to it better during
    removal.

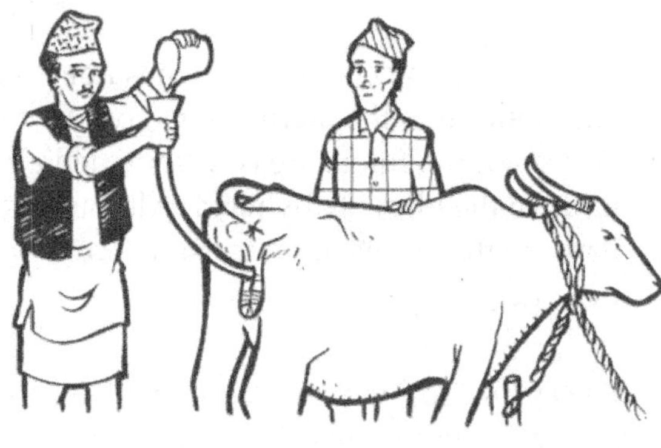

6. Flush the uterus with 1-2 liters of clean, warm,
    soapy water or disinfectant solution such as
    Potash, *Savlon*, Iodine, or Chlorohexidine. To
    flush the uterus, use a 1-meter long narrow tube
    or hose with smooth edges. If the cervix is open,
    insert the end of the hose into it. Or, if the cervix
    is closed, hold the end against the cervix. On the
    other end of the hose, place a funnel, and pour
    the solution into the funnel. Wait a few minutes
    for the animal to push most of the solution back out.

7. Place antibiotic boluses into the uterus. Even if the cervix is
    almost completely closed, the boluses can be broken up and
    the pieces pushed through the cervix. Almost any antibiotic
    will work such as tetracycline, sulfa or furazolidone. See page
    151. If boluses are not available, use 6 tetracycline capsules
    that contain 500 milligrams each (made for humans).

8. Give an injection of antibiotics.

Prevention
*   Allow the baby to nurse immediately after
    delivery. Nursing will release oxytocin in the mother's body,
    causing the uterus to contract and push the placenta out. The
    release of oxytocin also helps prevent a prolapsed uterus.
    Some veterinary doctors also give an oxytocin injection.

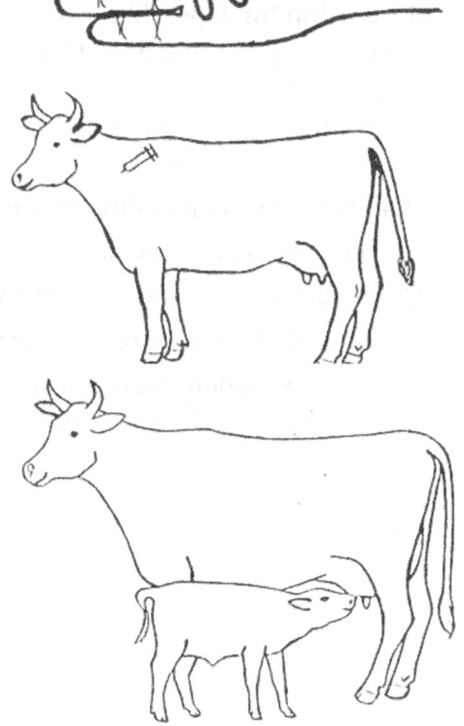

10.7.3.5 Metritis

Metritis means an infection of the uterus. There are two types:
- **Acute metritis**, which develops rapidly (usually following delivery), and can make an animal very sick.
- **Chronic metritis**, which lasts for a long time and doesn't usually cause severe illness but can lead to infertility.

Metritis can be caused by several things:
1. Infections which cause abortions, such as brucellosis or leptospirosis. See page 161.
2. Retained placenta.
3. Contamination of the uterus, often due to unclean conditions during delivery (dirty hands, equipment, bedding).

Symptoms
- Pus or other discharge from the vulva.
- Pain in the belly (especially with acute metritis).
- Fever (especially with acute metritis).
- Lack of appetite (especially with acute metritis).
- Infertility (in chronic cases).

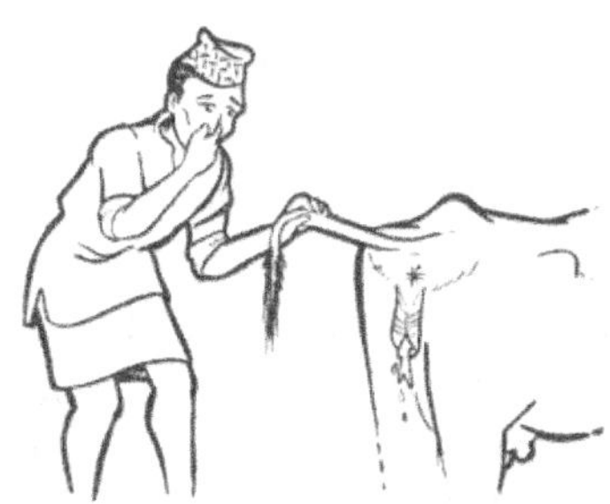

Diagnosis:
- Based on the symptoms

Treatment: An infected uterus is like an "infected wound." It needs to be cleaned, and antibiotics may be used to control the infection. See intra-uterine antibiotics. See page 151.
- *Acute metritis*, soon after delivery: treat as a retained placenta (clean uterus, insert antibiotics, and give antibiotic injection).
- *Chronic metritis*, long after giving birth: put antibiotics into the uterus using a long pipette (technicians trained in artificial insemination or "AI" know how to do this); or the AHA may simply give an injection of antibiotics.

Alternative: An effective and more natural alternative for treating metritis is to use a prostaglandin injection. See page 131. This brings the animal into heat repeatedly (called "short cycling") until she is cured. An injection of prostaglandin is given every eleven days from the beginning of her previous heat. The frequent heat periods use the animal's own defenses to treat the metritis.

Note: If an animal has a discharge from the vulva that consists of thick pus, she may have a "pyometra," a pus-filled uterus, which is difficult to treat. One recommended treatment is to bring her into heat using a hormone called "estrogen." See page 131. Then once in heat, put antibiotics into her uterus using a pipette. Alternatively, the animal can be "short cycled" using prostaglandins.

Caution: Estrogens and prostaglandins must be handled carefully since they can cause pregnant animals (and humans!) to abort.

10.7.4 Mastitis (Swollen Udder) (Lopsided, Hot Udder) (Bad Milk)

Mastitis means an inflammation of the udder. This usually means that the udder or teats are swollen, hot and reddened. Mastitis lowers milk production. The most common causes are injury to the udder or bacterial infection.

Symptoms of acute mastitis: The udder becomes **swollen**, **hot** and **painful**. The animal may become ill and stop eating.

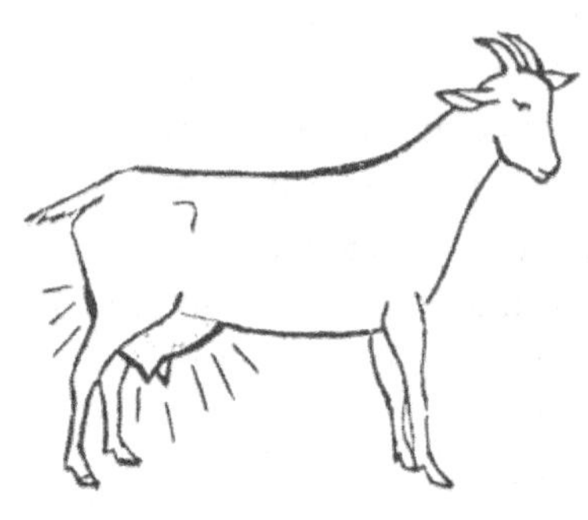

If an animal with mastitis is treated with antibiotics, then the milk should not be drunk for several days afterwards. If the owner decides to drink the milk anyway, then the milk should be carefully boiled first.

What to do if you suspect mastitis?
1. Examine the milk
Squirt some milk into your hand, a cup or a leaf and examine it closely. Check to see if it is watery, smells bad, or has lumps, pus or blood in it. Any of these symptoms indicates mastitis. **Note:** It is easier to see lumps if milk is squirted onto a dark colored surface (e.g. a black piece of paper or a dark green leaf).

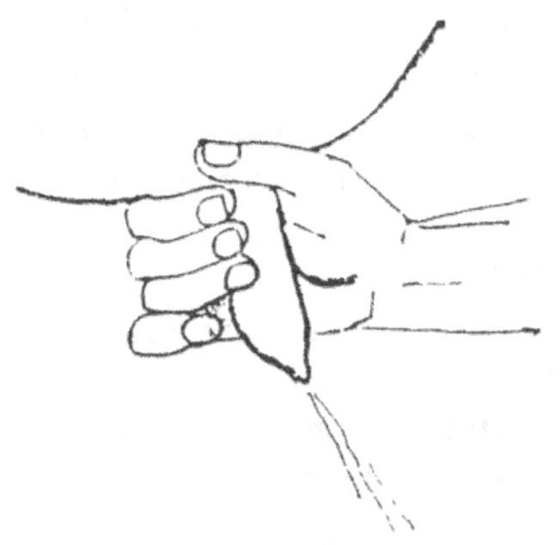

The milk can also be examined with a special solution called "mastitis solution." This solution is usually blue in color. Several milliliters of milk are mixed with several milliliters of solution. Then the mixture is swirled to see if it becomes thick, which indicates mastitis.

2. Take the temperature of the animal

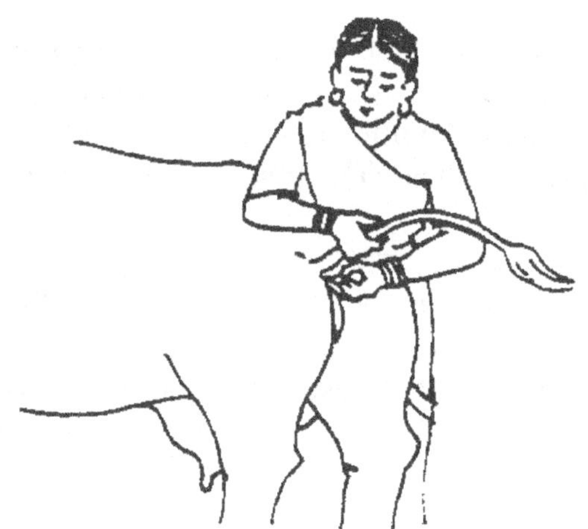

Table: Treatment of Mastitis

Milk is Normal		Milk is Not Normal (i.e. watery, smells bad, or has clots, blood, or pus)	
Animal does <u>not</u> have a fever	**Animal has a fever**	**Animal has a fever**	**Animal does <u>not</u> have a fever**
Often due to udder damage.	Mastitis plus toxemia.	Bacteria in udder plus toxemia	Bacteria in udder but no toxemia
<u>Treatment</u> Milk frequently[1] (may need to use teat cannula[2]). Apply warm, wet cloth.[3] Treat wounds on udder and teats.[4] Give food and water.	<u>Treatment</u> Milk frequently[1] (may need to use teat cannula[2]). Apply warm, wet cloth.[3] Treat wounds on udder and teats.[4] Give food and water. Antibiotics (IM or SC).	<u>Treatment</u> Milk frequently[1] (may need to use teat cannula[2]). Apply warm, wet cloth.[3] Treat wounds on udder and teats.[4] Give food and water. Antibiotics (IM or SC). Use Intra-mammary antibiotics if possible.	<u>Treatment</u> Milk frequently[1] (may need to use teat cannula[2]). Apply warm, wet cloth.[3] Treat wounds on udder and teats.[4] Give food and water. Do not have to give antibiotics IM or SC; unless unable to use intra- mammary antibiotics. Use Intra-mammary antibiotics if possible.

[1]***Milking frequently*** (at least 4 times daily) helps to decrease the pressure, (and pain) and flushes out the udder as well. If no milk will come out, then a clean teat cannula should be inserted into the teat so that milk can come out.

[2] See page 158, 'using a teat cannula.' **Caution:** NEVER insert sticks or pieces of straw into the teat to help the milk come out! Remove the cannula when not milking!

[3]***Applying a warm, wet cloth*** to the udder and teats helps to reduce swelling and pain.

[4]***Giving antibiotics*** helps to kill any germs in the udder.

[5]***Treating any wounds on the teats or udder*** helps to kill any germs that may invade the udder. Apply gentian violet, antibiotic ointment, Vaseline, or cooking oil to the wound.

Prevention:

Mastitis can be prevented by:

- Keeping animals clean, particularly after milking (when the teats are still open).
- Washing and drying the udder before milking.
- Dipping the teats in disinfectant solution immediately after milking.

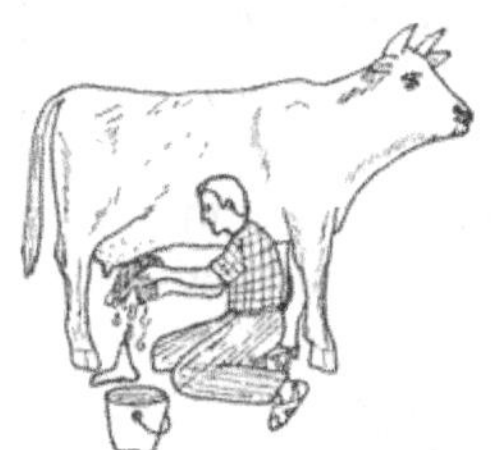 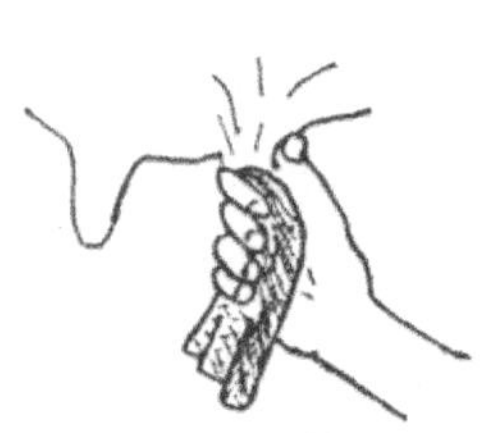 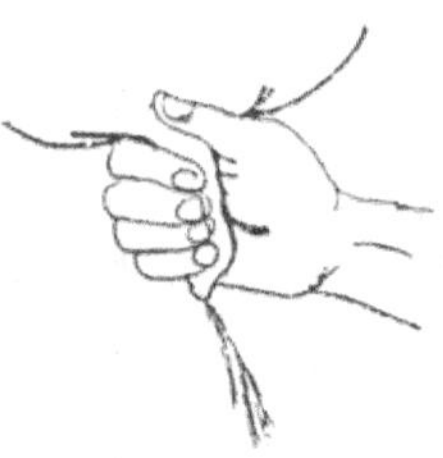 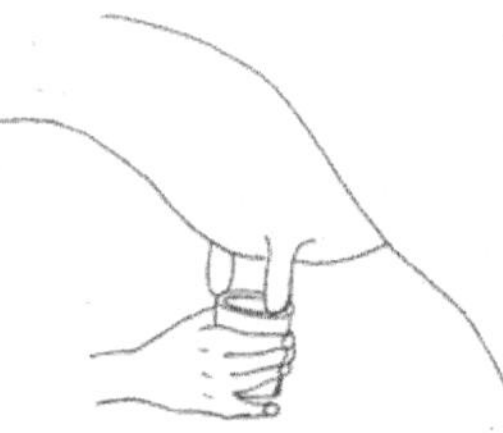

- Make young females gentle and accustomed to being milked by massaging the udder daily during the few months before giving birth. This will help prevent injury to the udder.

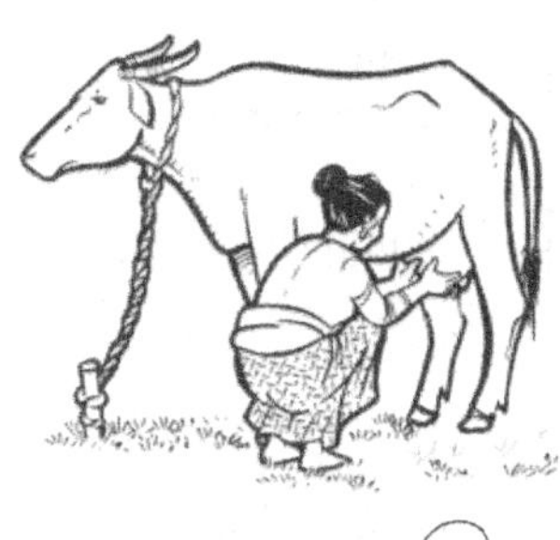

- Selecting milking animals from mothers that have good strong udders (and not poor udders that hang down low).

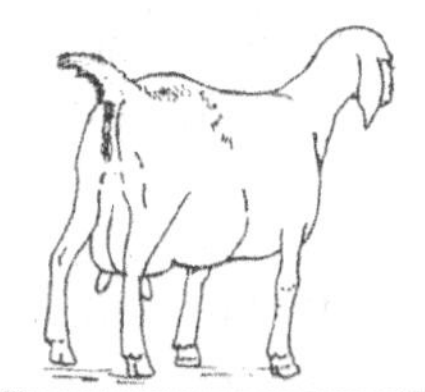

Note: Bad milk should not be drunk by either humans or the baby animals themselves. Bad milk should be thrown-away until it looks normal again.

How to Use Intra-Mammary Antibiotics

1. Milk the affected teat completely.

2. Clean the tip of the teat with disinfectant.

3. Insert the plastic cannula (that comes with intra-mammary antibiotic) into the tip of the teat.

4. Attach the tube of antibiotic to the cannula.

5. Squeeze the contents of the entire tube into the teat.

6. Remove the cannula and hold the end of the teat closed

7. Gently massage the medicine up into the udder.

Note: Intra-mammary antibiotics are more difficult to give than IM or SC injections. If no one is available who knows how to do this, then give an injection instead.

Caution: Read and follow the label on the intra-mammary tube. Some intra-mammary antibiotics contain steroids that may cause a pregnant animal to abort.

If a teat cannula is not used properly, it will push bacteria into the teat and cause infection.

1.   The cannula should be soaked in disinfectant for at least 10 minutes. If no disinfectant is available, then use locally-made alcohol or spirits. Some cotton should also be soaked in the disinfectant with the cannula.

2.   If the animal reacts or kicks when touching the udder, then restrain the animal in a crate. If the animal still moves too much, then restrain it with a rope tied around the abdomen in front of the udder or tie the legs in ways to prevent kicking. See pages 23, 26, 27.

3.   Wash your hands and clean your fingers (including fingernails) with disinfectant.

4.   Grasp the teat, holding it on the sides. Clean the end of the teat thoroughly with a disinfected piece of cotton wool.

5.   Then, hold the cannula at the base (NOT THE TIP!) and insert it into the teat.

6.   If the cannula accidentally touches the skin on the side of the teat, or if the animal moves and touches the cannula, clean the cannula and begin again.

7.   After the milk drains out, remove the teat cannula.

10.7.4.1 Chronic Mastitis

Sometimes an animal has mastitis that won't heal. The animal may not appear sick. However, the milk production may be decreased, and the milk may be abnormal or watery. This may be due to a germ that is resistant to the antibiotic used.

Treatment

If possible, submit a sample of milk to a laboratory to determine which antibiotic might work. Try to get a sample *before* treating with antibiotics.

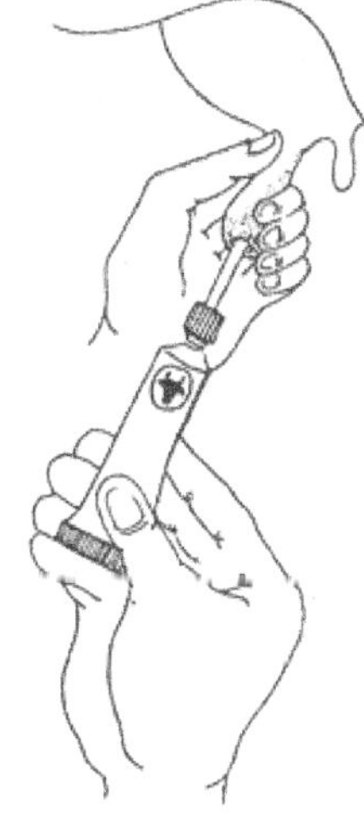

If it is impossible to test a sample in the laboratory, try treating with an antibiotic different than was previously used. An intra-mammary antibiotic is best, but if it is not available, use IM or SC antibiotics. Follow the label instructions which usually indicate treating for 4 days. Do not stop treatment early as this may increase the resistance to the germs.

10.7.5 Infertility and Abortions in Female Animals

Infertility is the failure to reproduce offspring. This can happen for many different reasons. For a review of infertility problems see page 164, general guidelines regarding breeding of livestock.

Taking a history and doing an examination is very important. This may reveal specific causes, such as whether the animal was exposed to any toxins, had a high fever, received certain medicines or vaccines, was injured, or has a poor diet.

The first step is to decide if the female animal is the reason for the infertility, or if the male animal is the reason.
- If the female animal has been bred by several different males, and still does not produce babies, then it is probably the fault of the female.
- If several female animals have been bred by the same male, and most of them aren't pregnant, then it is probably the fault of the male animal.

In female animals, there are two common types of infertility:
1. *No heat.* The female never shows signs of heat.
2. *Repeated breeding and abortions.* When the female comes into heat and is bred, but fails to become pregnant, the term used is repeated breeding. In fact, she may come into heat more often than normal. Or, the female becomes pregnant but never completes the pregnancy in a normal manner. This can happen if the baby dies in the uterus, or if it is born too early to live, and is called, "abortion." *The most common causes for infertility and abortions are:*
    - Infection
    - Malnutrition due to a poor diet, or parasites
    - Certain medicines and vaccines
    - High fevers
    - Injury
    - Toxins

10.7.5.1 No Heat!

What are the possible reasons why an animal may not come into heat?

Already pregnant! This is the most common reason why a female animal does not come into heat. Perhaps she was bred without the owner knowing it (e.g. she was loose and came into contact with a male or vice versa).
> Treatment: Wait to make sure the female is not pregnant. If possible, get a veterinarian or technician to perform a rectal examination and check for pregnancy. At the same time, they can check the ovaries and uterus for other problems.

The Owner Cannot Tell When the Animal Is In Heat. It is important to review with the owner how and when to recognize the signs of heat in her animals. See page 135.

"Silent Heat." Sometimes the female comes into heat but does not show the normal signs of heat. This happens more often if there is no male animal nearby.
> Treatment: Keep the female with, or near, a male animal during the breeding season. Even if the owner cannot tell if the animal is in heat, the male animal probably can.

Old Age: Check the teeth of the animal to estimate its age. If the animal is very old, explain this to the owner.
> Treatment: Old animals should be culled from the herd and replaced with younger animals. This should be done on a routine basis so that the herd of animals does not become old all at once. For example, 20 percent (1/5) of a herd of sows should be culled and replaced yearly, so that there is a proper mixture of older and younger animals.

Malnutrition / Deficiency: Some animals may lack something in their diet that prevents them from coming into heat. The most common cause is lack of enough energy in the diet (i.e. the animal is thin). The problem is made worse if the animal also has many parasites. In many tropical countries, the soil and plants lack a mineral called phosphorus. Animals suffering from phosphorus deficiency may not reproduce normally.

> Treatment: Feed animals a balanced diet and make sure that they have enough energy so that they aren't thin and sickly. See page 106. In addition, treat them for parasites.

> **Note:** Ask the government extension worker if any mineral deficiencies are common in your area. If so, consider feeding extra minerals based on the advice of a local specialist. Do <u>not</u> depend on expensive phosphorus or vitamin injections. Rather, feed vitamins and minerals with the food.

> **Caution:** Many livestock owners are exploited by vendors of vitamin injections or mineral products. In some cases, inexpensive local feed sources can provide the needed vitamins and minerals. Often, the more important problems are parasites and insufficient foods containing energy.

Too fat: Female animals that are too fat often fail to come into heat and get pregnant. They may also have trouble giving birth, or give birth to weak offspring.

> Treatment: Feed smaller quantities of a well-balanced feed until the animal loses weight.

Infection: Metritis may also cause infertility. See page 161.

Problems with the Ovaries or Uterus: If the possible causes mentioned above are eliminated, then there may be something wrong with the ovaries that prevents normal heat. An animal that has a deformity in its reproductive organs may fail to get pregnant, or may abort once pregnant. This is often the case when a cow gives birth to twins - one of which is male and one is female. In cattle, 95 percent of female twins do not have a fully developed reproductive tract and are infertile. In America, these female twins are called "free-martins."

10.7.5.2 Repeated Breeding and Abortions

Many of the causes for repeated breeding and abortions are similar and can be considered together.

Malnutrition (deficiencies)
This is due to a poor diet or parasites. See pages 51, 125,176, 196.

Cyst on the Ovary
A cyst is a fluid-filled lump that may develop on the ovary of a female. A cyst may produce hormones that disrupt the animal's normal heat cycle. The female animal may exhibit strange behavior, such as being in heat continuously, exhibiting male behavior, or never showing signs of heat. The following two types of cysts are most common:

Follicular cyst
Symptoms: The animal comes into heat, and then comes into heat again before she should.

Diagnosis: Based on symptoms. The cyst can be confirmed by a rectal exam (done by a skilled person).

Treatment: Give an injection of a hormone containing chorionic gonadotropin (also called HCG).
If this injection is not available, an old treatment is to use a pipette and put about 10 ml of 5 percent
iodine solution into the uterus.

Prevention: Cystic ovaries may be caused by injections of estrogen hormones, or by eating certain
forages that are high in estrogens. Seek advice of a skilled person if you suspect a problem of cystic
ovaries in your area. Consider culling animals with chronic cystic ovaries (especially if the problem
occurs more than once) since a tendency for cystic ovaries may be passed to the offspring.

Luteal cyst
Symptoms: The animal does not come into heat at all.

Diagnosis: Based on the symptoms.

Treatment: Give an injection of prostaglandin. If the treatment is effective, the animal should
come into heat within 3 days. If prostaglandin is not available, put iodine into the uterus as
described above.

Prevention: Consider culling animals with cystic ovaries (especially if it occurs more than once)
since a tendency for cystic ovaries may be passed to the offspring.

Infections
Metritis (infection of the uterus) has already been discussed as a disease of the uterus. See page 154.
Metritis is also a common cause of infertility. In addition to general metritis, many different germs
cause infections that result in infertility and abortions. Determining the exact germ, even with the help
of a laboratory, is often difficult. However, the following organisms are the most common causes of
metritis:
- In cattle, an organism called "trichomonas" can cause infertility or irregular heat cycles. Cattle
  transmit this to other cattle during breeding.
- In pigs a virus called "parvo" can cause infertility, abortions or mummified piglets.
- The following section describes two of the most common infections that cause abortions.

Brucellosis
Brucellosis is due to a bacteria called <u>Brucella</u> and may cause abortions, infertility, and inflamed
testicles of cattle, buffalo, goats, sheep, pigs, and dogs.

Brucellosis is also an important **public health disease** because it can cause "undulant" or "Malta"
fever in humans. The symptoms in humans include a fever that increases and decreases (i.e. undulant)
as well as headaches and general weakness. See page 281. Humans are infected by contacting the
placenta, drinking milk, or when slaughtering an animal for meat (particularly pigs).
Animals are infected when the organism enters their mouth through contaminated food or water,
or by having contact with infected animals, particularly their placentas. The bacteria then enter the uterus
and cause abortions during late pregnancy. The abortions may be followed by retained placentas and
subsequent infertility. *Brucella* bacteria are also present in the milk of infected animals.

Diagnosis: Diagnosis can be made from a blood sample or from culturing an aborted animal, the
placenta, or milk.

Treatment: None.

Prevention / Control:

- In many countries, government authorities require blood testing to identify infected animals which must then be slaughtered.

- In some countries a brucellosis vaccine is licensed and available, but an AHA must handle it properly and according to the label instructions and regulations of her country.

- Aborted animals, and the associated placenta, should be buried or burned. Keep other animals and humans from touching them.

- Humans should always boil milk before drinking it to kill *Brucella,* as well as other harmful organisms.

Caution: **Never** treat an animal with a retained placenta that just aborted without wearing a plastic glove. Always wash your hands and arms afterwards. If accidentally exposed to Brucellosis, take 500 milligrams of tetracycline, by mouth, four times a day for two weeks.

Leptospirosis
Leptospirosis causes disease in animals and humans. See page 287. Dogs, pigs, cattle, rats and wildlife serve as sources of infections. The organism comes out in the urine of infected animals. Animals and humans become infected by drinking contaminated water, or by contact with the urine of infected animals.

Symptoms: Young animals can become quite sick with fever, jaundice, and red urine (called hemoglobinuria). See page 246. Anemia, and possibly death may follow these symptoms. Adult animals may have abortions late in pregnancy, or lowered milk production with thick, yellow, blood-tinged milk yet with no inflamed udder. Sometimes there are no symptoms, particularly in pigs and adult animals that are not lactating.

Diagnosis: Diagnosis is often based on symptoms. It can be confirmed by a blood test.

Treatment: Treatment with tetracycline or streptomycin may help if done early in the course of the disease.

Prevention/Control: Simultaneous treatment with streptomycin and vaccination may help control an epidemic, if done early. Streptomycin stops the shedding of the organism in the urine. Rat control also helps.

Certain Medicines and Vaccines as a Cause of Abortions
Certain medicines and vaccines can cause abortions. This is why it is very important to read the label on all medicines before using them. If the label is difficult to understand, ask someone to help. Some common medicines that cause abortions in animals are:
- steroids, such as dexamethasone
- estrogens (used to make female animals come into heat)
- prostaglandins (used to make female animals come into heat)
- Carbon Tetra-Chloride (CTC) - used to treat liver fluke

High Fevers or Overheating as a Cause of Abortions
Overheating or any condition that causes a high fever in an animal may result in abortion or failure
to conceive. Some diseases that cause high fevers and hence abortion or failure to conceive include
hog cholera, African swine fever and erysipelas in pigs, foot and mouth disease in cattle, and anthrax
in any species.

> Treatment: In hot climates, it is always wise to avoid overheating by breeding animals,
> especially pigs, early in the morning or later in the evening. Provide protection from the
> sun and extreme heat. Do not overheat animals during transport, handling, castrating,
> vaccinating or worming. Consider transporting animals only at night. See page 62 for
> treatment of overheating, or a high fever.

Trauma, Stress, Injury as a Cause of Abortions
An animal that has had trauma or stress may be infertile, or experience early abortion. Stress or
trauma could be due to an accident or a fall, injury from other animals (particularly from horn
butting), rough handling, a long voyage, overcrowding, or lack of shelter from excessive cold,
mud, wind, sun, or heat.

Toxins as a Cause of Abortions
- Certain plants may contain toxins that result in abortion or infertility. For example, the tree
  called Leucena produces a toxin called "mimosine." Although the Leucena leaves provide rich
  forage, if these leaves are eaten in large amounts, they may result in infertility or abortion in
  certain species.
- Feed that is stored improperly, or becomes wet, may become moldy. his mold can produce a
  toxin called a "mycotoxin," which can cause infertility or abortion.
- Microorganisms that cause certain types of mastitis or other infections may produce toxins that
  poison the animal. This is called, "toxemia," and may result in abortion.

10.7.6 Infertility in Male Animals

Infertility in the male may be temporary as in the case of an overheated boar, or it may be permanent.
The male may simply have mechanical difficulties to breed a female because of leg or feet problems,
difference in size of the two animals, or abnormalities in his reproductive organs. There may be
problems in the quantity or quality of his sperm.

10.7.6.1 Overused Male

In some situations, the male is overused and is breeding too many females in a short period of time.
See page 165.

10.7.6.2 Too Fat

Male animals that are too fat may not be able to breed properly.

10.7.6.3 Lack of Exposure to Females

Breeding boars raised in isolation may also fail to perform well.

10.7.6.4 Swollen Testicles

The two most common reasons for swollen testicles are **infection** and **injury**. Infection is often due to
Brucella which causes the testicles to swell and then shrink, resulting in infertility. More rarely, a tumor
may cause the testicles to become larger than normal.

Symptoms/Diagnosis: The testicles will be enlarged, painful and hot, due to inflammation.
A chronic infection may cause abscesses to form in the testicles.

Treatment: Bathe the testicles in cold water. If the animal has a fever or other signs of infection,
give antibiotics such as penicillin or tetracycline. If the animal is in pain, give a painkiller such as
aspirin.

Control/Prevention: Do not buy animals that have unevenly shaped, small, or swollen testicles.
Do not buy animals from a farm that has a history of selling animals with testicle problems.

10.7.6.5 Broken Penis (Phimosis, Paraphimosis)
See page 247.

10.8 BREEDING GUIDELINES

10.8.1 Do not breed females that are too young or too small.
The age at which a female is ready to breed often depends on the quality of food she ate
when growing. It is often best *not* to breed a female during her first heat, particularly if
she is small, as this may result in birthing difficulties, small and weak babies, or small
litters (in pigs).

10.8.2 Do not breed animals that are too thin or unhealthy.
Thin or unhealthy animals (male or female) may abort, be infertile, or have small, weak
babies or litters. It is best to delay breeding a thin, unhealthy animal until it is recovered
or in better condition.

10.8.3 Breed females when they are "in heat."
Females must be bred when they are "in heat." Signs of heat vary in different animals.
See Table, page 135. Some animals should be bred only once during their heat (e.g. cattle,
buffalo, sheep and goats), whereas other animals should be bred more than once during their
heat (e.g. horses and pigs). See Table, page 135. Do not try to force animals to mate.
The female may injure the male if she is not in heat.

10.8.4 Daily observe females for signs of heat.
Looking for signs of heat should be done at least once daily. Often, animals more actively
show heat signs at dawn and dusk. Be sure to observe animals you think are pregnant, as
signs of heat in them indicate that they are no longer pregnant and need to be re-bred. Bred
animals should be especially watched near the time of their expected heat (i.e. 18-23 days
after breeding for most animals). If a female has trouble getting pregnant, or loses her
pregnancies repeatedly, she should be slaughtered, or at least not used as a breeding
animal since her fertility problem might be passed to her offspring.

10.8.5 Do not stress or overheat breeding animals.
Stress and overheating should be avoided in both female and male breeding animals
because it may make them infertile. If the female must be taken to the male, she should
be taken *before* she comes into heat. If she is already in heat, she should be walked
gently and during the cool time of the day. In boars, overheating may cause infertility
for two months.

10.8.6 Avoid inbreeding.

The breeding of two closely related animals is called "inbreeding." Inbreeding should be avoided because it results in less-healthy and less-productive offspring. See page 167.

10.8.7 Do not breed the male too often.

Male animals should not be "overused" by breeding too frequently. This results in semen with insufficient sperm in it. Overbreeding can especially be a big problem in seasonal breeders like buffalo where many females come into heat in a short period of time. As a general rule, boars should breed no more than once per day, and stallions no more than once every other day. For sheep and goats, there should be at least one male for every 50 females. For buffalo bulls, try to breed them no more than once per day. Contrary to common customs, it is not necessary to have a male buffalo breed the female two times on the same day!

10.8.8 Do not depend on only one male.

At least two males should be available for breeding, as there may be infertility problems in one of the males. Infertility should be suspected if females keep returning to heat following breeding.

10.8.9 Use a semen test if available.

To verify fertility, a semen test can be performed by a trained technician.

10.8.10 Keep records.

Carefully write down breeding dates. Do not depend on your memory!

10.9 GENETIC IMPROVEMENT

10.9.1 Importing Animals

Many livestock improvement projects import breeding animals to rapidly improve the productivity of the local breeds. There are advantages and disadvantages to importing breeding animals.

Advantages: Improvements in productivity of the livestock occur within a few generations.

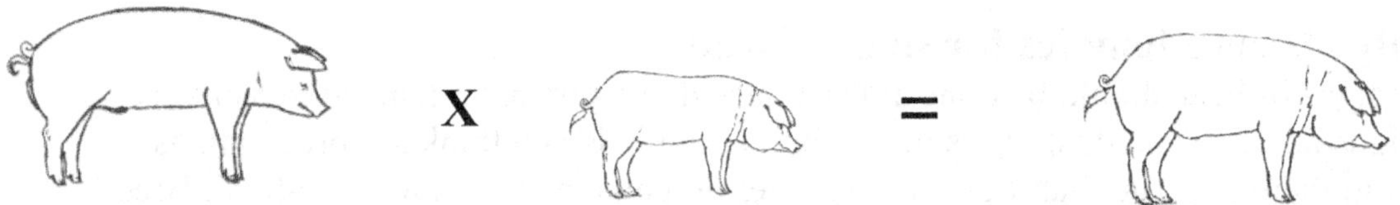

Disadvantages: Importing animals may be expensive and risky. The risk is that imported animals may become sick or die because they have less resistance to local diseases, or cannot adapt to local conditions, feeds, or management systems. Also, imported animals may cost more in terms of money, labor, feeding, treatment, and maintenance. Many livestock improvement projects have failed because the local livestock producers were not ready to provide the type of management or feed that imported animals require.

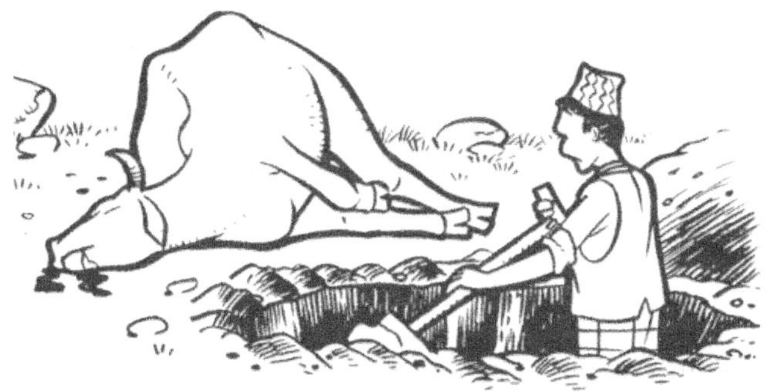

Carefully consider the advantages and disadvantages of importing animals, as well as the other options for genetic improvement.

10.9.2 An Intermediate Option: Limited Cross-Breeding

Some livestock improvement projects limit the number of animals imported by breeding only a few imported animals to local animals. For example, an improved male goat will be placed in a region to breed too many of the local female goats. The offspring are called, "half-bloods," that is, one-half foreign breed and one-half local breed. Half-bloods have the advantage of being adapted to local environment and also being more productive than the local animals.

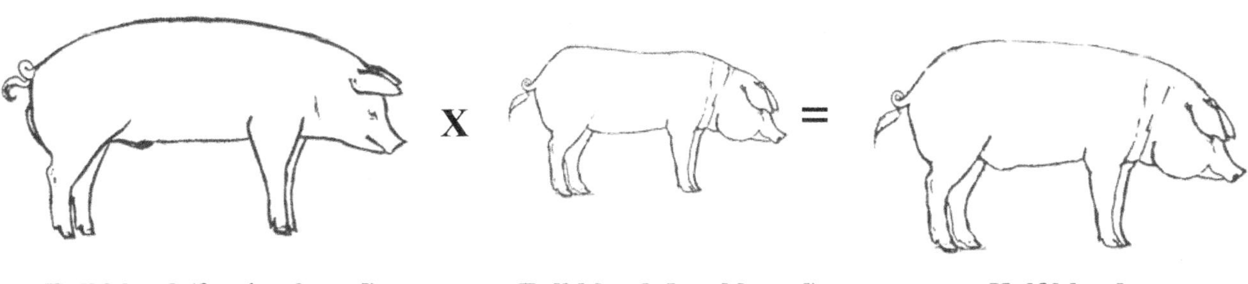

Full blood (foreign breed)   **Full blood (local breed)**   **Half blood**

As an alternative, the half-bloods can be bred back to one of the imported animals (one that is unrelated - to avoid inbreeding). The resulting offspring are then "three-quarter bloods", in other words, three quarters foreign breed and one quarter local breed. This strategy has worked well in many livestock projects.

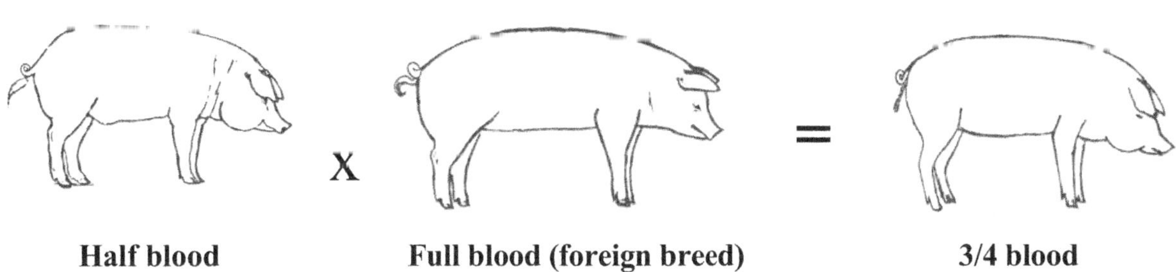

Half blood   **Full blood (foreign breed)**   **3/4 blood**

10.9.3 Other Options for Genetic Improvement

What are other options to improve the local livestock without importing animals?

10.9.3.1 Selection

Genetic improvement can be achieved by carefully selecting young animals for breeding based on the performance of their parents. This is called "**selection.**" If the parents grew quickly and produced well, their offspring are likely to do the same. Improvements by selection may be slower than if an improved animal is imported. However, the risks are less since the offspring are well-adapted to the local conditions.

10.9.3.2 Culling

Unproductive animals or those with defects should not be used as breeding animals. Instead, unproductive animals should be castrated before they are old enough to mate. The process of removing undesirable animals from the herd is called "**culling.**" Culling prevents a livestock producer from wasting resources on poor quality livestock.

10.9.3.3 Avoid inbreeding

Inbreeding is when two closely related animals are bred together. This is sometimes done deliberately to develop certain characteristics in the offspring. However, inbreeding is generally not recommended because there is a risk that offspring will have defects, or are weaker, smaller and less productive. There are three ways to avoid inbreeding:

Don't breed related animals to each other.
When the same males are used continuously in an area, these same males will most likely breed their mothers, sisters, or daughters, or their offspring may be bred to one another. The solution is to send these males to another area and bring in new ones.

Don't breed the sire

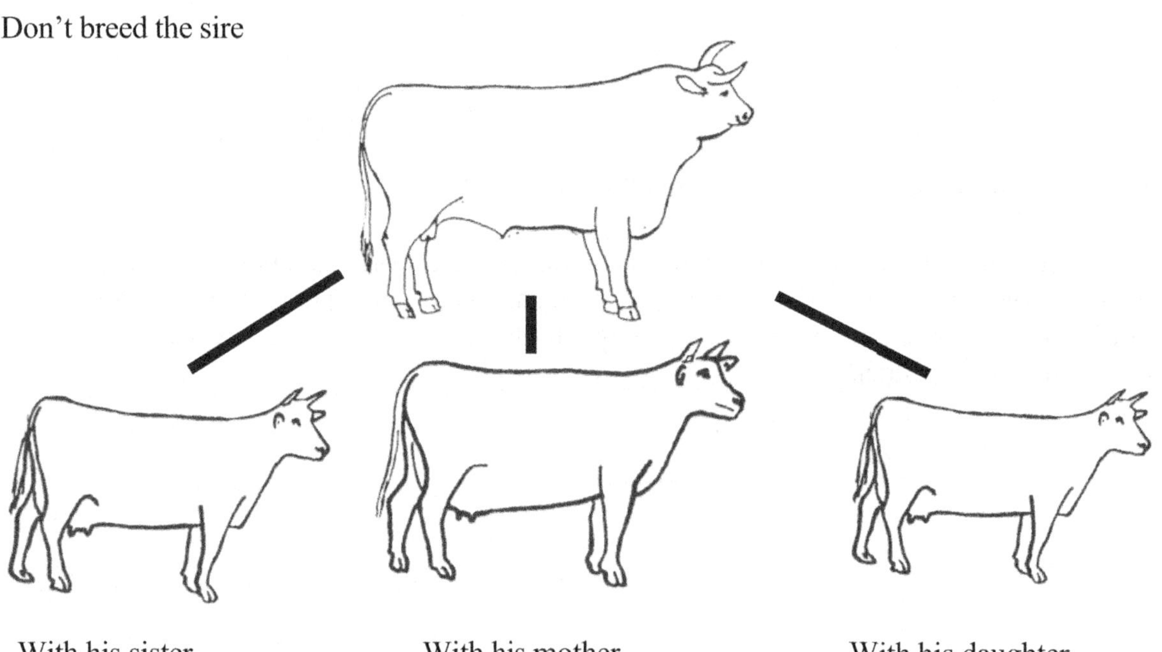

With his sister   With his mother   With his daughter

Don't leave animals loose or unattended.
Animals that run loose or are unattended may mate with their relatives or with poor quality animals. Also, if breeding took place while the animals were running loose or unattended, it is impossible to know who the father was. The solution is to avoid letting animals run loose or leaving them unattended.

Castrate young males that will not be used for breeding

Some male animals reach puberty at a young age, and if not castrated, may mate with their mother or sisters. The solution is to castrate young males that will not be used for breeding.

10.10 CASTRATIONS

Castration is the process of removing or destroying the testicles so that they become non-functional. Since it is a painful process, the authors recommend the use of local anesthetic to prevent pain. In some countries anesthesia may not be available and the castration must be done anyway. In those situations, the AHA must use their own judgment. There are three principle reasons to castrate:

1. Castration prevents a male from making other animals pregnant.
2. Castration makes the male less aggressive, easier to handle, and safer to be around.
3. Castration helps the animal to gain weight faster.

10.10.1 Best age for castration

Bulls can be castrated as young as 2-3 months of age. Goats and sheep can be castrated as young as 2-3 weeks of age. The advantage of castrating young animals is that it is least traumatic for the animal, easiest, and safest. The disadvantage is a greater likelihood of developing stones that block the urethra and prevent the animal from urinating. Horses and mules are usually castrated at 2-3 years of age. Although mules are sterile and cannot reproduce, they can still mate because the testicles produce testosterone. Uncastrated mules can be difficult to handle. Pigs are best castrated around two weeks of age.

10.10.2 Burdizzo method

Castration is best done in the field by using the "burdizzo", a special clamp which crushes the spermatic cord and blood vessels leading to the testicles, without cutting or wounding the scrotum skin. The crushing causes the testicles to shrink and stop producing sperm. The advantage of this method is that there is no open wound. The disadvantage is the need for a special instrument, and if the burdizzo is used improperly, the scrotum may become infected or the testicles might not shrink (so that the animal is not castrated).

There are different sized burdizzos: small ones for sheep/goats; and large ones for cattle/buffalo. On a large animal, closing the burdizzo requires some strength and may require a helper. Or one handle of the burdizzo may be placed on the ground or on the technician's knee. A burdizzo should never be used on a horse. The spermatic cord must be crushed at different levels (see diagram below) to ensure that the blood vessels which travel down the center of the cord and supply the scrotum with blood won't be crushed. If you crush these blood vessels, the entire scrotum may fall off and infection may occur.

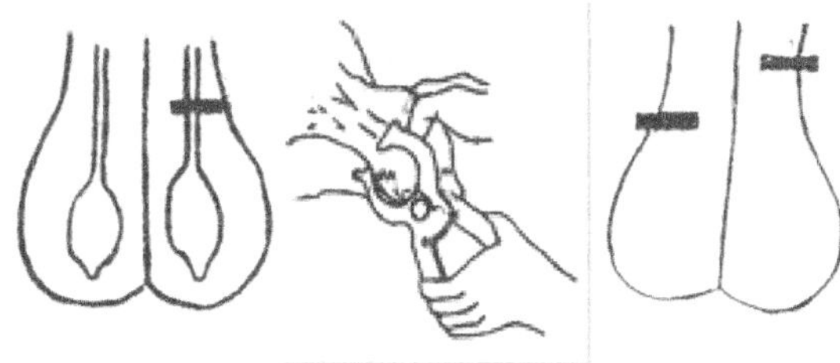

A burdizzo crushes the spermatic cord and vessels without breaking the skin. Crush each side at different levels to avoid crushing the blood vessels in the middle that supply the scrotum.

Burdizzo method for bulls, goats, and sheep:
- Restrain the animal.
- Grasp the spermatic cord.
- Hold the spermatic cord tightly against the side of the skin to prevent it from slipping sideways.
- Close the burdizzo until it clicks shut over about 1/3 of the skin covering the cord. Avoid crushing the center part of the cord which contains vessels supplying the scrotum with blood.
- Hold the burdizzo closed for several seconds and then release.
- For extra assurance, crush the cord again about one cm above (or below) the first crush.
- Repeat the procedure for the spermatic cord on the other side. However, crush the cord at different levels on the other side to ensure that blood will continue to reach the scrotum. **Do not crush all the skin across both cords at the same level, since this will crush the blood vessels and the whole scrotum will die and become infected.**
- Apply anti-fly ointment onto the area which has been crushed to prevent maggot infestation.

10.10.3 Open method

Using the open method, the scrotum is cut and the testicle is removed. The advantage of this method is that it works well, is easy to perform, and requires no special instruments. The disadvantage is a risk that the wound may get infected with maggots or bacteria. The animal may also bleed a lot after the cord is cut, causing weakness and even death. ***Important note:*** Be sure to make a large incision and, after castration, to exercise the animal to ensure good drainage and to minimize swelling. Be as clean as possible by washing your hands and the area of castration with soap, clean water and disinfectant. Use a clean, sharp cutting instrument.

Open method procedure for bulls 6 months or younger

- Obtain a clean, sharp knife.
- Secure the animal with ropes.
- Wash your hands and the animal's scrotum with soap, clean water and disinfectant.
- Use disinfectant and water to clean the scrotum. If possible, use local anesthetic.
- Grasp the end of the scrotum, pull it tightly, and cut off the lower 1/3 of the scrotum.

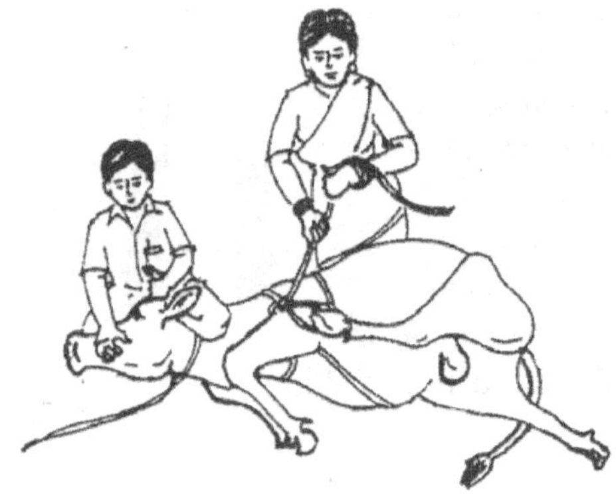

1. Restrain the animal

**2. Wash your hands and the area of
the animal to castrate**

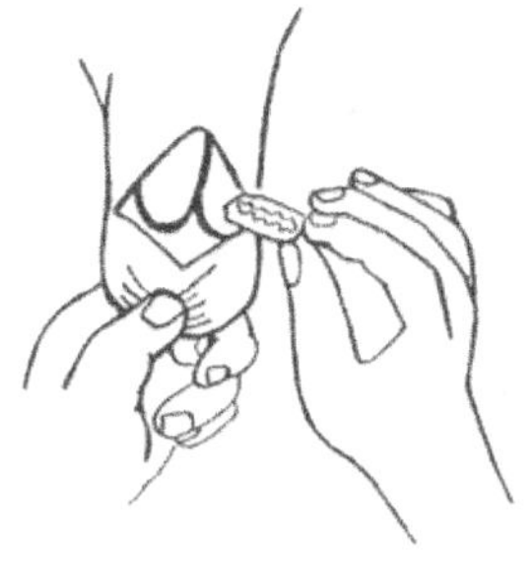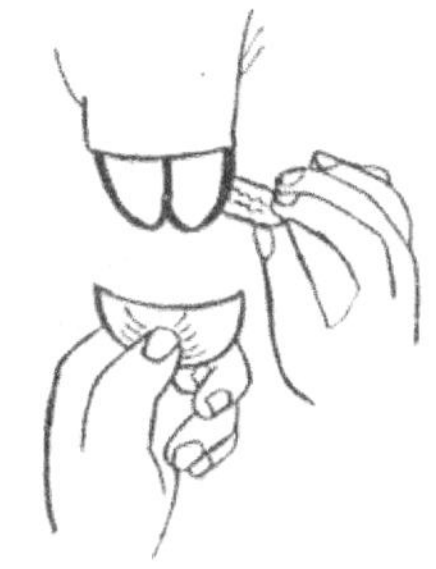

3. Make an incision….   **4...and remove the lower 1/3 of the scrotum**

- Grasp the testicle and pull on it steadily until the cord breaks.
- If any fatty tissue is hanging out of the scrotum, cut it away.
- Use anti-fly ointment to prevent maggot infestation.
- Exercise the animal for 1-2 weeks to decrease the swelling and help the
  wound to drain properly.

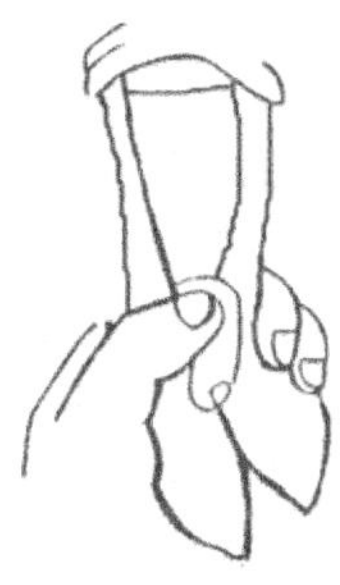

Open method procedure for young sheep and goats (6 months or younger):

- Hold the animal tightly on its side.
- Wash your hands and the animal's scrotum with soap, clean water and disinfectant. Use local
  anesthetic if possible.
- Grasp the scrotum and make two incisions parallel to the middle line of the skin (make them
  low enough on the scrotum so that they can drain properly).
- Cut deep enough to expose the shiny white covering (tunic), but do not cut it.
- Grasp the testicle and pull it steadily until the cord breaks.
- If any fatty tissue is hanging out of the scrotum, cut it away with a knife or scissors.
- Use anti-fly ointment to prevent maggot infestation. Exercise the animal for 1-2 weeks to
  help drainage and healing.

Open method for older bulls, sheep and goats (older than 6 months):

(The open method in older animals carries more risk of bleeding problems)

- The procedure is the same as the open method in
  animals six months or younger, except for the
  following:
  - Apply a clamp to the cord (if available).
  - Release the clamp and tie a suture around the
    cord where it was clamped.
  - If a clamp is not available, simply tie a suture tightly
    around the cord twice
  - Cut the cord below the tie.
- The rest of the procedure is the same as for young animals.

Elastic band method (not generally recommended)

This method consists of a small rubber band that is applied by a special instrument, around the
scrotum of small kids and lambs at about one week of age. The band cuts off the circulation and
the whole scrotum falls off eventually, usually without infection. However, infections can occur,
particularly in areas at risk for tetanus. This method is less preferable.

Castration of Horses

- Horses should be castrated around 2-3 years of age - after they have had enough time to fully develop, but before they become difficult to handle.
- Burdizzos should *not* be used on horses or mules since their scrotal sacks are shorter, making it difficult to properly locate and crush the cord. Therefore, the open method should always be used.
- Horses and mules are prone to tetanus. They should therefore be protected beforehand with tetanus toxoid. They should also be given a long-acting penicillin injection at the time of castration.

The Procedure
- Give a sedative such as *Rompun* (if it is available and can be properly given).
- Cast the horse and tie its legs securely (see chapter on restraint).
- Wash your hands and the animal's scrotum with soap, clean water and disinfectant.
- Give local anesthetic (if available) in two different places, as follows:
    - Inject about ten ml of a two percent solution subcutaneously along the line of the proposed incision for each testicle. The incisions should extend the entire length of the testicle (parallel to the middle line of the scrotum and about 2 cm to either side of this line).
    - Inject about 10 ml of local anesthetic into the cord itself (inject high up on the cord) of both testicles.
- After waiting a few minutes for the anesthetic to begin to work, make two incisions along the line where the local anesthetic was injected subcutaneously. Make the incisions the entire length of the testicle (otherwise it will not drain well afterwards). The incisions should be made deep enough to go through the skin but not into the shiny white coat that surrounds the testicle (called the tunic).
- Apply traction to the testicles to free them from the surrounding tissue.
- Cut through the tunic so that the testicle pops out.
- Expose the cord of the testicle by pulling on it gently (without breaking the cord).
- Tie a suture around the cord (including the white coat). This can be repeated 2-3 times, to be sure the cord is well tied so that it doesn't bleed after it is cut.
- Cut the cord below the sutures using a hot metal iron (if available). Cutting with a hot metal iron helps control the bleeding   If a hot iron is not available, clamp the cord (to crush it) below the sutures. After clamping for 1-3 minutes, cut the cord below the clamp marks.
- Repeat the procedure for the other testicle.
- Cut away the tunics of both testicles to facilitate good drainage and prevent infection.
- Remove any loose tissue that hangs from the incision.
- Give the horse an injection of long-lasting penicillin to prevent tetanus.
- Release the ropes and carefully help the horse get up without injuring itself.
- Observe the horse for several hours to check for bleeding.
- Walk the horse daily for the next two weeks to reduce swelling and help drainage.
- If the incisions close-up, or get infected, the horse must be cast again, the incisions must be opened and cleaned, and the horse should be given another injection of penicillin.

Note: The key to avoiding infection is cleanliness and good drainage. This is accomplished by good washing and disinfecting, making long incisions, removing extra tissue (such as the tunic), giving penicillin and exercising the animal (to minimize swelling).

Procedure to castrate a horse

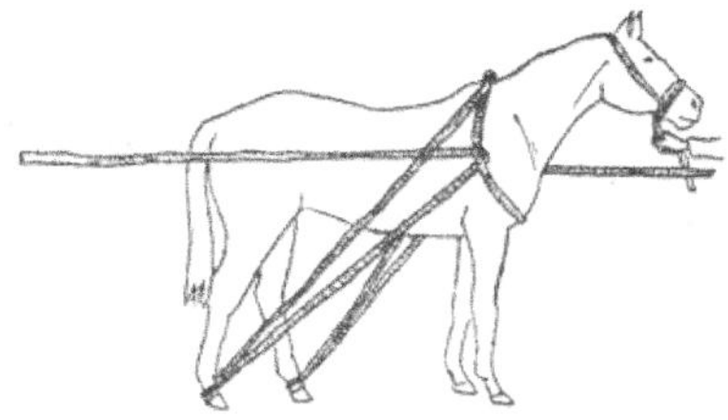

1. Cast the animal properly

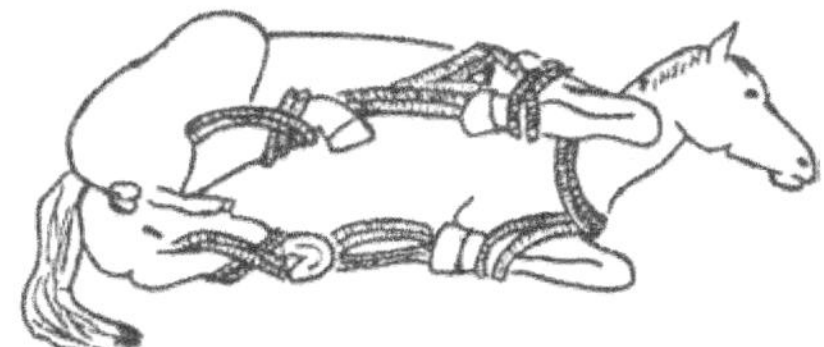

2. Tie its legs securely

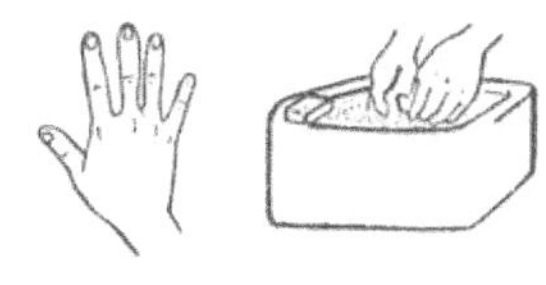

3. Wash your hands and the area to be castrated

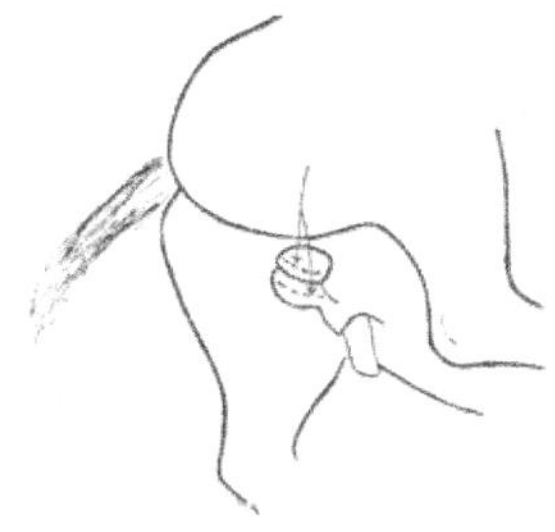

4. Give local anesthetic in two lines.

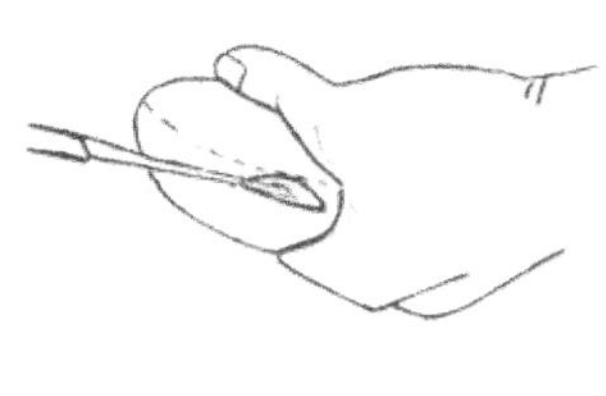

5. Cut the scrotum the entire length of the testicle

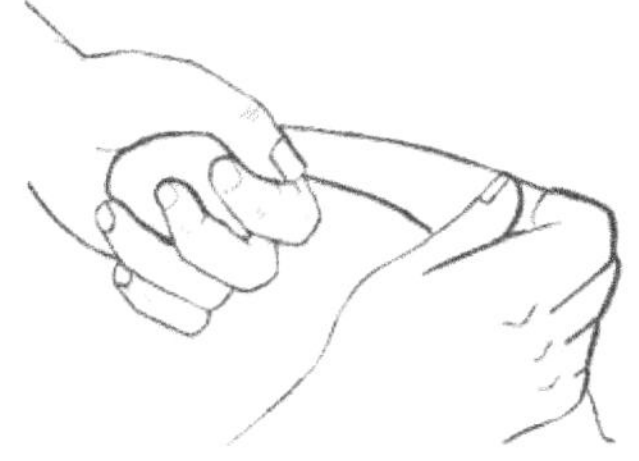

6. Extract the testicles

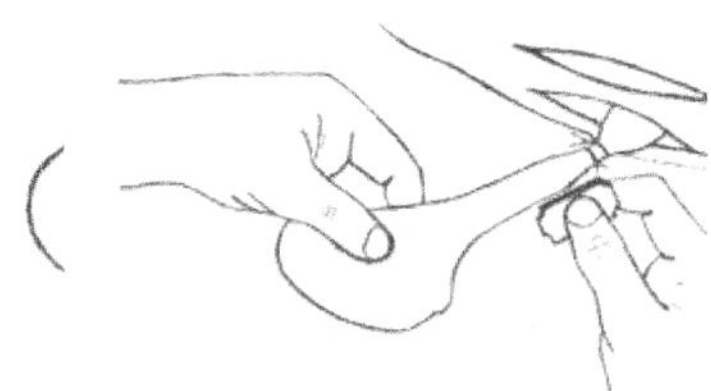

7. Cut the tunics and "pop" the testicles out

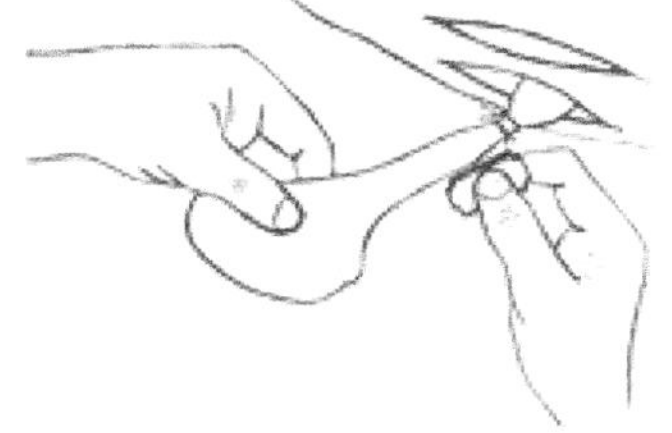

8. Crush the cords and cut below the crushed area

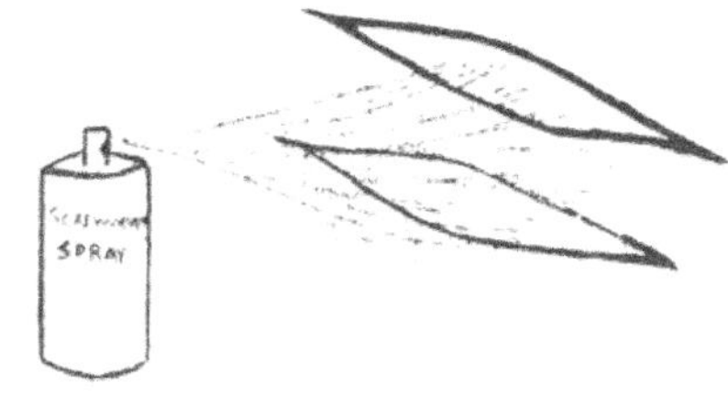

9. Treat the area with an anti-fly product to protect against screwworms

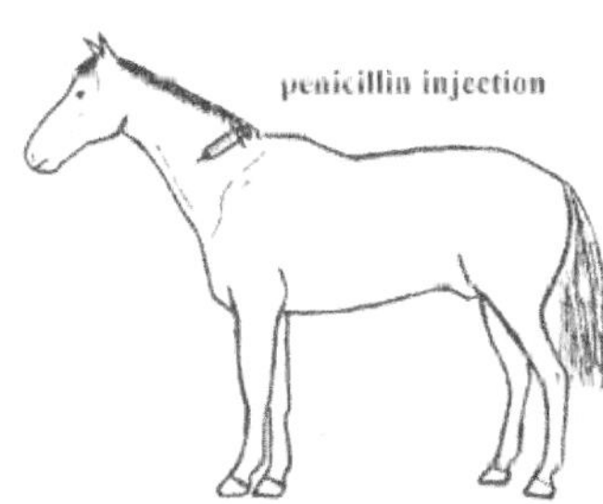

10. Give the horse an antibiotic.

11. Exercise the horse for five days after injection of castration to minimize swelling.

Castration of Pigs - Introduction

- Most people prefer to castrate male piglets for several reasons:
    - To prevent the risk of having boars around that are not needed for breeding (they can injure other animals or people).
    - To prevent boars from breeding their sisters, mothers and daughters, which would result in in-breeding.
    - To encourage fast growth.
    - To prevent unpleasant taste and odor in the meat (boars should be castrated at least one month before slaughter).
- It is best to castrate male piglets around two weeks to two months of age, since castration is less traumatic in younger pigs.

Castration Procedure for Young Piglets

- Have one person hold the piglet firmly by the hind legs above the hock. If necessary, the piglet can be squeezed firmly between the holder's legs.

- Feel the scrotum to check whether it may contain intestines (i.e. a hernia). If a hernia is present, do not castrate the pig, but find someone who knows how to treat hernias.

- Wash your hands and the animal's scrotum with soap, clean water and disinfectant.

- Draw the testicle into a pocket of scrotal skin by grasping it between the thumb and fingers. Make an incision through the skin of the scrotum and into the testicle itself. The incision should be parallel to the midline of the scrotum, and it should be about 1/2 to one centimeter away from the midline. This incision should be long enough to press the testicle out through the cut.

- Pull the testicle out and cut the cord near the body (or the cord may simply break as it is pulled). The other testicle can be removed in the same manner by making another incision on the opposite side of the midline. Make sure that the incisions are low enough for good drainage when the pig is standing; this will help the wound to heal more quickly.

- After the operation, all blood from around the incision should be washed away. If not, the blood will attract flies and later the wound will be filled with maggots. Put *Himax* ointment, *Lorexane Cream*, or another pesticide around the wound in order to keep the flies away. The piglet should also be kept away from dirty, wet areas until the wounds heal.

Castration of Older Pigs

- Castrating older boars carries a greater risk of bleeding and infection. As with older cattle, it is best to use local anesthetic. The blood vessels should be tied with cat gut (some people use fishing line or similar material). Be sure to make long incisions to encourage drainage. Make the pig walk during the week following castration to reduce swelling and to encourage drainage. Give the pig an injection of long-acting penicillin to prevent infection, including tetanus. Apply medicine to the wound daily to prevent maggot infestation.

10.11 ARTIFICIAL INSEMINATION (A.I.)

Artificial insemination includes the process of collecting semen from the male and, **at the correct time**, depositing this semen into the female's reproductive tract. If done correctly and at the proper time, the sperm from the male and the egg from the female join to create a baby.

Semen Collection: Semen contains many sperm and fluids from various glands. Semen Collection must be done in a way that keeps the sperm alive and healthy. The first step is to collect the semen from the male. Usually the male is put with a female animal that is in heat. Then when he mounts, his penis is directed into a container that is shaped like a vagina (called an artificial vagina). His semen then goes into a small bottle connected to the end of the "artificial vagina." The semen is put into a special solution to keep the sperm alive and healthy and to dilute the semen (since the semen from one collection contains enough sperm for many females).

Semen Storage: The diluted semen can be used immediately; or it can be frozen and stored for many years in a tank containing a special freezing chemical called "liquid nitrogen." A special machine is necessary to make liquid nitrogen. The tank must be checked routinely and more liquid nitrogen added regularly since the chemical evaporates whenever the tank is opened. If not checked regularly, the liquid nitrogen may evaporate completely causing the sperm to die.

Breeding the Female: When it is time to breed the female animal, the stored semen must be carefully warmed up; and then put into a long, skinny pipe (called a pipette). The pipette containing semen is inserted into the vagina of the female; and on into the cervix. When the tip of the pipette is just through the cervix, the semen is pushed out of the pipette (like giving an injection with a long needle). The sperm move through the uterus and into the oviduct where they may join with an egg.

Time of Breeding: The female must be inseminated near the time of ovulation (i.e. when the egg is released from the ovary). This is different for each species, but generally occurs near the end of the heat period. For instance, it is best to breed cows about 8-12 hours after heat.

One common problem is that some farmers do not recognize signs of heat, making it impossible to correctly time the artificial insemination. Or the animal may already be bred by a male animal (instead of by artificial insemination).

Successful artificial insemination requires that farmers recognize signs of heat. For **"heat detection,"** See page 133 and 164.

Advantages of A.I.:

• Fewer male animals are required. The semen collected at one time from a male can be diluted and used on several female animals.

• It may save money because an individual farmer does not need to keep, and feed, a male animal to serve just a few female animals.

• Semen can be brought from far away without having to bring in live animals. This may be important in remote places where transport is difficult. It will also prevent the possibility of bringing in new diseases carried by live animals.

• Through the use of AI, one can prevent the transmission of many venereal diseases.

• One can start a cross-breeding program without importing breeding stock which are often not adapted to the local conditions and become sick.

Disadvantages of A.I.:

• Owners must properly recognize the signs of heat in the female animal, or expensive semen may be wasted by using it at the wrong time.

• Special equipment and materials are required on a regular basis. Specifically, liquid nitrogen must be available or the semen will become warm and the sperm will die. This is a big problem in many developing countries.

• A trained AI technician must be available to put the pipette of semen into the animal.

• Efficient communication systems and transport are often needed to get the female animal bred at the right time. This is difficult in remote areas where most messages and supplies are carried by people who walk from one place to another.

10.12 METABOLIC DISORDERS RELATED TO PREGNANCY

Hypocalcemia - "Milk Fever"

- See page 270.

Ketosis in Cattle

- See page 253, 271.

Hypomagnesemia / Grass Tetany

- See page 272.

Pregnancy Toxemia in Sheep

- See pages 258, 277.

Systems of the Body and Associated Veterinary Problems

11.0 Digestive System

REVIEW

Any problem that interferes with **movement** of food through the digestive system, **breakdown** of food, or **absorption** of nutrients, will prevent proper use of food by the body. If the problem continues, eventually the animal will become thin and sickly, and suffer from **malnutrition**. See pages 125, 191.

> **Digestion** is the process of food being broken-down into smaller substances and absorbed from the digestive system into the body.

Function of the Digestive System
- To break-down food into smaller substances which are called nutrients.
- To pass nutrients to the blood.
- To carry the undigested food to the rectum so it can pass from the body as manure.

In other words, the following must happen:
- The food must **move properly through the digestive tract**;
- The various glands and organs must **secrete the proper digestive juices (enzymes)**;
- The digestive juices (and sometimes the good microorganisms) must **break the food down into small substances called "nutrients"**;
- The nutrients must be **absorbed into the bloodstream**.

TWO MAJOR GROUPS OF DIGESTIVE SYSTEMS FOR LIVESTOCK

Treatment of digestive problems depends on the type of digestive system an animal has.

Grass-eaters

Grass-eaters have digestive systems that are adapted to eating large quantities of grass and other roughages (although they can also eat grains and other feeds). Grass-eaters include cattle, buffalo, sheep, goats, llamas, camels, horses, ponies, and mules.

Non-grass eaters

Non-grass eaters can digest some young, tender, green grass and vegetables, but digest mature grasses poorly. They mainly need other kinds of food, such as grains, vegetables, and meat to survive. This group of animals includes pigs, chickens, dogs, cats, and most birds. They have what is called a "simple stomach."

BENEFICIAL MICRO-ORGANISMS - DON'T KILL THEM!

Grass-eaters are able to eat large quantities of rough grass because they have beneficial micro-organisms (bacteria and protozoa) which live in their stomachs and intestines. Grass-eaters that chew their cud are called ruminants. They include sheep, goats, cattle, buffalo, yaks, camels, and llamas. When they chew their cud, they mix the beneficial micro-organisms with the grass they have eaten. Similar micro-organisms also live in the large intestine of horses and rabbits.

These beneficial micro-organisms are responsible for digesting the rough part of grasses and leaves. In addition, they also produce some protein and B-vitamins which help the grass-eaters' bodies to grow and remain healthy. If the beneficial bacteria and protozoa die, grass-eating animals will not be able to digest their food properly. For instance, if an AHA feeds antibiotics (by mouth) to a grass-eating animal, these beneficial micro-organisms may die, and the animal may get indigestion.

Digestive tract of a ruminant

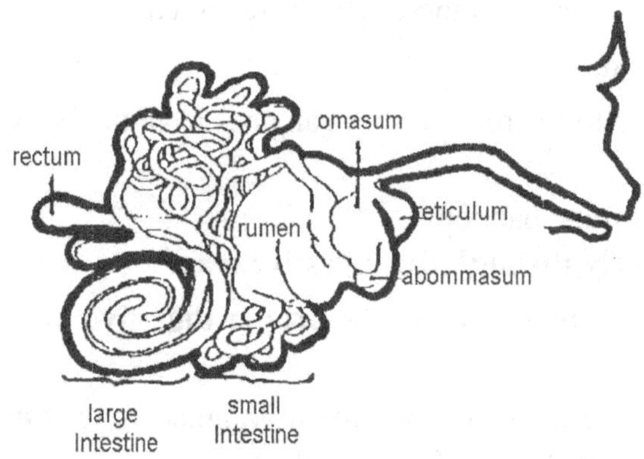

Digestive tract of a non-ruminant

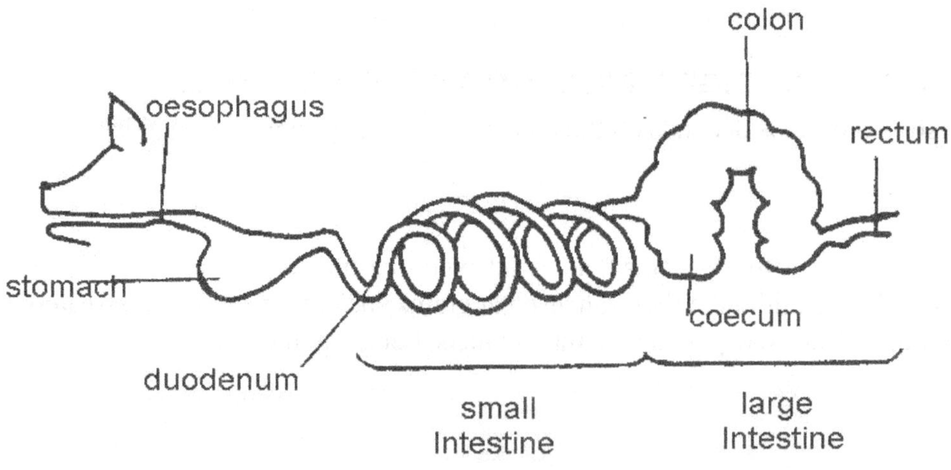

Digestive System Problems

11.1 LACK OF APPETITE (ANOREXIA)

The following problems may cause an animal to lose its appetite, and quit eating.

Sore Mouth: An animal with a sore mouth cannot eat properly.

Bad Food: An animal often will not eat food that tastes bad, is rotten, or is too salty. Similarly, if the food container is dirty and smelly, the animal may not eat.

Pain: Pain in any part of the body may cause an animal to eat less. Parasites, injuries, infections, constipation, and other problems can cause pain.

Bad Teeth: An animal with bad teeth cannot eat properly.

Lack of Water (dehydration) will cause an animal to lose its appetite.

Fever: An animal with a fever will usually quit eating normally. Similarly, an animal that is too hot will not eat properly.

Summary:
If an animal is not eating, and does not want to eat, usually one of the above problems can be identified.

11.2 PROBLEMS OF THE MOUTH (BITING, CHEWING AND SWALLOWING DISORDERS)

The lips, the teeth, and the tongue, are all necessary for proper biting, chewing, and swallowing. If an animal has saliva dripping from its mouth, or if it takes food into its mouth but cannot chew and swallow it, examine its mouth very carefully.

Before examining the mouth of an animal, take a proper history to make sure that it does not have rabies! An animal with rabies may appear to be choking on something, or unable to swallow. See pages 52, 251, 253. If in doubt about rabies, always wear plastic gloves to protect against the saliva of the animal.

Examination of the Mouth of Livestock and Horses

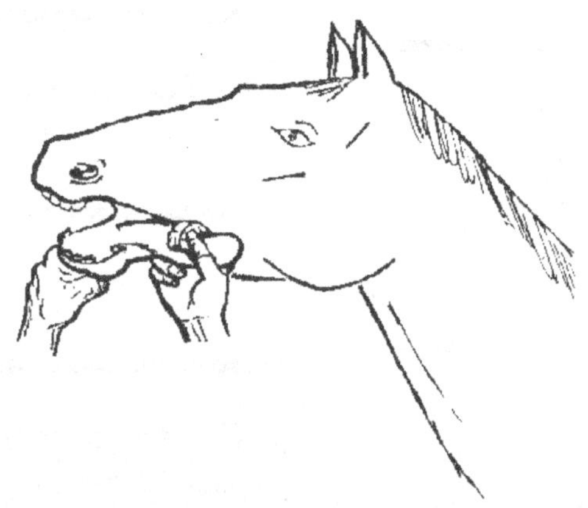

After making sure that the animal does not have rabies, do the following:

1. Put the animal in a crate, or cast it.
2. Grasp the tongue firmly, gently pull it out of the mouth, and examine it. Look for sores and infections in the mouth.
3. Place the tongue to one side between the molar (rear) teeth to prevent the animal from gritting its teeth or accidentally biting you (usually an animal won't bite its own tongue).
4. Carefully slide your hand over the top of the tongue and back to the throat. The hand should be kept in the middle of the mouth - as far away from the teeth as possible.
5. Feel carefully to determine if there is a sore in the throat, or if the animal has something caught in its throat.

General Treatment of Biting, Chewing and Swallowing Problems:

When an animal has a problem swallowing, or chewing, give it **soft food.** For example, give the animal a watery paste of cooked grain that does not require much chewing and can be easily swallowed.

11.2.1 Mouth Infection (Stomatitis)

An infection of the mouth is often called 'stomatitis.' A disease that also affects other parts of the body - such as Foot and Mouth Disease (a virus) can cause it. A foreign body such as a piece of sharp grass or wood that causes an infected wound in the mouth may also lead to a case of stomatitis.

Symptoms: Difficulty eating or swallowing, along with excessive salivation.
Diagnosis: Based on symptoms and examination of the mouth.
Treatment: If the wound becomes infected, rinse the mouth with a disinfectant like Potassium Permanganate solution or salt water. If the infection is severe, antibiotic injections should also be given. Penicillin is usually effective against stomatitis. Feed soft food.

11.2.2 Teeth Problems

Sometimes animals are not able to chew their food properly because of problems with their teeth. They can become very thin and sickly. The following four causes are among the most common:

1. The animal's upper and lower teeth may not be properly aligned to chew well.

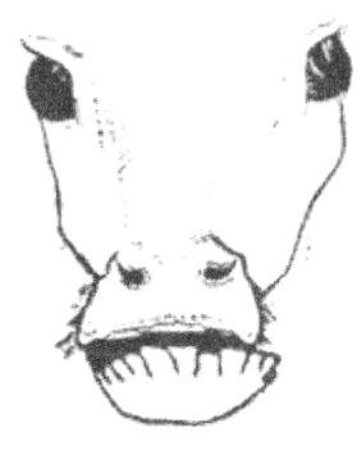

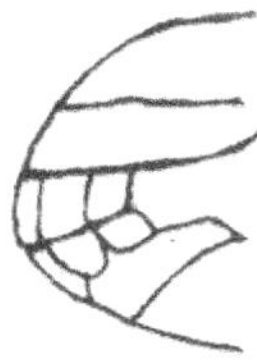

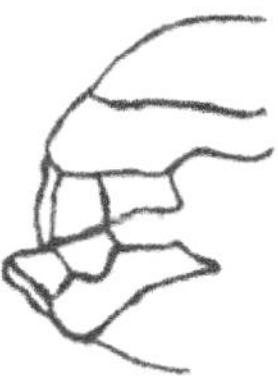

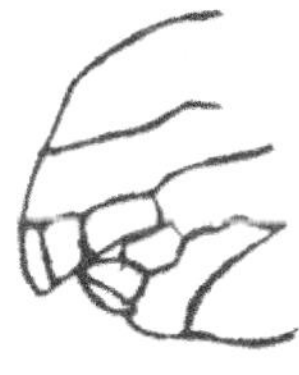

Cow with crooked mouth	*Horse with normal teeth*	*Horse with underbite called "monkey mouth"*	*Horse with overbite called "parrot mouth"*

Treatment of teeth that are not aligned properly: There is no treatment. The condition can be managed by feeding soft, high quality food. The animal should not be used for breeding because this condition may be passed on to future generations.

2. Painful, missing or infected teeth are more common in older animals, particularly on those which have been overgrazed on sandy soils. Teeth problems are also caused by calcium / phosphorus deficiencies, especially during the time of tooth development. In general, teeth problems can be reduced by providing mineral mixes and by preventing animals from overgrazing pastures.

The animal's teeth may be worn down or missing (especially a problem in old animals, particularly those that have grazed on sandy soil).

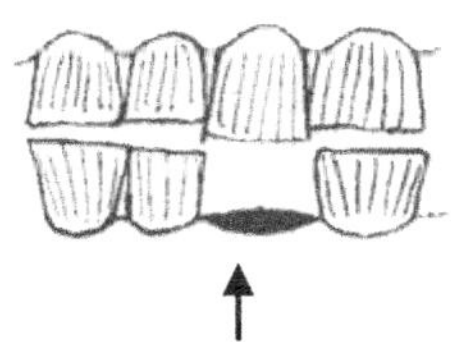

Missing molar

Symptoms: Difficulty eating or swallowing. Salivation.

Diagnosis: Check the teeth to see if one is rotten or broken, or if teeth are worn away.

Treatment for infected, painful teeth: It may be necessary to restrain the animal and remove the rotten tooth with a forceps or pliers. If the animal has a fever, give it antibiotic injections. Penicillin is usually effective. Feed soft food.

- Removal of the infected teeth. This is often difficult unless the animal is anesthetized or properly casted and restrained (See pages 18, 21, 26, 27.)

- **Anesthetize or cast the animal** and securely restrain it to avoid injury to itself and to you.

- **Hold the mouth open** with a mouth speculum or block of wood. Be careful not to damage the tongue.

- **Grasp the affected tooth** with a pair of pliers and wiggle it until it is loose enough to remove; then remove it.

Treatment of worn or missing teeth: There is no treatment. Old animals in this condition should be culled from a herd. The problem might also be managed with high quality feed and drinking water.

3. The animal's gums may be infected or rotten.

> **Treatment for infected, painful gums:** If the animal has a fever, give it antibiotic injections. Penicillin is usually effective. Feed soft food.

Infected gums

4. **The special case of horses.** The upper jaw of horses is wider than the lower jaw. This may cause the inner edge of the lower back teeth (molars) and the outer edge of the upper back teeth (molars) to become sharp.

Symptoms:	The horse may have sores on its cheeks and tongue, and much food may drop out of its mouth when the animal eats. Horses with sharp teeth often become thin.
Diagnosis:	Based on symptoms.
Treatment:	File the outer edge of the upper molars and the inner edge of the lower molars with a file (called a "float").

Upper and lower jaw showing
where the teeth become sharp (arrows)

Floating a horses teeth

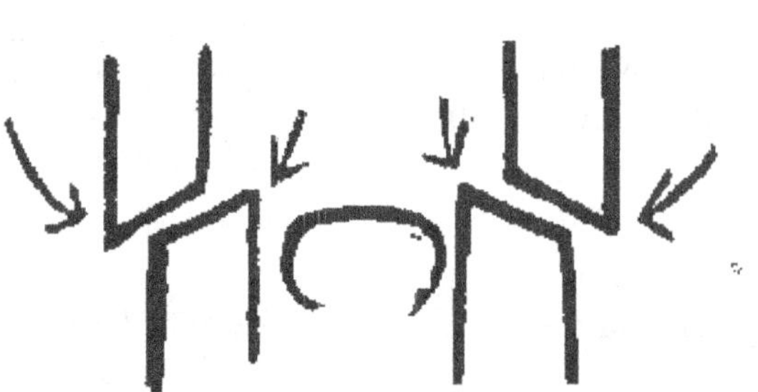

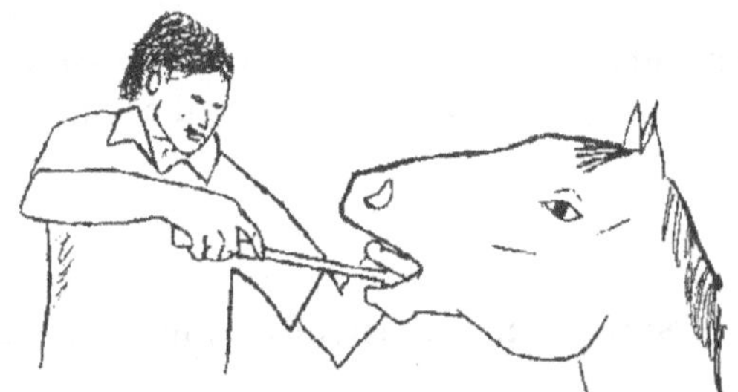

11.2.3 Infectious Diseases of the Mouth

Wooden Tongue and Lumpy Jaw

These are two separate, chronic diseases. They occur mainly in cattle, but are also seen in sheep and goats. Both of these diseases cause problems with chewing and swallowing.

Wooden tongue is caused by a bacterium called <u>Actinobacillus</u>. The bacteria enter through a small wound in the surface of the tongue. For instance, grass with sharp seeds may cause wounds on the tongue of livestock. These wounds can then become infected with <u>Actinobacillus</u> and the tongue becomes hard and swollen - like a piece of wood.

Lumpy Jaw is also caused by a bacterium. This bacterium is called <u>Actinomyces</u>. The bacteria enter through wounds in the gums, and affect the bones in the jaws of the animals. These wounds may then develop into bumps which have pus in them.

Symptoms: The animal finds it difficult to chew its food and swallow. The tongue or jaw becomes very swollen, and the animal becomes thin because it cannot eat properly.

Diagnosis: Based on the symptoms.

Treatment:
- Animals with Wooden Tongue make amazing, quick recoveries when treated with sodium iodide. For an average cow, give 125 ml of 20 percent sodium iodide, intravenously. If sodium iodide is not available, treat with combined pen-strep injections, or with penicillin injections, for approximately one week.
- Animals with Lumpy Jaw often do not respond well to treatment, and often require a long course of treatment with antibiotics and sodium iodide. Unless the animal is very valuable, it is better to consider selling it for meat.

Orf

This condition is also called **Contagious Ecthyma** or **Sore Mouth**. It is an acute viral disease of sheep and goats. Usually young animals are affected.

Symptoms: Sores develop on the skin of the lips, and may extend into the mouth. The sores may develop pus in them. Affected animals often stop eating, and saliva drools from the mouth. Sores may also develop on the feet, near the coronary band. These sores cause the animals to limp. Young animals are more often affected (since older animals are usually more immune). It is contagious, so many young animals in contact are often affected at the same time.

Diagnosis: Based on symptoms

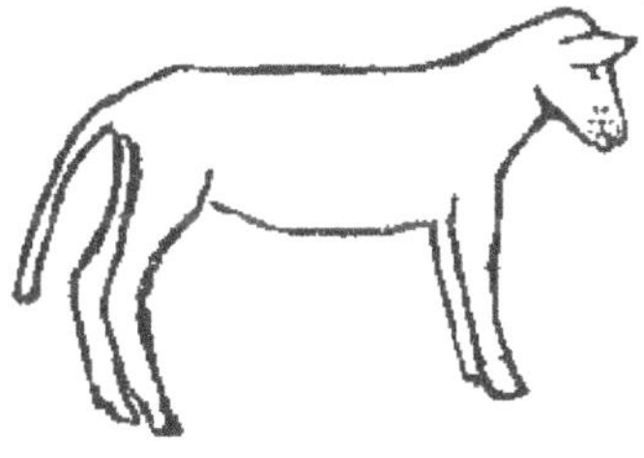

Treatment: The animals usually recover well without treatment, but young animals may
need to be coaxed to eat. If sores are severe, then wash out the mouth with an
antiseptic like potassium permanganate solution. If the sores become infected
and filled with pus, give penicillin injections. Gentian Violet or antibiotic/fly
ointments work well when applied to sores on the lips.

- Note: An AHA should wear gloves because Orf can also spread to people.

Foot and Mouth Disease

This is a disease of ruminants and pigs. It may cause sores in the mouth which prevent livestock
from eating properly. It also causes animals to develop sores near the feet, so they become lame and
unable to walk properly. See pages 49, 51, 223.

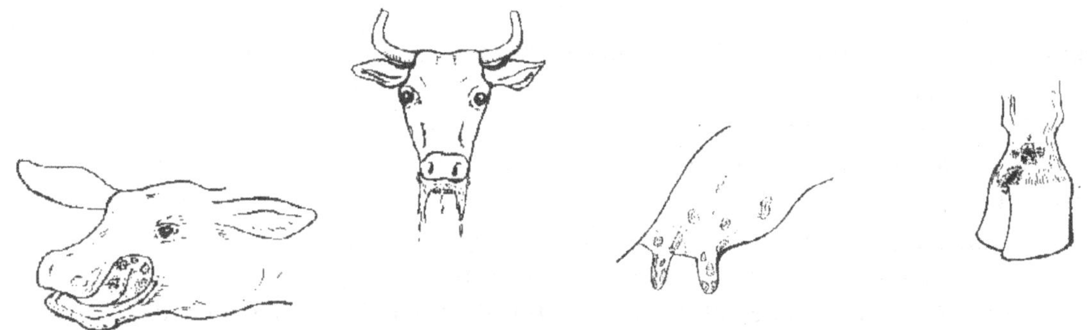

11.3 THROAT PROBLEMS

Sometimes an animal will be unable to swallow properly because it has a wound, or something
caught in its throat. This might occur if the animal eats something like a mango seed or avocado
pit, or if medicines are forced down its throat improperly.

11.3.1 Wounds in the Throat

Symptoms: The animal may drool and will not even swallow fresh green grass when offered
it. (First, take a proper history to make sure that it does not have rabies!
Then examine the animal's throat as described above.)

Diagnosis: Sometimes a small piece of wood, metal or other object will be found in the
animal's throat. Other times only the wound left from such an object will be found.

Treatment: Grasp the object and pull it out as gently as possible. Sometimes large pieces of
rotten tissue will come out with the object. Then, give an antibiotic injection (such as
penicillin) for 5 - 10 days to help with the infection.

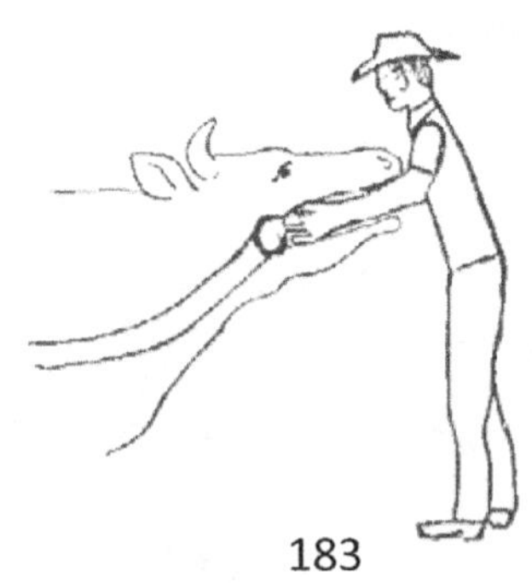

11.3.2 Blocked Esophagus ("Choke")

As the food is swallowed, it passes down the esophagus (the food-pipe) on the left side of the neck, and into the stomach. Sometimes the food becomes stuck in the esophagus and will not pass on to the stomach. The technical name for this is an "esophageal obstruction", or "choke."

> **Symptoms:** The animal will quit eating and often saliva will run from its mouth. Ruminant animals will begin to bloat rapidly, and the animal may shake its head and act agitated because it cannot swallow. Sometimes, the food may be seen, or felt, as a lump in the esophagus on the left side of the neck. Choke may occur when an animal eats a whole piece of fruit or vegetable (such as a mango, avocado, or potato).

> **Diagnosis:** Take a good history and rule-out rabies as a possibility. Try to feel the lump of food under the skin on the left side of the neck. Try to pass a stomach tube down the esophagus. If the tube stops abruptly before reaching the stomach, something is probably blocking the esophagus.

> **Treatment:** Massage the lump by hand or with a smooth stick, or try to push it down the esophagus with a stomach tube.

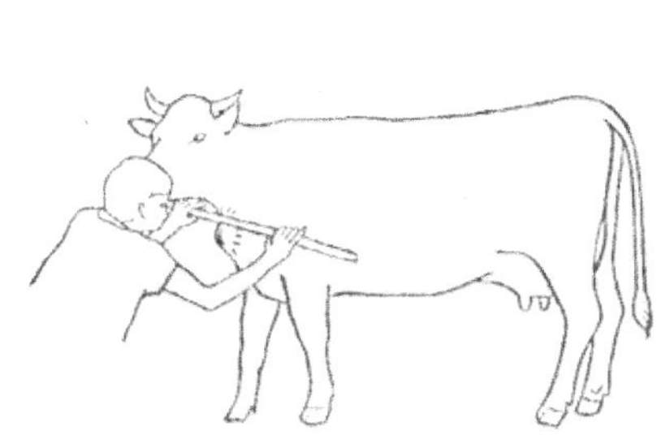 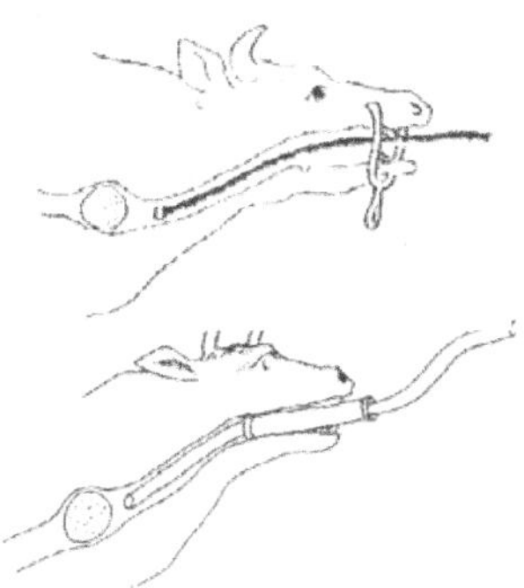

If this is unsuccessful, your only choice is to wait and, in the meantime, treat the animal's other symptoms (such as bloat). Hopefully, the lump will pass to the stomach on its own.

Prevention: It is best to prevent this problem by:
- avoiding those feeds that may cause choke;
- cooking things like potatoes before feeding them; and
- not grazing in areas where they may eat avocados, mangos or other things that could cause choke.

11.4 STOMACH PROBLEMS

The problems associated with the stomach vary depending upon type of stomach the animal has (e.g. ruminant or non-ruminant).

11.4.1 Stomach Problems in Ruminants

Overeating

Whenever an animal eats too much of anything (even good food), it can cause problems, such as bloat, diarrhea, indigestion, and/or laminitis (sore feet). If the animal has overeaten on grain, this should be considered an emergency.

Symptoms: Symptoms vary according to the substance eaten. See the following sections.

Treatment: As seen in the section on First Aid, page 80, the main treatment is to **get the food out of the digestive tract as rapidly as possible**. Because it is difficult for ruminant animals to vomit, it is easiest to feed medicine that will make them have diarrhea (like magnesium sulfate). The diarrhea then empties the digestive system.
Large animals: Feed 250 gm magnesium sulfate dissolved in water.
Small animals: 25 gm magnesium sulfate dissolved in water.
Some people feed local medicines which cause animals to vomit which may work even for ruminant animals.

Prevention: Regular provision of fresh drinking water may help to prevent overeating.

Bloat (Tympany)

Bloat occurs when too much gas collects in the animal's stomach (i.e. the rumen and reticulum).
This may happen when there is a sudden change in diet, particularly to more rich food (such as green, leafy forage or grain), when the animal eats poisonous plants, or when the animal has choke. The gas may build up to such an extent that the animal cannot breathe properly and may die unless the gas is rapidly removed.

Animals can die very quickly from bloat.

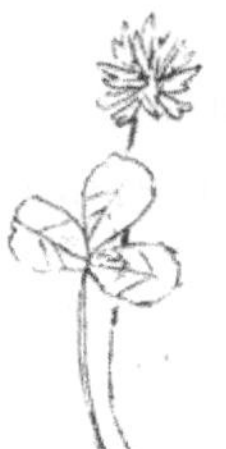

Causes of Bloat
- Choke
- Sudden change in diet.
    - corn and other grains
    - tree fodder
    - legumes (like clover)
    - rich grasses
- Eating poisonous plants

Note: Clover tends to make a gas mixed with some watery bubbles so that the animal cannot burp properly. This is called "frothy bloat."

Symptoms: (This is an **acute** disease)
1.	The animal's rumen is swollen and looks like a balloon. It is usually swollen on the left side, but in severe, acute cases the whole stomach looks swollen.
2.	In severe cases the animal will have difficulty breathing, and saliva may come from its mouth.
3.	There will <u>not</u> be a high fever.

Note:	Some animals always look like they are slightly bloated. This is called <u>chronic bloat</u>. It is not a problem that will cause an animal to die suddenly.

Diagnosis:

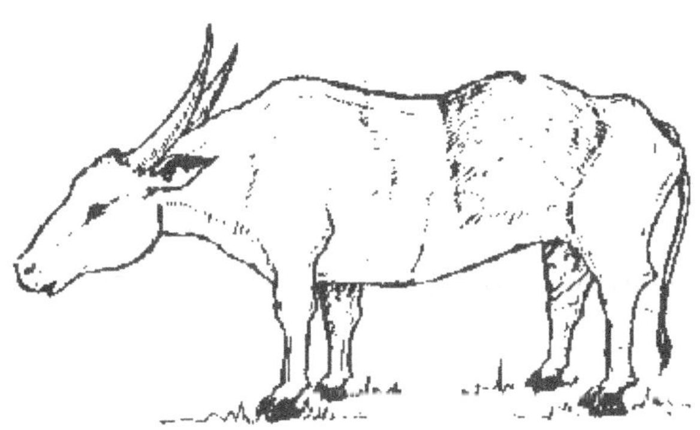

1.	Tap the animal's left side near the rumen. It will sound like a drum because it is filled with air.
2.	Check the animal for "choke."
3.	Verify whether there was a sudden change in diet, or the possibility that the animal ate some poisonous plants.

Treatment of Serious Bloat Cases:

The animal already has much air in its stomach and is having difficulty breathing. (If the animal is already lying down, it can die within minutes.)

  Warning! - If an animal is already gasping for breath, do not try to feed medicine because it may go into the animal's lungs!

1.	If possible, keep the animal on its feet and keep its head uphill. Quickly pass a **stomach tube** or flexible hose into the stomach. See page 60. Move the tube around in the stomach until the opening of the tube enters the gas pocket. You will know when this happens because much gas will rush out.
2.	If the animal is near death, and the gas cannot be successfully removed by a stomach tube, the rumen can be punctured on the left side with a knife or a special "trochar." If a special trochar is not available, **do not hesitate** to use a knife or other sharp object..
3.	Feed medicine as described below. After the problem with gas is relieved, if the rumen was punctured, do <u>not</u> suture it shut. Instead apply ointment to prevent infection and flies.
4.	Give antibiotic injections (penicillin) for 5 days to prevent infections of both the skin and the abdomen.

Site of insertion of trochar or knife into rumen (in emergencies only!)

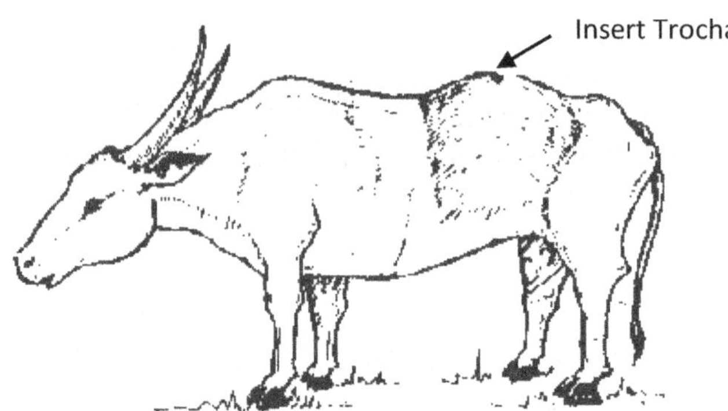

Place the trochar inside the cannula and rapidly force both through the skin at the indicated place on the left side of the animal. Then remove the trochar and the gas will rush out through the cannula. Leave cannula in place until the gas is gone, and then remove it also. If using a knife, simply stab through the skin at the proper site, and the gas will rush out.

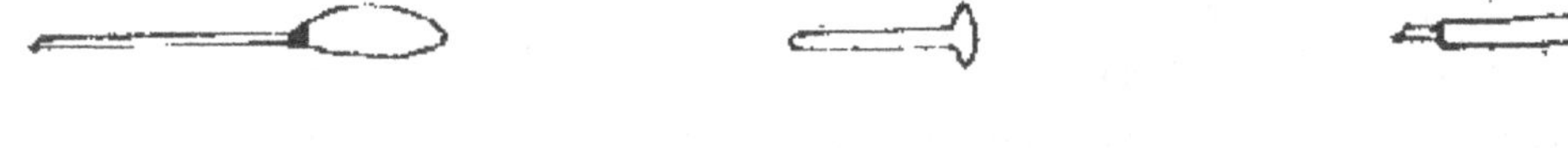

Trochar	Cannula	Trochar inside of cannula

Treatment of Less Serious Cases of Bloat

In less serious cases, the animal has already eaten the food. However, the animal is not gasping for air, still has some energy, and can move.

1. If possible, use a stomach tube to remove the gas.
2. Using the stomach tube, feed some oil (cooking oil or mineral oil) or some special bloat medicine. If using a stomach tube is not possible, carefully feed the medicine using a bottle or a piece of bamboo. If no bloat medicine or oil is available, feed the animal soapy water.
3. Some people also feed magnesium sulfate. The magnesium sulfate will cause the animal to have diarrhea and get rid of the food causing the gas. It will help to prevent the animal from bloating again.

    Dose for large livestock: 250 gm magnesium sulfate

    Dose for small livestock: 25 gm magnesium sulfate

Cooking oil or Mineral Oil

Animal:	Buffalo, cow, ox, goat, sheep, etc.
Dosage:	Large animals: 1 - 4 liters
	Small animals: 1/4 - 1/2 liter
Frequency:	Every 2-4 hours until recovery

Control/Prevention of Bloat:
- Avoid sudden changes in diet.
- Avoid grazing animals in areas where they might eat poisonous plants or things that cause bloat.
- Allow animals to drink water before feeding them.

Impaction / Constipation

Constipation is the term used for an unusually hard stool. The cause may be eating dry food without enough water, or not eating enough roughage.

Impaction is the term used when the stomach or intestine is packed with solid food which cannot move through the digestive tract. Like constipation, this usually happens when an animal lacks water or roughage. Constipation, if not treated in time, may progress to an impaction.

Symptoms: The animal has no appetite, does not chew its cud, has no stool, may appear uncomfortable, and may strain to defecate, but without success. If you press against the animals left side (against the rumen), it feels very hard and does not sound like an air-filled drum (i.e. bloat) because it is filled with solid material.

Diagnosis: The diagnosis is based on symptoms and a history of eating dry food without enough water or roughage.

Treatment: Ordinary cooking oil, or mineral oil, is a very effective treatment. For a big   animal, 1 - 4 liters of oil should be fed with a stomach tube or bottle. If the oil is too expensive, then try giving magnesium sulfate. See page 188. Provide several buckets of water. Since the animal may not want to drink, give the water by stomach tube, bottle, or bamboo tube. Treatment may be repeated twice daily. Offer fresh, green grass to help stimulate the digestive tract.

Treatment:
-Water!
-Mineral or cooking oil
-Magnesium sulfate
-Fresh, green grass

Control/Prevention: Animals should always be given lots of fresh water to drink. Fresh, green grass or other roughages are also necessary to keep the stomach moving properly.

Stomach Pain in Ruminants
(Indigestion in Ruminants)

Sometimes an animal quits chewing its cud and is not
eating properly. This often occurs after an impaction.
Also, it is often caused by **pain in the "belly"** from
various causes:
-Sudden changes in food.
-Constipation.
-Bad or rotten food.
-Parasites.
-Overeating grain.
-Feeding antibiotics.
- "Hardware Disease" (accidentally eating a sharp
object). See below on this page.

> **Indigestion** can also be caused by
> **feeding too many antibiotics** to a
> ruminant animal. These drugs kill the
> good microorganisms. Or,
> indigestion can be caused by **eating
> too much grain** all at once. This re-
> sults in acid production; and the good
> bacteria may die.

Symptoms: The animal quits eating and chewing its cud. It often has pain in its stomach and may even grunt with pain. There may be extra gas in the rumen.

Diagnosis: Based on physical exam and history

Treatment:

1. Treat any other obvious medical problems.
2. If the animal grunts with pain, and has a fever, use antibiotic injections. (Penicillin) to treat the infection in the rumen.
3. Provide fresh, green grass.
4. If possible, give Vitamin B injections to stimulate the appetite. See page 312. However, Vitamin B injections are expensive and it may be cheaper to simply give tasty, green grass.
5. Some stomach stimulant or other similar local medicine can be given to help the animal's appetite.
6. Seriously affected animals which have not been eating for a long time, can be treated by feeding several handfuls of grass from the rumen of a healthy animal. This grass contains the proper micro-organisms which will start growing again in the sick animal's rumen. This grass can be obtained from a place where animals are cut for meat; or one can take the grass from the mouth of a healthy animal when it is chewing its cud. This can then be fed by stomach tube to the sick animal. This process is called a rumen transplant.

Control/Prevention: Indigestion can be prevented by feeding antibiotics properly; by regularly feeding medicines for parasites; and by controlling what animals eat.

Hardware Disease

Sometimes an object, like a sharp piece of wire, is accidentally swallowed. This object can then scratch or puncture the wall of the stomach, causing pain and infection. Eventually, the wire can poke through the stomach and into the heart resulting in rapid death. Hardware disease is often a problem where recent house-building has taken place (and hardware such as nails and wire were left at the site), and where machines are used to cut the grass. The machines will cut up wire into small pieces, making it easier for the animals to accidentally swallow a piece when they are grazing.

Treatment: If these animals can be referred to a veterinary doctor, sometimes
an operation can be performed and the wire removed; or a magnet can be placed
in the stomach to attract the hardware and keep it from puncturing the stomach wall.

- If the animal has a fever, give penicillin injections as described in the
  section on treatment of stomach pain.

11.4.2 Stomach Disorders in Non-Ruminants

Colic in non-ruminants

Colic is a common term meaning pain in the belly (i.e. the stomach or intestines).

This is a **very common problem in horses** but is also seen in other animals.

Colic has many causes including excess gas, constipation, impaction, lack of
proper blood circulation to the intestines (due to parasites), or twisting of the intestines.

Symptoms: Symptoms of colic include lack of appetite, restlessness, rolling, kicking
at the belly, sweating, rapid heartrate (due to the pain), inability to pass manure,
and sitting like a dog.

Diagnosis: Primarily based on symptoms. An experienced veterinarian may do a
rectal palpation to feel for excess gas or an obstruction in the digestive tract.
However, this is a risky procedure for an inexperienced person.

Treatment: The animal should be given pain killers like aspirin, xylazine,
Paracetamol or *Novalgin*. See Medicine Chapter. The animal can also be
fed some oil (cooking or mineral oil, liquid paraffin) or magnesium sulfate.
The animal should be walked to help stimulate its digestive tract (and possibly
pass some manure or gas) and to keep it from rolling and thrashing. Once the
animal recovers somewhat, it should be fed worm medicine.

Prevention/Control: Give worm medicine regularly, according the needs of the
geographical area. Avoid sudden changes in feed.

Vomiting

This is more of a problem in non-ruminants (except for horses which cannot vomit). It can
occur as a result of eating rotten food or poison, or because of a block in the digestive tract.

Symptoms/Diagnosis: Determine the cause of the vomiting. The history is often helpful,
especially if the owner knows what the animal has eaten.

Treatment: The treatment depends upon the cause. In the case of poisoning or bad food, the
animal may vomit and empty its stomach. Magnesium sulfate can also be fed to help
cause diarrhea which will help the animal get rid of the poison. For a blocked
digestive tract, there is little you can do except feed some magnesium sulfate or
oil to help dissolve the obstruction.

11. 5 INTESTINAL PROBLEMS

Intestinal problems of both ruminants and non-ruminants can be considered together.

11.5.1 Diarrhea

This is a complex problem with many causes. The most common cause of diarrhea in livestock in developing countries is related to **internal parasites**. Parasites can damage the liver as well the lining of the stomach and intestines.

> **Causes of diarrhea in livestock**
>
> - Parasites
> - Dirty food or water
> - Sudden change in diet

> **Problems associated with diarrhea**
>
> Acute Diarrhea -> Dehydration
>
> Chronic Diarrhea -> Malnutrition

The main problem associated with acute diarrhea is **dehydration.** The main problem associated with chronic diarrhea is **malnutrition**.

Dehydration occurs when too much water leaves the body and the body's cells cannot work properly, nor can the blood move properly. Any animals with acute diarrhea (including people) should be checked for dehydration and given plenty of fluids. See page 55. Even animals with chronic diarrhea should have lots of fresh water to drink.

> **Treatment of Diarrhea**
>
> **(General)**
>
> 1. **Fluids** are the most important treatment. Many animals can be saved by simply giving enough water to drink.
> 2. Parasite medicines
> 3. Kaolin or similar medicines to slow down the diarrhea.
> 4. Antibiotics (if animal has a fever also).

Acute Diarrhea

Background: Livestock usually get acute diarrhea from:
- A sudden change in diet.
- Eating food or water that contains bacteria or viruses.
- Eating foods that are difficult to digest.
- Eating poison or dangerous plants.
- Certain parasites (coccidiosis).
- (Rarely) by drinking too much milk, other rich food, or colostrum.

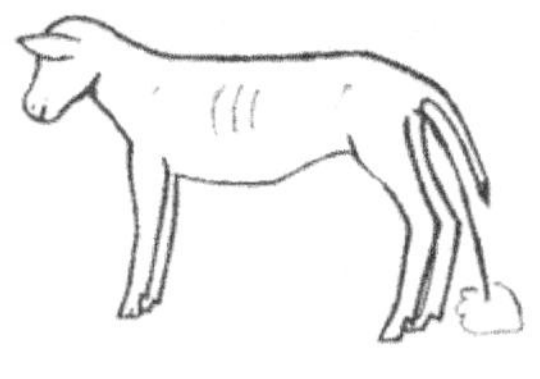

- Young goats and sheep that are left home during the day while the mothers graze commonly get diarrhea. This happens because they become thirsty and hungry, and then drink dirty water or eat old food.
- Pigs can get diarrhea after being fed rotten food.

Symptoms: The animal gets diarrhea and may have a fever. Sometimes (but not always) there may be blood in the diarrhea. The animal may act sick and quit eating.

Diagnosis: The AHA must decide whether this diarrhea is simply due to a change in food, or whether it is an infectious diarrhea. This is based on the history (what did the animal eat); whether or not there is a fever; whether or not the animal appears really sick.

1. If the animal acts sick and has a fever, the diarrhea is probably caused by bacteria or viruses. Exception: Newborn or very young animals (e.g. pigs, calves, lambs, kids, foals) often become cold and listless when they have diarrhea, and the cause is usually a bacterium or virus (or both).
2. If the diarrhea has red blood in it, suspect coccidiosis. This is seen especially in young cattle, in young sheep and goats, in chickens and in rabbits. See page 297.
3. The animal may not act sick and may not have a fever. This diarrhea is probably due to a change in feed or too much rich feed.

Treatment:

1. Fluids. (See page 105) Even very sick baby animals can be saved with fluids given by mouth. Its best to give small amounts of fluid frequently until the animal starts to make urine normally again.
2. Kaolin and similar medicines may help stop the diarrhea.
3. Antibiotics. These are important to give to the animals which have diarrhea and fever at the same time. Sulfadimidine is effective, cheap and easily available. (It may also work against coccidiosis.)
    Caution: Feeding antibiotics by mouth to adult grass-eating animals may kill the good micro-organisms in their stomach resulting in indigestion. Therefore, only feed antibiotics by mouth if the grass-eating animal has severe diarrhea and a high fever. See page 189.
4. Coccidia Medicine: See page 298.

Control/Prevention: The most important factor is sanitation. Animals should always have clean, fresh water to drink. The food should be fresh, and it should not be fed from the floor.

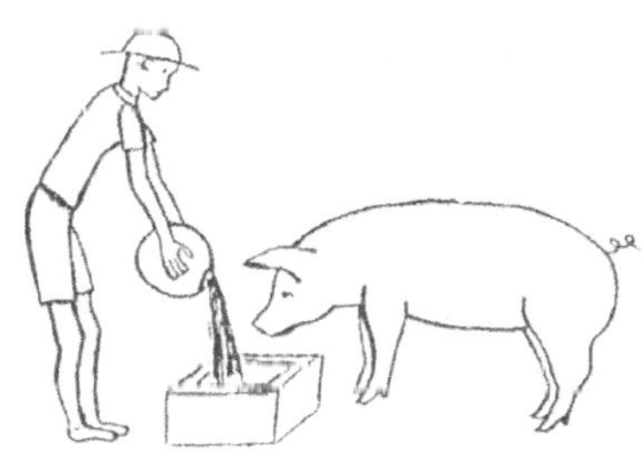

Chronic Diarrhea

> **Background:** The most common reason for chronic diarrhea is **parasites**.

> **Symptoms:** The animal has diarrhea; and may have had problems with loose stools for a long
> time. Sometimes the diarrhea occurs every day; and sometimes it is intermittent.

> **Diagnosis:** Diagnosis is usually based on symptoms and history. When taking the history,
> verify when the animal last received parasite medicine and how frequently it has been
> given. Also, ask about the duration of the diarrhea. If it has been going on for months,
> the internal organs may already be permanently damaged. Then the animal may never
> get well, no matter how it is treated. At that time, it is important to warn the owner and
> ask them why they did not come earlier. (Remind them of the need to treat their other
> animals regularly for parasites.)

> **Treatment: Water** is the most important treatment. Specific treatment depends on what
> parasites are most common in the area, the species of the animal, and the age of the
> animal. See Chapter 9 for details on treatment of parasites.

> **Control/Prevention:** See section on internal parasites. The most important thing to
> remember is simply: ***Prevention is better than Cure.***

Bloody Diarrhea / Dysentery
By definition, diarrhea with blood in it is called **dysentery**.

Chronic dysentery is often due to parasites.
Symptoms and Diagnosis: The animal has a history of chronic diarrhea with blood in it.
Often the animal has not been fed parasite medicine regularly.
Treatment: Treat the animal for the most likely parasite, according to its age and how it is kept.

Acute dysentery may be due to:
- Parasites (especially coccidia).
- Bacteria and viruses (bad food).
- Poisons or poisonous plants.

Symptoms: The animal gets diarrhea which contains blood. The animal may have a fever,
be lethargic and quit eating. If the animal has dark, bloody things that look like
intestines in its diarrhea, it is very serious.
Diagnosis: The diagnosis is based on symptoms and a good history. Find out whether the
animal may have eaten poison, or some poisonous plant. In addition, take the
temperature and examine the diarrhea.
Treatment: The same as other types of acute diarrhea - except that it is more serious and
should usually be treated with antibiotics. If the animal is young, be sure to treat it with
coccidiosis medicine. Also, give fluids and kaolin.
Control/Prevention: Sanitation is important! Shepherds should be extra diligent during the
rainy, wet season. Animals must not be allowed to graze fodder that may be dangerous
to them.

11.5.2 Blood in the Stools (without diarrhea)

If the **stools are red or black** in color, then there is bleeding into the digestive tract. This can be caused by many reasons, including poisons and rich foods. In livestock it is most serious if blood is accompanied by diarrhea.

If the bloody stools look very black, then the bleeding is happening in the stomach or in the beginning of the small intestine. If the bloody stools look more red, then the bleeding is closer to the rectum, probably in the large intestine.

If there is a wound in the wall of the stomach or the intestine, this wound is called an **ulcer**. Blood can come out from these ulcers. Wounds can also be caused by parasites - but then the animal usually has diarrhea as well.

Symptom/Diagnosis: See blood in stools.
Treatment: Give the animal some feed that is not too rich, but is easy to digest (like tender green grass).
Control/Prevention: All animals should regularly be given medicine for parasites.

11.6 INFECTIOUS DISEASES OF THE DIGESTIVE SYSTEM

11.6.1 Infectious Diseases Affecting the Stomach and Intestines:

Enterotoxemia / Pulpy Kidney / 6- Month Disease

This is an infectious disease caused by a bacteria <u>Clostridium perfringens</u>. This disease mostly affects sheep, goats, pigs and horses. Young animals seem to be more often affected. These bacteria live in soil, manure and the intestines of ruminants and produce toxins (poisons) that normally cause no problems. However, when an animal eats a lot of rich food (milk, rich pasture or different grains), the bacteria may reproduce quickly and make a lot of toxin which gets into the blood and makes the animal very sick.

Symptoms: Often the animal is found dead before symptoms are even noticed. Sometimes, the animal may breathe rapidly, stagger, and convulse, as well as have a fever, diarrhea (sometimes with blood), and/or bloat. Death can follow shortly. When the dead animal is cut open, parts of the intestines may be filled with a reddish, watery diarrhea. The kidney may also look soft and rotten.

Diagnosis: Diagnosis is usually based on the symptoms and history. In some countries, special lab tests can also be done to confirm the diagnosis. There is usually a history of eating a lot of rich food. The problem is more common in "improved breeds" which might be given better quality feed. In pigs, the disease occurs during the first few weeks of life. It can also occur in young lambs 2-10 months of age, particularly when the new green grass is just coming out. This is why it is called 6- months disease, because it happens twice a year.

Treatment/Control: Treatment of sick animals is very difficult. Often, no matter what is done, the animals die. Piglets can be given 1 cc of penicillin in the mouth, once daily for 3 days. Mildly ill animals can be treated with magnesium sulfate and stomach stimulants. Control is very difficult unless a vaccine is available. In many countries, a vaccine is available that is given to pregnant mothers (especially goats) and also to young animals at about 1 month of age. It usually must be repeated (follow the instructions on the vaccine package).

If milking goats are fed so that they give lots of milk, their babies may be more susceptible to this disease.

Rinderpest

This is a very infectious disease caused by a virus. It is the one of most feared diseases in the world because it is highly fatal. Cattle, buffalo, pigs and other animals with split hooves can get this disease.

In some countries, the disease was controlled for many years by vaccination. However, the disease resurged when the vaccination stopped.

The virus is spread in the feces, in the saliva and in the breath of sick animals. Although it affects several systems in the body, it seems to mostly affect the digestive system.

Symptoms: The animal begins showing symptoms within 3-15 days of contact with the virus (i.e. an incubation period of 3-15 days). Symptoms include high fever, discharge from the eyes and nose, lack of appetite, followed by diarrhea, dehydration, labored breathing and often death. Small red wounds develop on the lips, nose, mouth and tongue which can become infected (and make the breath smell bad).

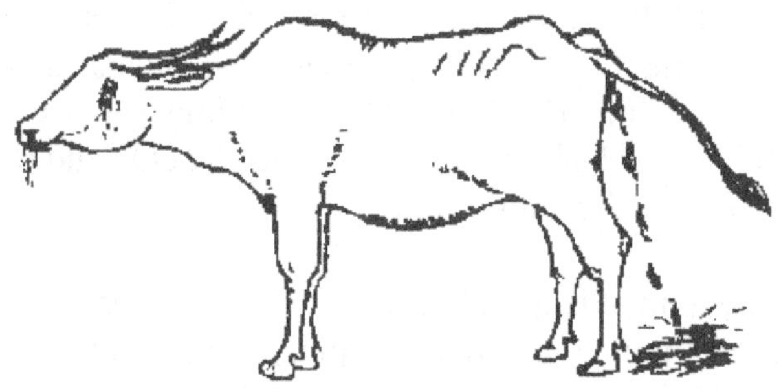

Diagnosis:

When a dead animal is examined, the abomasum is very red and has many wounds (ulcers) on it. The mouth, pharynx, and vagina may also have wounds in them and have a bad smell to them. The liver and spleen may be swollen.

Treatment/Control: Treatment of sick animals does not work. Most sick animals simply die. If they do recover, then they have immunity for the rest of their lives. In areas where Rinderpest occurs, all young animals reaching 6 months of age should be regularly vaccinated. The vaccine should give animals immunity for the rest of their lives. In areas where no vaccination has been done, young animals will not receive Rinderpest antibodies from their mothers' colostrum. Therefore, these young animals should be vaccinated along with the other animals, even before they reach 6 months of age.

Anthrax

Anthrax is an acute infectious disease that can affect almost all mammals. It is caused by a bacteria, <u>Bacillus anthracis</u>. It usually causes death in cattle, buffalo, sheep and goats. However, affected pigs and horses become sick but often do not die. Animals get anthrax from the soil or from eating blood or bone products from infected animals (e.g. blood meal). Once the blood from an infected animal mixes with the soil, the soil is contaminated, and the bacteria (spores) can live there for years. Anthrax is a **public health disease**. It spreads easily to humans when they handle the meat, blood or wool of infected animals. See page 95.

Symptoms: Sometimes the animals die so quickly that no symptoms are seen. However, the dead animal may have black blood coming out of its nose, mouth or anus. If the animal has not yet died, it may have a high fever, difficult and rapid breathing, a swollen throat, and black blood around mouth or throat. If pigs in an area seem to develop swollen throats for no apparent reason, and then often recover, suspect anthrax. Anthrax is sometimes hard to distinguish from HS.

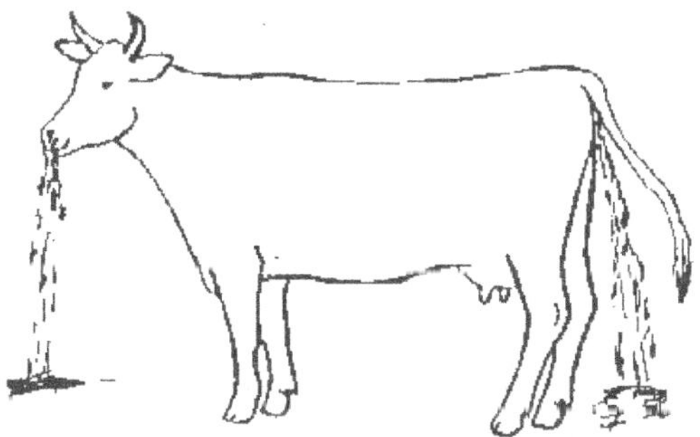

Cow with anthrax; bloody nasal discharge and bloody diarrhea

Diagnosis: Based on the symptoms. It is also possible to make a thin blood smear. Stain the smear with several drops of new methylene blue, and examine it with a good microscope (the microscope must have a good light). Then, the AHA can see the bacillus with the capsules or spores.
Caution! Once the blood is exposed to air, anthrax spores develop. A person who inhales these spores may develop anthrax in the lungs. Persons handling the meat or blood of an infected animal may also develop anthrax. If you suspect an animal has died of anthrax, avoid cutting it open since you will contaminate the soil indefinitely and risk getting anthrax yourself.

Treatment: If the animal is just breathing hard, treat it with tetracycline, just like pneumonia. For pigs with swollen throats, treat with tetracycline or penicillin.

Prevention: Vaccines are available in many countries. Carefully follow the instructions on the package insert to know how to care for and administer the vaccine.
Caution: Vaccinating against anthrax *during* an anthrax outbreak is risky for an AHA. Animals that are already incubating the organism at the time of vaccination may still get sick from anthrax and die. The owner may then believe that the vaccine killed the animal and request some repayment for the loss of the animal. Try to vaccinate the animals in the area *before* an outbreak begins. This is often difficult. Some farmers tend to wait until they hear of an anthrax problem and then want to vaccinate during an outbreak.

Swine Fever
This is a viral pig disease also called **Hog Cholera**. It is a very dangerous, rapidly contagious disease.
It affects the whole body but is put in this section because it causes diarrhea also.

> **Symptoms:** Symptoms begin with a fever, then progress into diarrhea and weakness. The pigs
> may also develop a discharge from the eyes and nose; and become weak and wobbly in
> the hind legs. Most pigs die within a week, although a few may recover.

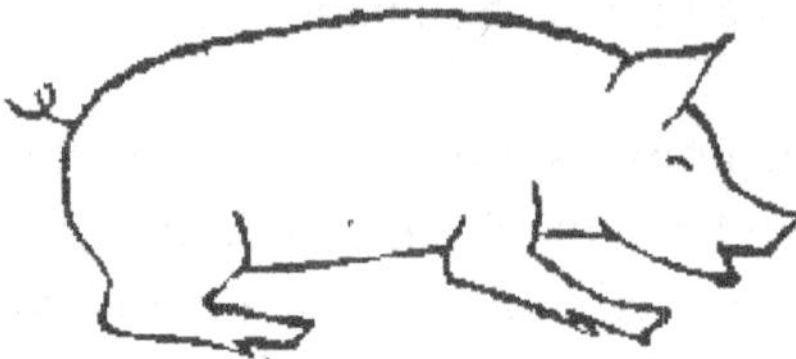

Sow with hog cholera (high fever resulting in open-mouth breathing).

> **Diagnosis:** A tentative diagnosis is based on the history and symptoms, and confirmed by post
> mortem specimens and observations. During the post mortem exam, small ulcers can
> often be seen in the large intestine near where it joins the small intestine. Usually the
> history will indicate that most pigs in an area are becoming rapidly and seriously ill.

> **Treatment:** None.

> **Prevention/Control:** Check with veterinarians or the Ministry of Agriculture for available
> vaccine.   In most countries, this disease must be reported immediately to the district
> veterinarian. All sick pigs should be strictly isolated. People from the outside should not
> go near them because this disease can be spread on food, on clothes, and even by birds.

Liver Disease
Liver Disease is difficult because it usually happens along with other problems. However, it can be
considered as part of the digestive tract.

> **Symptoms:** Animals suffering from **Acute Liver Disease** get quite ill and quit eating. This is
> seen more often in humans and dogs than livestock or horses.   Liver disease in livestock
> is usually chronic and may result in permanent liver damage. Chronic liver disease is
> most often due to liver flukes, immature larvae of large roundworms, or eating poisonous
> plants. An animal with liver disease may also have a swollen throat.

> **Diagnosis:**   An animal with liver disease may have "jaundice" resulting in yellow coloring
> under its eyelids, on the whites of its eyes and on its gums. Diarrhea may also be present.
> If the animal has already died, the liver may be hard and crumble easily.

> **Treatment:**   Liver damage is usually permanent. However, the extent of the damage is
> difficult to know. The AHA should treat the animal for liver flukes (if it is a known
> problem in the area) and other parasites. Some liver fluke medicines may affect the
> liver (especially CTC). Learn which liver fluke medicines are available in your area
> and try to use those which do not affect the liver.

> **Control/Prevention:** Treat regularly for parasites

Systems of the Body and Associated Veterinary Problems

12.0 RESPIRATORY SYSTEM

Review

When an animal breathes, air enters its mouth or nose. Oxygen, one of the gases in air, is essential for life. The body gets its energy from the nutrients in food, but needs oxygen in order to do this.

From the nose to the lungs, the respiratory system provides the passageway that allows oxygen and other gases to enter the body. After oxygen reaches the lungs, it moves inside red blood cells. These cells carry oxygen to every part of the body, which uses the oxygen and produces carbon dioxide ("used" gases). "Used" gases are then transported by red blood cells back to lungs. When the animal breathes-out, the "used" gases are then sent outside the body.

When it is too hot, the body also cools itself by using the respiratory system. Even if an animal, like a working oxen or a sow, is not sweating much, it can cool itself by giving off warm air as it breathes. This is why animals breathe faster, or with their mouths open, when the weather is too hot, or when they have a fever.

Function of Respiratory System
-Brings fresh air (oxygen) to body -Removes used air (carbon dioxide) from body -Keeps the body cool

Any part of the respiratory system, from the nose to the lungs, can be affected by various disease conditions. This chapter will consider only the most common respiratory problems affecting livestock.

Most Common Problems of the Respiratory System
-throat infections -lung infections -chronic lung damage -poisoning -allergic reactions

12.1 SYMPTOMS OF RESPIRATORY DISEASE

Procedure:

I. Stand quietly and observe the animal from a distance. A healthy animal breathes almost effortlessly. However, if any of the following signs are seen, there may be a respiratory disease:

Symptoms:

-Increased respiratory rate
-Difficult breathing
-Eye and nose discharge
-Coughing and sneezing
-Swollen throat
-Swollen stomach
-Fever

1. **Increased respiratory rate** (can also increase from overheating, pain or fear)
2. **Difficult breathing**
    * Flaring of the nostrils
    * Open-mouth breathing
    * Breathing with the neck extended
    * Jerky movement or extra effort of the rib muscles
    * Well-developed line of muscles across the animal's ribs (also called "heave-line" and is associated with a chronic respiratory problem; also called "heaves" in horses).

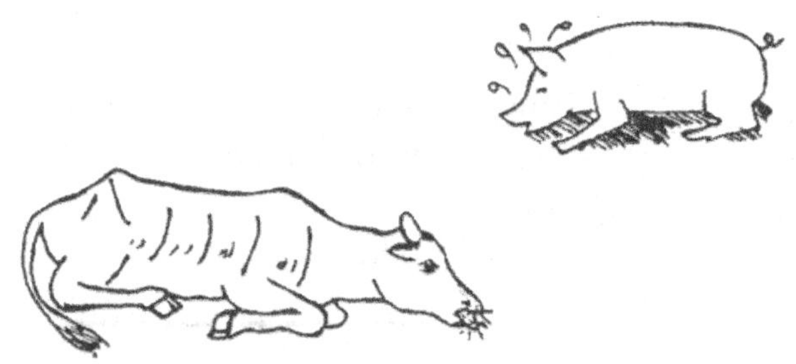

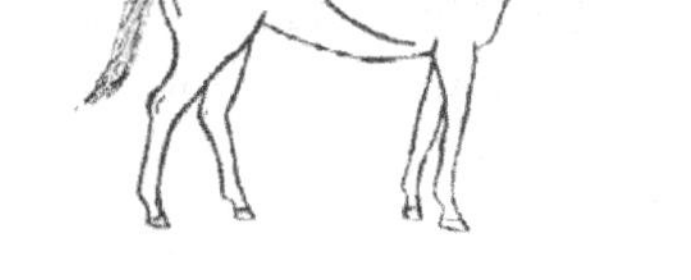

Horse with "heave-line" across its abdomen.

3. **Discharge** from nose and eyes.
4. **Coughing and sneezing.**
5. **Bloated abdomen** - Many animals that are having difficulty breathing (especially cattle and buffalo) may look slightly bloated. This is not because of a stomach problem. Rather, when they breathe rapidly, some of the air goes to their rumen instead of to their lungs. In fact, many farmers complain that their buffalo or oxen is "bloated" when the real problem is in their lungs or throat!
6. **Swollen throat.**

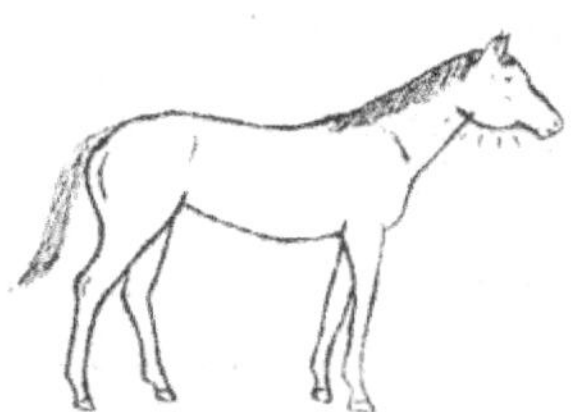

II. Move close and examine the animal carefully, including whether it has a fever.

12.2 DIAGNOSIS OF RESPIRATORY DISEASE:

A proper history is especially important when deciding how to treat an animal with respiratory disease.

In general:

- Animals with chronic respiratory problems do not get well easily - and they are often expensive to treat.
- Acute respiratory problems can usually be treated more effectively than chronic respiratory problems.

1. Take a history. Is it acute or chronic?
2. Examine the animal carefully and thoroughly. Remember to take the temperature.
3. Use the following chart to guide the choice of treatment.

<u>**Signs of Respiratory Disease**</u>
- Increased Respiratory Rate.
- Difficult Breathing.
- Discharges from Nose and Eyes.
- Coughing and Sneezing.
- Swollen Throat.

---

1. Take History - Acute or Chronic??

Acute (less than 4 days)		Chronic (more than 4 days)	
2. Take Temperature		2. Take Temperature	
Acute with Fever	Acute with No Fever	Chronic with Fever	Chronic with No Fever
Diagnosis	Diagnosis	Diagnosis	Diagnosis
Bronchitis/ Pneumonia	Poison	Old Pneumonia	Liver Fluke/ Other Parasites
H.S.	Allergy	Tuberculosis	Lungworm
Anthrax		Throat Infection	Emphysema
			Tuberculosis
Treatment:	Treatment:	Treatment:	Treatment:
Tetracycline	Magnesium Sulfate or other poison medicine	Tetracycline	Parasite medicine
	Antihistamine/ Steroids	(Recovery is difficult!)	(Recovery is difficult!)
	Antibiotics		

12.3 CONTROL / PREVENTION OF RESPIRATORY DISEASE

General Principles:

There are **many causes of respiratory problems**. However, a good farmer can do certain things that will prevent livestock from becoming ill with respiratory disease:

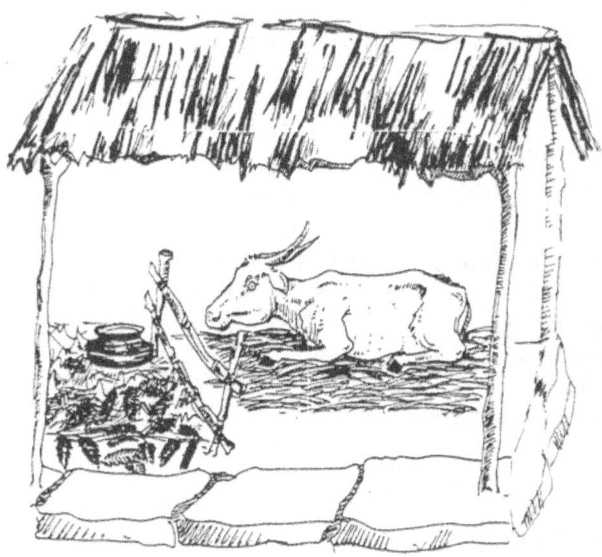

1. **Protect livestock from very hot and very cold temperatures**. Make the sick animal as comfortable as possible. Provide shade and extra water in hot weather, and shelter from cold and wind in cold weather. Exposure to difficult temperatures makes animals weak, and they become ill with common microorganisms that do not normally cause disease.

2. **Provide fresh air**, even in very cold weather. Animals should be protected from the wind, but should not be shut inside a barn with all doors and windows closed.

3. **Separate sick, coughing animals** from healthy animals to prevent disease spread.

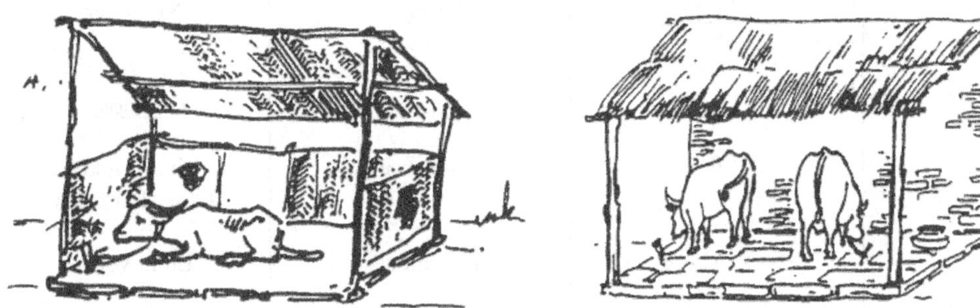

4. **Treat regularly for parasites. Lungworms** and **immature large roundworms** often damage the lungs, allowing harmful microorganisms to cause a respiratory infection.

5. **Keep livestock well-nourished**. Animals that are already **weak** from **malnutrition** and/or **parasites**, are more likely to develop respiratory problems.

6. **Vaccinate for diseases commonly found in the area.**

12.4 RESPIRATORY SYSTEM DISORDERS

12.4.1 Swollen Throat

Causes:
-Chronic parasite problem.   See chapter 9.
-Infectious diseases:
    Hemorrhagic Septicemia.   See page 205.
    Anthrax.   See page 196.
    Strangles in horses.   See page 208.
-Object, wound or infection in throat. See page 183.

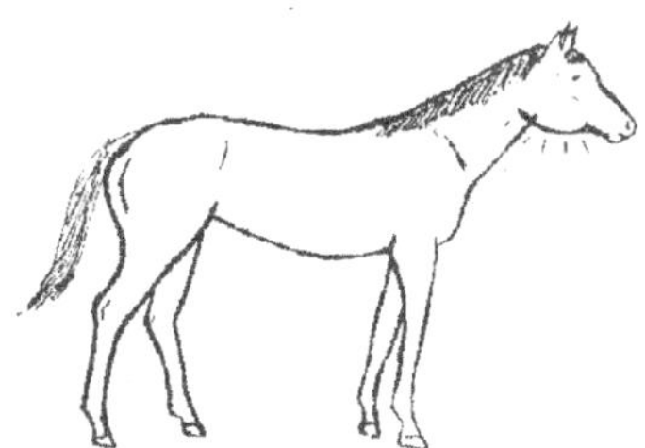 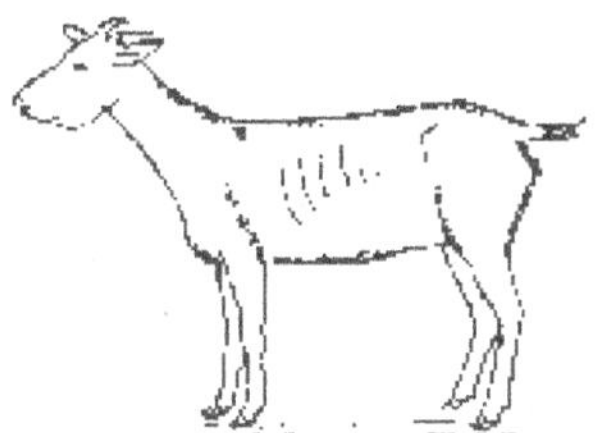

Symptoms:
-Often associated with cough.
-Fever (if caused by infectious disease).
-If caused by infectious disease, then usually other respiratory symptoms are also seen.
-If the animal coughs when the AHA holds the throat, this is a sign of an infection in the throat.

Treatment:
1.   If there is no fever, then simply treat for the most likely parasite (e.g. liver fluke, small roundworms and/or lungworm).
2.   If associated with infectious disease, treat the specific disease.
3.   If the animal has something in its throat, remove it and treat with antibiotics.

12.4.2 Blood from the Nose or Mouth

Sometimes an animal may have blood around its nostrils or around its mouth. This is most often due to bleeding in the nose or throat. However, it can also be from bleeding deeper down in the lungs, causing the animal to cough up blood (e.g. an old abscess in the lungs that finally ruptures and causes bleeding).

Symptoms/Diagnosis: Determine if the bleeding is from one nostril or from both nostrils. If the bleeding is from one nostril, then there may be parasites (leeches or maggots), a wound or a tumor in that particular nostril. Look for swelling. Find out if leeches are a common problem in your area.

If bleeding is from both nostrils and the animal is breathing very hard, then suspect that the bleeding is in the lungs. This is a very serious condition and there is little an AHA can do.

Treatment:

For maggots.	See pages 118-119.
For nasal leeches.	See page 112.

For bleeding from the lungs: keep the animal quiet and offer plenty of water to drink.

Control/Prevention: See sections on leeches and maggots.

12.4.3 Bronchitis

This is usually a mild respiratory problem resulting from an infection in the lungs. It is usually an acute problem but can become chronic if not treated properly.

Symptoms/Diagnosis: The respiratory rate is usually increased and there is a slight change in the way the animal breathes. A slight cough is also common, sneezing may occur and a nasal discharge develops. A fever is also present.

Treatment: The animal should be treated with antibiotics. Tetracycline is the best antibiotic for killing the common microorganisms that cause respiratory problems.
The animal should be treated for 3-5 days with the antibiotics.

12.4.4 Pneumonia

This is usually a more severe respiratory problem. It is usually an acute disease. It is also caused by an infection in the lungs. Animals can die very quickly if not treated.

Symptoms/Diagnosis: The respiratory rate is usually very rapid and the animal appears very sick, often "gasps" for breath, and has a high fever. There may also be a cough and the throat may appear swollen.

Treatment: The animal should be treated with antibiotics. An injection of tetracycline is the best. However, if no one is available to give an injection, then tetracycline boluses can be used. Treatment must be continued for 3-5 days, even if the animal gets better sooner.

12.4.5 Lungworm

The presence of lungworm can often look like pneumonia or bronchitis. However, the animal usually does not have a fever. See pages 332-333. The presence of lungworm makes the animal more susceptible to other lung problems like pneumonia.

12.4.6 Emphysema

This is a chronic problem affecting the lungs. The lung tissue has been damaged and does not work properly. In livestock, emphysema is fairly common in buffalo, cattle, and horses. The cause is not clear. It may be associated with **chronic liver fluke** problems, tuberculosis, or result from pneumonia. In horses, it may be related to an allergy.

Symptoms/Diagnosis: The respiratory rate is rapid but there is usually no fever. The animal tires quickly when walking. Usually the animal has difficulty exhaling, since the lung tissue has lost its elasticity. This may be seen as extra abdominal effort or extra effort of the muscles along the ribs each time the animal exhales. There may also be a "heave line" which is extra muscle development along the ribs to help the animal exhale.

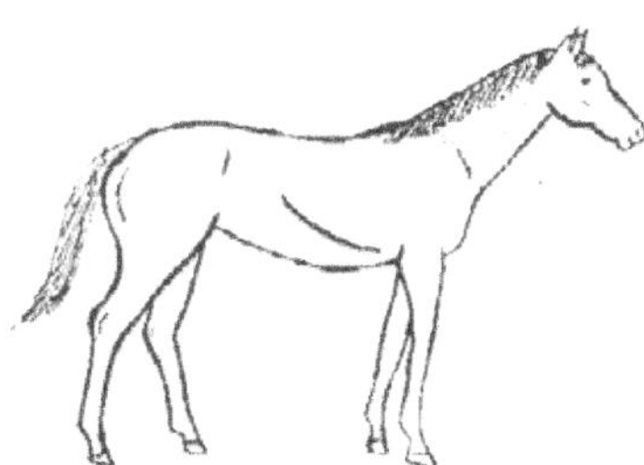

Treatment: Usually treatment is not very effective. Treat for parasites. Affected livestock might still produce milk if they do not exert themselves much, and if food and water are carried to them. Sometimes horses improve with antihistamine treatment and a well-ventilated environment.

12.4.7 Poisonings

Some types of poisonings cause respiratory problems. See page 81. For example, some plants contain cyanide, which causes difficult breathing. The animal will salivate and breathe rapidly. The history will usually indicate the possibility of eating poisonous plants.

12.4.8 Allergic Reactions

Some animals get a reaction when they eat certain plants, or are bitten by certain insects, or snakes. This reaction may cause the entire head to swell to the point that the animal cannot breathe properly. See page 82.

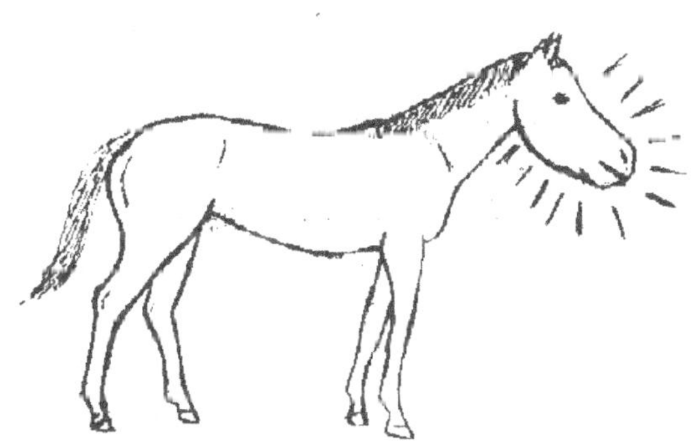

12.4.9 Hemorrhagic Septicemia

Hemorrhagic septicemia (HS) is also called "septicemic pasteurellosis." It is an acute, infectious disease, which mostly affects cattle and buffalo. Buffalo seem most easily affected and young animals die very quickly. HS really affects the whole body, including difficulty in breathing.

HS is caused by a bacteria, <u>Pasteurella multocida</u>. This bacteria lives in the throat of animals that have had the disease and recovered. The bacteria are then spread in the saliva and nasal droplets of the animal. The organism of HS produces a toxin that travels throughout the body and causes severe illness.

Animals that have just traveled a long distance, or are stressed and weak for some other reason are susceptible to HS. It is also called "Shipping Fever" since it often occurs shortly after animals have been shipped under difficult conditions.

Symptoms:
-     Sudden death.
-     High fever (104-107 degree F).
-     Swollen throat (sometimes the entire head may appear swollen).
-     Difficulty breathing and swallowing.
-     Saliva dripping from mouth.
-     Stomach may be swollen due to difficulty in breathing.
-     Diarrhea sometimes with blood.

Diagnosis: Diagnosis is based on symptoms and a history of no vaccination against HS. Sometimes HS is very difficult to distinguish from anthrax. However, in anthrax, black blood is often seen coming from the mouth, nose or anus, and the spleen may be enlarged on post mortem examination.

Often, more than one animal is affected since the disease is very contagious and can spread throughout an entire village.

Examine the dead animal: Often there are little spots of bleeding under the skin, on the intestines and in the heart. A yellow, sticky fluid is often seen in the tissues of the swollen throat. This same fluid may be seen around the heart, lungs, and intestines. A blood smear should be taken from the blood in the heart or the spleen and examined in the laboratory.

Treatment: In some outbreaks of HS, treatment may be unsuccessful. Tetracycline injections in high doses might work, especially if given early in the course of the disease. If tetracycline is not available, then use any other antibiotic you may have.

Vaccination/Control: It is important to immediately separate sick animals from healthy animals. It is also important to keep susceptible animals separated from animals that may be carrying these bacteria in their body. (For this reason, it is often recommended to kill animals that have recovered from HS.)

Many government veterinary services provide vaccines against HS (there are several HS vaccines available). It usually takes at least one week from the moment of giving the vaccine to protect the animal. Therefore, it is best to vaccinate beforehand and not wait until an outbreak begins.

An AHA should carefully explain to farmers that the vaccination requires 2-4 weeks to protect the animal. A farmer will then understand that if their animals die within the week after vaccination, it is because the vaccine had not yet started to work.

12.4.10 Tuberculosis (TB)

This is a **chronic, infectious disease** found in most species of animals, and in people. Because it can be spread between livestock and humans, it is called a "**Public Health Disease.**" TB is caused by a bacteria called <u>Mycobacteria</u>. There are three main kinds of these bacteria: the bovine kind (cattle and buffalo), the human kind, and the bird kind. Livestock and humans can become infected with all three kinds.

People and animals with TB in their lungs usually develop a chronic cough, become thin, and slowly die. TB organisms can also live in other parts of the body including the digestive system, the reproductive system, and the udder. The symptoms may vary depending upon the part of the body affected. In cattle, the organism tends to settle in the lungs, whereas in poultry, it goes to   the intestinal tract. In many countries, no one really knows how many livestock have TB. In other countries, the problem is well documented in both people and animals.

Spread of disease:
1. **By air:** Infection is usually spread by breathing in drops of saliva when a sick animal (or person) coughs. This is a big problem in cold countries where cattle are kept in closed barns for many months during cold weather. If there is not good ventilation in the barn, the cattle will be more likely to breathe contaminated air.

2. **By food or water:** Occasionally infection can take place by eating food which has the   bacteria in it. For instance, drinking the milk from infected cows may infect pigs, calves and people. When an infected animal drinks, the saliva from its mouth may contaminate the water. Another animal that drinks from the same water source may become infected.

Symptoms: The symptoms depend upon where the organism is in the body. There may be rather vague symptoms or no symptoms at all. Sometimes the animal gradually becomes thin, develops a chronic cough, and if producing milk – has low milk production. If the organism has also affected the intestinal tract, the animal might have diarrhea.

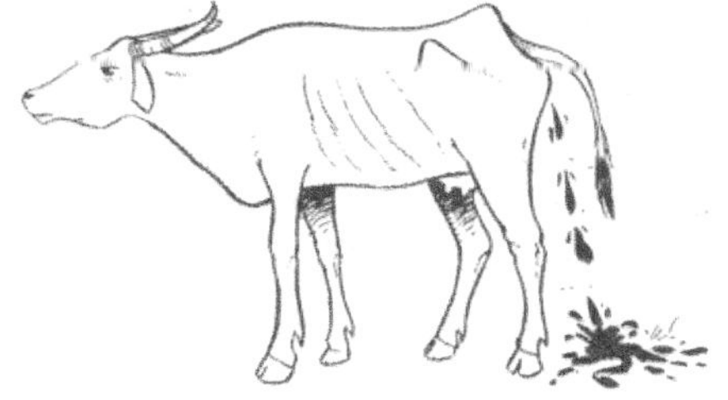

Post Mortem: Wherever these bacteria end up, they begin to form a type of abscess. These abscesses are called **"tubercles."** Tubercles may be as tiny as a speck of sand. Or, they may be as large as an egg. Sometimes these tubercles contain thick pus; and sometimes they may be hard like rocks. Eventually these tubercles ruin the tissue so much that the organs don't function normally.

1. **Respiratory TB**: Tubercles begin to grow in the lungs. The animal will cough and become thin.

2. **Digestive System TB:** Tubercles may form around the organs of the digestive system, (such as the intestines), sometimes causing diarrhea.

Diagnosis: Observe the symptoms. During post mortem examination, try to preserve a piece of tubercle and its surrounding tissue in 10% formalin or 50% glycerin. A lymph node near the tubercle is also a good specimen to collect and preserve. The specimens can then be sent to a veterinary laboratory for diagnosis. The government veterinarians may also want to do some special testing of other animals in contact with affected animals to determine how many animals actually have the disease.

Treatment: It is not recommended to treat livestock with TB. They should be killed to keep the disease from spreading.

Control: According to the law in some countries, all animals must be tested with tuberculin. If an animal has a positive test or is confirmed to have tuberculosis, it cannot be sold. Rather it is killed to keep the disease from spreading. By strict testing of all animals and slaughtering those with TB, the disease can be controlled.

In countries where TB is a significant health problem, the World Health Organization (WHO) recommends that all human babies be vaccinated at birth with BCG. Similarly, any person with a chronic cough should have their saliva tested for TB. In addition, all milk should be thoroughly boiled; and all meat should be well cooked to prevent transmission of the disease.

12.4.11 Ephemeral Fever:

This is an acute viral disease of cattle that occurs sporadically; and sometimes several animals can be affected at about the same time. It is also known as **"3 Day Sickness."** It is seen mostly in the rainy season and is thought to be spread by insects. Most animals recover on their own with no treatment.

Symptoms: Affected animals have a sudden high fever, difficulty in breathing, lack of appetite, as well as lameness and stiffness (sometimes the animal refuses to stand). Lactating animals will experience a major drop in milk production. Other symptoms may be shivering, discharge from the eyes and nose, excess salivation, difficulty swallowing, and extra fluid under the skin, particularly around the joints.

Diagnosis: The diagnosis is difficult and based on symptoms. Symptoms can include a combination of lameness, fever and difficulty breathing, as well as the tendency for most animals to recover on their own.

Treatment/Control/Prevention: No treatment is available. Efforts should be made to keep the animal as comfortable as possible. Give the animal aspirin or any other medicine that relieves pain and reduces fever. If the animal cannot stand, be sure to provide for soft ground and provide it with water, shade (in hot weather) and protection from the wind (in cold weather).

12.4.12 Strangles

This is an acute infectious disease of horses. It is caused by a bacteria, Streptococcus, which affects mainly young animals. It causes abscesses in the lymph nodes of the neck, which may eventually burst and drain through the skin or nostrils. The pus from these abscesses contains the bacteria which spread to other horses when eating food contaminated by the pus.

Symptoms: Affected horses have a loss of appetite, a high fever, and pus draining from the nose. The throat area is usually swollen and very painful, and the horse often extends its neck to relieve the pain. Abscesses develop around the throat which break open and drain through the skin and nose. Once the abscesses open and drain, the animal gets well quickly.

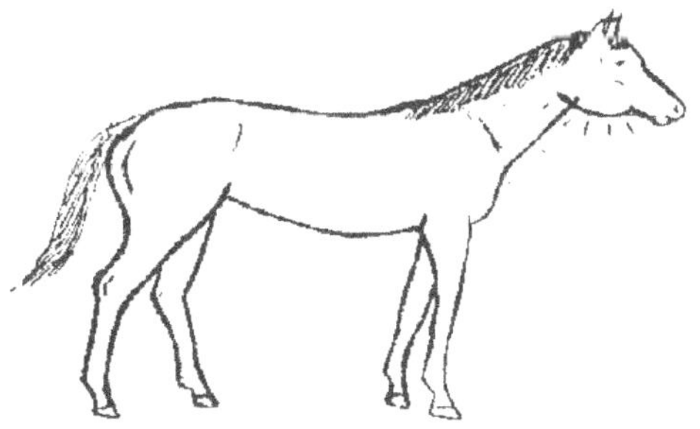

Diagnosis: Diagnosis is usually easy and based on symptoms.

Treatment: Use penicillin as soon as signs are seen and continue until the horse is well. Try to place a hot compress on the abscess (be careful because the area is very painful) to ripen the abscess so that it can be lanced and drained as soon as possible. See abscesses, page 220.

Prevention: Horses diagnosed with strangles should be isolated so that other horses do not become contaminated by the pus.

13.0 MUSCULAR SYSTEM

REVIEW:

The function of the muscular system is to allow movement of the body and the internal organs.

For a muscle to work properly, several things are required:
1. A nerve to bring it messages.
2. Nutrients and oxygen which are brought to it through the blood.
3. Veins to carry the used-up nutrients away.
4. Regular exercise in order to remain strong and healthy.

13.1 MUSCULAR SYSTEM DISORDERS

13.1.1 Atrophy / Paralysis

When a muscle does not work, it shrinks and weakens, which is called **atrophy**.

Injuries as a cause of atrophy

A common reason for atrophy is injuries.
1. Paralysis. This is the term used when a limb cannot move. This is often due to damage to the nerves that are connected to the muscle, or damage to the main nerve (spinal cord) in the backbone.
2. Serious injury to bones or joints (e.g. fractures or arthritis) may make the animal unable to use its muscles, and then the muscle shrinks (i.e. atrophy). If the animal recovers, and begins to use its muscle, it may regain its normal size again. For a complete discussion of paralysis, see page 259.
3. Atrophy may result from an injury to the muscle itself, to the tendons which attach to it, or to the blood vessels which go to and from the muscle.

Nutritional deficiencies as a cause of atrophy

Certain vitamins and minerals (e.g. vitamin E and selenium) are necessary for muscles to function properly. If vitamin E and/or selenium is deficient in the diet of young calves and lambs, the muscles cannot work properly. In these cases, paralysis can occur without any sign of injury.

13.1.2 Lumps and Bumps

Abscesses/Hernias/Seromas

Sometimes an animal will be seen with a lump on its side or on its belly near the umbilicus, or near the scrotum. This can be from several causes: an abscess, a hernia or a seroma/cyst. For more details, see page 220 under the "Skin System."

13.1.3 Diseases of the Muscles

There are many diseases caused by the bacteria <u>Clostridium</u>. Two of these diseases, called **Blackquarter (Blackleg)** and **Malignant Edema,** are closely related and have similar symptoms.

Blackquarter (BQ) (Blackleg)

This is an acute, infectious disease that is quite common in some geographic locations. It is seen mostly in cattle. However, a similar disease is also seen in buffalo, sheep and, very rarely, in pigs.

The bacteria that causes this disease (<u>Clostridium chauvoei (feseri)</u>) is found in the intestines of animals and in the soil. This bacteria forms a protective shell (spore) that allows it to survive for a long time in the soil. The bacteria pass through the wall of the intestine and enter the blood, and then travel to the muscles where they can cause the disease. These bacteria can also enter through wounds in the skin.

This disease is seen mostly in young cattle between 6 months and 2 years of age. It is also seen in sheep, usually after shearing.

Symptoms:
- Lameness – usually one of the first symptoms.
- Rapid onset; sometimes sudden death (i.e. within 1-2 days).
- Grunting due to pain.
- Swelling – possibly of one leg, neck, back, or on the side.
- High temperature.
- Rapid breathing.
- No movement of the rumen.
- The skin of the affected area becomes dark and dry. Air (gas) collects in the muscles and under the skin. When the swelling is pressed a crackling sound is often heard due to the air and gas.

Diagnosis: A blood smear from the muscle swelling should be made and examined by the district veterinarian. (This blood smear will help to distinguish BQ from anthrax.) Do not do a post-mortem in case it is Anthrax. However, if you do cut into a muscle affected by BQ, it will appear black and dry, and will smell bad.

Control and Prevention:
- Bury dead animals more than one-meter-deep to prevent the jackals and wild dogs from digging them up. If possible, a layer of lime should be put directly on the body before it is covered with soil and stones. 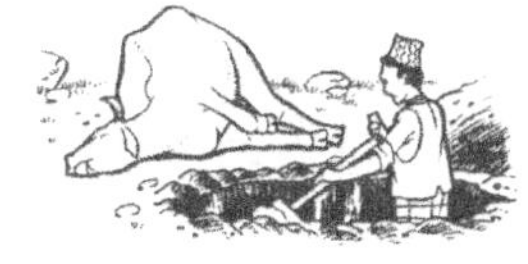

- In areas where BQ is found, all cattle between the ages of 6 months and 3 years should be vaccinated. If at all possible, sheep should also be vaccinated. 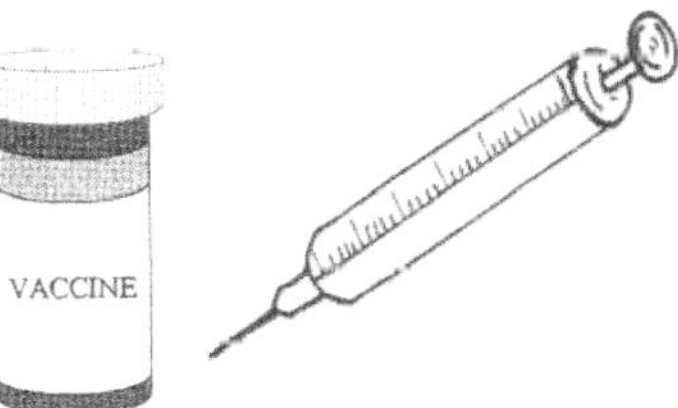

Treatment:

- Penicillin and other antibiotics like Tetracycline can be used in high doses to save some animals if they are treated early, but most animals die even with treatment.

Malignant Edema

This is an acute, infectious disease, difficult to distinguish from Blackquarter. Malignant edema is most common in cattle and sheep but, unlike Blackquarter, it can also be seen in pigs and horses.

The bacteria, <u>Clostridium septicum</u> is found in the intestines of animals and in the soil. It forms spores that can live in the soil for a long time. The bacteria usually enter the body through wounds caused by accidents, tail docking, castrations, and unclean vaccinations. Similarly, the uterus can become infected if the person assisting with the delivery has dirty hands or arms.

Symptoms: Similar to Blackquarter except that less air (gas) collects under the skin. Instead the swellings may contain more jell-like fluid.

Diagnosis: Same as for Blackquarter.

Control and Prevention:

- Bury dead animals as with Blackquarter.

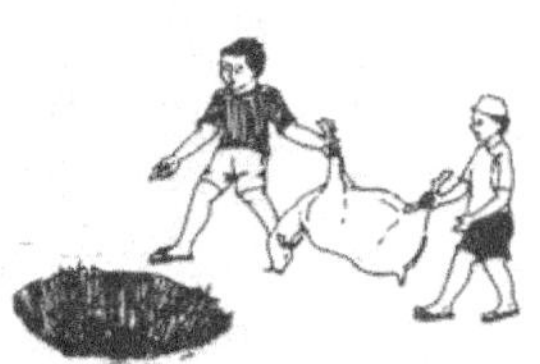

- In an area where BQ/Malignant Edema is found, all animals, especially sheep, should be vaccinated.

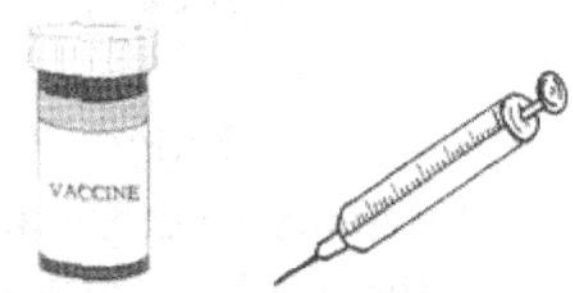

- All deliveries, castrations and vaccinations should be done in a clean manner.

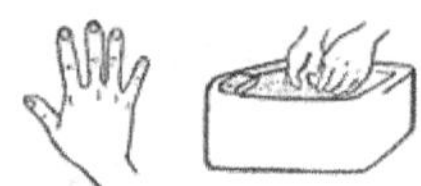

Treatment:

- Penicillin and other antibiotics like Tetracycline can be used in high doses to save animals if they are treated early. Most animals die even with treatment

Tetanus (Lockjaw)

Tetanus is an acute, infectious disease found throughout the world. It is caused by a bacteria, <u>Clostridium tetani</u>, which often starts growing in deep wounds. The bacteria make a kind of poison, called a toxin. This toxin travels throughout the body and affects the nerves. Then the muscles do not work properly, but instead become stiff and go into spasms. For a complete discussion of tetanus, see page 258 (Nervous System).

Systems of the Body and Associated Veterinary Problems

14.0 Skin System (Including Horns and Hooves)

INTRODUCTION:

The skin completely covers the body. The body is always making new skin so that as old skin is rubbed off, there is new skin underneath. The skin also contains sweat glands, blood vessels, lymph vessels and nerve fibers. Horns and hooves are both part of the skin. For both horns and hooves, the hard tissue develops from the soft skin. This skin contains special cells that produce the hard tissue. If these cells are damaged, then the hoof or horn will not grow properly.

Function of the skin:
- The skin **protects** the internal organs from bacteria and other harmful things.
- The skin helps to **regulate body temperature** (the sweat glands help to do this).

14.1 TYPES OF FRESH WOUNDS

There are three main types of wounds: 1. sharp cuts and tears; 2. scrapes (abrasions); and 3. puncture (deep) wounds. Wounds that were made with a very sharp instrument will often bleed more. Deep puncture wounds are more susceptible to tetanus. Wounds that involve a joint are very serious and the animal may have permanent damage to the joint even if the wound heals.

14.2 TREATMENT OF FRESH WOUNDS

> **Most wounds heal naturally if they are kept clean and dry.**

1)   Properly restrain the animal, being careful to avoid any further injury.

2)   Control any excessive bleeding. See page 78.

3)   Examine the animal to make sure there is nothing else wrong with it, that there are no other wounds, and that there are no fractures at the site of the wound.

4)   Wash your hands with clean water and soap.

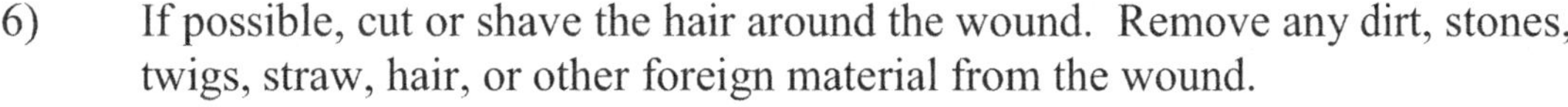

5)   Wash the wound with clean water and soap.

6)   If possible, cut or shave the hair around the wound. Remove any dirt, stones, twigs, straw, hair, or other foreign material from the wound.

7)   Rinse the wound with a dilute antiseptic solution such as potassium permanganate, *Savlon*, iodine, bleach, or regular soap. Do not use concentrated solutions since they may damage the wound further and delay healing.

8)   Decide if the wound should be sutured (see page 214 on criteria to suture a wound). Remember that almost any wound will heal without suturing. However, the advantage of suturing is faster healing and less disfigurement.

9)   If there are screwworms in the area, cover the wound and surrounding area with a product effective against screwworm. See page 120.

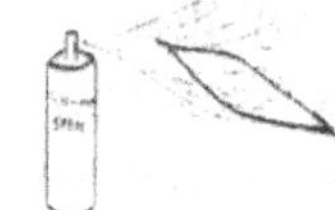

10)   If the wound is a deep puncture wound, and hydrogen peroxide or antiseptic solution is available, pour or squirt some as deep into the wound as possible. This will make it less susceptible to tetanus infection.

11)   If antibiotic ointment or spray is available (for people or animals), cover the wound with it.

12)   If possible, place a bandage on the wound to keep it clean. Almost any material can be used to bandage the wound as long as it is clean. A bandage should never be too tight or it will damage the tissue around it.   Depending on the severity of the wound, the cleanliness of the environment, and how easy it is to handle the animal, the bandage should be changed every one to three days. At the same time, the wound should be examined, washed and disinfected.

13)   If injectable antibiotic is available (penicillin is preferable), give it for at least one week or until the wound is dry and non-inflamed. This is especially important if there is tetanus in the area, the environment is dirty, or the wound is deep or might involve a joint.

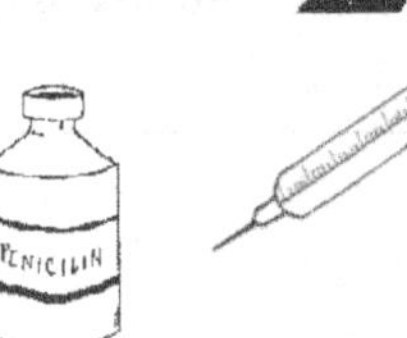

Important note: *a wet, dirty bandage is worse than no bandage at all!* If the environment is wet and dirty, the wound needs cleaning daily, and the bandage changed at the same time. If this is not done, the wound is likely to get infected.

14.3 SUTURING / STITCHING

Definition:

"Suturing" a wound is the same as "sewing", or "stitching" it closed.

Only certain types of wounds can be sutured successfully. In fact, if some wounds are sutured, they are more prone to infection. Therefore, do not try to suture a wound unless it meets the following six criteria:

Six criteria to suture a wound:
1. It must be a **fresh** wound and it must be sutured within 12 hours of when the wound occurred.
2. It must be **clean**.
3. It must be **gaping** (spread open). Do not suture a deep puncture wound since it will be more prone to infections, particularly tetanus.
4. The **tissue** around the wound **should be healthy**. If the tissue around the wound is badly bruised and damaged, then the blood supply to the wound will be damaged. In this case, if the wound is sutured, it will not heal well.
5. **Someone** must be available who **knows how** to suture.
6. The **essential equipment** must be available.

Equipment Needed

Essential
-Soap and clean water
-Disinfectant (local drinking alcohol will also work)
-Metal, glass, or plastic container for disinfectant and instruments
-Suture kit (see following page)

Optional
-local anesthetic
-clean needle and syringe for injecting local anesthetic

Kit for suturing

Needle holder: To hold the needle during suturing. Other forceps or pliers can be used if a needle holder is not available.

Rat-tooth forceps: To hold and manipulate tissues.
Tweezers can be used if a rat-tooth forceps is not available.

Other forceps: To clamp tissues and vessels. Several types of forceps are available such as "Krile" forceps, Allis tissue forceps, Mosquito forceps. It is useful to have one to two pairs of forceps available to hold tissues and clamp blood vessels that are bleeding.

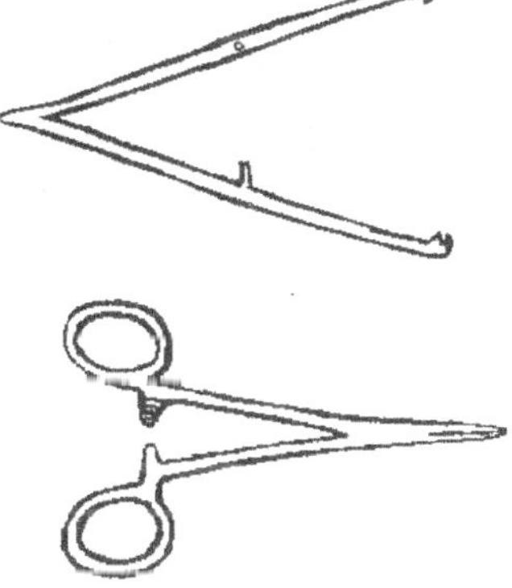

Suturing needles: To suture the skin or other tissues. There are two types:

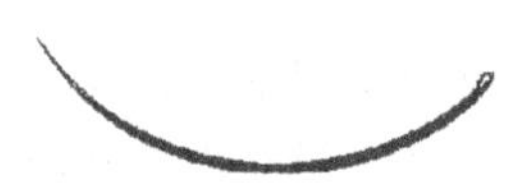

1. ***Cutting needle:*** has a sharp, three-cornered tip to pass easily
   through the skin.
2. ***Round (tapered) needle:*** has a sharp, but smooth tip to pass
   through muscle and other soft tissue.

Suture material (i.e. thread): There are various materials that can be used and can be divided into those that are eventually absorbed by the body and those that are not:

1. ***Absorbable sutures*** *(e.g. catgut):* For internal use because they eventually are absorbed. Absorbable sutures are not usually used on the skin because they irritate the skin too much. Absorbable sutures remain strong for about 7-10 days. However, if the wound is infected, the sutures may weaken after almost 3 days.

2. ***Non-absorbable sutures*** *(e.g. silk, cotton, nylon, horse hair)*: These materials are generally used for the skin and should be removed after the wound heals (otherwise, they may cause an infection). Non-absorbable sutures are generally strong. Each has their advantages and disadvantages. For example, silk suture is usually easy to manipulate, but can serve as a wick by absorbing anything wet, resulting in possible infection. Nylon causes the least inflammation and less infection. However, it is more difficult to manipulate. Also, because nylon is slippery, the knot can become untied if not secured well.

Ideally, suture material should be sterile or soaked in alcohol before use. Suture material comes in various sizes usually marked as follows from thickest to thinnest:

3   2   1   0   00   000   0000

Thickest ⟵——————————⟶ Thinnest

For large animals, usually sizes 0-2 are used. For small animals, usually sizes 00-1 are used.

14.3.1 Procedure for Suturing:

1. Control bleeding by applying pressure or clamping any visible blood vessels that are bleeding. If a bleeding vessel is large, consider tying a suture tightly around it to stop the bleeding.

2. Choose an appropriate needle (cutting or taper and correct size). A cutting needle is easier for thick skin.

3. Choose the appropriate type and size of suture material. In some places, local fiber (e.g. horse hair) is used successfully as suture material.

4. Place the material (needle, suture, needle holders) in disinfectant or alcohol for at least 20 minutes.

5.	Shave and clean the wound and surrounding area thoroughly. First use soap and water and then use non-irritating disinfectant. Be sure to remove all debris from the wound.

6.	Consider using local anesthetic. If the wound requires numerous stitches, local anesthetic will decrease the likelihood of injury to the animal or people handling the animal while suturing (e.g. when suturing a wound on the leg or face of a horse). See page 217 on the use of local anesthetics.

7.	Use an appropriate type of suture pattern (see following section).

8.	After suturing the wound, complete the following steps.
   * Clean all blood from around wound and allow it to dry.
   * Apply antibiotic ointment, powder or spray, as well as anti-fly ointment, powder or spray to protect the wound.
   * Give an antibiotic injection such as long-lasting penicillin.
   * Bandage the wound, if possible, to keep it clean.
   * Instruct the owner to keep the animal in a clean, dry area.

9.	After 7 - 10 days, check the sutures and the wound.
   * If healed, cut the sutures and remove.
   * If not healed, clean carefully. If there is a minor infection, remove some sutures to allow drainage from the wound. Give antibiotic injection.
   * If very infected, or a minor infection appears to be worsening, remove all sutures, open the wound to allow maximum drainage and leave the wound to heal as an "open wound" with daily cleaning and bandaging. Give antibiotics also.

14.3.2 Types of suture patterns

Simple interrupted suture pattern: This pattern works well for muscle and skin. It is very strong but it takes more time to complete than other suture patterns.

* Push the needle through one side of the layer of tissue (use needle holders, if available) near the edge of the wound.
* Push the needle through the layer of tissue on the other side of the wound.
* Pull the suture tight enough to bring edges of the wound together (but not so tight that the wound is "puckered" or "wrinkled").
* If using nylon suture, be sure to tie it in at least three knots to prevent untying.
* The stitches should be approximately 5mm apart in small animals and 10mm apart in large animals.

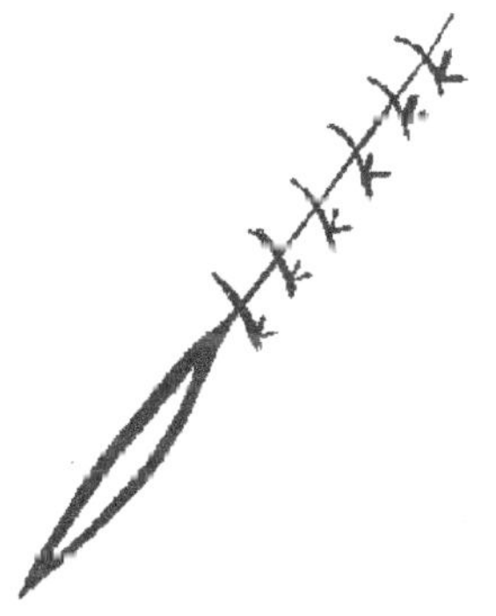

Simple continuous suture pattern: This pattern works well for muscle and skin also. It is not as strong as interrupted sutures but can be completed more rapidly.

- Push the needle through one side of the layer of tissue (with needle holders or pliers, if available) near the edge of the wound.
- Push the needle through the layer of tissue on other side of the wound.
- Continue this process without tying a knot until you reach the end of the wound, drawing the suture tight enough to pull the edges of the wound together (but without "puckering" or "wrinkling").
- Each suture should be 5 mm apart for small animals, and about 10 mm apart for large animals.
- At the end of the wound, check the whole line of stitches. They should be tight enough to pull each side of the wound together so that the sutured wound lies flat and smooth. If not, adjust the sutures (i.e. tighten or loosen them accordingly).
- Tie a secure knot. Tie nylon with at least three knots because it is slippery and easily becomes untied.

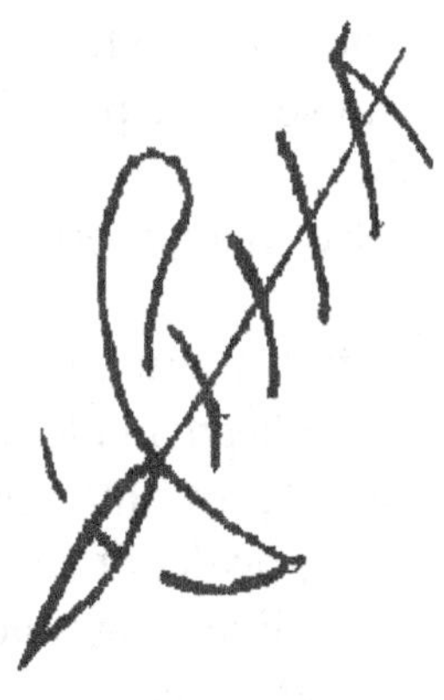

Mattress suture pattern: This is a good, strong suture pattern for thick skin on animals like cattle and buffalo and can be completed rapidly.

- Push the needle through one side of the layer of tissue near the edge of the wound.
- Push the needle through the layer of tissue on the other side of the wound.
- Push the needle through the layer of tissue again on same side.
- Push the needle on through the layer on the other side of the wound also.
- Pull the suture so that the skin comes together.
- Tie securely, (tie nylon at least three times.)
- Repeat the process to the end of the wound.

14.3.3 Local Anesthesia for Suturing

Local anesthetic is used to reduce suffering of the animal while suturing or during minor operations. It is usually injected under the skin, making it numb so that the animal feels little to no pain. Because the animal does not feel pain, it moves or reacts less to the needle sticks, allowing the work to be completed more efficiently and safely.   However, the first injection of the local anesthetic itself is a painful thing (but less so than multiple needle sticks when suturing)! Therefore, small wounds are often sutured, and abscesses are often opened without using local anesthetics.

Several local anesthetics are available including lidocaine, Novocain, lignocaine, and bucaine. These local anesthetics are usually available in about 2% solutions. If they are more concentrated than this, then dilute them with distilled water to about 2%.

Procedure:

- Clean the skin with soap and a disinfectant.
- Clip/shave the hair from the injection site (or from the edges of the wound) and clean the wound properly (as described in the preceding section on suturing a wound).
- Use a needle about two inches long and 18 or 20 gauge in diameter. **Be careful** to properly restrain the animal and warn everyone around the animal that it may react to the pain when the needle is inserted.
- Starting from the wound edge, insert the needle about one inch directly into the tissue under the skin. Once the needle is inserted, begin injecting the anesthetic while simultaneously withdrawing the needle slowly so that the anesthetic is given in a trail along the edge of the wound. Inject along the entire edge of the wound where the sutures are to be placed. It should require about two cc of anesthetic for every inch or so.
- Once the needle is completely withdrawn, insert it again in the same manner, but this time, insert the needle in an area that is already numb (so that the animal feels less pain). Continue spreading the local anesthetic along the edge of the wound.
- Wait for several minutes and test the skin by pricking it with a needle (but be careful that the animal does not injure anyone!). When the animal no longer reacts (i.e. the edge of the wound seems numb), the suturing can begin.

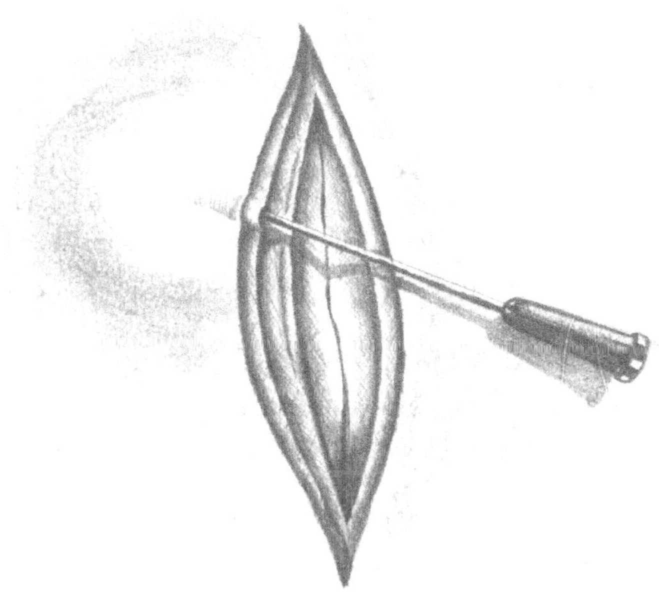

Place local anesthetic along the wound edge, to decrease the pain during suturing.

14.4 BLEEDING WOUNDS / HEMORRHAGE: THIS IS AN EMERGENCY.

See pages 78-79. First Aid.

14.5 TREATMENT OF CHRONIC WOUNDS

1.   Shave around the wound and clean it. Remove all dead tissue, pus and maggots or
     screwworms. (See disinfectants and antiseptics.)

     - *Remove all worms*: A wound will not heal if it contains maggots or screwworms.
       Therefore, to remove them, phenol/camphor (mothballs) can be crushed and mixed with
       water, and then poured in the hole where the worm has entered. Although the mothballs
       do not dissolve very well in water, they work well anyway and are often locally available.
       Chloroform, kerosene, spirit, and turpentine also work.

     - *Remove all debris and establish good drainage:* It may be necessary to soak the wound
       or use hot compresses for several days to decrease swelling, soften the tissue, remove
       old, dead tissue/debris, and open the wound to establish good drainage. If the wound is
       already draining pus, insert a piece of cloth soaked with antiseptic to keep the wound
       open and draining for a few days.

2.   Never try to suture a chronic wound. Leave it open to drain and then heal.

3.   Once the drainage has stopped, apply antibiotic ointment, powder, or spray to protect against
     infection.

4.   Apply ointment, powder or spray to protect against maggots or screwworms.

5.   If the wound seems to be infected, give an antibiotic injection like long-acting penicillin.

6.   Provide good supportive care. That is, keep the animal in a clean, dry environment away
     from other animals, and provide high quality food and clean, fresh water. If the animal
     appears to be in a lot of pain, give it a painkiller medication.

If at any time a thick scab forms and the wound appears inflamed, red or sore at the edges, there may
be an infection. To check this, pull off a corner of the scab and apply gentle pressure to the wound
(but be careful to prevent injury if the animal reacts to the pain). If pus oozes out from under the
scab, gently remove the entire scab and clean the wound thoroughly. If it appears that the wound
may need to drain for a few days, insert a piece of cloth soaked with antiseptic to keep the wound
open and draining. Once the wound has adequately drained, apply antibiotic cream. Check, and
clean the wound daily until it begins to heal properly.

14.6 WOUNDS FROM WILD ANIMAL BITES

Treat animal bite wounds as acute or chronic wounds, depending upon when the bites occurred.
Remember that animal bite wounds become easily infected and are often quite painful.

14.7 BURNS

Burns can be caused by heat, fire, explosions, electricity and sometimes chemicals. Surface burns (i.e. those affecting only the surface of the skin) are usually not a serious problem. Deep burns, however, can involve the entire layer of skin, the sub-cutaneous tissue under it; and sometimes even muscles and bones. Deep burns can result in serious infections, loss of body fluids, and even death. For most burns, the most important treatment is to keep the affected area clean to avoid infection   while the tissues heal.

Take the following immediate actions when a burn occurs:
- Apply cold water immediately to the affected area. Rinsing with lots of cold water is particularly important for a chemical burn.

- Rinse the affected area with a mild, non-irritating disinfectant solution.

- In a dirty environment, apply an antibiotic ointment and, if possible, a bandage to keep the wound clean. In a clean environment, consider not bandaging, rather expose the wound to fresh air while it heals.

- If necessary, give the animal an antibiotic injection to help prevent infection.

- Provide good nursing care such as high quality food, clean drinking water and a clean, dry environment away from other animals.

- Check the wound at least every two days for infection. If you suspect an infection, gently remove some scabs to check for pus. If there is pus, wash the wound thoroughly, apply antibiotic cream to the wound and give the animal an injection of antibiotics.

14.8 LUMPS AND BUMPS

(Abscesses, Hernias, Seroma or Cyst, Hematoma, Cancerous Growths)

Sometimes an animal will be seen with a large bump on its side or on its belly near the umbilicus; or there may be smaller bumps within the muscle itself. These lumps and bumps may be due to one of the following which are often difficult to distinguish:

1. **Abscess-** an abscess is simply a pocket of pus. This is usually the result of a small wound which later becomes infected. Sometimes the wound is so small that it goes unnoticed until an abscess forms. Abscesses can be a problem particularly in goat herds. It is advisable to avoid buying goats from a herd with abscess problems.

Circles indicate common places for abscesses in goats

2. **Hernia**- hernia is the term used when one part of the body pushes through a muscle and into another part of the body.

- For example, if an animal is hit on its side, the muscle can tear. Then the intestines from inside the belly protrude through the muscle tear resulting in a bump under the skin.

- The belly, at the umbilicus, is a common place for a hernia to occur. Normally, after a baby is born and the umbilical cord is no longer needed, the surrounding muscles close around it. However, sometimes a small hole remains and the intestines protrude through the hole. This is called an "umbilical hernia."

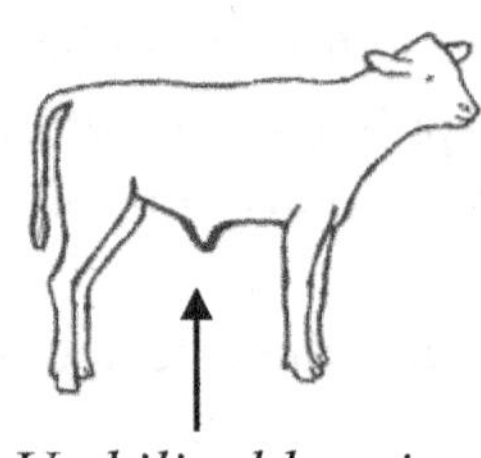

Umbilical hernia

- Hernias also occur in the scrotum of male animals, called a scrotal hernia. That is, the intestines push their way through a hole in the body wall into the scrotum of the animal. This can cause problems during castration, especially in pigs. If the scrotum is cut open in an animal with a scrotal hernia, the intestines might be cut by mistake. For this reason, it is important to always feel the testicle carefully before beginning a castration.

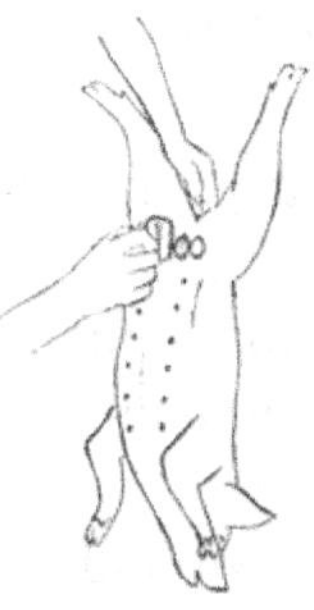

- **Hernias are dangerous** because if the intestines or the stomach get stuck in the hole, they may be damaged permanently and can even cause death.

3. **Seroma or Cysts** - A seroma or cyst is like an abscess, but instead of being filled with pus, it is filled with a watery fluid.

4. **Hematoma** - A hematoma is like an abscess, but instead is filled with blood. These usually happen as the result of injury and the rupture of a blood vessel.

5. **Cancerous growth**- Cancer is a complex disease that happens when cells in the body begin to multiply abnormally. Sometimes these cells grow together in the same place and form a large bump in the skin or in the muscles. These lumps of cancer tissue are called "tumors." There is no good treatment for most types of cancer unless the bump can be surgically removed. Sometimes the cancer cells spread throughout the body which eventually results in death.

- **"Bovine Leukemia"** is an example of a cancer in cattle that spreads throughout the body. It is caused by a virus which grows in the lymph nodes and causes them to enlarge. These enlarged lymph nodes can be seen and felt under the skin. There is no treatment.

- **Venereal tumors** in dogs are another example of cancerous growth. This tumor is spread during breeding. The tumor begins as a small growth that eventually develops into a large, red mass. In some countries, these tumors are surgically removed.

Examination and treatment of lumps:

- *Take a careful history:* When an animal has a lump, take a careful history to try to distinguish a hernia from other causes of lumps. If the animal has fallen or been hit, yet there is no wound, then it might be a hernia.

- *Examine the animal:* Feel carefully for a break in the muscles around the edge of the lump. Also try to reduce the lump (i.e. push the contents of the lump back inside the body). If you can feel a hole in the muscles and/or you can reduce the lump, then it is probably a hernia.

- *Check for heat (inflammation):* If you cannot push the lump back inside, feel the swelling carefully for excess heat (i.e. inflammation). If it is hot, then it might be an abscess (although old abscesses are not often hot).

- *Prepare to insert a needle:* Shave the hair over the bump. Then, clean it with soap and water and disinfectant solution.

- *To identify the liquid in the lump, insert a sterile needle through the skin and into the lump:* If watery, clear fluid comes out of the needle hub, then the lump may be a cyst or an abscess that is not ready to be cut open (because there is no pus yet). If blood comes out, the lump may be a hematoma which will usually disappear over time and does not need to be cut open.

- *Apply hot compresses for 3-4 days:* If it is an abscess, the hot compresses will help it to "mature" (i.e. develop pus). After 3 or 4 days, try the same procedure of cleaning the area and inserting a needle to check the liquid.

- *If pus, cut open the abscess:* Once you detect pus, then you can assume that the lump is an abscess. An abscess should be cut open at its lowest point and as widely as possible to maximize drainage. The better the drainage, the faster it will heal. Do not bother to use a local anesthetic before cutting, but instead cut as rapidly as possible. Press around the abscess to remove all pus; then rinse the inside of the abscess thoroughly with clean water or disinfectant solution.

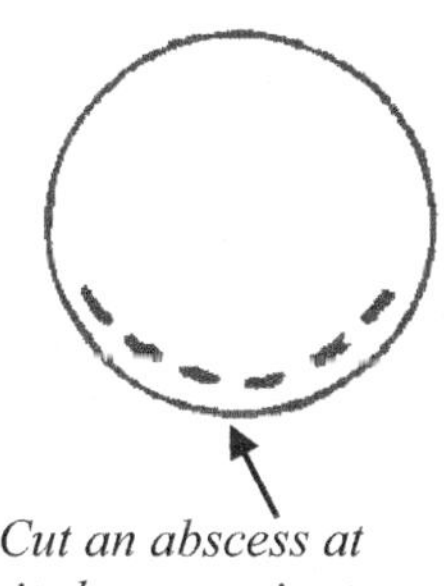

Cut an abscess at its lowest point to maximize drainage

- *Keep the cut abscess open and draining:* Once an abscess is cut open, keep it open and draining for several days. Flush the abscess with clean water or disinfectant daily for several days to remove the pus. If the abscess begins to close early and trap some pus inside, insert a thin piece of cloth or cotton gauze soaked in disinfectant. It will keep the incision open and draining.

- ***Protect against maggots or screwworm:*** Apply a spray, ointment or powder to protect against maggot or screwworm infestation.

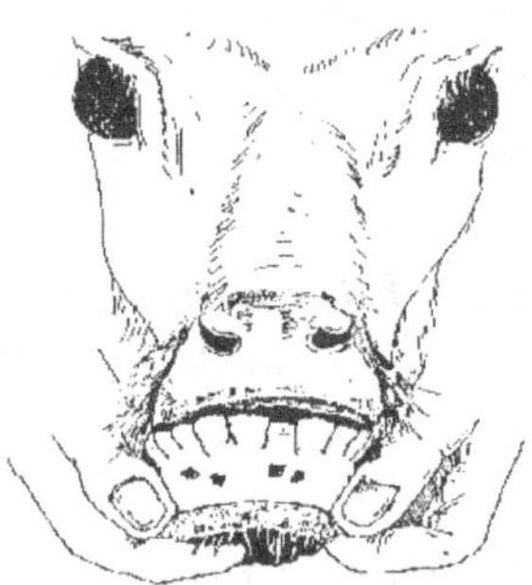

14.9 ULCERS/VESICLES

Sometimes a small sore may develop without any obvious injury on the skin, lips, gums, tongue or vulva. These problems have been covered in other places but will also be mentioned here.

- A **vesicle** is a small bubble in the skin that is filled with fluid. Vesicles can form as a result of burns, insect bites, allergies, and infectious diseases like Foot and Mouth Disease or Pox.

- An **ulcer** refers to a hole in the skin which can be shallow or deep. An ulcer may develop after a vesicle bursts (sometimes the vesicle is not noticed).   Deep ulcers can become chronic and take a long time to heal.

*Vesicles on the gums
can become ulcers*

- The main treatment for vesicles and ulcers is to keep them clean to prevent infection. Generally, it is best if ulcers can be kept open so that the air can help them to heal. However, it may be wise to cover an ulcer with a bandage (if possible) in order to prevent infection if the environment is dirty, or if there are many flies.

- If an ulcer becomes infected and has pus, etc., then the ulcer should be treated as an infected wound. See page 219.

14.10 CRUSTY SPOTS

Several disease conditions can cause crusty spots and sores on the skin of livestock.

Warts

- Warts are dry, crusty bumps that occur on the skin, mainly in younger animals, and are caused by a virus. They are seen most often in cattle, horses, dogs, and occasionally rabbits.

- Most animals develop resistance to the wart virus with increasing age and the warts eventually disappear on their own. Sometimes the resistance fades away and the animal gets warts again. However, resistance will then develop again and the warts will disappear.

  Cattle: Warts usually appear on the head, neck, shoulders, ears and sometimes on the belly or back. Warts might also appear on the penis of young bulls and the vulvas of young cows which may interfere with breeding.

Horses: Warts usually appear on the nose and lips, and disappear after a few weeks.

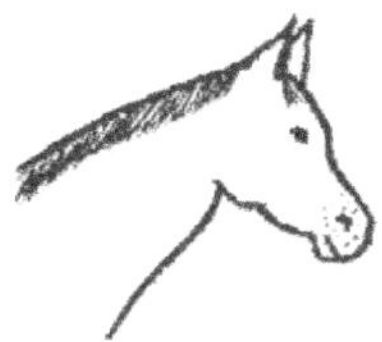

Dogs: Dogs get two kinds of warts. One kind appears in the mouth and often results in infections of the mouth. The other is exterior and looks like warts on cattle.

Treatment / Control of Warts: This disease gets well on its own. No treatment is necessary. Try to control the disease by keeping animals infected with warts separate from other animals.

Pox

Pox is the word used to describe a group of diseases that produce bumps in the skin and eventually scab-covered, crusty sores. These diseases are caused by viruses that are spread directly from animal to animal, and sometimes indirectly by insects.

Cattlepox: Two different kinds of pox affect cattle.
- One is more serious than the other but both of them cause sores on the udder and teats. These sores are painful, and milking becomes very difficult. The sores heal without treatment but it may take 1 or 2 months. People can also become infected by milking cattle which have open sores. However, people also recover on their own.

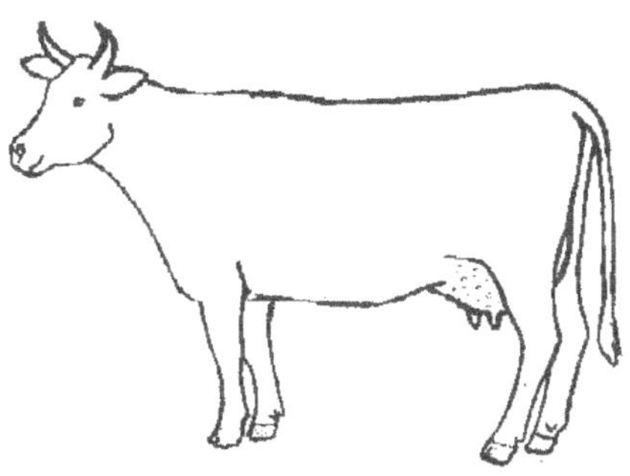

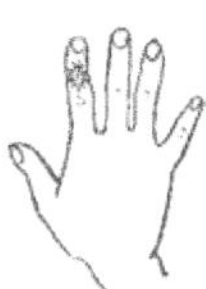

- A similar virus causes lumps in the skin and in the lining of the digestive system, the respiratory system, and the reproductive system. This disease is called "**lumpy skin disease**." The lumps often fall off and the area underneath may become infected (which eventually heals).

Sheep pox and Goat pox: These are two similar diseases caused by viruses. The symptoms in goats are not as serious as in sheep.
- **Symptoms:** The eyelids become swollen; pus and mucus come from the nostrils; and crusty sores develop on the nose, ears, and other areas which are free of long hair or wool. When the scab is removed from these sores, a "star-shaped" scar remains.

- **Treatment:** None except supportive care. Most animals recover on their own.
- **Prevention and Control:** Vaccines are available in some countries.

Swine pox: This is a mild disease causing crusty sores on the skin of pigs. Later the scabs drop off and the pigs look "spotted." Most pigs recover easily without treatment.
- **Prevention and Control:** Controlling lice is important to prevent the spread of this disease.

Sore-mouth (Contagious Ecthyma)

This is a similar disease but causes sores mainly around the mouth. It can affect the ability of the animal to eat.

Ringworm

This contagious skin disease is caused by a fungus and causes dry, crusty sores. See page 123.

14.11 BROKEN HORNS

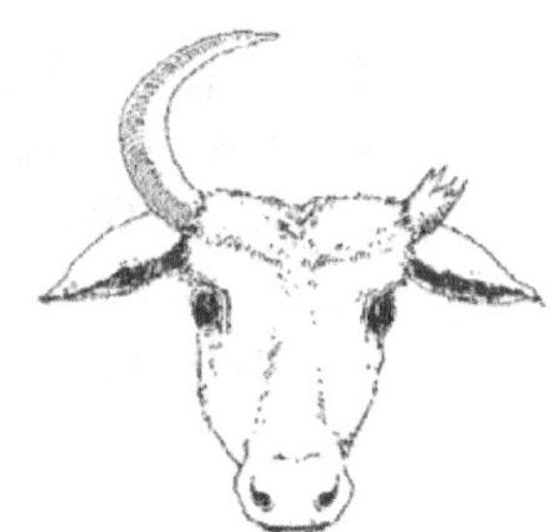

A normal horn in most livestock is partly hollow. The top 1/3 of the horn is solid; and the bottom 2/3 of the horn is more hollow and has blood vessels in it. Livestock may break their horns fighting or getting caught in something (and then trying to break loose). If the outer, hard coat of the horn is scraped off or the tip of the horn is broken, the condition is not usually serious. However, if the bottom 2/3 portion of the horn is broken, two serious problems may result, both of which require rapid treatment:
- Serious hemorrhage (blood loss) can occur.
- The hole from the horn opens right into the head of the animal (i.e. its sinuses). If maggots infest the wound, the animal will probably die.

Treatment of Broken Horns:
1. If the tip of the horn is broken, it can be filed to make it smooth.
2. If the hard, outer covering has come off, the bleeding should be stopped. This can be done with pressure or by using potassium permanganate crystals on a damp piece of cotton wool. The cotton wool is held in place until the bleeding stops. Then protect the injury against maggots or screwworm.
3. If the bottom 2/3 of the horn is broken, the horn should be removed at its base to allow it to heal.
4. If a piece of special "embryotomy wire" or dehorner is available, it can be used to cut through the base of the horn. If not available, then a regular saw can be used. (A hack saw works well.)

- Cut the hair around the base of the horn; and clean with disinfectant.
- Use about 5 - 10 ml of local anesthetic around the base of the horn.
- Cut the skin around the base of the horn.
- Using a piece of embryotomy (fetotomy) wire, place the wire in the skin incision; and start cutting by pulling on the handles attached to the wire.
- Once you start cutting, do not stop or the wire or saw may become stuck and break.

- Near the end of the cut, when only the skin is remaining, an assistant should support the horn so that the skin does not tear with the last few cuts.
- To control the bleeding, use potassium permanganate crystals, apply a hot metal iron for several seconds, or clamp the bleeding vessels with forceps or pliers.
- Apply a thin layer of cotton in the holes of the animal's skull to prevent flies from laying eggs in the skull. The cotton wool must be thin to allow air to reach the wound and dry it. Gentian violet (if available) works well on the wound itself and keeps it dry.
- Apply maggocide / screwworm ointment, powder, or spray around the wound to prevent maggots.
- Remove the cotton wool and check after 3-4 days. If there are signs of infection (i.e. pus), clean the area thoroughly and give antibiotics.
- Apply new cotton wool to the holes, gentian violet (if available), and a product to prevent maggot / screwworm infestation.

14.12 METHODS OF DEHORNING:

Some people prefer that their animals do not have horns to avoid injuries to people or other animals, and to provide more space (e.g. at a feeding trough). The growth of horns can be prevented by destroying the cells that produce the hard, horny tissue. These cells are found in the skin surrounding the horn. The process of removing the horns is called **dehorning**. It is usually easiest and least traumatic to dehorn animals when they are young. If dehorned properly, the horns will not re-grow. It is advisable that someone experienced in dehorning show you how to do it the first time.

- **Larger animals:** For animals older than 6 months, the above method described for cutting off broken horns with embryotomy wire can be used to cut off the entire horn - whether it is broken or not. A "dehorner" can also be used (if available), or a saw.

dehorner   *saw for dehorning*

- **For younger animals:** Either cutting, or burning with a hot iron, or a combination of the two can be used. In very young animals (less than 1 week), caustic soda can be applied to prevent the horn from developing.

Use of a Hot Iron

- This can be used in some places on animals under two months of age. It must be done very carefully with goats because it is easy to apply the hot iron for too long and cause permanent brain damage. If left on for too short of a period, the horn may grow back or develop a "scur" (i.e. a deformed, stunted horn). With experience, one learns how long to leave the hot iron in contact with the skin.

- There are rods that heat up with electricity, made especially for dehorning. An AHA can make one of these by attaching a wooden handle to an iron cylinder. The end of the cylinder is heated until red hot and then placed around the emerging horn bud to burn the skin (i.e. the skin cells around the base of the horn which cause the horn to grow). The hot iron should be left in place for only a few seconds; and should be rotated slightly.

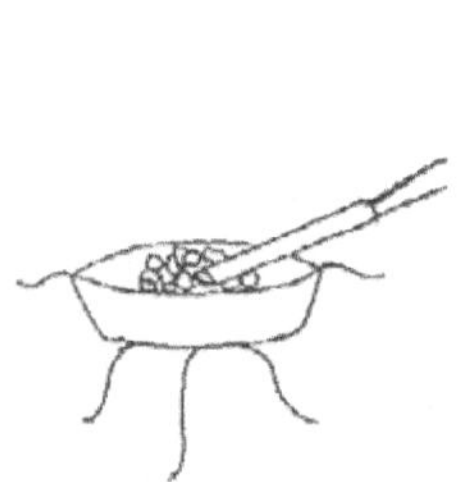

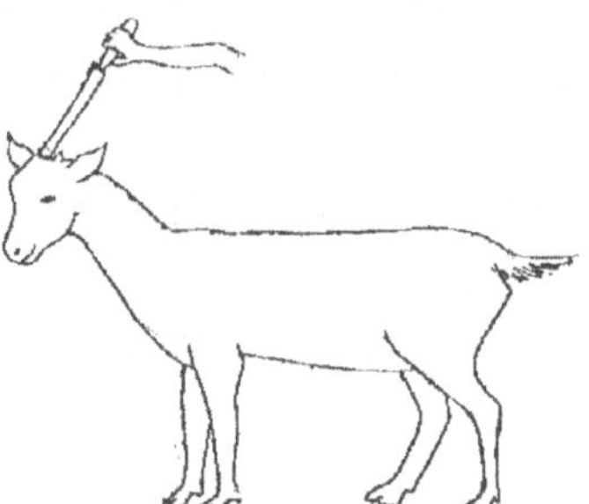

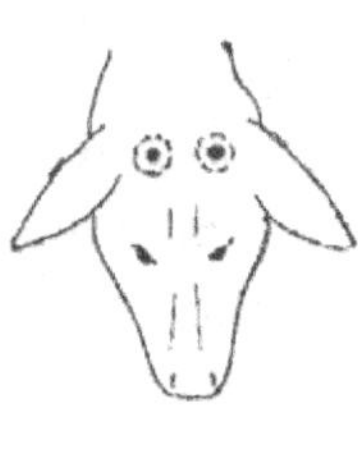

Heating the metal
cylinder over coals

burning the tissue
around the horns

burned tissue
around the horns

- After burning, the animal should be observed closely for several days to ensure that it does not bump its head and cause bleeding.

Cutting

- This method is also used on young animals.

- The emerging horn, often called a "horn bud", is cut off using a sharp knife or a small, cylinder-shaped knife called a "debudder." If one carefully removes both the horn and about 1/2 cm of tissue around the horn, then the horn should not grow back.

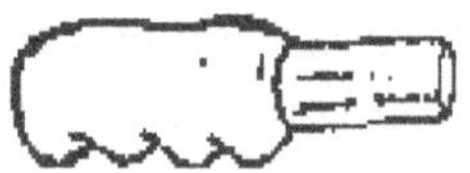

debudder

- The bleeding can be stopped by burning the skin with hot metal, by clamping the bleeding vessels with forceps, or by using potassium permanganate crystals.

Use of caustic soda

Caustic soda is a chemical that causes tissue to die. It comes as a paste or in a solid form that looks like a pencil. By applying it around the emerging horn, the cells that produce the horn die, and the horn stops growing and falls off.

- The calf should be young (about one week).
- The hair around the newly-growing horn should be clipped. (This allows it to be seen easily.)
- The tip of a caustic soda pencil is then applied to this area with firm pressure and moved in a circular direction around the emerging horn. Or, the gel can be applied according to instructions.
- Continue to apply caustic soda until a shallow hole has been produced and all bleeding stops.
- Avoid using an excessive amount of caustic soda, since it may get wet and run down the face and cause damage to the skin or eyes.
- Do not press too hard with the pencil. If you do, the skin will break and the tissue will be damaged more than necessary.

14.13 HOOVES AND THEIR CARE

The hoof is formed by special skin cells that are
found at the coronary band.   If the cells at the
coronary band are damaged due to injury or disease
(e.g. foot and mouth disease), the hoof may become
deformed or cracked. Lameness may also result.
See page 236.

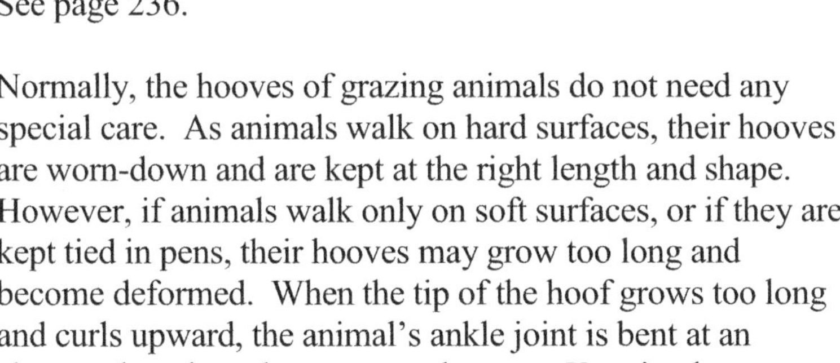

coronary band

Normally, the hooves of grazing animals do not need any
special care. As animals walk on hard surfaces, their hooves
are worn-down and are kept at the right length and shape.
However, if animals walk only on soft surfaces, or if they are
kept tied in pens, their hooves may grow too long and
become deformed. When the tip of the hoof grows too long
and curls upward, the animal's ankle joint is bent at an
abnormal angle and may cause damage. Keeping hooves
trimmed properly will prevent many kinds of foot and
lameness problems.

Trimming Hooves

Various instruments can be used to trim hooves, including knives, saws, special hoof-trimmers,
and files.

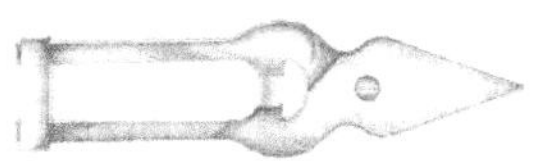

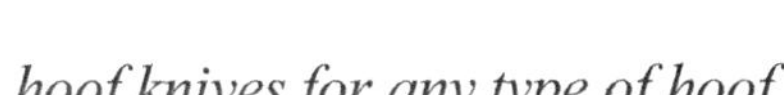

hoof trimmer for goats and sheep

hoof knives for any type of hoof

The hoof should be cut short-enough and in the proper shape so that it sets evenly on the ground,
the ankle is kept at a proper angle, and the animal can walk normally. The animal must be properly
restrained during the process or it may become frightened and hurt itself. Horses can be trained to
stand still while their hooves are worked on and trimmed. However, cattle and buffalo must usually
be cast. Some gentle goats and sheep can be restrained by lifting their foot during the trimming
process. Others must be turned-up on their bottom.

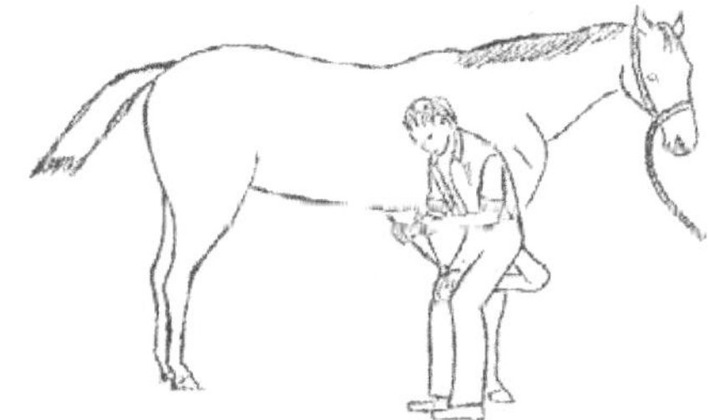

Position for trimming the front foot of a horse

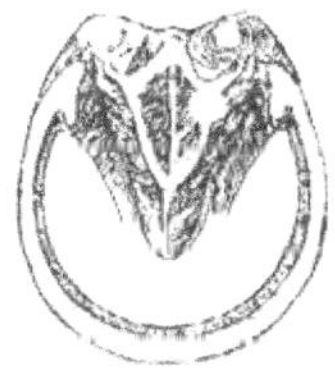

*Shape of a well-trimmed horse hoof
(view from the bottom of hoof)*

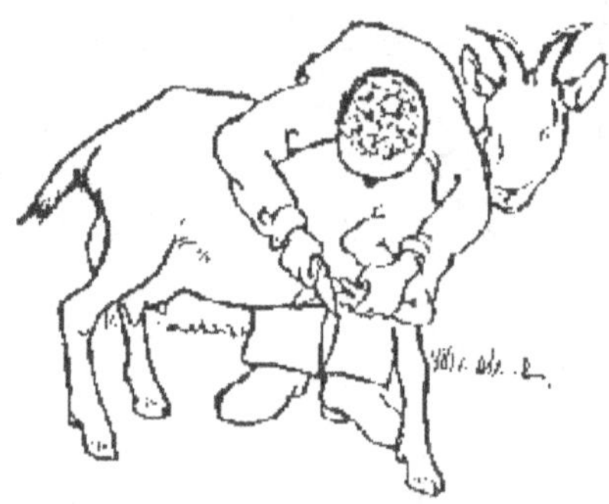

*Position for trimming
the front foot of a goat*

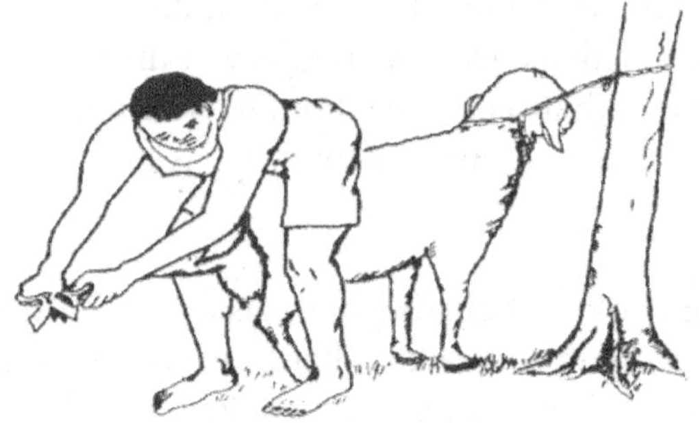

*Position for trimming
the back foot of a goat*

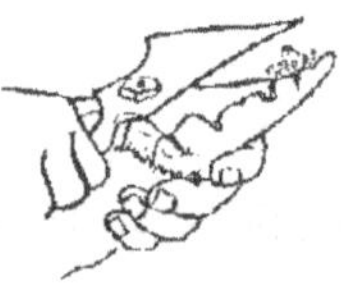

*Trimming a goat
or sheep hoof*

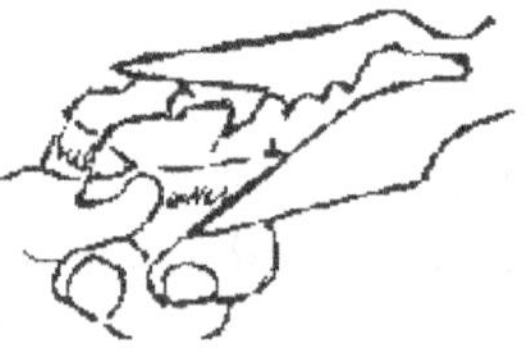

*Trimming a goat
or sheep hoof*

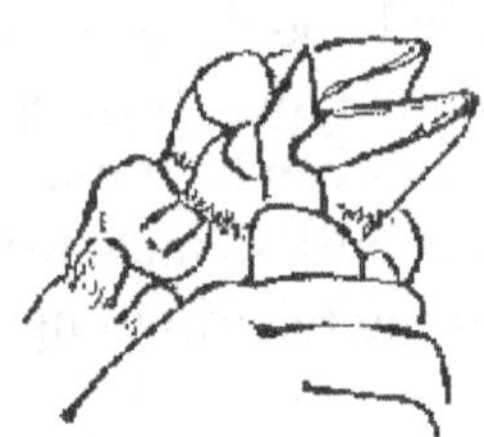

*Trimming a goat
or sheep hoof*

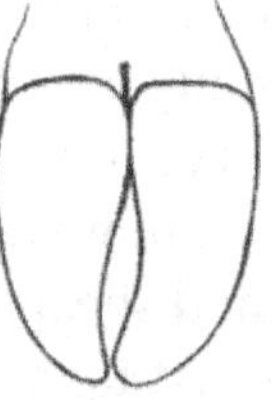

*Normal shape of a well
trimmed goat, sheep, cow,
llama and alpaca hoof
(view from bottom of hoof)*

14.14 FOOTROT

Footrot is a severe infectious condition affecting the feet of sheep and goats (also occasionally cattle and buffalo). It is caused by two bacteria working together: <u>F. necrophorus</u> and <u>B. nodosus</u>. These bacteria cause infections that start between the toes. Then the hoof starts to "rot" until the sides of the hoof separate from the bottom of the hoof.

Symptoms:
- Severe lameness, such that the animal may not even want to stand up.
- Poor condition and weight loss since the animal does not eat properly.
- Red, swollen tissue around the coronary band and between the toes.
- Sores between the toes that may smell badly and ooze pus.
- Hoof wall separating or splitting.

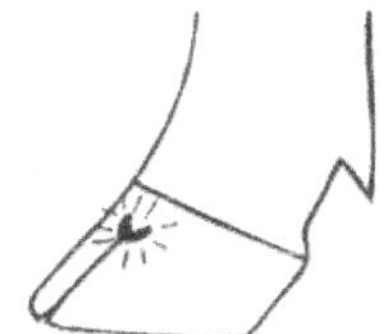

Diagnosis:
- Based on the history and the symptoms.

Treatment:
- Trim the hoof well and clean the wounds. This requires trimming the hoof sometimes until it bleeds. All pockets of pus must be opened and dead tissue removed.
- Pack the open wounds with cotton soaked in a disinfectant. Bandage the foot.
- Antibiotic injections will help control the severe infections (pen/strep often works well).
- Keep the animal in a clean, dry environment.
- Change the bandage whenever it becomes wet or dirty.

Prevention/Control:
- The animals can be walked through a foot bath of 10% formalin.
- Keep the animals in a clean, dry environment.
- Trim the hooves regularly.
- Do not buy animals from herds that are known to be infected

15.0   Skeletal System

15.1   DEFORMITIES OF LEGS

Deformed or Bent Legs at Birth

Some animals are born with deformed legs, in which the legs bow out or bow in, or the animal cannot straighten the leg. Sometimes, the deformity prevents the animal from standing. If the joints in the leg are not stiff; and if it is possible to straighten the legs with slight force, then the problem may be treatable.

Treatment: The same types of splints can be used here that are described in the section on broken legs. See page 233.

- Gently straighten the leg as much as possible. This will help to stretch the tendons that may be contracted.

- Before appying a splint, put ample padding around the leg so that sores do not develop under the splint.

- Apply the splint and tie it securely in place.

- Lift the animal to the standing position 3 or 4 times every day.

- Remove the splint every 2 or 3 days and check for sores under the splint. While the splint is off, massage the affected leg while bending and straightening it to stretch the tendons and keep the joints from becoming stiff.

- Each time the splint is replaced, the leg should be straightened as much as possible to its normal position.

- If there is no improvement after two or three weeks of treatment, the animal will probably never have normal legs.

Stiff legs

Sometimes the joints of a baby animal are very stiff and hard; and they cannot be moved at all. There is no good treatment for this problem.

15.2 LAMENESS

Sometimes an animal cannot walk properly. The term for this general condition is "lameness." If an animal cannot move at all, the condition is called "paralysis."

Lameness can be acute or chronic. In either case one must always check first for a fracture.

Lameness with Fractures

A fracture is a broken bone. A fracture is often accompanied by injury to the surrounding tissues, including blood vessels and nerves. Fractures can result from falling, colliding with something, or being hit by something.

Lameness is usually due to:
1. **Injury** to:
   - -Bone,   See page 233.
   - -Muscle,   See page 209.
   - -Hoof,   See page 236.
   - -Skin,   See pages 235-236.
   - -Nerve,   See pages 209, 259.

2. **Bone or joint infection**,
      See page 234.

3. **Mineral deficiency**,
      See page 242.

4. **Inflammation of the joints**,
      See page 238.

Fractures can be divided into three types:
1. **Simple fracture**: The bone is broken in only one place, and there is no wound in the skin.
2. **Compound fracture**: The bone is broken in more than one place, but there is no wound in the skin.
3. **Open fracture**: A wound in the skin, resulting in the bone being exposed, accompanies the fracture (either simple or compound) and infection may result.

Examination of Fractures: When a fracture is suspected, handle the animal carefully to avoid further injury to the animal or to the people handling it. Sometimes, the animal may be very frightened or stressed by the pain and won't become calm until the fracture is stabilized. Examine the fracture thoroughly. Check for wounds, bleeding and whether a joint may be involved in the fracture. Examine the entire animal for other injuries.

Some fractures are difficult to diagnose without the aid of an x-ray. An x-ray is a picture of the bones taken by a special machine. However, even without an X-ray machine, the following signs can help to diagnosis fractures:

- Severe pain or local tenderness, resulting in the animal limping, not bearing weight on the affected limb, not standing up, or reacting strongly when the affected area is manipulated.
- Deformity or abnormal angle of the bone.
- Local swelling.
- Crackling noise when the affected area is manipulated - due to the broken bone ends rubbing against each other.

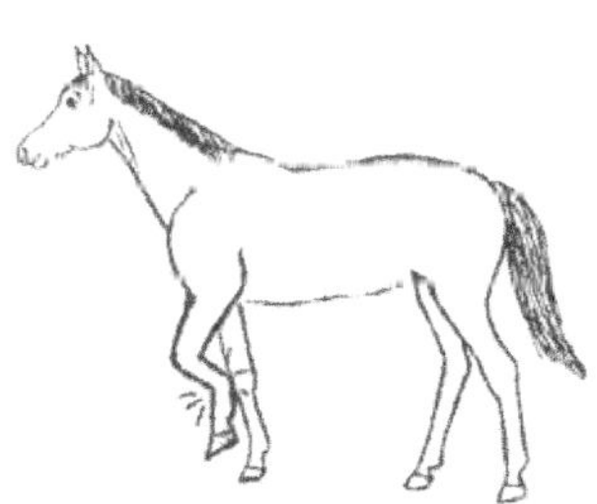

General Treatment of Fractures

Most fractures will heal if the fractured ends are placed close to each other and immobilized. However, infection or involvement of a joint may complicate healing. The following steps should be taken to treat a fracture:

1. "Clean the wound" asso-ciated with the fracture.

2. "Set" the broken bones.

3. "Fix" the broken bones.

4. "Provide supportive care" for the animal until it recovers.

1. "**Clean the wound**" (if there is one). Open fractures require special care to avoid serious bone infections. The wound must be thoroughly washed and cleaned. Antibiotic cream should be applied topically. The wound should be protected from flies. Penicillin injections should be given to prevent infection.

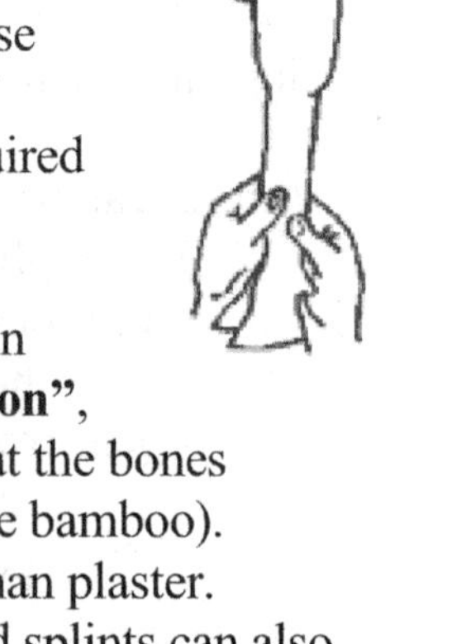

2. "**Set**" **the bones:** In any fracture, the broken ends of the bones should be adjusted so that they are properly aligned, and as close as possible to each other. This is called **"setting"** the fracture. Sometimes setting the bones is difficult because the muscles contract and pull the bones out of alignment. Several strong people may be required to align the bones.

3. "**Fix**" **the bones:** Once the bones are set, they must be "immobilized" (i.e. held in place so that they do not move while healing takes place). This is called **"fixation"**, or "fixing the fracture." There are many different ways to "fix a fracture" so that the bones cannot move. One easy method is to use **splints** made from strips of wood (like bamboo). Wood splints are less expensive, more easily available, and more lightweight than plaster. They can be easily made, but do get ruined when wet (like plaster does). Wood splints can also be removed easily and replaced to check and treat wounds associated with the fracture. A bandage should be applied under the splint for padding, and extend beyond the edges of the splint. The bandage should be sprayed or sprinkled with insecticide powder to prevent maggots/screwworms, particularly if there is a wound.

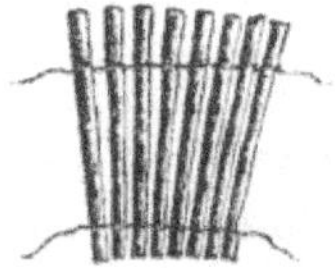 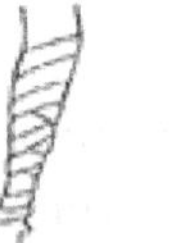 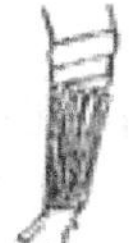 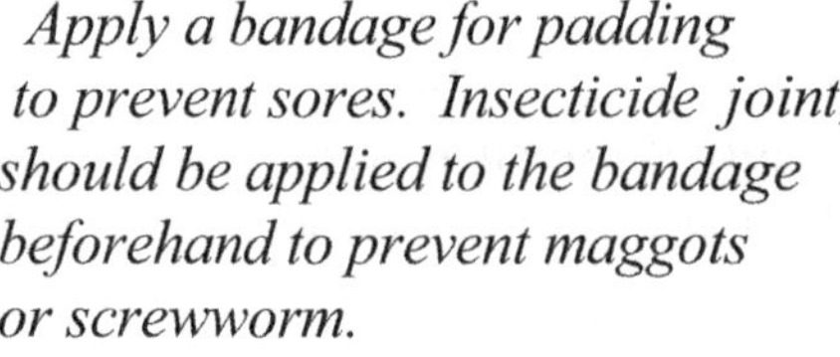

| Splint made from bamboo or wood. | Apply a bandage for padding to prevent sores. Insecticide joint, should be applied to the bandage beforehand to prevent maggots or screwworm. | Apply the splint, including the above and below the fracture. The bandage under the splint should extend beyond the splint. |

4. "**Provide supportive care for the patient**": See page 234. This means regularly checking the splint, turning the patient over periodically, providing high quality food, clean drinking water, and adequate shelter away from other animals that might cause more injury or stress.

Supportive Care for a Fracture Patient:

See page 78 for general information on First Aid. In addition, the following are guidelines that apply specifically to fracture patients.

1. **Time required:** In general, a splint should remain on small animals for at least one month, and on large, heavy animals for at least two months. However, the time required may vary considerably depending upon the following factors:
   - *Age of the animal:* Young animals heal faster than old animals.
   - *Size of the animal:* Small animals heal faster than large animals. Large animals may sustain permanent muscle damage if they cannot stand up and are lying down for longer periods on a hard surface without moving.
   - *Temperament of the animal:* It is more difficult to properly treat and care for an excitable animal with a fracture than one that is easy to handle.
   - *Type of fracture:* Simple fractures heal faster than open or compound fractures.
   - *Location of the fracture:* Fracture of large bones, or high on a leg take longer to heal than small bones, or fractures further down. Fractures that involve a joint may take longer to heal, and the animal may develop arthritis due to permanent joint damage.
   - *Ability to properly set the fracture:* Fractures that are poorly aligned may take longer to heal.
   - *Ability to immobilize the bone:* Fractures that are not properly immobilized will take longer to heal.
   - *Blood supply:* Fractures that have a good blood supply heal more rapidly than those without a good supply.
   - *Infection:* An infected bone, soft tissue, or joint will delay healing, or even prevent it.

   Consideration should be given to all of these factors before treating a fracture. Several factors together may considerably increase the time for healing or even prevent healing. In this case, the owner may prefer to slaughter the animal.

   - Keep the animal on soft ground and turn the animal over from side to side several times daily: This prevents them from getting any wounds on their skin from laying in the same position. It also helps blood flow to the fractures which encourages faster healing. The animal (especially big, heavy ones) should be kept on soft ground particularly if it cannot stand up. Otherwise, the pressure of its own body may cause permanent muscle damage.

2. **Lift the animal:** If possible, the animal should be lifted to its feet at least once per day. The animal can then support itself for a while on its other legs. This will help the animal's blood circulation and muscles.

3. **Provide good food, water, shelter and protection from other animals:** Animals that are healing from a fracture need high quality food, clean, fresh water, and good shelter from heat, excessive sun, or cold. They also need protection from other animals that might injure it.

4.   **Watch/smell for maggot infestations, wound infections or dying tissue:** Wounds should be observed daily for possible maggot infestations or wound infections. As a preventive measure, the bandaging and wound itself (if there is one) should be sprayed or dusted with insecticide powder or liquid that is effective against maggots/screwworm. The bandage and splint should be applied correctly to avoid circulation cut-off. Animals with open fractures should receive antibiotic injections such as penicillin.

Nevertheless, if the animal suddenly stops eating, has a fever, smells bad (i.e. rotten smell coming from the area of the fracture) or seems to be in unusual pain, the splint should be removed immediately. Then examine the fracture for possible infection, maggot/screwworm infestation, sores, or poor blood circulation. Poor blood circulation may result from the splint or bandage being too tight, or pressing against an important blood vessel. It also may result from not enough padding under the splint. Sometimes the arteries which supply blood to the bone and surrounding tissues are permanently damaged by the same accident which broke the bone. If the arteries are permanently damaged, the fracture may never heal.

Dislocation of Joints

Sometimes the bone itself is not broken but instead the bones come out of their proper position within a joint. This is called a "dislocation." If the muscles and tendons which hold the joint in place have also been torn (i.e. not just stretched), then the condition may be serious.

Treatment of dislocations: First, try to push and pull the joint back into the correct position. (If there is a grating sound when moving the bones, it means there is a fracture also.) Then treat the animal like a fracture patient:
1.   For joints in the upper leg, simply rest the animal and give it proper daily care.
2.   For joints in the lower leg, hold the bones in place with the use of a splint.
3.   Provide good supportive care as for a fracture patient.

Lameness without Obvious Fractures

Lameness due to Wounds:

Lameness may be due to wounds almost anywhere on the leg. Depending on the nature of the wound, it might be possible to suture it. See pages 213-214.

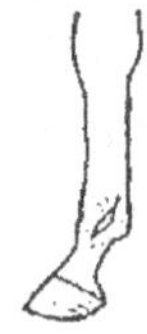

Treatment: All wounds should be cleaned thoroughly, and any maggots or screwworms should be removed. Ointment or spray should be applied to prevent maggots or screwworms.

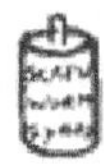

If the wound is infected, then an antibiotic injection should also be given (particularly if there is a risk of tetanus).

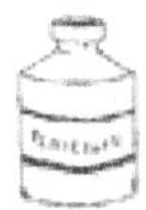

Lameness due to Wounds or Abscesses around the Hoof

One of the most common causes of lameness is a wound or abscess in the hoof or near the hoof. (The hoof is part of the Skin System but it is included here with other lameness problems.)

Examination of Hooves

- The hooves of horses, goats, and sheep can often be examined while the animal stands, by lifting the foot off the ground. For cattle/buffalo, each leg can be hoisted with a rope, or the animal should be cast.

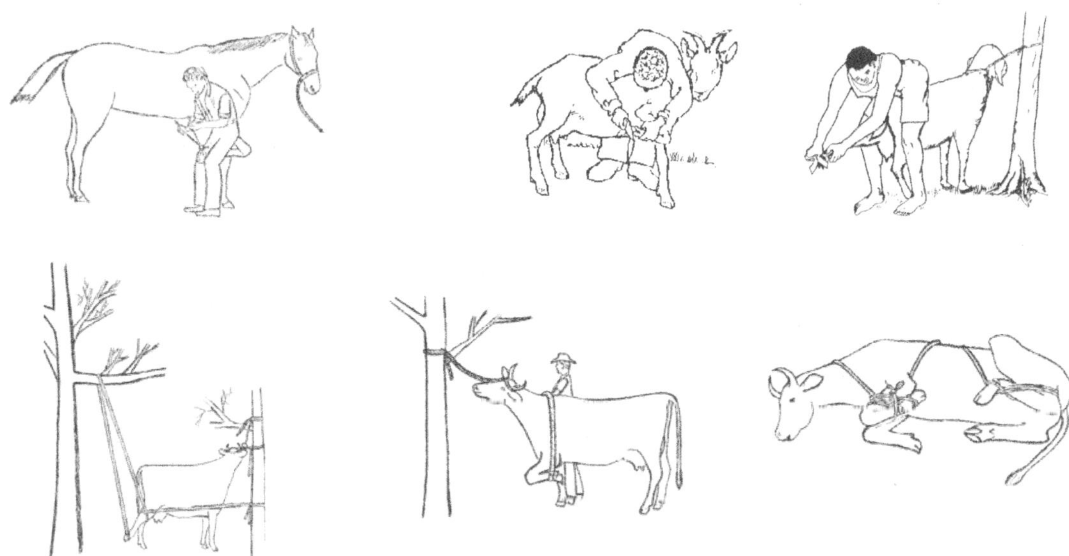

- After the animal is cast, the hoof is cleaned thoroughly and pressed in various places to see if any certain spot is sore (i.e. upon pressing a sore spot, the animal will quickly withdraw its leg).

- Next, look for small dark spots on the bottom side of the hoof which may indicate an abscess or a bruise, particularly at any spots that are sore. These spots should be carefully trimmed with a hoof knife until they are open and shallow. If pus comes out, it is an abscess. If blood comes out, it is a bruise.

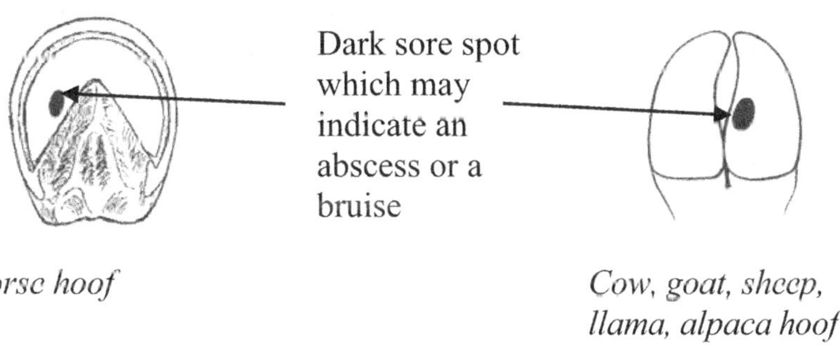

Horse hoof

*Cow, goat, sheep,
llama, alpaca hoof*

- On the bottom-side of a horse's hoof, push on the soft, triangular part called the "frog." If pus comes out, there is an infection within the frog. See next page for details of treatment. Keep the animal in a dry, clean area.

- In animals with a cloven hoof, the space between the toes should be carefully examined for any wounds due to a foreign object (e.g. a stick).

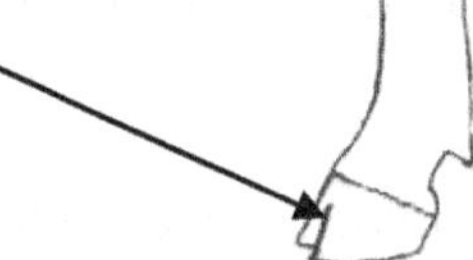

- The coronary band should be examined for any wounds.

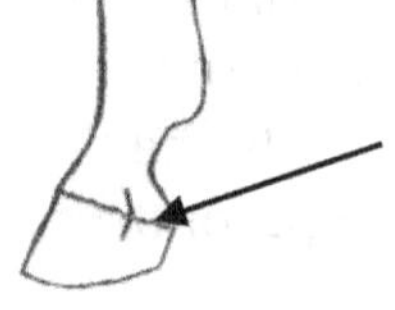

- The entire hoof should be examined for cracks or splits. If severe enough, this could cause lameness and, more rarely, infection.

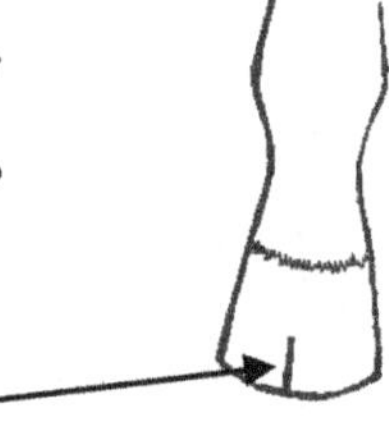

Treatment:

- **Abscess or infected frog**: The most important treatment is to trim the hoof or frog to allow good drainage. If possible, the animal's foot could also be soaked in Epsom salts (if available) or disinfectant. Keep the animal in a dry, clean environment. If the problem doesn't begin to improve within 2-3 days, give the horse an injection of long-acting penicillin.

Trim an infected frog to allow for maximum drainage

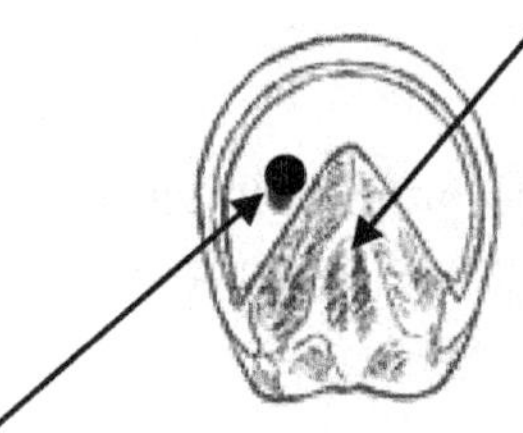

Open any abscess to allow for maximum drainage

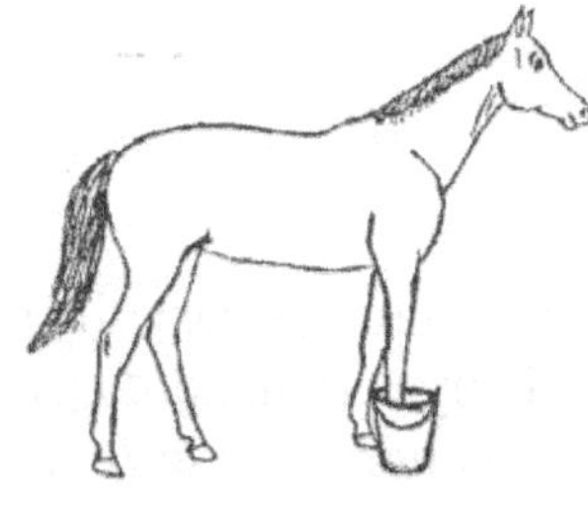

If possible, soak the animal's foot in Epsom salts, or dilute disinfectant

- **Bruise:** The most important treatment is rest. Keep the animal off stony, hard surfaces while it is recovering. If the animal is in pain, painkillers can be given also.

- **Wounds:** Wounds should be cleaned, maggots/screwworms removed, and insecticide against *maggots*/screwworms applied to prevent further infestation. If there is evidence of infection, then an antibiotic injection should be given (e.g. penicillin). If the coronary band is affected, it should be taken seriously since permanent damage in this area may result in a deformed or cracked hoof. Make every effort to prevent infection, and encourage healing as rapidly as possible.

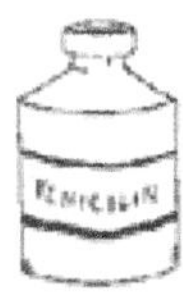
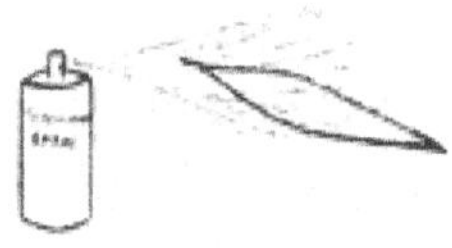
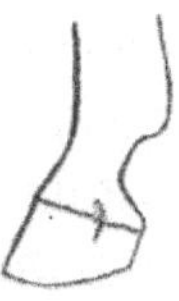

- **Cracked** *hoof*: Treat a cracked hoof by first trimming the hoof to a normal shape. Then file a horizontal groove at the top of the crack to prevent it from becoming longer. Also, file a "V" shape at the bottom of the crack so that the crack doesn't touch the ground.

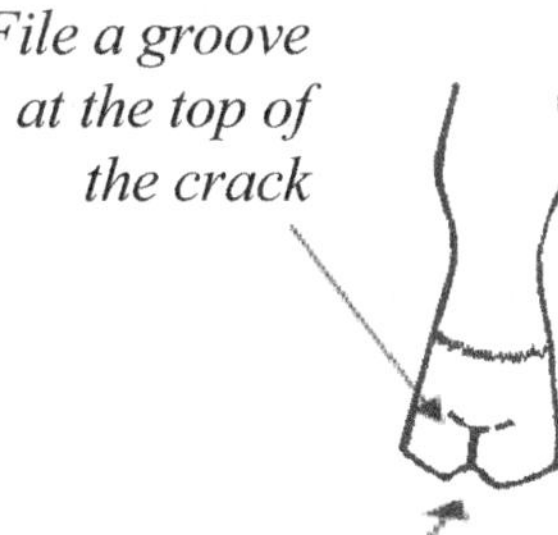

File a "V" shape at the bottom of the crack so that
the crack doesn't touch the ground

Lameness due to Sprains and Strains

When a muscle, tendon or ligament is twisted or stretched too much or worked too hard, it may become sore and swollen and cause lameness. We call this a **strain** or a **sprain**.

> **Treatment of Sprains:** The main treatment is rest. Also, pain killers can be given. Liniments may also be applied (see medicine section below), and the affected area can be soaked in cold water (e.g. a cold stream). Keep the animal on soft ground.

Lameness due to Arthritis

It is not uncommon to see old oxen, cows, and buffalo with painful and enlarged joints. This condition is called **arthritis** and most villagers are familiar with it. There are two basic types of arthritis:

- infectious arthritis
- non-infectious arthritis (also called degenerative arthritis).

Infectious arthritis is most commonly seen in baby animals as a result of an infection of the navel. This condition is called **"navel ill."** See pages 53, 56.

Non-infectious arthritis/degenerative arthritis is seen in older animals due to the normal wear and tear process. The cartilage in the joints begins to degenerate and does not provide the usual cushion. The result is a lame animal with enlarged joints.

> Younger animals may also have degenerative arthritis due to an injury to a joint, or excessive work and strain. Fat, or heavy animals suffer more from arthritis probably due to the weight on their joints. In addition, animals with poor leg conformation tend to get arthritis at a younger age due to the increased stress on their joints.

> Animals that stand on hard surfaces such as concrete all the time may develop arthritis. Eventually, an animal with arthritis may become so painful that the animal is unable to walk, and the muscles begin to waste away.

> **Treatment:** There is no real treatment for this disease. Only the symptoms can be treated by painkillers.

Prevention:

- Proper treatment of any wound/injury that involves a joint may help to prevent arthritis in the joint.
- Do not house animals on concrete all the time. Do not overwork animals.
- Don't purchase or breed animals with poor conformation to their legs. Bad conformation may be passed on to their offspring.

Body Conformation

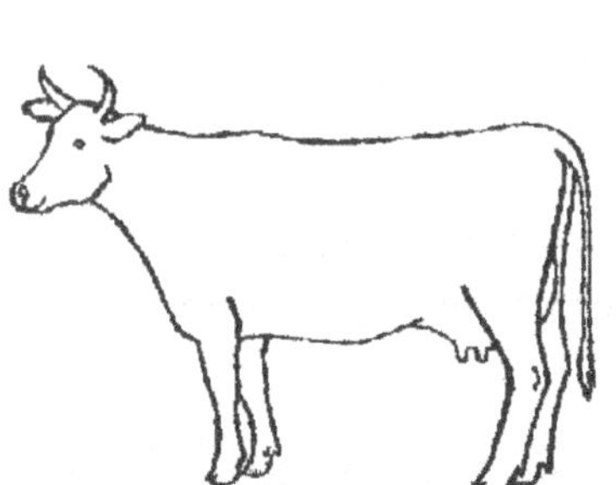

Good leg conformation

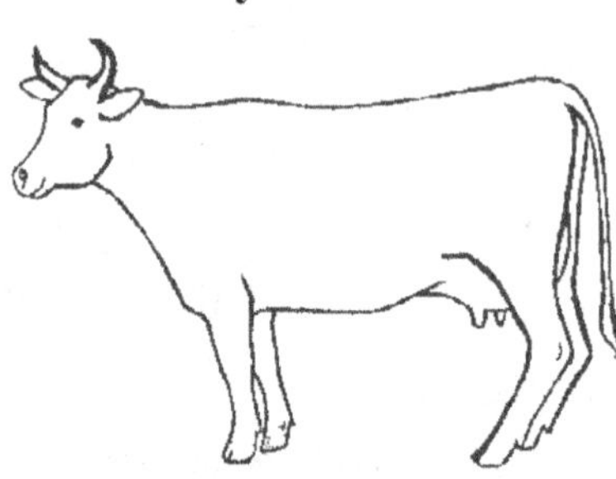

Bad leg conformation
(Back legs too angled)

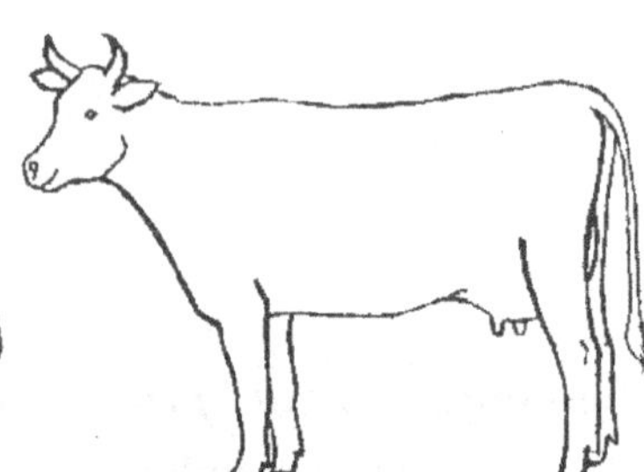

Bad leg conformation
(Back legs too straight)

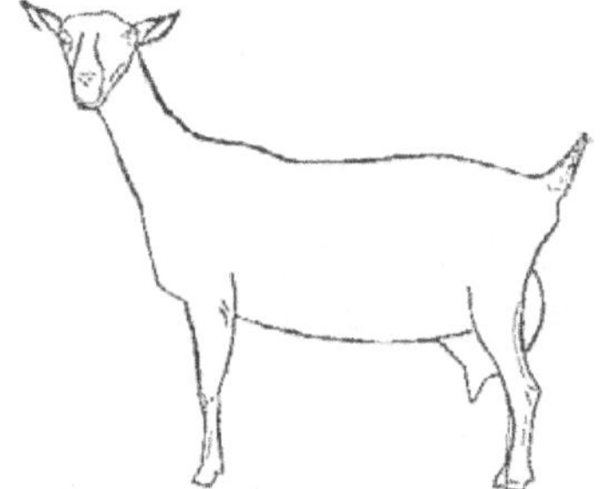

Good overall
conformation

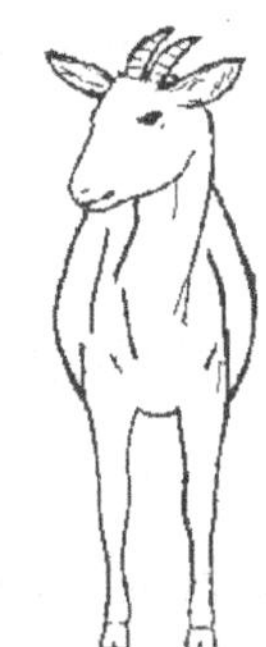

Good leg
conformation

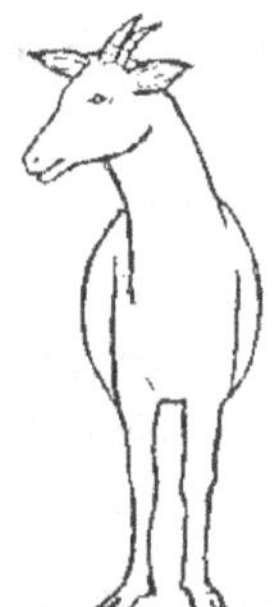

Bad leg
conformation

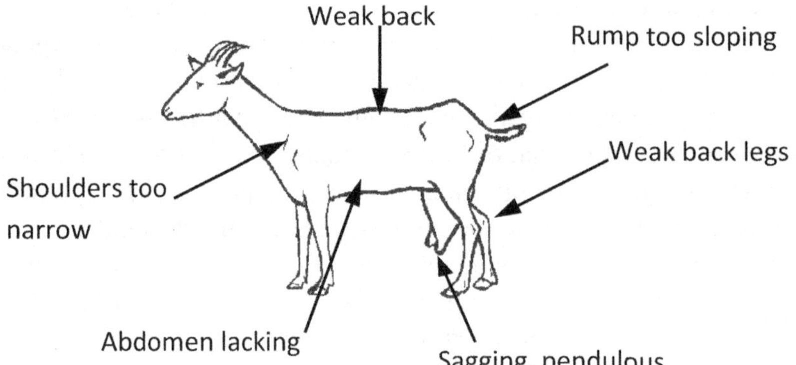

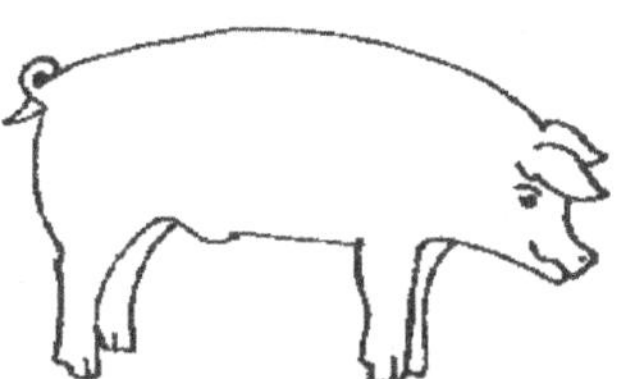

Good leg conformation

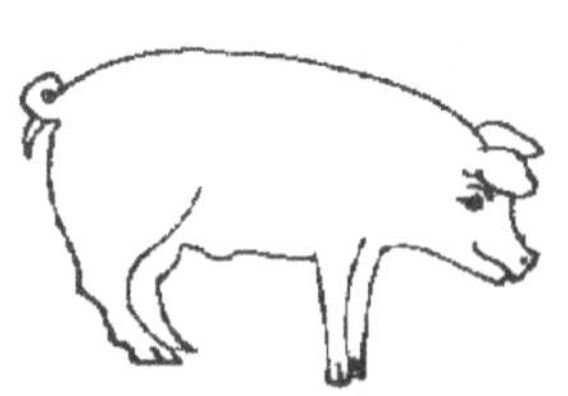

Bad leg conformation
(weak back legs)

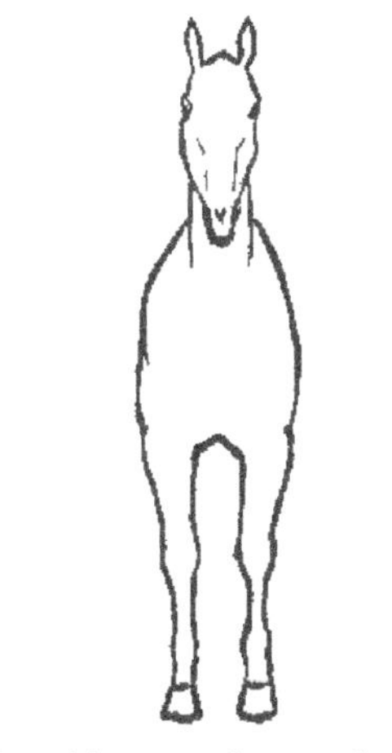

Good leg conformation

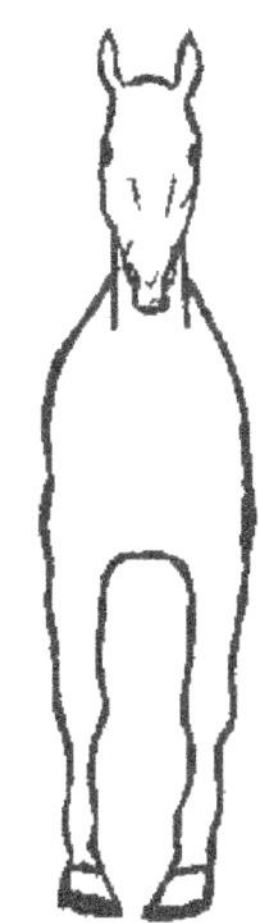

Bad leg conformation
(toes point in)

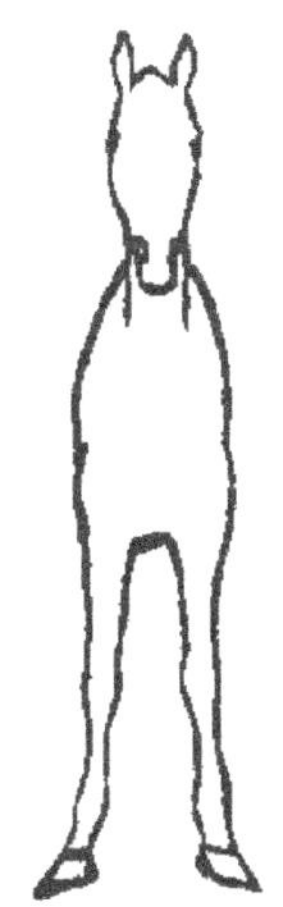

Bad leg conformation
(toes point out)

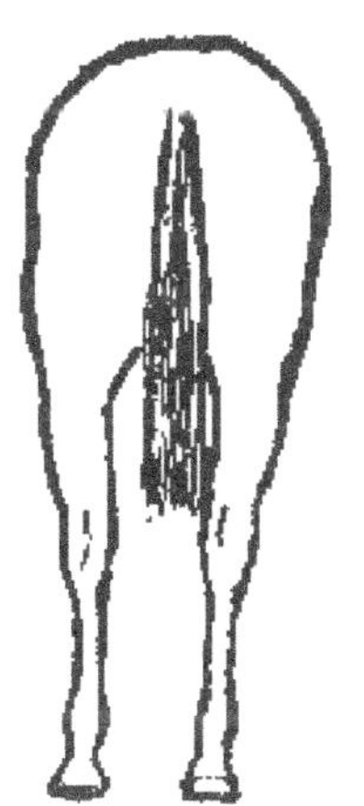

Good leg
conformation

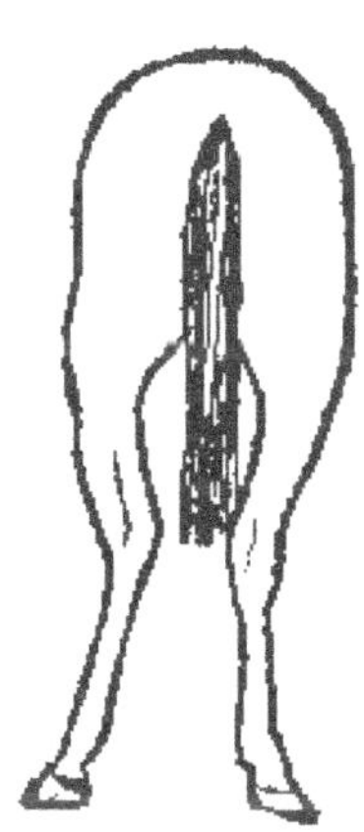

Bad leg conformation
(toes point out)

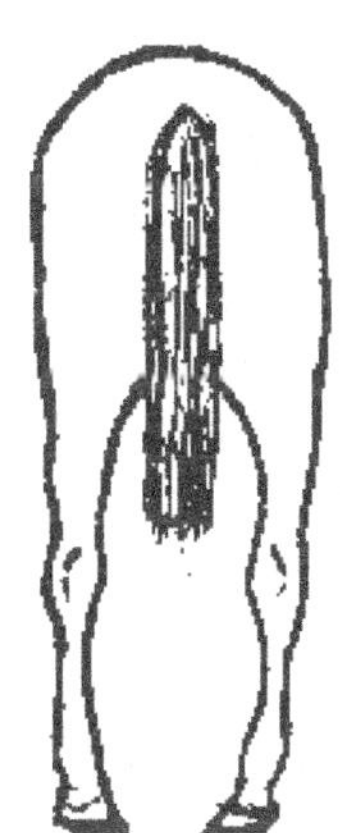

Bad leg conformation
(toes point in)

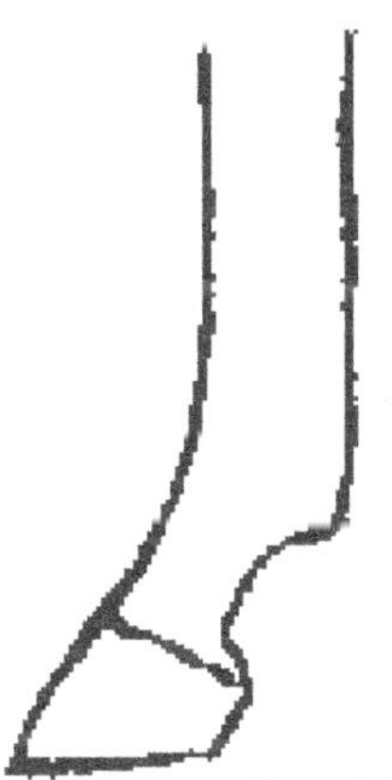

Good leg & hoof
conformation

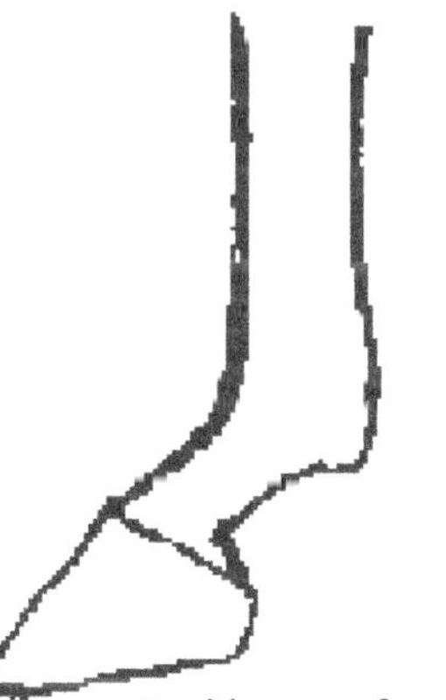

*Bad leg conformation
(too sloping)*

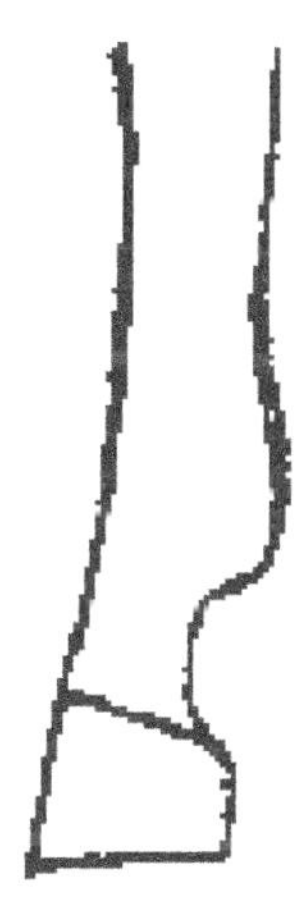

*Bad leg conformation
(too straight)*

Other faults commonly found in horses' skeletal system:

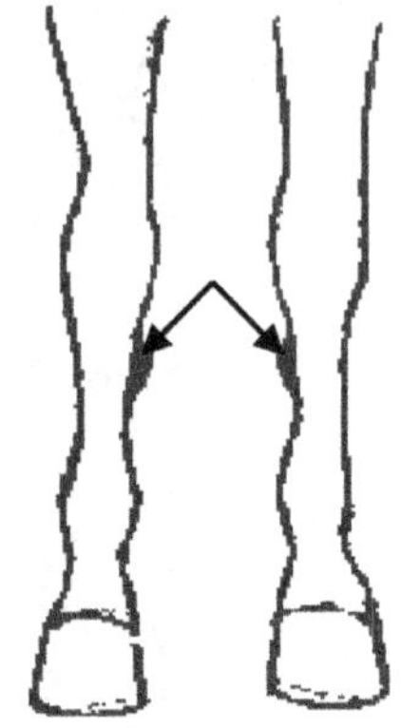

Splints (inflammation and possibly fracture of the splint bone)

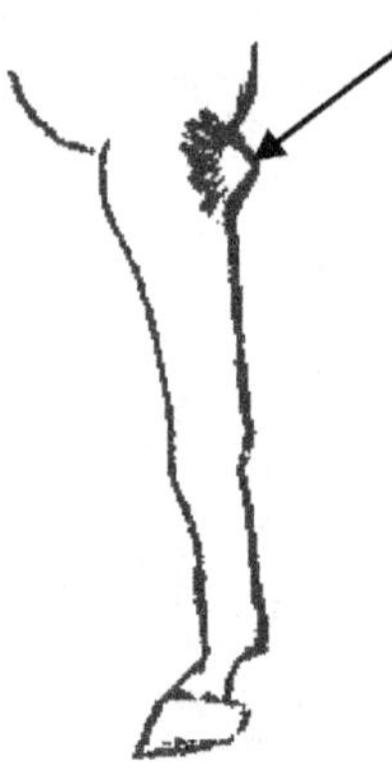

Capped elbow (injury to the elbow joint of front leg

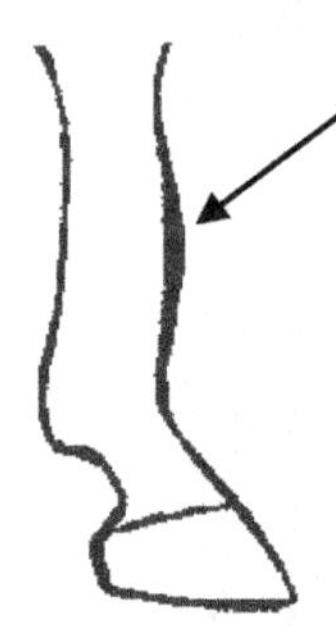

Bucked shin (weakness of the shin bones and/or too much work on hard surface)

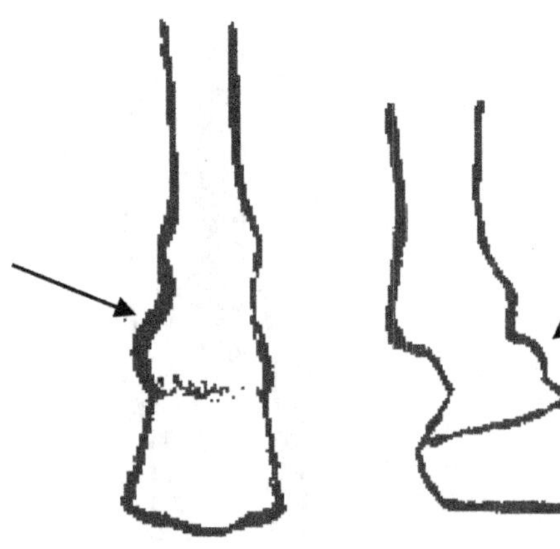

Arthritis in pastern joint

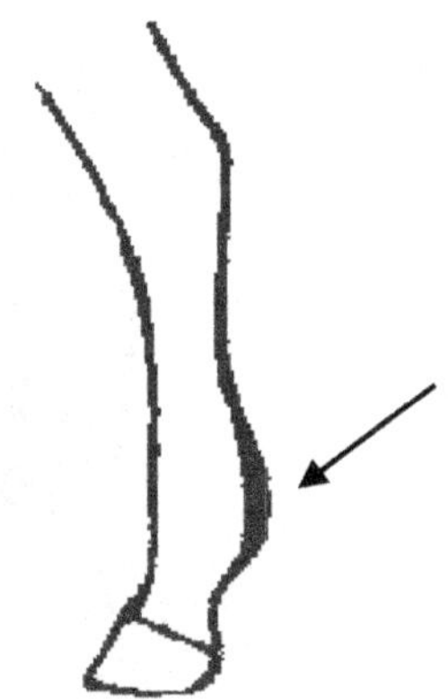

Bowed tendon (tendon is inflamed & maybe torn)

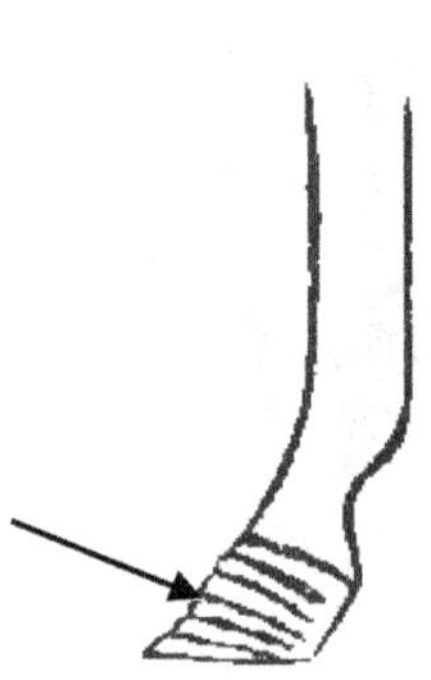

Deformed hoof (history of laminitis)

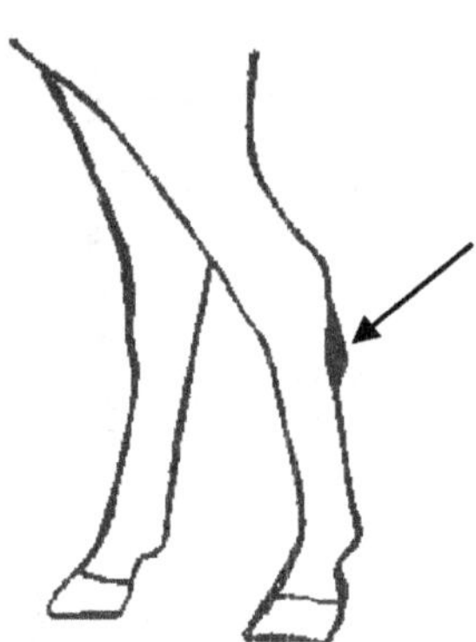

Curb (injured ligament)

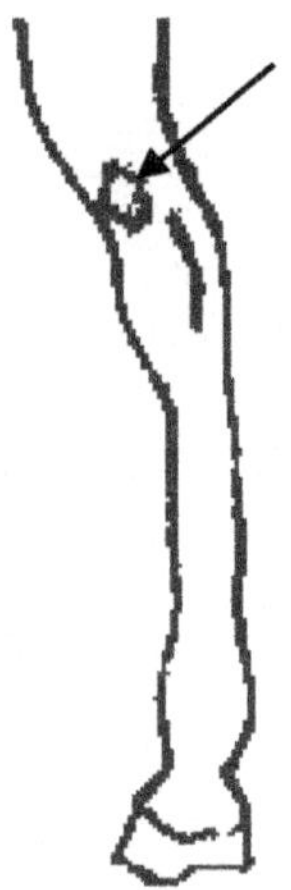

Windpuffs (extra joint fluid due to stress on the joint)

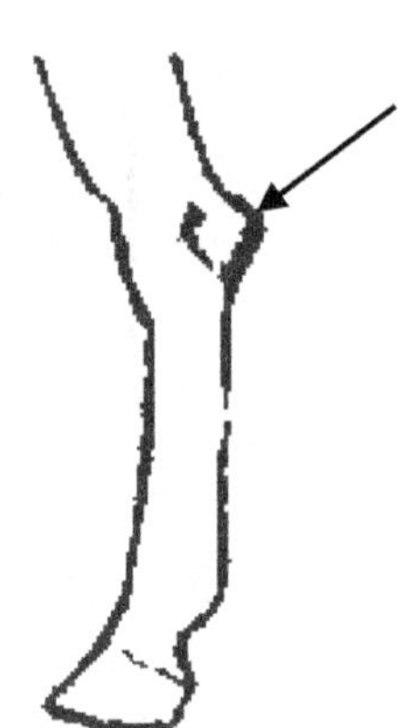

Capped hock (inflammation usually due to a previous injury)

15.3 LAMENESS DUE TO NUTRITIONAL DEFICIENCIES

If many bones and joints are crooked or deformed, then the animal may have a nutritional problem. For details regarding mineral deficiencies, See pages 306-310. In general, deficiencies of calcium / phosphorus and Vitamin D can cause problems with lameness.

- **Calcium deficiency** is very rare. It may be seen in racehorses, in cattle that are being fattened with lots of grain, in young sheep, in lactating sows that are being fed only grain and no mineral supplement, and in high-producing dairy cows right around calving. (For **milk fever**, See pages 148, 270.)
- **Phosphorus deficiency** is much more common because phosphorus is deficient in many types of soil. See page 309.
- **Vitamin D** is also essential for the body to be able to use calcium and phosphorus properly. Therefore, Vitamin D deficiency can also be associated with phosphorus deficiency or encountered in animals that are housed inside and never exposed to sunlight.

15.3.1 Rickets

The most common deficiency associated with bones in **young, growing animals** is called rickets. It is caused by a lack of phosphorus and/or Vitamin D. Young animals become lame with swollen knees. They also develop bumps on their ribs. Their backs become arched and they are reluctant to move.

15.3.2 Osteomalacia

Osteomalacia means "soft bones" and is usually due to a chronic phosphorus/vitamin deficiency in **adult animals.** Mostly pregnant or milking cows suffer from this disease and they become lame and stiff. It may also cause infertility.

> **Treatment:** Suspected cases of rickets and osteomalacia should be given mineral supplements (e.g. bone meal) to eat. See page 306-308. Be sure that the animal is exposed regularly to some sunlight (or if possible, give it vitamin D to eat). **Do not bother treating rickets or osteomalacia with intravenous calcium or phosphorus. Rather, provide these minerals in the diet.**

15.4 INFECTIONS OF THE BONE

An infection of the bone is called "osteomyelitis." Bone infections are not common in livestock or horses except following injuries, particularly an "open" fracture. Osteomyelitis might also occur after an injury in which a sharp object has punctured the skin.

Symptoms:

- Hot, swollen, and painful in the affected area
- Fever
- Possible drainage of pus

Note: An animal might also have a chronic drainage of pus due to a piece of dead bone (e.g. an old fracture). When taking a history, ask the owner if the animal had an injury in the area of the draining pus (even if it occurred several months ago).

Treatment: Give penicillin injections and be sure to remove any foreign object that has penetrated the skin. The penicillin will also help protect against tetanus. If there is a chronic drainage of pus due to dead bone, the dead bone must also be removed, otherwise, the drainage won't stop.

16.0 URINARY SYSTEM

INTRODUCTION

- The kidneys clean the blood and make urine. They also regulate the water and salt content in the body.
- Urine is made in the kidneys and passes into the bladder via the ureters.
- The urine travels from the bladder to the outside of the body via the urethra.
    - The urethra in females is large and empties into the vagina.
    - The urethra in males is small and easily blocked. It is located within the penis. See page 247.

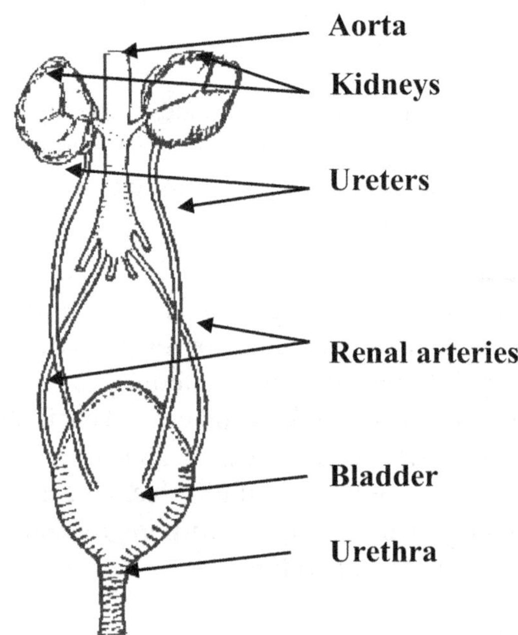

16.1 URINE COLOR

If an animal drinks a lot of water, then it makes more urine and the urine is more dilute. Conversely, an animal that does not drink much water has less urine, which is more concentrated (i.e. bright yellow in color). Therefore, the appearance of an animal's urine, can provide an indication of how much water it is drinking. If the urine is bright yellow, then the animal has not drunk enough water. If the urine is pale yellow, then it has had enough to drink.

> In general, the amount of urine an animal makes depends upon how much water it drinks.

There are also some diseases that make the color of the urine change. For instance, if an animal has hepatitis, then the urine can be a muddy, brown color (although hepatitis is very rare in livestock and horses). An animal that has eaten certain poisonous plants, or that has an infection in the urinary system may have red urine (i.e. due to blood in it).

16.2 SICK ANIMALS NEED TO DRINK WATER, TOO

In some cultures, there are beliefs that animals with certain types of illnesses should not receive water. However, sick animals need to make urine just like healthy ones. Otherwise, toxins from the body build up, making the animal even sicker, causing the kidneys to stop working, and even causing death. Therefore, whether an animal is well or sick, it must be given plenty of fresh, clean drinking water.

16.3 REDWATER

"Redwater" is a common problem related to the urinary system and indicates that the urine is red in   color. It is important to determine the cause of redwater before using expensive medicines for treatment. There is a simple field test to help distinguish certain causes of red-colored urine. See page 287. The term for blood cells in the urine is "hematuria."

16.3.1 Hematuria in Cattle and Buffalo

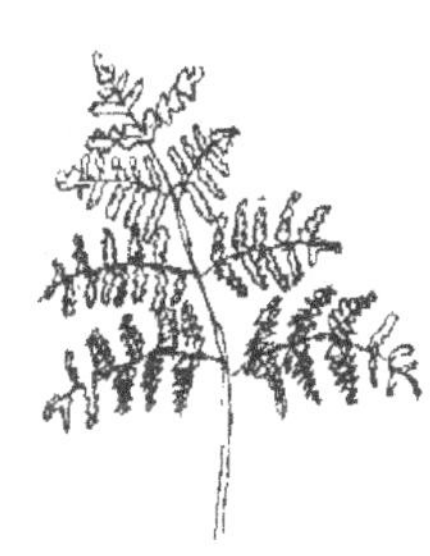

Wounds in the urinary tract. Anything that causes bleeding in the urinary tract may cause redwater. Eating large amounts of bracken fern over an extended period of time (e.g. 2-3 months) may result in a **chronic disease,** particularly, in cattle and buffalo (and less commonly sheep). The bracken fern causes bleeding to occur inside the body. These symptoms may appear long after the animal has stopped eating the bracken fern, and may be associated with bladder cancer.

Note: Animals do not normally eat bracken fern, but will if they are hungry enough (e.g. during a drought when there is little fodder).

Symptoms: The main symptom is red-colored urine. The animal may also have a fever. The condition is chronic and the animal gradually becomes thin. Sometimes an animal may appear to recover, only to relapse at a later date.

Diagnosis: The diagnosis of hematuria is based on observing red blood cells in the urine with a microscope. Even without a microscope, one can collect urine in a container, let it sit for at least one hour and look for red cells to appear at the bottom of the container. The diagnosis of bracken fern poisoning is based on a history that the animal ate bracken fern.

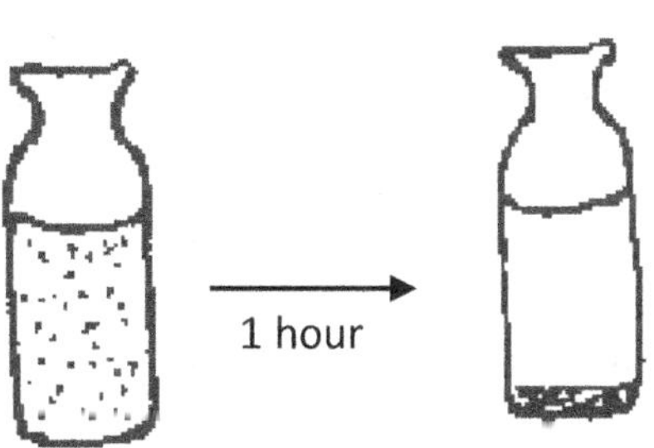

urine sample collected   *blood cells*
in a clear container   *settle to bottom*

Treatment: Treatment options are limited. The AHA can give the animal plenty of fresh drinking water and rest. If the problem is already chronic, the animal is less likely to recover. Penicillin might help if the animal has a low-grade fever (assumed to be an infection that is complicating the problem). Local herbal diuretics (i.e. which cause the animal to make more urine) might also be helpful.

Prevention: Be especially careful during periods of drought (i.e. when animals are more likely to eat poisonous plants), by not allowing animals to graze in areas where there are known toxic plants like bracken fern.

16.3.2   Hematuria in Pigs (Bloody Urine)

In pigs, the problem of hematuria is seen most often in female pigs within three weeks of breeding. The bloody urine results from an infection by an organism <u>Corynebacterium suis</u> in the bladder and kidneys. Most boars (approximately 80%) have this organism in the tissues around their penis. If the sow or gilt is even slightly injured or irritated during breeding, the organism can go up into her bladder and kidneys, resulting in infection and bloody urine.

Treatment: A week-long course of antibiotics, such as tetracycline or penicillin, given to the female pig usually clears up the problem temporarily. However, several weeks or months later, the problem may recur. The sow gradually becomes thin. It is best to slaughter the sow soon after she has been treated for this condition (i.e. after the antibiotic residues are no longer in her meat, and before the problem recurs or she gets thin).

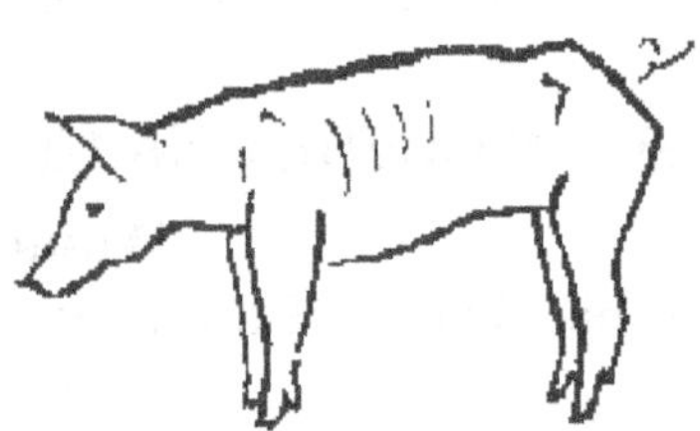

Thin sow after chronic hematuria

Prevention: There are no proven methods to prevent this problem. In herds with a chronic problem of hematuria, the sheaths around the penis of all the breeding boars can be flushed with 1 gram of tetracycline every six months. This can be done by emptying several tetracycline capsules (e.g. four capsules of 250 milligrams or two capsules of 500 milligrams) into 100 ml of water and gently flushing the fluid into the sheath around the penis using a syringe (with no needle!). This treatment has not been studied in a controlled clinical trial, but experienced veterinarians believe that it is effective in decreasing the problem in a herd.

16.3.3   Babesiosis: (Piroplasmosis, Tick Fever, Texas Fever)

Babesiosis is a disease caused by small organisms, called <u>Babesia</u>, that live in the red blood cells. Babesia cause the red blood cell to burst, and the red color from the burst cell appears in the urine.

Babesiosis is spread by the bite of ticks. A tick drinks the blood of an animal that already has Babesiosis. When the tick bites another animal, it transfers the <u>Babesia</u>.

Symptoms:
- The animal becomes suddenly ill with a fever and stops eating. The respiratory rate is fast and the pulse is rapid.

- Sometimes the animal develops nervous symptoms which might appear like rabies.

- Most animals (except horses) have red-colored urine.

- Because the red blood cells have broken open, the animal also develops anemia. The eyelids and the gums become pale like any other animal with anemia. If the animal does not die from fever and infection, it might die later from anemia. In a dead animal, the spleen will be large and filled with blood.

Diagnosis:
A tentative diagnosis can be made by the symptoms and knowledge that Babesiosis is a problem in the area.

As a simple field test, a sample of urine can be collected in a container and allowed to sit for at least one hour. In animals with hematuria, red blood cells will appear at the bottom of the container. But in animals with Babesia, no blood cells will appear at the bottom of the tube (because the cells have already burst). Instead, the urine is uniformly red in color due to a component of the red blood cell called "hemoglobin" that is present in the urine. The condition is therefore called "hemoglobinuria."

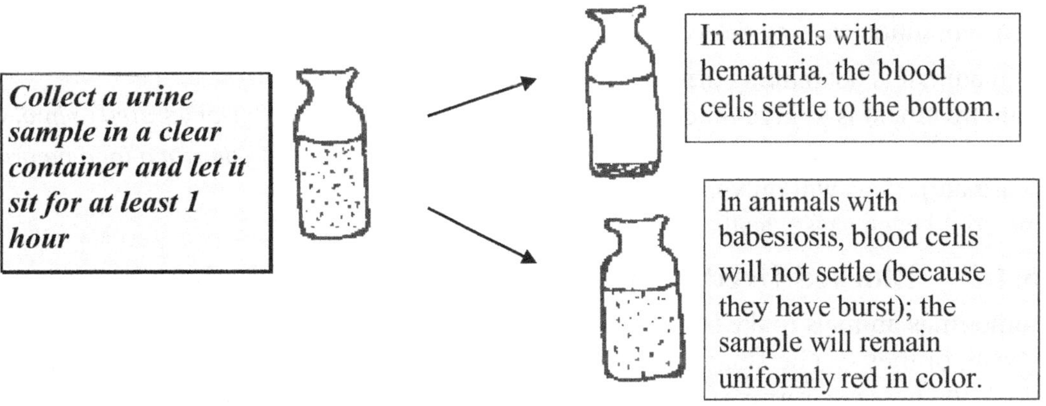

The diagnosis can be confirmed by examining a blood smear from a drop of blood. That is, the blood smear can be sent to a laboratory and examined under a microscope. The Babesia organism can be seen inside the red blood cells. If there is no access to a laboratory to confirm the diagnosis, you should still treat the animal based on its symptoms of Babesiosis. A good response to treatment will also help confirm the diagnosis.

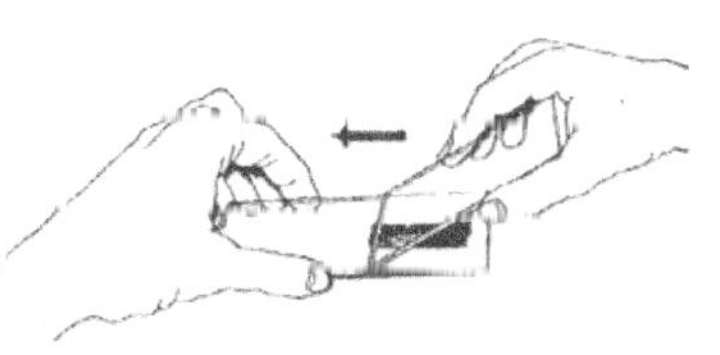

Treatment: There are special drugs to treat Babesiosis (e.g. *Berenil*). Good nursing care (e.g. good food, water, and shelter) is also important since the animal may be very ill.

Control: Controlling ticks will help decrease the spread of Babesiosis. Animals may be vaccinated against Babesiosis (however the vaccine is not available in many countries). Sometimes an AHA has no good way of preventing the disease.

Note: Animals that recover from Babesiosis usually develop resistance to it. However, new animals lacking this resistance may die if brought into an area with Babesiosis. If you purchase new animals, be ready to rapidly treat them upon the first symptom or they may become gravely ill and die.

16.3.4   Other Causes of Redwater

In addition to bracken fern, there may be other local plants that cause the urine to become red. Ask other AHAs or veterinarians about the poisonous plants in your area.

16.4   "NO URINE!" / ANURIA

An animal owner may complain that his/her animal's "urine is closed down." Your job will be to determine whether the urethra is blocked (and therefore urine cannot come out) or whether the animal is not making any urine.

16.4.1   Dehydration

The most common reason for lack of urine is dehydration. Be sure to take a proper history and find out whether the animal has some condition causing dehydration (e.g. diarrhea).

If an animal is not making urine because of dehydration, the main treatment is to give fluids. See page 268. **Note:** Do not give a dehydrated animal a "diuretic" (i.e. a drug that causes it to urinate). This will only make the animal more dehydrated and could even cause death.

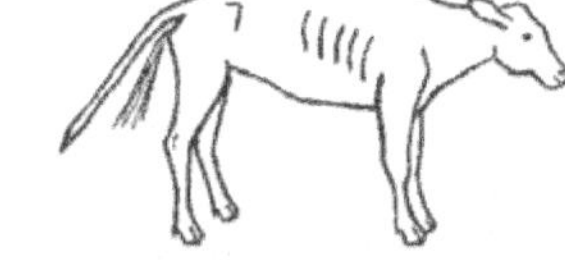

Dehydrated animal with diarrhea (and no urine)

16.4.2   Blocked Urethra: (Stones, Calculi, Urolithiasis)

Sometimes animals make hard "stones" in their bladder called "calculi." They can be large like a bean, or they can be small like sand. The stones sometimes become stuck in the urethra and block the passage of urine. A blocked urethra occurs most commonly in male animals because the urethra is small, especially that part of the urethra within the penis. A blocked urethra due to calculi is most common in male animals that have been castrated at a young age.

Treatment: Treatment of a blocked urethra requires some special instruments, and training. A narrow plastic tube, called a "catheter", is passed up the urethra in the penis until the catheter meets the stones. Then, by gently pushing on the catheter, the stones may become dislodged. If you do not have a catheter you can gently massage the penis. This may help the stones to become dislodged and pass from the urethra.

Note: Sometimes, a diuretic is given in hope that the increased amount of urine may cause enough pressure to dislodge the stone. However, this practice is not always effective and may result in a burst bladder.

16.5   BROKEN PENIS: (PHIMOSIS; PARAPHIMOSIS)

When a bull pursues a cow in heat, he tries to mount and insert his penis into her vulva. If he misses her vulva, it is possible for his penis to become bruised, broken, or swollen. The penis of a stallion or bull can also swell up from other injuries, like being kicked by another animal. The swelling may impede the blood flow to the penis causing the tissue to die.

- If the penis swells up while it is extended, then sometimes it cannot retract. This is called **paraphimosis**. If a retracted penis swells up, then sometimes it cannot extend. This is called **phimosis**.

    Symptoms / Diagnosis: The penis and/or the tissue around it will be swollen. In some cases, the animal may have trouble urinating. The animal's whole belly may become swollen. If the tissue of the penis dies, an infection may start, or the area may become infested with maggots.

    Treatment: Treatment is not easy. Surgery is usually not possible.

    - The penis and the surrounding tissue should be thoroughly washed. All black, dead tissue must be removed.

    - Animals should be given antibiotics. Long-acting penicillin is a good choice because it also protects against tetanus.

    - Any maggots should be removed and the affected area treated with a product effective against maggots or screwworm.

    - For paraphimosis, when the penis is stuck outside the body and cannot go back in, try to reduce the swelling and gently push the penis back into the sheath. The swelling can be reduced by bathing the affected area in cold water, applying ice or a cloth soaked in magnesium sulfate, and/or giving the animal *Lasix*. If the penis comes back out again, then gently push it back in and place a suture in the sheath to keep the penis retracted for a few days. Once this is accomplished and the swelling has diminished, the suture can be removed. If the penis cannot be pushed back into the sheath, then it must be bathed regularly to keep the tissue from drying out and to reduce swelling.

    - For phimosis, when the penis is stuck inside the body, try pulling gently to extend the penis. Sometimes it is necessary to massage the penis near the scrotum, and even higher in case it is   stuck there.

16.6 RUPTURED BLADDER

Sometimes the urethra is completely blocked by stones or swelling so that the animal cannot urinate at all. Then the bladder gets bigger and bigger and the animal will be in pain. It will try to urinate but be unable to. Finally, the bladder may burst and the urine goes into the belly, around the stomach and intestines. Most animals die from this condition.

    Diagnosis: The animal tries to urinate but cannot. The animal is also in pain.

    Treatment: There is no good treatment for this. Therefore, if a male goat or buffalo is completely blocked, you may want to cut it for meat before the bladder ruptures.

16.7 CYSTITIS

This is a general term used for an infection of the urinary bladder.

    Symptoms: The animal may have a fever, will urinate frequently and may have pus or blood in the urine. The animal may also strain and appear in pain when trying to urinate. If pus is seen in the urine, a proper history must be taken. This is because an animal with a uterus infection will also have pus in the vagina (which may also appear in the urine).

    Diagnosis: Based on symptoms. Or, you may take a urine sample and examine it with a microscope for the presence of white blood cells.

    Treatment / Control: Antibiotics should be given; and the animal should be given lots of water to drink. Some people also put a few grams of magnesium sulfate, or other salt, into the water for   the animal to drink. This makes the animal thirsty so that it drinks lots of water, and then it will urinate more than usual. This helps to flush out the organisms and rinse the wounds that may be in the bladder. Other drugs like *Lasix* and local medicines may also help the animal to urinate more.

17.0 Nervous System

Introduction:
Nervous system problems are challenging to diagnose and treat because different problems may have similar symptoms. In addition, a certain nervous system problem may have different symptoms in different animals! This book divides nervous system problems into the five main groups below, even though there is overlap among the groups.

For all nervous problems, **taking a history** is very important. For instance, it's useful to know that an animal may have first acted aggressively or abnormally excited, even though by the time you are examining it, it is paralyzed. Or, a history may provide critical information such as exposure to poisons, or being bitten by an aggressive dog. Also important is an **examination of the animal's environment** (including where it was in the past month) as well as a **thorough physical exam**.

FIVE GROUPS OF NERVOUS SYSTEM PROBLEMS

1. Strange, aggressive, excited or crazy behavior, see page 250.

These animals often develop convulsions, coma or paralysis later.

-Rabies	Page 251.
-Poisons	Page 83.
-Object caught in throat	Page 184.
-Liver problem/ failure (horse)	Page 197.
-Low blood sugar/ ketosis (cow)	Page 253.
-Salt poisoning (pigs)	Page 269.
-Milk fever	Page 270.
-Grass tetany	Page 271.
-Vitamin A deficiency	Page 311.
-Pseudo-rabies	Page 252.

2. Walking in circles, blindness, or pushing head against objects, see page 256.

-Listeriosis	Page 280.
-Parasites (in brain)	Page 338.
-Vitamin A deficiency	Page 311.

4. Stiffness, trembling, convulsions and coma, see page 83.

The following problems often end like this:

-Poisons	Page 83.
-Tetanus	Page 258.
-Rabies	Page 251.
-Pseudo-rabies	Page 249.
-Milk fever	Page 270.
-Grass-tetany	Page 272.
-Salt-poisoning	Page 313.

3. Tilted head, see page 257.

-Ear infection	Page 257.
-Parasite (in brain)	Page 338.

5. Paralysis, see page 259.

-Injury or trauma	Page 288.
-Parasites (in spinal cord)	Page 121.

17.1 STRANGE, AGGRESSIVE, EXCITED OR CRAZY ANIMAL

Several different problems will cause an animal to act strange or crazy. *If rabies is a problem in an area, then it must always be considered as a possible diagnosis.* However, not every animal that acts strange has rabies. In some parts of the world, rabies is very rare or not found at all. Sometimes it is tricky to deal with the situation of a strange-acting animal, because not only is the diagnosis difficult, but the animal may be dangerous, and there may be panic in the community about the situation.

> **Be careful!** An animal with a nervous system problem may be more likely to cause injury to people or other animals.

Problems That Cause Animals to Act Strange or Crazy

- **Rabies!**
- Poisons (plants or some kinds of insecticides)
- Bone or other object caught in the throat making swallowing difficult
- Liver failure due to liver fluke or other cause
- Low blood sugar / ketosis (cattle)
- Salt poisoning in pigs
- Grass tetany
- Milk fever
- Vitamin A deficiency
- Pseudo-rabies

What to do?

1. Take a proper history. Be sure to ask the following questions:

   - Was the animal bitten recently (also look for bite wounds)?
   - Was the animal recently injured (look for signs of any injury)?
   - Were, or are there any other animals in the area with similar symptoms (if so, examine them also)?
   - Was a known rabid animal in the area recently?
   - How long has the animal had these symptoms?
   - Was there any known contact with insecticides, poisons or poisonous plants (ask where the animal has been housed or grazed in the past month, and go check the area)?
   - If pigs are affected, ask whether there was any shortage of water? (Is there salt in the feed?)
   - What kind of food has the animal received in the past three months?
   - Did the animal recently give birth? Is it lactating now?
   - When was the animal last treated with deworming medicine?

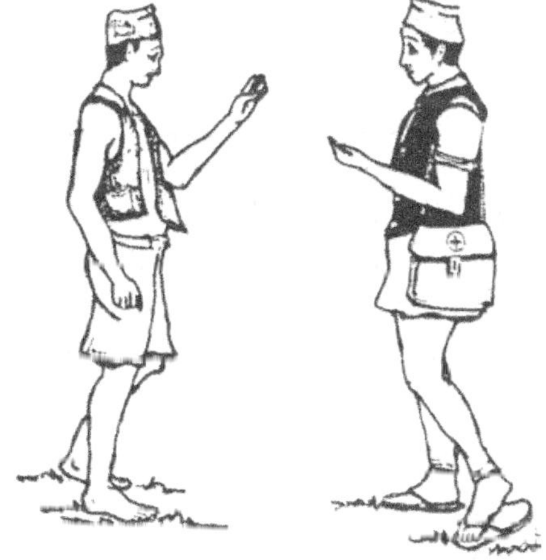

2. Thoroughly **examine the animal.**
If there is any chance that the animal may have rabies, wear
plastic gloves (or plastic sacks) on the hands when examining
the animal.

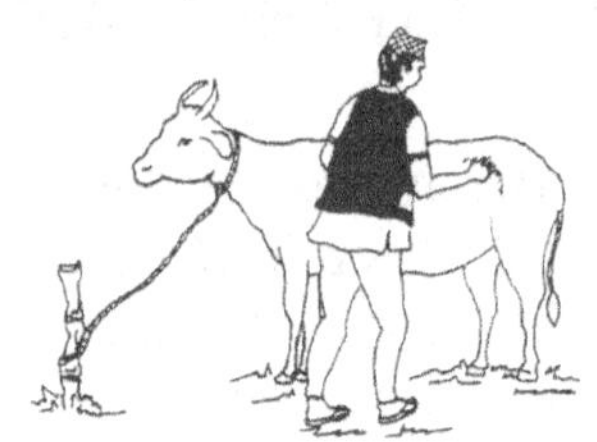

Note: If any people in the area have been bitten by a strange
acting animal, inform the nearest medical officer.

17.1.1 Rabies

What should an AHA do when an animal acts strange or crazy? What should they do after a wild dog
has run through a village biting livestock and people? These are common situations for AHAs in areas
where **rabies** is a problem.

Rabies is caused by a virus that affects the nervous system of all livestock, horses and people. (It does
not affect poultry.) It is a frightening public health disease because after an animal or person gets sick
from it, there is no treatment, and the disease is nearly 100% fatal.

Rabies is spread through the **saliva of rabid animals,** often by
biting. Certain animals are known to spread rabies, such as dogs,
skunks, bats and raccoons.

The rabies virus moves from the bite wound to the brain, using the
nerves as a pathway. This process usually takes 3 – 8 weeks, but in some cases, can take more than six
months. Then the animal may begin to act strangely, appear weak, especially in its hind legs, and (due
to paralysis in the throat muscles), drool, stop eating,
and have a very odd-sounding voice.   An animal
with rabies may seem to have something caught in
its throat.

Caution: Many AHAs have been
exposed to rabies when examining an
animal's throat because the animal
appeared to have something caught in its
throat!

When is the animal contagious?
The animal is contagious at the same time it has
symptoms.

How do I determine whether someone was exposed?
Anyone who was in contact with the animal's saliva or nervous tissue (e.g. the animal's brain tissue)
should be considered "exposed", especially if the saliva or nervous tissue was in contact with a
wound or mucous membrane (i.e. tissue around the eye, in the nose, or mouth) of the person.

What can be done following exposure to rabies?
If exposed to rabies, wash the exposed area with soap and water (soap kills the rabies virus), and if
possible, rinse with disinfectant. Then seek post-exposure rabies vaccination *immediately*. **Do *not*
wait for symptoms to appear.** If a person or animal receives post-exposure rabies vaccinations *before*
symptoms begin, the virus can be stopped before it reaches the brain, and the animal's or person's life
can be saved. Once rabies symptoms appear, the person or animal will die.

Symptoms: Symptoms vary. *However, all animals show some change in behavior and most stop eating.*
Cattle often appear to have weak back legs. In general, an animal will show either "**furious rabies**" or "**dumb rabies.**" "Furious rabies" means that the animal acts aggressively. "Dumb rabies" means that the animal acts dull, listless, and weak. Sometimes their lower jaw may even hang open. All animals eventually become paralyzed and die. Most animals die within 4 or 5 days after the first symptoms appear.

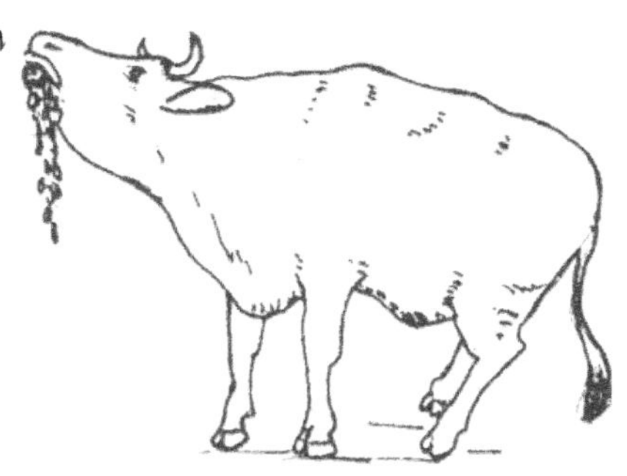

If the animal is still alive 14 days after the first symptoms appear, then the animal probably does not have rabies.

Diagnosis: A tentative diagnosis can be made based on symptoms and history. If there is a history of being bitten, and if rabies is common in the area, then assume that the animal has rabies. The diagnosis can be confirmed by carefully removing the animal's brain (i.e. using gloves to avoid exposure to the brain tissue) and having a laboratory do one of the following three tests:

1. *Fluorescent antibody:* an accurate and rapid test, but one that requires fresh brain tissue that has been stored in ice.

2. *Mousebrain inoculation:* an accurate test that requires fresh brain tissue, but is less rapid than the fluorescent antibody test.

3. *Negri body test:* less accurate test (i.e. can miss some rabies cases), but the advantage is it does not require fresh brain tissue. That is, the brain can be placed in a solution of 50% glycerine or 10% formalin and transported long distances. However, since the test is less accurate, persons bitten by an animal should receive anti-rabies vaccination even if the test is negative.

    In many remote areas, laboratory tests are impossible, and the following measures should be taken.

Measures to take regarding a suspect rabies case (with   no access to a laboratory for confirmation):

1. The bite wounds on the victim (livestock or human) should be thoroughly and immediately washed with water, soap and, if available, disinfectant. Use gloves when washing these wounds to avoid further exposure to the rabies virus.

> **Wash all bite wounds thoroughly with water, soap and, if available, disinfectant!**

2. All people bitten should begin post-exposure rabies vaccination as soon as possible. **Note:** If the bites are near the head, then it is even more urgent to receive post-exposure injections since the virus will travel more rapidly to the brain.

3. If the animal is acting deranged and aggressive, it should be killed as soon as possible to prevent further suffering and spread of rabies. At the same time, ensure that everyone exposed to the virus completes the series of post-exposure vaccination. Otherwise, catch the animal and chain it inside a secure pen to

observe for 14 days. Continue to give the animal food and water. If it is still alive
after 14 days, then rabies can be ruled out as the diagnosis and those persons receiving
the post-exposure vaccination can stop doing so. If the animal becomes paralyzed
and dies during the 14-day observation period, assume a diagnosis of rabies. Ensure
that everyone exposed to the virus completes the post-exposure vaccination series.

Vaccinations for Rabies

There are many different kinds of vaccines used throughout the world. However, they
are divided into two groups:

1. **Pre-exposure vaccines** are injections that are given at regular intervals (e.g. annually) before
    possible exposure to rabies. Consult a local veterinary officer for further information about
    what rabies vaccines are available in your area for livestock.
    For wildlife, there are effective pre-exposure vaccines that can be given by leaving it in
    some food for the wildlife to eat.
2. **Post-exposure vaccines** are a series of injections that are given after possible exposure
    to a rabid animal. This series is usually effective in preventing rabies *if* it is given *before*
    symptoms begin in the person/animal exposed.

    > **Control / Prevention:** All dogs in the area should be vaccinated regularly with **pre-
    > exposure** rabies vaccine. AHAs and their community can organize a vaccination clinic
    > for all dogs. They can request help from the government vets.

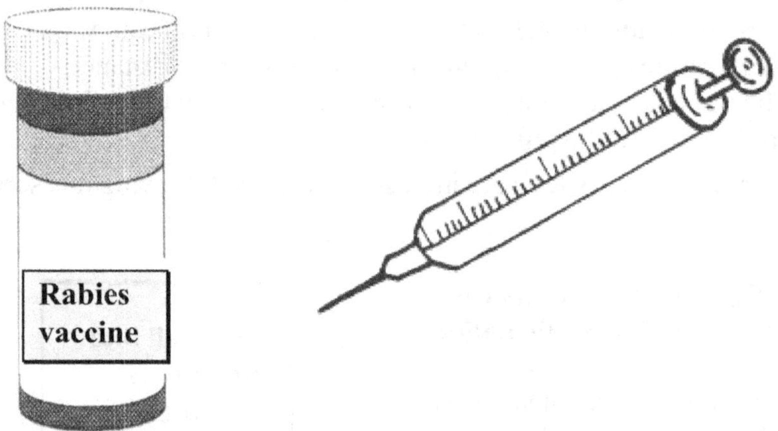

17.1.2 Ketosis/Acetonemia in Cattle and Sheep ("Crazy Cow",
"Pregnancy Toxemia" or "Low Blood Sugar")

This is not an infectious disease. It occurs in cows within a few weeks after calving and in sheep
(and sometimes cows) during late pregnancy. When it occurs in late pregnancy, it is often called
"pregnancy toxemia", and mainly effects ewes that are carrying twins or triplets. Cows or ewes that
are fat during early pregnancy are especially prone to ketosis. In cows, ketosis after calving is usually
a complication of another problem such as mastitis, metritis, pneumonia or stomach problems which
causes the cow to stop eating, resulting in low blood sugar (i.e. "ketosis"). In sheep, ketosis results
because the ewe is not eating enough calories to keep up with the energy demands of 2-3 fetuses in
addition to her own body. See pages 271, 272.

Symptoms/Diagnosis: Symptoms can be vague. Most cows and sheep with ketosis stop eating and become listless. However, cows or ewes may be affected neurologically (i.e. act a bit crazy). Milk production decreases also.   Ewes (or cows) with pregnancy toxemia often die.

Treatment for ketosis in cows:
1. Give 500 ml of 50% glucose, IV.
2. Give propylene glycol or glycerol twice daily.
3. Treat any other problem the cow may have.

Treatment for pregnancy toxemia in ewes (and sometimes cows)
1. Give propylene glycol or glycerol twice daily.
2. Consider performing a caesarian section to remove the fetuses, particularly if the mother is valuable. If done late enough in pregnancy, the fetuses might also survive.
3. Give high quality food and water to encourage the animal to begin feeding (an AHA can even grind the feed fine and give it through a stomach tube).
4. Provide good shelter.

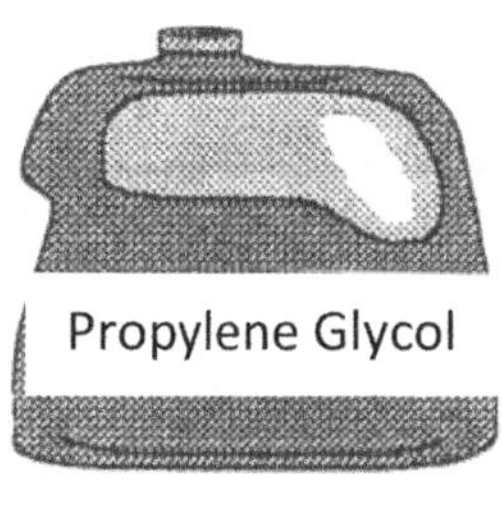

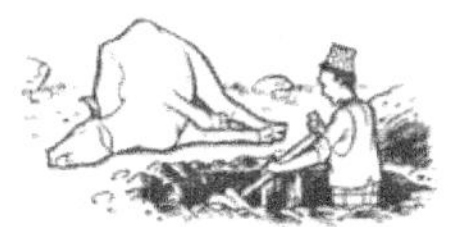

Note: Pregnancy toxemia is difficult to treat; the animal will probably die, particularly if it is not treated early.

Prevention/Control: Do not allow ewes or cows to get too fat during pregnancy. Be sure to give enough feed during late pregnancy. If a newly- calved cow becomes sick with mastitis, metritis, etc., treat her immediately.

Note: Sometimes, it can help to make the flock of sheep walk a bit. Observe carefully for symptoms in any of the sheep, then treat immediately.

17.1.3 Common Toxicities and Poisonings

Summary

The word **"toxicity"** is the same as a poisoning. It means that an animal has taken into its body a certain substance than it cannot handle (i.e. a poison), resulting in harmful, or "toxic" effects in the body. Some substances are not toxic in small quantities, but only at larger doses. A toxin in the blood is called *"toxemia."* The symptoms of toxicity vary depending upon the type of toxic substance taken into the body. It is beyond the scope of this book to review all toxicities, but some of the most common ones are included in the chapters related to the system affected. The most important thing to do when you suspect toxicity is to take a careful history. Examine the area where the animal has been (for toxic plants, rat poisons, etc.), verify the food, water, and any medications it has received (including the quantity or dose). Ask if there are other animals in the area with the same symptoms. Conduct a thorough examination of the affected animal.

Examples of different types of toxicities:

Salt poisoning is a condition found most commonly in pigs. Normally, the body needs salt to stay healthy. However, if the pig does not receive enough water while eating a normal amount of salt in its diet, the salt actually begins to act like a poison in the body because it becomes too concentrated. The pig trembles, has convulsions, and may even die. See pages 55, 269, 313.

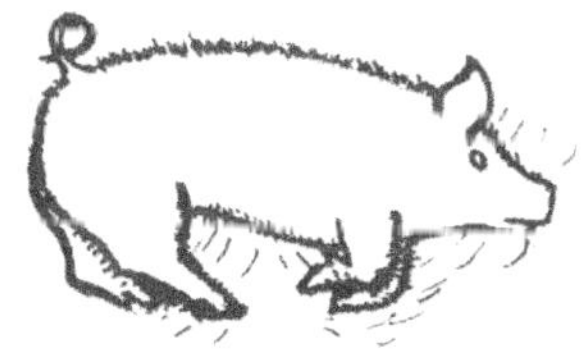

Snake-bite poisoning is a different kind of toxicity. The poison from snakes, even in small amounts, causes harmful effects in the body.

Toxemia is a condition resulting from various diseases like hemorrhagic septicemia, metritis, mastitis and navel infections. The bacteria make toxins that travel in the blood and act like a poison to the body. These toxins affect many different organs and the animal can become very sick in several different systems at the same time. This is a very serious condition that often results in death.

Common Toxicities and Poisoning
In Livestock

Livestock commonly suffer from poisonings due to:

- Eating too much rich food (grain overload)   See page 185.

- Eating poisons (plants and others)   See page 80.

- Snake and insect bites   See page 82.

- Touching or eating some kinds of insecticides   See page 83.

- Eating mineral mixes, or salty food, without enough water   See page 55.

- Toxemia from infectious diseases like hemorrhagic septicemia, metritis, mastitis, navel infections, etc.   See page 267.

17.2.1 Circling Disease (Listeriosis)

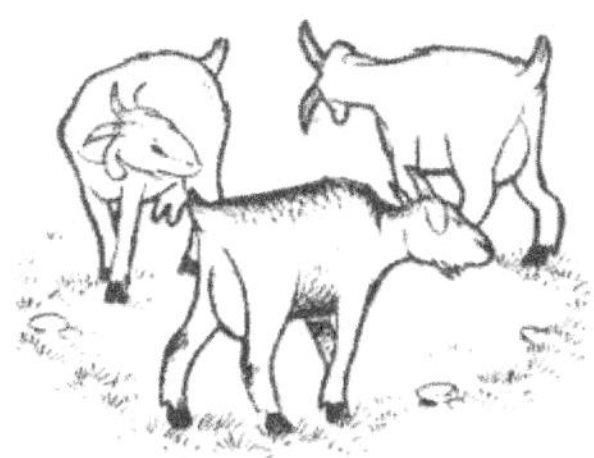

This disease is seen mostly in ruminant animals. It is caused by a
bacteria that is often associated with feeding rotten silage. It is also a
Public Health disease because it can cause abortions and death in
people if they eat/drink unpasteurized cheese or milk, or touch an
aborted fetus or placenta from the affected animal. (See page 280).

Symptoms/Diagnosis: This disease can be confused with rabies (See page 251), with
Vitamin A deficiency (See page 311), with Gid (See page 338) and with a deep ear
infection
(See page 257).

1. Animals are weak and depressed. They have a fever.
2. Animals act like they are blind. Their head is tilted. They may walk in circles.
   They may press their head against the wall. The muscles of the face are often
   paralyzed.
3. Eventually the sick animals collapse and die.
4. Once an animal is very sick, it usually dies – even with treatment. Goats and
   sheep die quickly, within 2 or 3 days. Cattle live longer, perhaps up to two
   weeks.
5. Sometimes animals with Listeriosis do not show any of these symptoms – they
   simply have abortions.

Treatment: Animals can survive if treated with
penicillin before they become too sick. If penicillin is not
available, use tetracycline.

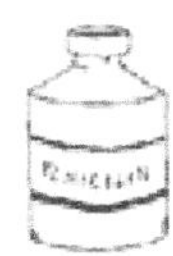

Prevention/Control: Spoiled silage should not be fed. The placenta and dead babies
from abortions should be buried. Remember, people can get this disease. Therefore, the
placenta and aborted fetus should be handled with plastic gloves.

17.2.2 Parasites in the Brain

Some parasites have immature forms that may move into the brain of the animal. When this
happens, the animal often appears blind, walks in circles, or presses its head against the wall, etc.
Examples are:

Tapeworm cysts in the brain ("Gid")　　　See page 338.
Broken horn with maggot infection　　　See page 225.

17.2.3 Vitamin A Deficiency

Vitamin A deficiency can cause animals to be blind at night. Some animals, especially cattle, will
stumble and walk strangely.

17.3 TILTED HEAD

Various diseases will cause animals to walk with their head held in a funny position. Although they may act strange, these animals are usually not aggressive like some animals with rabies.

17.3.1 Ear Infection

An ear infection is called **otitis**. A severe ear infection that has spread to the inner ear often causes the animal to tilt its head. Animals with inner ear infections are often alert and will usually eat and drink.

See Chapter 20.

Control of ear mites is important for the prevention of ear infections – especially in rabbits. See Chapter 9. Injuries and bites from other insects can also cause ear infections. It is important to treat simple ear infections before they spread deep into the ear.

Symptoms:
- Animals with infected ears often shake their heads and scratch their ears.
- Pus or blood may come from the ear.
- In severe infections, the head becomes tilted.
- There may be a fever.

Diagnosis: Based on symptoms.

Treatment:
For *simple infections* (the head is not tilted)
- Clean the outer ear with a diluted disinfectant/ antiseptic solution. (Do not pour liquid in the ears of horses, mules or donkeys.)
- Use antibiotic ointment (eye ointment works well) or benzyl benzoate.
- Give antibiotic injection if there is a fever.

For *severe infections* (the head is tilted):
- treat with tetracycline or penicillin (IM) for about two weeks.

Control: Treat for mites, ticks and other parasites.

17.3.2 Parasite in the Brain

See "Gid."   See page 338.

17.4 STIFFNESS, TREMBLING, CONVULSIONS

17.4.1 Convulsions and Coma

Many problems start with the animal acting excited and trembling; then the animal develops stiffness and convulsions. Many of these animals become unconscious and die. History taking is very important in these cases.

The following problems often end in convulsions and coma:

-Poisons	See page 83.
-Tetanus	See page 258.
-Rabies	See page 251.
-Pseudo-rabies	See page 249.
-Milk fever	See page 270.
-Grass-tetany	See page 271.
-Salt poisoning (pigs)	See page 313.

17.4.2 Tetanus (Lockjaw)

This is an infectious disease found throughout the world. It is caused by a bacteria, <u>Clostridium tetani</u>, which grows in wounds or other places that have no access to air. The bacteria are found in the feces of people and animals, as well as in the soil.

If these bacteria enter into deep wounds, uteruses, umbilical cords, or castration wounds where there is no air, they multiply and produce a "toxin" (poison). The toxin travels throughout the body and affects the nerves.

Horses are very sensitive to this disease. Cattle, sheep, goats, and pigs get it sometimes. People can get this disease if the tetanus organism enters a wound or the uterus. Newborn babies can get this disease if the umbilical cord is handled in a dirty manner and the mother of the newborn was not vaccinated with tetanus vaccine (called Tetanus Toxoid).

Symptoms: Symptoms start about one week after the bacteria enters the body. Sometimes no wound is seen.

1. Lack of appetite.
2. Stiffness of muscles in tail, ears, jaws, neck and legs. In pigs, the ears and tail will stand straight up.
3. Third eyelid comes out over the eyeball. (It looks like a red cover coming from the inner edge of the eye.)
4. Convulsions or tremors, particularly in response to loud noises.
5. Infected wound(s), umbilical cord or uterus.
6. Death due to starvation, lack of water or suffocation because the breathing muscles are affected.

Diagnosis: Based on symptoms.

Treatment:

1. Thoroughly clean and disinfect any wound.
2. Give large doses of penicillin IM or SC; and put antibiotics (especially penicillin) in the wound.
3. In some countries an anti-toxin is available to inactivate the toxin (that remains in the body even after the tetanus organism is dead). However, the dose needed to treat a large animal with anti-toxin usually makes treatment unfeasible.
4. Provide clean food and water. Help the animal to eat and drink if necessary.

Control/Prevention: Tetanus is difficult to treat; but it can be prevented.

1. **Tetanus Toxoid Vaccination:** In some countries, all horses are vaccinated with Tetanus Toxoid. In developing countries, this is usually available for pregnant women; but is often unavailable to give to livestock or horses. If available, give according to the instructions on the label.

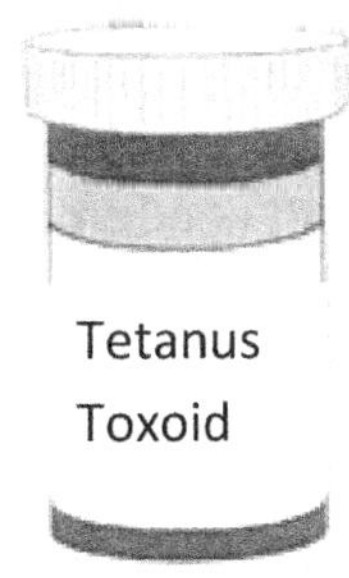

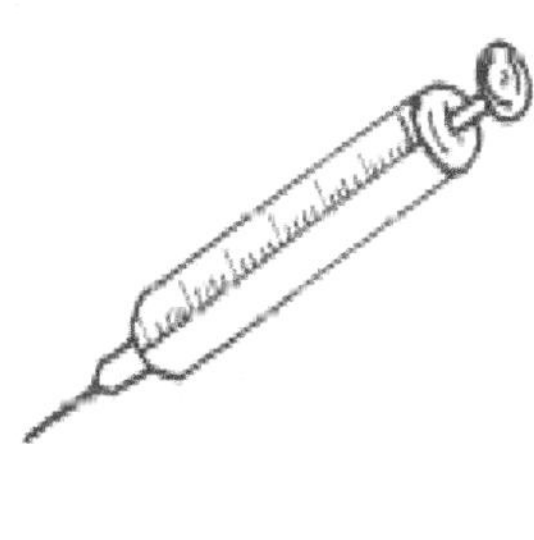

2.   **When castrating,** be clean and careful. If tetanus is a big problem in your area, give horses and pigs long-acting penicillin injections when castrating them.

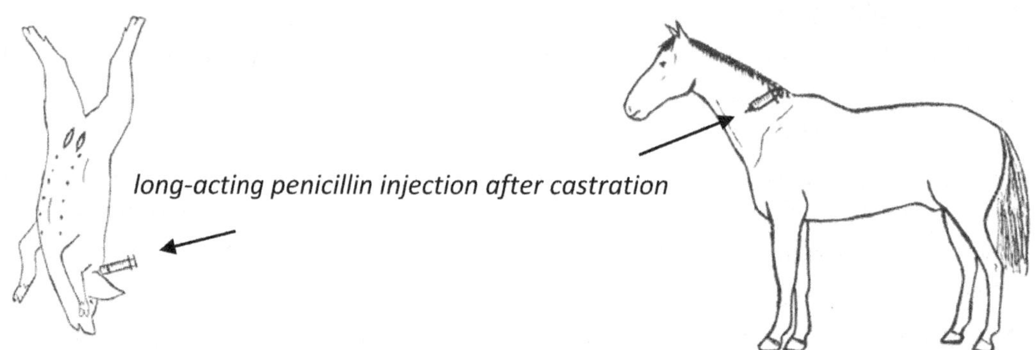

17.5.0 PARALYSIS

For an animal to move its body parts, the muscles must be working properly. In addition, the nerves which go to its muscles must also be working properly.

Paralysis is the term used when an animal cannot move a certain part of its body. It is often caused by damage to the nerves.

Symptoms/Diagnosis:

1.   Paralysis due to **injury**: Sometimes just one leg is paralyzed, but more often both hind legs are paralyzed and the animal cannot get up. This is often due to an accident where the animal has fallen and damaged the spinal cord. Or, it may be due to nerve damage in the legs during delivery.
Note: Heavy animals that cannot stand up for some reason, may suffer permanent damage to nerves or muscles that are crushed by its own body weight (especially if lying on a hard surface like concrete).

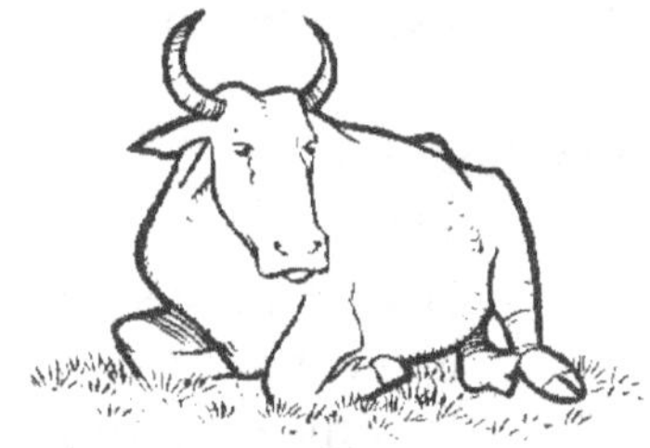

2.   Paralysis due to **nutritional deficiencies:**
a.   **Acute:** This can be due to calcium deficiency at the time of calving (See page 270); or magnesium deficiency when eating lush grass (See pages 272, 310).
b.   **Chronic:** A thin, malnourished animal may simply get thinner and weaker. Eventually it becomes unable to walk or move.

3.   Paralysis following **unknown causes:** Sometimes, it is impossible to determine the reason for the paralysis.

Treatment: For all conditions, the treatment is basically the same (See page 148, "downer cow"). If the backbone is damaged, there is no treatment. The AHA can only give good supportive care, pain killers/anti-inflammatory medicines (like aspirin) when the animal seems uncomfortable. Wait several weeks to see if the animal improves on its own.

18.0 The Circulatory, Blood and Lymphatic Systems

18.1 THE CIRCULATORY SYSTEM

18.1.1 Review of the Circulatory System

The circulatory system moves blood to all parts of the body. Blood carries food and water to the cells of the body, and also removes waste material. The circulatory, respiratory and blood systems work together to provide oxygen to the cells of the body. Oxygen is essential to keep the cells alive and functioning. The circulatory system is made up of the heart, arteries, veins and capillaries.

Diagram of the circulatory system

Note: Major arteries are shaded. Major veins are white.

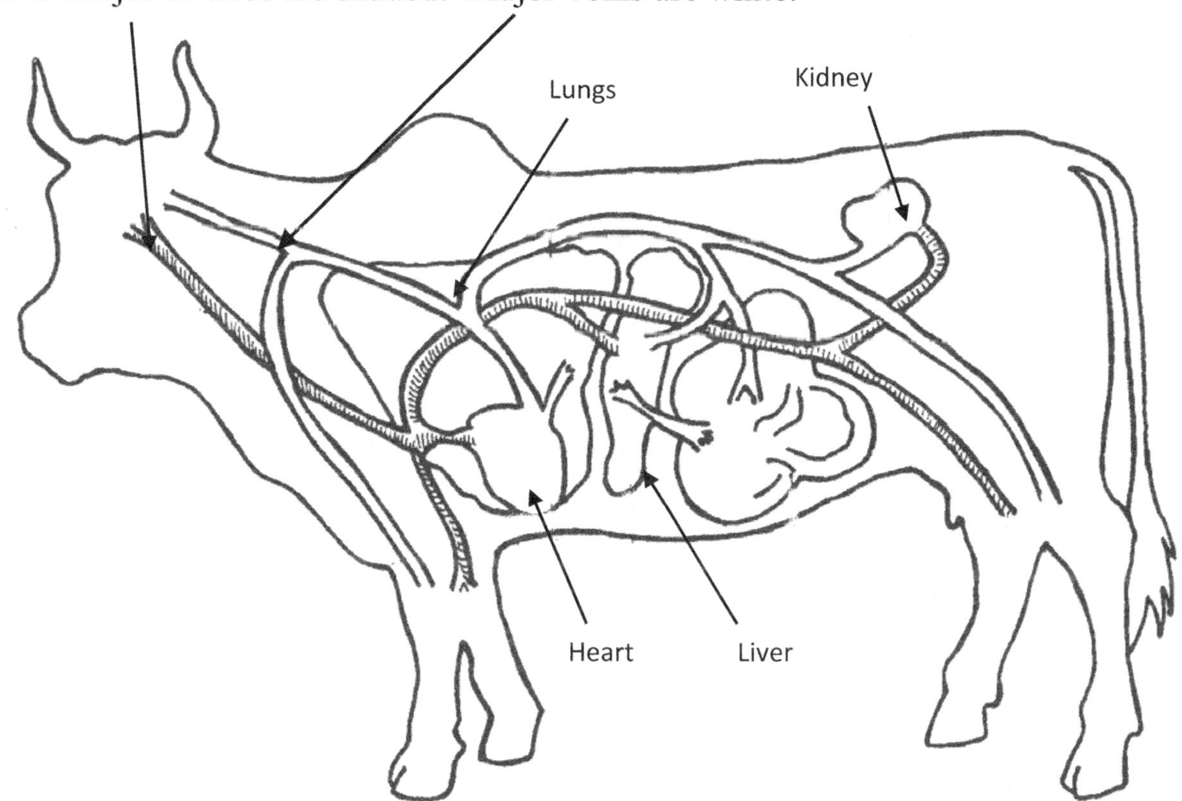

Problems Associated with the Circulatory System

Common problems of the circulatory system are few. Problems such as heartworms (common in dogs) are not covered in this book.

Hardware Disease

If the heart stops pumping blood, an animal will die almost immediately. Heart failure in livestock is most commonly associated with accidentally eating a nail or wire (i.e. hardware). Once eaten, the hardware may penetrate the stomach wall and diaphragm and then poke the heart. This condition is called "hardware disease" and is covered in the digestive system. See page 189.

Shock

This is the term for the circulatory system failing to function properly. Shock may result from blood loss, a severe infection, an internal abscess that suddenly bursts, or injury. It is covered under First Aid. See page 85.

18.2 THE BLOOD SYSTEM

18.2.1 Review of the Blood System

The blood system consists of red blood cells, white blood cells, platelets and plasma (blood water).

Function of the Blood System:

- To carry food and water to the tissues.
- To carry oxygen to the tissues.
- To remove carbon dioxide and other waste products from the tissues.
- To protect the body against bacteria and toxins (Immunity, See page 89).
- To provide necessary materials to the glands (to make secretions).
- To distribute hormones and enzymes.
- To transport heat throughout the body.
- To stop bleeding by making the blood clot.

18.2.2 Problems Affecting the Blood System

Anaemia (Anemia)

Anemia is a condition of "thin blood" due to insufficient red cells in the blood. The thin blood cannot carry enough oxygen to the tissues of the body. Anaemia is usually caused by internal and external parasites, as well as any chronic disease or organism that destroys the red blood cells (such as Babesia).

Symptoms: Symptoms are discussed in the parasitology section. See page 329.
- Pale color under the eyelids (instead of a healthy pink color).
- Sometimes extra fluid collected under the jaw (bottle jaw).
- Lack of energy.

Diagnosis:
- Without special laboratory equipment, diagnosis is based on symptoms.
- In the laboratory, a technician can count the number of red cells in a blood sample. Or a technician can measure the amount of hemoglobin (the substance that is in the red blood cells).

Treatment:
- Treat for internal parasites.
- If present, treat for external parasites.
- If present, treat any chronic conditions.
- Feed the animal well balanced rations.

Control:

- Regular treatment for worms and flukes, and control of external parasites, will prevent most problems.
- A good diet is important to prevent anaemia.

Blood Cancer

There are certain types of cancer that affect blood cells. One type is "leukemia" and may be diagnosed with a blood test. Leukemia interferes with the body's ability to build up immunity. There is no good treatment for livestock with leukemia. See page 273.

18.3 THE LYMPHATIC SYSTEM

18.3.1 Review of the Lymphatic System

The lymph system consists of the lymph nodes and the lymph vessels.

Function of the Lymphatic System

- The lymphatic system communicates with the circulatory system. It takes water and fluid from the tissues and carries them back into the blood.

- The lymphatic system also helps protect the body. It works together with the white blood cells to remove various germs that enter the body.

Lymph Nodes

Lymph nodes (also called lymph glands) are located throughout the body, including the neck, between the back legs, the chest, and abdomen. Lymph nodes act as a filter, removing dead cells and organisms (like viruses and bacteria) which should not be in the blood. White blood cells also multiply in the lymph nodes.

If any lymph node is enlarged, there is probably an infection somewhere in the body, or more rarely, cancer. When cutting open a dead animal, check for enlarged lymph nodes. To diagnose some diseases, it is important to collect lymph nodes and put them in formalin or alcohol (i.e. collect specimens). The specimens should then be sent to a laboratory for examination. If possible, ask the laboratory exactly what specimens should be collected and how.

Meat Inspection

When animals are slaughtered, the meat is often inspected for any sign of disease that may spread to humans. The inspector first checks the lymph nodes for any signs of infection. Usually the meat cannot be sold if there are signs of infection.

19.0 Endocrine System

19.1 REVIEW OF THE ENDOCRINE SYSTEM

The endocrine system consists of glands and hormones. Glands are situated throughout the body and produce "hormones." A hormone is a chemical substance that, once produced by a gland, enters the blood stream, and travels throughout the body. Hormones act as "chemical messengers" to control the work of different organs. Reproductive hormones are covered in Chapter 10. See page 131. Other hormones control growth, blood pressure, chemical balance in the blood and tissues, as well as coordination of many systems within the body. This chapter is about that part of the endocrine system which affects the work of AHAs.

Posterior Pituitary Gland and Oxytocin

Oxytocin is a hormone made by the posterior pituitary gland in the brain. When a baby animal starts to nurse, the mother's pituitary gland releases oxytocin that affects the uterus and the udder. Oxytocin has two main functions:

1. It causes the muscles of the uterus to contract during delivery (to push the baby and placenta out).
2. It causes milk to be released from the udder into the teats (called "milk letdown") so that milk will flow easily.

Practical Uses of Oxytocin: Sometimes oxytocin injections are given to pigs during delivery to hasten the birth of all the piglets. Oxytocin is also used to help expel the placenta and other secretions from the uterus or, after treating a prolapsed uterus, to make the uterus contract.

The Thyroid Gland and Goiters

The thyroid gland consists of two parts, one on each side of the windpipe, just below the larynx. The function of the thyroid gland is to take iodine from the blood and use it make hormone called "growth hormone." This hormone is necessary for normal development of the brain and body.

"Goiter" is the term for an enlarged thyroid gland. A goiter results from iodine deficiency. The thyroid gland enlarges in an effort to make enough growth hormone, despite the lack of iodine. Goiter (or iodine deficiency) is more serious for fetuses and young animals resulting in stillbirth (i.e. dead at birth), stunting, weakness, and mental retardation. If baby calves, lambs or kids are born dead, always check for goiter. If you find goiter, give "iodized salt" (i.e. salt treated with iodine) to pregnant mothers. See page 310.

Adrenal Glands and Steroids

The adrenal glands are two small glands located near the kidney. The hormones made by the adrenal glands are commonly called: "steroids", "corticosteroids", or "cortisone."

Steroids, Corticosteroids and Cortisone
AHAs must understand about these hormones because they are made into injections that are often used and abused in veterinary medicine. They are commonly referred to as "steroid" injections. Dexamethasone is a common type of steroid used in veterinary medicine to reduce inflammation and treat allergic reactions or shock. See page 85.

Caution: Steroids reduce the animal ability to fight infection and can cause an animal to abort. Do not use steroids on an animal that has an infection, or is pregnant.

20.0 Organs of Special Sense

REVIEW

Sensory nerves bring general sensations from all parts of the body to the brain. The four major organs which give special senses are:
>   the tongue, for the sense of taste.
>   The nose, for the sense of smell.
>   The eye, for the sense of sight.
>   The ear, for the sense of hearing.

20.1 TONGUE

The tongue is important not only for tasting, but also for licking, chewing, swallowing and vocalizing. Diseases of the tongue are covered in the chapter on the Digestive System. See page 182.

20.2 NOSE

The nose is important for smelling, breathing, and enhancing the appetite.

20.3 EYE

The eye is a complex and delicate organ. It is protected by the surrounding bones, eyelids, eyelashes, eyebrows, and tears. Light enters the eye through the cornea (the outer surface) and then an opening (called the pupil), then passes through a lens which helps clarify or focus what is being seen. The light then hits the back of the eye called the retina which sends the message (of what is being seen) through the optic nerve to the brain for interpretation. It is the job of the pupil to allow the correct amount of light into the eye. When there is plenty of light, the pupil constricts to allow only a small amount of light to come in. When there is little light, the pupil opens wide to allow in the maximum amount of light.

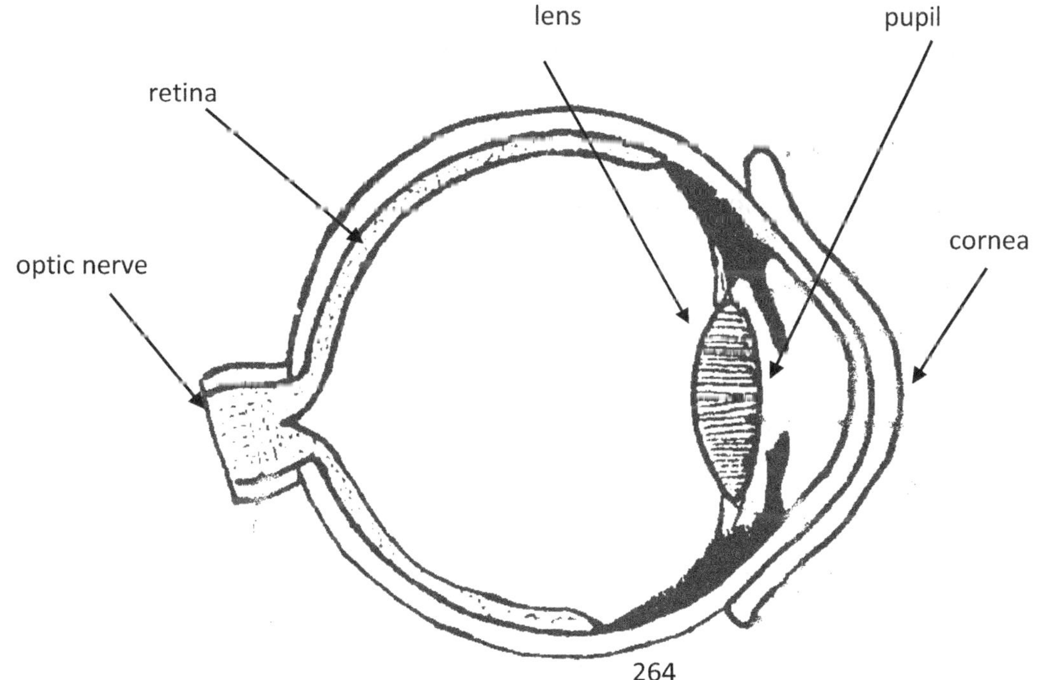

20.3.1 Injury or infection of the eye

Injury or infection of the eye will result in excessive tears, blinking, discharge and/or cloudiness of the eye. Inflammation of the pink tissue surrounding the eye is called "conjunctivitis." In cattle, a certain fly can carry a bacteria that causes "pink eye." In some places, cattle get cancer of the eye, particularly eyes with white hair surrounding them. See page 85.

Diagnosis:
- Properly restrain the animal and wash your hands.

- Examine the eye for any foreign materials that may be lodged in it. Also check for scratches or ulcers on the cornea (front surface of the eye). A scratched or ulcerated cornea is *very* painful and will cause much blinking, sensitivity to light, tears and sometimes swelling (sometimes the animal won't even open the eye). An injured cornea may also appear cloudy. Sometimes a scratch on the cornea may be difficult to see even though it is causing immense suffering to the animal. If available, a certain dye (called "fluorescein") can be placed in the eye to help detect any scratches (i.e. the dye causes any scratch to appear bright green).

- If there is no evidence of injury, examine the conjunctiva (i.e. pink tissue around the eye). If it is red and discharging a lot of mucus, it may be infected.

- Try to determine whether the condition is acute or chronic (i.e. ask the owner how long the problem has existed). Chronic problems are more difficult (sometimes futile) to treat.

- Cattle with cancer of the eye (called "cancer eye") have heavy crusts, invading the tissue surrounding the eye, and on the surface of the eye.

Treatment of an infected or injured eye:
- Properly restrain the animal.
- Rinse the eye with boiled (but cooled) water. If available, add boric acid to the water at a ratio of 1 ml boric acid to 100 ml water. Use clean cotton wool or other clean, soft material to clean around the eye.
- Remove foreign materials, if possible.
- Treat with antibiotic ointment, or drops that are made especially for eyes (i.e. usually labeled "ophthalmic" or "for use in eyes"). Ointment should be applied at least twice daily, and drops at least 6 times daily (i.e. drops are less practical for treating livestock).
- Keep the animal in a place that is shady or dark since sunlight is very bothersome to an injured eye.

Note: There is no treatment of "cancer eye."

Caution:
- Only use ointments or drops that are made especially for the eyes.
- Never use steroid ointment in an injured or infected eye since steroids may make the problem worse.

20.3.2 Removal of worms from the eye

- Dilute a sterile local anesthetic with distilled water to make about a 0.5% solution
  and squirt several ml into the eye. Then wait several minutes and flush the eye out
  with distilled water. The worms should be washed out with the distilled water.
  See page 86.

20.4 EAR

The ear is divided into 3 parts:

1. The <u>outer ear</u> consists of the part of the ear seen, on the outside of the head, as well as
   the opening into the ear itself.

2. The <u>middle ear</u> consists of a membrane, called the "ear drum", which vibrates when
   sound comes to it, and tiny little bones which are connected to the ear drum. The
   middle ear is also connected to the throat by a small duct.

3. The <u>inner ear</u> consists of the inside part which is directly connected to the brain.

20.4.1 Otitis

An infection of the ear is called otitis, which is usually due to bacteria. Otitis is not
very common in livestock or horses, but can result from wounds or insect bites.
Ear mites also   cause infections, especially in rabbits. See page 257.

Symptoms:
- The animal often shakes its head and scratches the ear because it itches.
- In severe infections, blood or pus may come from the ear.
- The animal may also have a fever.

Diagnosis:
Based on symptoms.

Treatment:
- Thoroughly wash the ear with clean water or a diluted disinfectant/ antiseptic solution
  (dilute hydrogen peroxide also works well). **Exception:** Do not pour liquid in the ears
  of horses, mules, donkeys.
- Dry the ear using a cotton swab or clean cloth.
- Use antibiotic ointment or benzyl benzoate in the ear.
- Give an antibiotic injection if the animal has a fever.

21.0 Miscellaneous Disorders

This chapter includes conditions that do not pertain to one particular "body system." It also includes some diseases that are less common.

21.1 CONDITIONS AFFECTING MORE THAN ONE SYSTEM

21.1.1 Toxemia

A toxin is a substance that acts as a poison in the body. The word "toxemia" refers to a toxin in the blood which causes severe illness in many body systems and sometimes even causes death. Toxemia may result from diseases or conditions such as HS, metritis, mastitis or navel infections. See pages 154-5, 196, 205. The AHA should try to determine the cause of the toxemia.

Symptoms/Diagnosis:
- Poor circulation evidenced by a rapid, weak pulse.
- Dark-red or purplish color to the gums around the teeth, the skin inside the vulva, or at the conjunctiva (i.e. the tissue surrounding the eye).
- Sometimes a fever at first; but as the toxemia progresses, the animal's body temperature may drop below normal.
- Rapid breathing.
- Usually some underlying condition that is causing the toxemia.

Note: Offer the animal water to drink. If the animal drinks, this is a good sign that the toxemia may not have progressed far.

Treatment: Toxemia is life-threatening. It is particularly serious if the animal's body temperature has dropped below normal.
- Try to decide the main cause of the toxemia (e.g. metritis, mastitis etc.) and treat the underlying condition.
- If unable to determine the underlying condition causing the toxemia, yet the animal is still alert and in reasonable condition, treat with large doses of antibiotics such as tetracycline or penicillin.
- An animal with toxemia usually recovers or dies rapidly. If the animal begins to recover, offer high quality food, and water frequently.

21.1.2 Dehydration: Water Deficiency

Water is the most important nutrient and makes up about 50% of the animal's weight. The Water in the body is mixed with sodium chloride (salt), and other minerals (also called "electrolytes) such as potassium and calcium. When the body loses water (e.g. from diarrhea, vomiting, sweat), it also loses some of these good minerals, or they become out of balance with each other. This imbalance may cause problems with the functioning of the body's cells, blood flow, the heart beat and the kidneys. If the kidneys fail to function, wastes build up in the blood. The animal then develops signs of toxemia, becomes unconscious, and dies. A heart that beats abnormally may result in death also.

Some animals obtain water through the forage they eat. However, most animals must also drink water to survive. Sick animals, mother animals that are giving milk and baby animals especially need fresh, clean drinking water.

Symptoms of Dehydration:
* Dry mouth and nose.
* Lethargy.
* Dark urine or decreased urine production.
* When a fold of skin is pinched and then released, the skin does not return quickly into place (i.e. it's not "elastic"). See page 49.
* Sunk in eyeballs (a sign of severe dehydration).

Diagnosis: Based on symptoms.

Treatment:

The main treatment for dehydration is <u>water</u>. However, some body minerals may have been lost in the diarrhea or sweat. Oral Rehydration Solution (ORS) helps to replace these minerals and restore the dehydrated animal to health. If ORS is not available, give plain, clean water.

ORS packets for Small Animals
* In many countries, inexpensive "Oral Rehydration Salt Solution" (ORS) packets are usually available for humans (at health posts or pharmacies). Some countries make their own packets Other countries obtain packets supplied by UNICEF which is marked in big letters on the packets. These ORS packets can be used for animals. Prepare it according the instructions. Usually empty the contents of the packet into a liter of fresh, clean water.

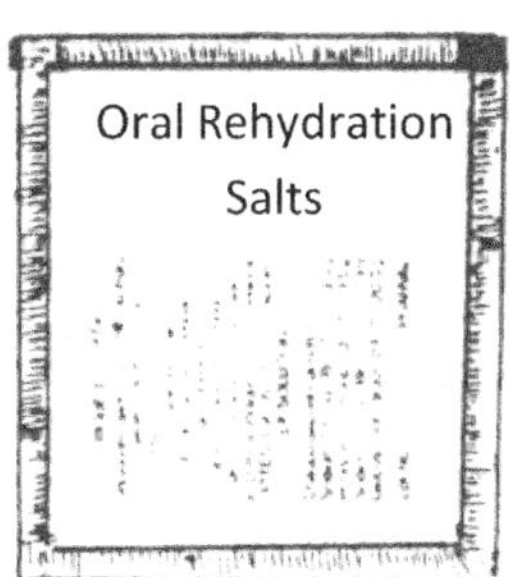

Warning!! Never mix the ORS without enough water. Making it too concentrated may worsen the animal's condition.

HOMEMADE SOLUTION (especially for large animals)
* If ORS packets are not available, ORS can be prepared by mixing two tablespoons of sugar and one teaspoon of salt in a liter of clean water. If possible, squeeze several drops of lime or lemon juice (to provide potassium) into the solution.

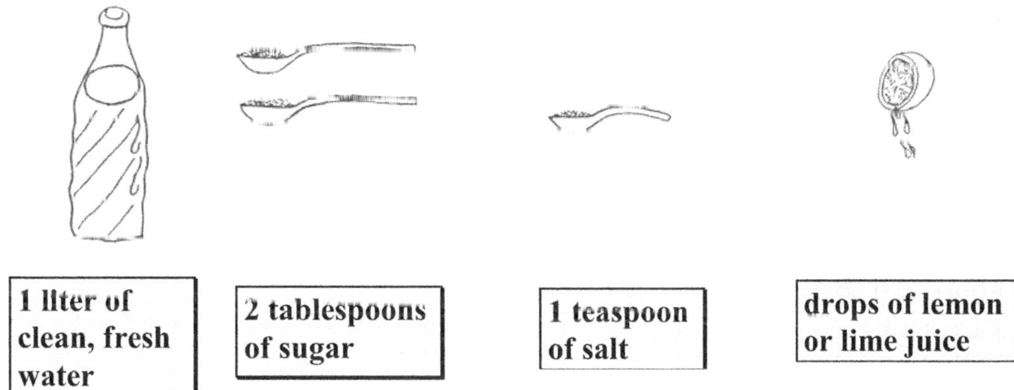

Ways to improve homemade ORS

- If rice flour is available, use 2 tablespoons instead of sugar. Rice flour is usually less expensive, provides some energy and helps thicken the diarrhea.
- If sodium bicarbonate (baking powder) is available, replace the teaspoon of salt with 1/2 teaspoon of bicarbonate and 1/2 teaspoon of salt.

Amount of Fluid to Give

How much ORS should be given? In theory, the animal should be given at least as much ORS as the quantity of its diarrhea.

> The more severe the diarrhea, the more ORS should be given.

How to Give the Fluids

- If the animal is too weak to drink, then it must be force fed. Small animals or babies (e.g. kids or lambs) can be fed the fluid slowly. Use a small spoon or syringe (without the needle) allowing the animal time to swallow. A dehydrated animal is often weak and must be handled gently. The fluid should be given slowly, allowing the animal time to swallow. Larger animals can be force fed the fluids using a stomach tube. See page 66.
- IV fluids may also be given by someone who knows how. IV fluids should be given slowly while at the same time monitoring the heart for irregular beats. If the heart begins beating irregularly, then stop giving the fluids. Begin again slowly once the heart beats normally.

Prevention of Dehydration:

- When an animal has diarrhea, begin giving water or ORS immediately (i.e. don't wait until the animal is dehydrated).
- Help sick or weak animals to drink.
- Supply clean, fresh water for animals to drink.

21.1.3 Water Deprivation or Salt Poisoning (Salt Toxicity) In Pigs

Pigs that receive salt in their diets but not enough water may develop a condition called "salt toxicity," "salt poisoning" or "water deprivation." The latter name is more appropriate since pigs usually develop this condition when they are receiving normal quantities of salt, but inadequate amounts of water.

The problem can begin within hours of water deprivation. Salt toxicity most commonly occurs when there is a change in management, and water is overlooked, the water source is interrupted, there is an electrical current in the water, or when feeding whey or other milk by-products that are high in salt content.

Symptoms:

- thirst and constipation.
- staggering.
- blindness.
- trembling and convulsions.
- laying on their sides and paddling.
- loss of consciousness, and death within a few days.

Note: The symptoms of "water deprivation" are similar to those of rabies, pseudorabies, hog cholera, African swine fever and edema disease.

Diagnosis:
- Based on clinical signs and a history of water deprivation.

Treatment:
- There is no good treatment.
- Giving water to animals that already have symptoms of water deprivation often makes the symptoms worse.
- Some AHAs administer a drug called "valium" which is an "anti-convulsant", in combination with "furosemide" which is a "diuretic." Diuretics are a class of drugs that rid the body of extra fluid and certain salts. In some instances, this treatment might help.

Prevention:
- Prevention depends upon good, alert management that will react rapidly when there is a lack of water.
- If there will be an inevitable shortage of water, do not give pigs salt or any feed with salt in it, until the problem is resolved.

21. 2 SOME DISORDERS RELATED TO PREGNANCY

21.2.1 Hypocalcemia – "Milk Fever"

Hypocalcemia occurs just prior to, or after delivery, particularly in high producing dairy cows, buffalo, goats, and sheep. When a large amount of calcium is mobilized to produce milk, the levels of calcium in the blood may drop too low, which makes the muscles and heart weak. Normally the body stores about 90% of its calcium in the bone but it cannot release the calcium quickly when milk production first starts. Milk fever can rapidly result in death if not treated quickly.

Symptoms:
- weak and sometimes unable to stand.
- body temperature lower than normal.
- constipation (sometimes).
- bloat due to inability to burp properly (sometimes).

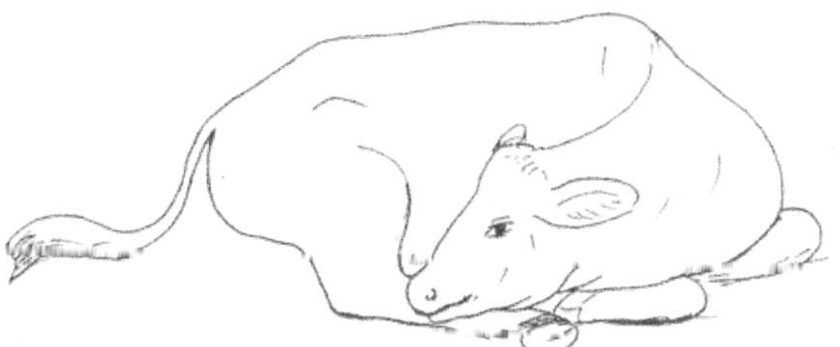

Diagnosis:
- From the history and symptoms.

Treatment:
- If very serious and near death, give IV calcium gluconate (i.e. a solution especially made for this problem), according to instructions on the bottle.
- If less serious (still standing but weak), then give calcium gluconate subcutaneously in 3 or 4 places where the skin is loose (neck, behind front leg, etc.). Give the amount listed on the bottle directions.
- Milk the cow a little, but not completely, until it is recovered from Milk Fever.

Warning: Give IV calcium slowly. Monitor the heartbeat as you give the calcium. If the heart starts beating irregularly, then immediately stop giving the calcium. When the heart beats normally, begin giving the calcium again, but very slowly while monitoring the heart beats.

Prevention:
• During the last part of the gestation period, do not give feeds containing high levels of calcium (like 271occidi or alfalfa hay).

21.2.2 Ketosis in Cattle

Ketosis is also called post-parturient acetonemia, crazy acetonemia, dyspepsia or slow-fever. It is usually seen from a few days to several weeks after calving. It is a secondary disease because the animal quits eating due to other causes (e.g. mastitis, metritis, milk fever, retained placenta). This causes the blood sugar levels to decrease. When this happens, most high producing dairy cows begin "burning" fat that is stored in their bodies. Then they may begin showing signs of ketosis. See page 253.

Symptoms:
• The odor of ketones may be present in the breath or urine.
• Anorexia (i.e. will not eat), and constipation.
• Sudden drop in milk production.
• Lethargic, or nervousness and trembling.
• Staggering, inability to rise.
• An underlying problem such as milk fever, mastitis, metritis or a displaced abomasum may also be present.

Diagnosis:
• Based on the symptoms and history.
• Special urine sticks are available that can confirm ketosis. When the stick is dipped in the urine, it immediately turns a specific color.

Treatment:
• Give 500-1000ml of 40% glucose solution IV.
• If the animal improves, then it probably had ketosis. Continue the treatment for ketosis by also giving propylene glycol (200-500 ml orally) daily, for several days.
• Treat any other underlying conditions.
• If the animal does not respond, then re-examine the animal.

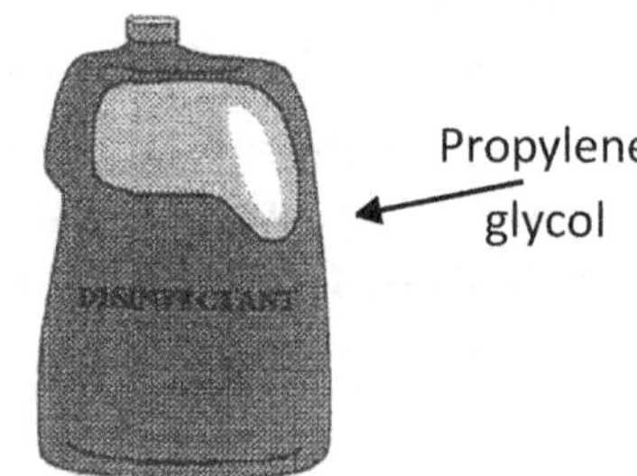

Prevention/Control:
• Do not allow pregnant cows to get too fat since this increases the risk of ketosis.

21.2.3 Pregnancy Toxemia in Sheep (ketosis in pregnant sheep)

This is also called "Twin Lamb Disease" because it is most commonly seen in ewes carrying twin or triplet lambs. Pregnancy toxemia usually occurs during the last few weeks of gestation, when the fetuses are growing rapidly and are taking lots of glucose from the mother's body. The mother's blood glucose drops, and her body begins burning fat. The by-product is a build-up of ketones in the blood. This problem may be triggered when something disrupts the mother's food intake (e.g. illness, suddenly moving or stressing the ewes, a storm). See pages 253, 254.

Symptoms:
- The odor of ketones may be present in the breath or urine.
- Weakness; inability to stand.
- Anorexia (i.e. will not eat).
- Nervous symptoms like walking in a circle, twitching, blindness, head pressing against immovable objects.

Diagnosis:
- Based on symptoms and history.

Treatment:
- No treatment is highly effective except an emergency operation to rapidly remove the lambs, or a dose of dexamethasone to induce the mother to give birth.
- Give IV glucose (200 ml of 40%).
- If early in the course of the disease, give the ewe glycerol or propylene glycol by mouth until she improves.

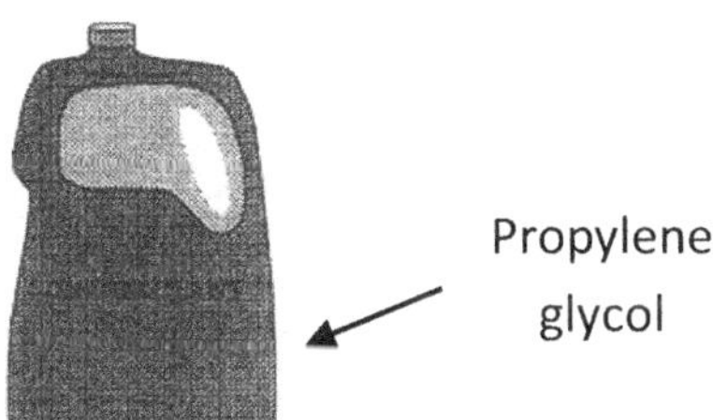

Prevention/Control:
- Do not allow ewes to get fat in early pregnancy.
- Give pregnant ewes regular exercise.
- In late gestation make sure that ewes get enough carbohydrates.
- If one or more ewes gets pregnancy toxemia, increase the amount of grain to all of the pregnant ewes. Consider giving them a dose of propylene glycol (if available), and watch them closely for symptoms so that treatment can begin early.

21.3 MISCELLANEOUS NON-INFECTIOUS DISEASES

21.3.1 Hypomagnesemia / Grass Tetany

This is also known as "grass staggers." It is seen in high producing dairy cows grazing on lush green grass or wheat pasture, particularly those fertilized with nitrogen and potash. This grass usually has a low magnesium content which may cause magnesium deficiency. Sometimes it is also associated with hypocalcemia in dairy cows that are pregnant.

Symptoms:
- similar to ketosis.
- staggering.
- the animal may fall down and thrash its legs frantically (i.e. tetany).
- muscle tremors.

Diagnosis:
- Based on symptoms and history (and knowledge that this is a problem in your area).

Treatment:
- Give IV a commercial mineral solution that contains both calcium and magnesium. (According to the instructions on the label.)

Prevention/Control:
- In areas where this is a problem, animals must be given extra magnesium in their diet. There are many ways to do this, such as feeding magnesium oxide or mixed magnesium compounds. Consult with a local veterinary officer.

21.3.2 Cancer

Cancer is a condition when certain body cells multiply abnormally. These abnormal cells are called "cancer cells" and may spread throughout the body via the blood or lymph system. Cancer cells that spread to other parts of the body are called "malignant." Cancer cells that don't spread are called "benign." Malignant cancer cells tend to invade organs like the liver, brain, heart, and lungs, which may eventually kill the animal. A group of cancer cells collected in one place is often called a "tumor."

Cancer is called by different names depending on the type of cell that multiplies abnormally. For example, cancer of the white blood cells is called leukemia, of lymph nodes – lymphoma, of certain skin cells – carcinoma, of bone cells – osteosarcoma. Certain types of cancer are more common in certain types, breeds, or families (bloodlines) of animals, as well as in certain geographical areas. In addition, certain viruses can cause cancer.

In general, no effective and inexpensive treatment is available for malignant cancer in livestock or horses. The animal will die slowly (or can be euthanized or slaughtered). Tumors can be surgically removed which can cure benign cancer or, if done early on, prevent malignant cancer cells from spreading.

Attempting to stop cancer cells from multiplying is done by using x-rays (called "radiation therapy") or by using certain chemicals (called "chemotherapy"). However, this is not usually feasible in livestock or horses.

21.3.3 Bovine Leukemia (Lymphoma)

In certain countries, bovine leukemia is one of the most common types of cancer in livestock. It is caused by a virus and can be spread throughout a herd by injecting many animals with the same syringe and needle. Symptoms are often vague and general, making the problem difficult to diagnose. Affected animals may have enlarged lymph nodes and may become frequently ill. There is no treatment.

21.3.4 Squamous Cell Carcinoma

Squamous cell carcinomas are one of the most common skin tumors. In cattle, they tend to occur around the eye, particularly where the hair is white in color, and can completely deform/destroy the eye, or the area around the eye. In horses, this cancer tends to occur around the eye or genital tract (vulva in mares and penis in stallions/geldings), and progress slowly. There is no effective treatment, although surgical removal of the affected area may help. In cattle, the affected eye is often removed and the animal can continue to produce milk or reproduce for an extended period.

21.3.5 Melanoma in horses

Melanoma occurs in gray-colored horses. It tends to begin around the area of the vulva
and then usually spreads to internal organs. The horse may lose weight and have various
symptoms (e.g. colic) depending upon which organs the cancer cells invade.

21.3.6 Bladder Tumors

These tumors may occur in cattle from eating **Bracken Fern** over a long period. Once
this tumor has started to grow in the bladder, there is no medical treatment for it.
However, the animal may occasionally improve on its own, for a while. See page 244.

21.3.7 Venereal Tumors in dogs

These tumors are spread through the breeding process. They start out small and
become a large, red mass. In some countries, these are successfully removed surgically.

21.4 MISCELLANEOUS INFECTIOUS DISEASES

21.4.1 Atrophic Rhinitis

This is an infectious disease of pigs that destroys the nasal bones, and sometimes
deforms the jaw bones of pigs. There may be several causes of this problem, but
one principal cause is a bacteria called "Bordctclla bronchiseptica."

Symptoms:
- Symptoms may begin with sneezing, but later the nasal and jaw bones may become
  deformed and the animal may not be able to chew properly.

Diagnosis:
- Based on symptoms (i.e. a deformed snout) or, when the animal is slaughtered,
  evidence of destroyed/deformed nasal bones.

Treatment:
- There is no treatment once the animal has a deformed snout.

Prevention:
- Controlling or preventing a problem in a herd involves a combination of good sanitation,
  good ventilation, and sulfonamides in the feed. In some countries, vaccine is available.
  Farmers should avoid buying pigs from a herd with a problem of atrophic rhinitis.

21.4.2 Erysipelas

Erysipelas is a bacterial disease of pigs. There are two forms of the disease: acute and chronic.
It is found in most countries of the world.

Symptoms:

Acute form:
- High fever
- Heavy breathing
- Hot and swollen joints
- Skin discoloration (red and purple),
  particularly on the ears, snout and abdomen
- Diamond-shaped, raised, reddish areas on the
  skin all over the body (particularly the back and sides)
- Death within 6 days

Chronic form:
- Diamond-shaped raised reddish areas on the skin all over the body
- Tips of the ears and tail may die and fall off
- Lameness due to arthritis
- Fatigue, heavy breathing, and bluish color (instead of a healthy pink) due to damage to
  the heart valves
- Sometimes sudden death related to damage of the heart valves

Treatment:
- Penicillin is the drug of choice. If unavailable, try using tetracycline.

Prevention/Control:
- Vaccines are available that can decrease the severity of the illness or protect pigs up
  to the age they are slaughtered. Breeding pigs should be re-vaccinated every year.

21.4.3 Trypanosomiasis

Trypanosomiasis in livestock is caused by a group of protozoa
(Trypanosomas) found in parts of Africa. It is usually a chronic
disease seen in cattle, sheep, dogs, pigs, camels, horses and most
wild animals. It is spread by a biting insect called the tsetse fly.
Some local animals are fairly resistant to the organism because
they have thick skin and the flies cannot successfully bite them.
There are about 12 different species of trypanosomas. Four of
the most important are: T. congolense, T. vivax, T. brucei, and
T. simiae.

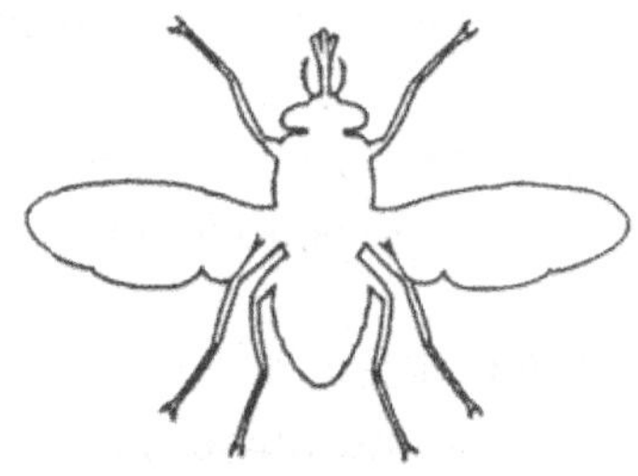
TseTse Fly

Symptoms:
- Fever   Anemia and weakness
- Abortion   Swollen lymph nodes
- Weight loss   Reduced milk production

Diagnosis:
- Thin and anemic
- The parasite can be seen by examining a blood smear with a microscope

Treatment:
- There are several drugs available for trypanosomiasis (e.g. *Berenil*). However, trypanosomes often become resistant to them. If trypanosomiasis is a problem in your area, find out which drugs are effective from the Ministry of Agriculture or a reliable local veterinarian or AHA. Follow carefully the instructions for use.

Control/Prevention:
- Control can be achieved through controlling the insect. See page 118.

21.4.4 Distemper

This is a highly contagious viral disease of dogs that causes both respiratory and nervous system problems. Distemper is found all over the world and is easily spread by drops of saliva in the air, or on contaminated objects. Most dogs are exposed as puppies and many die. Young dogs are particularly susceptible to distemper if they have not been vaccinated.

Symptoms:
- Fever for 1 – 3 days which goes away, and then returns for a week.
- Loss of appetite and energy.
- Often thick discharge from the eyes and nose, and the eyes appear red.
- Possibly diarrhea.
- Dogs that recover from these initial symptoms may then get nervous symptoms which can be fatal. The symptoms include twitching, seizures, and wandering.

Diagnosis:
- Based on clinical signs, especially in young dogs.

Treatment:
- Good supportive care.
- Paracetamol may help to reduce the fever.

Control / Prevention:
- Effective vaccines against distemper are available in many countries.

21.4.5 Peste Des Petits Ruminants (PPR)

Peste des Petits Ruminants (PPR) is also called "pseudorinderpest." It is an acute, viral disease of small ruminants that causes fever, sores in the mouth, intestinal infections, and pneumonia. The PPR virus is closely related to the virus causing rinderpest. It seems to affect sheep, goats and certain species of deer, and can be confused with rinderpest or contagious pneumonia. Although cattle may be infected with the virus, they do not usually become sick, and they do not transmit the disease. PPR is common in Africa   and the Middle East. It has recently caused problems in Asia also.

Symptoms:
- Animals develop a high fever and a dry muzzle.
- There may be a watery nasal discharge, followed several days later by a discharge of pus which gives a bad odor.
- Sores are also found in the mouth and, upon slaughter or necropsy, throughout the digestive system.
- Diarrhea.
- Pneumonia.
- Sometimes death within 21 days.

Postmortem Findings:
- Rotten sores are found in the mouth and throughout the stomach and intestines.
- Pneumonia.

Diagnosis:
- Based on symptoms and postmortem findings.
- If possible, diagnosis should be confirmed by isolating the virus in a laboratory.

Treatment:
- There is no specific treatment. However, the use of antibiotics and anti-parasite drugs may decrease the number of animals that die.

Prevention:
- PPR vaccine may be available. If not, rinderpest vaccine is effective. During an outbreak, you have two options:
  1. Vaccinate in a circle around the affected geographic area (but not in it).
  2. Vaccinate in the area of the outbreak but only vaccinate healthy-looking animals.

Caution:
- Vaccinating within the area of the outbreak may save more animals. But, it has risks; the community may blame the AHA for any animals that become sick after vaccination. Therefore, if you decide to vaccinate in the outbreak area, you must communicate very well with the community. You must explain that animals already incubating the virus at the time of vaccination may still become ill and die (from the disease and NOT from the vaccine). You must also explain that the vaccine takes several days before it is effective, and the animal may get the disease beforehand.
- *Do not use the old GTV Vaccine (Goat Tissue Virus Vaccine) for Rinderpest. It may actually make the situation worse.*

21.5 SUDDEN DEATH

Sometimes an animal dies suddenly – with no symptoms seen by the owner. There are several reasons for this and they have been covered in other sections:
- Poisons. See page 81
- Acute Diseases like Anthrax, Blackquarter or Hemorrhagic Septicemia.
- Heart failure due to a wire in the heart or some other reason. See page 189.
- Grass tetany. See page 271.

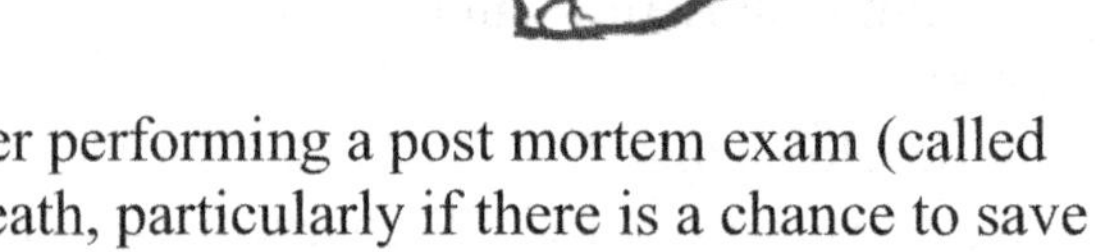

As always, take a careful history. Consider performing a post mortem exam (called a "necropsy") to determine the cause of death, particularly if there is a chance to save other animals with the same condition.

Caution: If you suspect that the animal died from anthrax, (the animal has dark blood coming from the mouth, nose or other body parts), do not cut it open. See page 196.

22.0 Public Health Diseases

In this book we use the term *Public Health Diseases* to refer to diseases that affect both the health of livestock and humans, and are caused by infectious micro-organisms. The technical name for a disease that can spread from animals to humans is a *zoonotic disease.*

22.1 LEPTOSPIROSIS

Leptospirosis was already mentioned as a disease causing abortion in domestic animals. See page 162. The bacteria (called <u>Leptospira</u>) that causes leptospirosis may also cause disease in people. People who work with infected animals or who are in contact with water that is contaminated by the urine of infected animals are most likely to get leptospirosis. This would include slaughterhouse workers, animal caretakers, and AHAs, as well as people who work in rice paddies, sewers, mines, and sugar cane fields. Leptospirosis might also affect people who drink or swim in water where infected dogs, rats or other animals have urinated.

Symptoms
- Sudden onset of fever, headaches, conjunctivitis, muscle pain, nausea/vomiting, and diarrhea. More severe cases could have jaundice, pinpoint hemorrhages on the skin, and/or kidney problems which could be life threatening.

Diagnosis
- Special laboratory tests are required.

Treatment
- In severe cases, supportive care may be needed. This includes re-hydration, control of a high fever, as well as treatment of kidney failure and/or electrolyte imbalances in the blood.
- The sick person must rest and drink plenty of water. General symptoms (headache, fever, muscle pain) may continue, or reappear, for up to 1 to 2 months after the first symptoms have appeared.
- Antibiotics (e.g. doxycycline) should be given, although sometimes the antibiotics themselves may initially cause a sudden rise in fever (due to destruction of the leptospira organisms).

Prevention / Control
- Animal owners and slaughterhouse workers should be warned about the disease and how to take proper precautions (i.e. wear protective clothing to avoid direct contact with tissues and urine).
- In an area where leptospirosis is known to occur, avoid exposure (i.e. drinking, bathing, or swimming) in ponds and streams.
- Drinking water sources should be protected from animals' urine.
- Lowlands should be drained, if possible.
- Practice good rodent control, including good food protection and garbage disposal.
- A vaccine for people and livestock is available in some countries.

22.2 HYDATID TAPEWORM

<u>Echinococcus granulosis</u> is a tapeworm in which the adult worm is found in the dog's intestines, even though it does not make dogs sick. The tapeworm lays eggs which pass out in the dog's feces. If these eggs are eaten by grazing sheep/goats, pigs, buffalo, or cattle, then cysts will develop in these animals. People also become infected by accidentally contacting dog feces, and then touching their hands to their mouth.

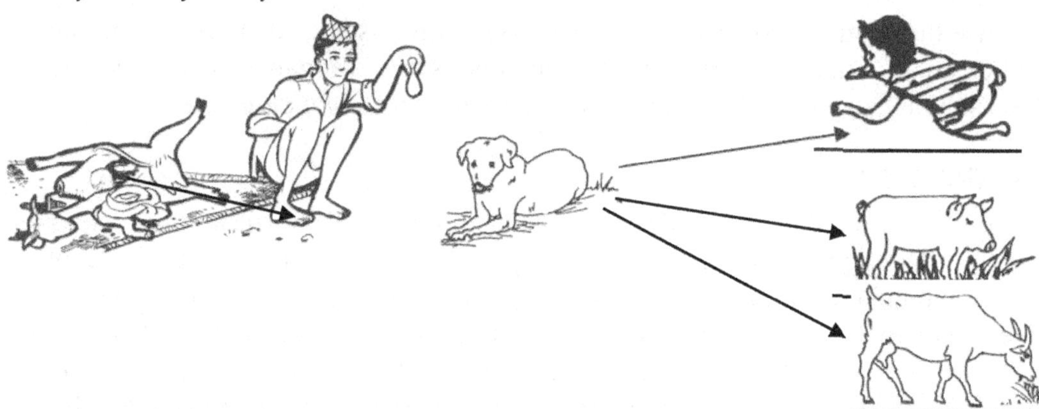

These cysts can grow large and destroy the tissues around
them. For instance, a person may suffer from lung or liver disease. X-rays are taken which
show large cysts in or near the lung or liver. At this time a difficult surgery is required to
remove the cyst and to save the life of the patient. This disease continues in nature when
animals with cysts are killed for meat. If these cysts are discarded and a dog eats them, the
cycle starts all over again.

These cysts are a major public health problem in some countries. This condition is referred to as
"**hydatidosis**", **echinococcosis** or **hydatid cyst disease**. Hydatidosis is most commonly seen in
areas where shepherds keep close contact with sheep, and where they also have close contact
with dogs.

Symptoms/Diagnosis

- The symptoms in people depend upon the location of the cysts (often in lungs, liver or
  brain). Diagnosis can be made with x-rays and a history of the disease in the area.

Treatment

- Surgery is the most common treatment. Some new parasite medicines also seem to work.

Prevention/Control

Several methods are available to control this disease:

- People should wash their hands after handling dogs or dog feces.
- Regularly treat dogs with medicine for tapeworms. This will prevent the spread of
  tapeworm eggs or segments in the dogs' feces. Praziquantel is a new medicine that is
  safe and effective and should be given every 6 weeks. However, it does not kill the eggs
  in the stools. Therefore, the stools following the first treatment must be disposed of carefully.
- When livestock are slaughtered, the cysts must not be fed to dogs. They must be buried or
  burned.

22.3   TRICHINOSIS

Trichinosis is caused by a small worm called <u>Trichinella</u>. Trichinosis is a disease of wild
animals and livestock (particularly pigs) and may also infect people. Infection occurs by
eating under-cooked meat (or garbage) that contains the trichinella cysts. Once eaten, the
cysts shed their outer coating and develop into adults which produce eggs. The eggs hatch to
larvae which enter the blood stream and form cysts in muscles and organs. The cysts appear
as small (up to 1mm long), white, lemon-shaped capsules.

Symptoms

- While in the intestine, the larvae may cause vomiting, pain and diarrhea. (Symptoms appear approximately 4 days after eating infected meat.)
- While entering the muscles and tissues (7 to 10 days after eating infected meat), the larvae may cause muscle pain, headaches, chills, fever, and swollen eyelids. More rarely, there can be a rash, as well as respiratory and neurological signs.
- Symptoms usually last about 10 days, but sometimes muscle pain can persist for months.

Diagnosis

- Based on the history of eating raw or improperly cooked meat.
- Special laboratory tests are available to diagnose trichinosis.

Treatment

- There is no good treatment except symptomatic treatment (e.g. pain control).

Prevention/Control

- This disease has been effectively controlled in some countries by cooking garbage before it is fed to pigs, and by not allowing pigs to run loose (to eat raw garbage).
- Meat inspection also helps to reduce the problem. Some countries examine meat under a special microscope to check for trichinella infection.
- To prevent the disease in people, all meat should be cooked at a temperature of at least 70 C. Freezing meat also kills the trichinella worm.

22.4   LISTERIOSIS

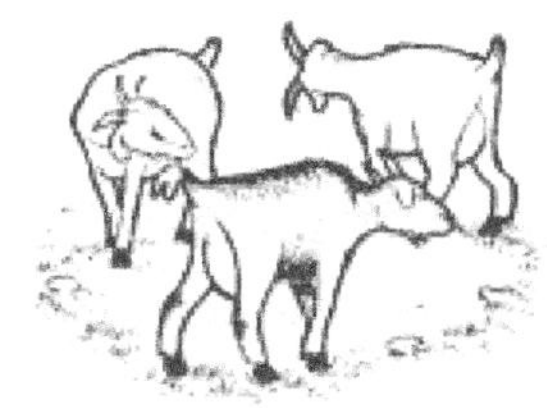

Listeriosis was already discussed as a nervous system disease in livestock called **Circling Disease**. See page 256. It was also mentioned as a cause of abortion and death in people.

Listeriosis is caused by a bacteria (<u>Listeria</u>) that is commonly found in the digestive system of many livestock and people. Usually this bacteria causes disease in babies less than one month of age, and in older people who are weak for various reasons. Sometimes the disease causes pregnant women to become sick, and their babies may be born dead or die shortly after birth. Although the bacteria are found in healthy people, cases of Listeriosis are sometimes associated with drinking unpasteurized milk or eating cheese from infected animals.

Symptoms/Diagnosis

- Babies are either born dead or die shortly after birth. Adults that are weakened by cancer or other conditions may develop a serious flu-like condition.
- Diagnosis is made by culturing the organism from the blood or cerebral-spinal fluid (i.e. fluid surrounding the spinal cord and brain). A special technique is required to get this type of specimen.

Treatment

- If Listeriosis is suspected, people should be given antibiotics. Ampicillin works well.

Control

- Good sanitation and pasteurization of milk and cheese products are important. Animals that have aborted should be isolated from other animals. The dead baby and placenta should be buried or burned, and people should avoid direct contact with the fetus or tissues (i.e. wear plastic gloves when touching tissue).

22.5 RABIES

Rabies is covered in Chapter 17. See page 251-253.

Treatment

- If an animal or person has been exposed to rabies, the most urgent and important thing to do is to wash the contaminated area thoroughly with soap and water. The rabies virus dies easily in the presence of soap.
- The next most urgent thing to do for a person exposed to rabies is to receive a series of anti-rabies injections. These are available in many countries from the Ministry of Health.

Prevention

- In most countries, dogs are the most common source of rabies transmission. If this is the case where you are working and there is a problem of rabies, a vaccination campaign for dogs should be conducted. Also, loose and wild dogs should be rounded up and impounded, or euthanized. These are the two most effective strategies for controlling rabies in most countries.

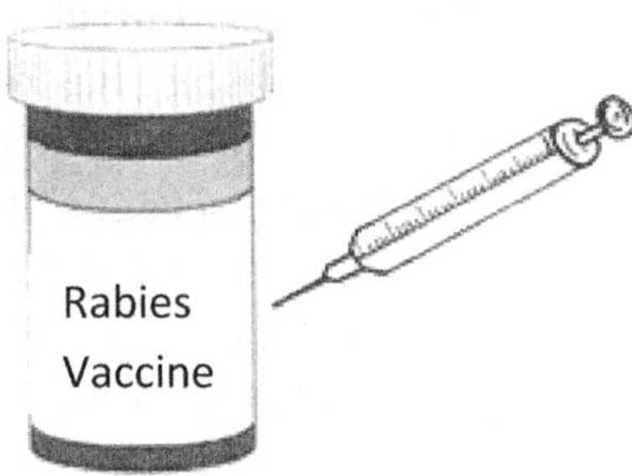

22.6 BRUCELLOSIS

Brucellosis was covered in the Chapter10. See page 161.

Treatment

- Persons accidentally exposed to Brucellosis should take 500 milligrams of tetracycline, by mouth, four times a day for two weeks.

Prevention /Control

- **Never** treat an animal with a retained placenta that just aborted without wearing a plastic glove/sleeve. Always wash your hands and arms afterwards.
- In many countries, government authorities require blood testing. Infected animals must be slaughtered.
- In some countries, a **Brucellosis** vaccine is licensed and available for cattle, but it must be handled properly according to the label instructions and regulations in your country.
- Aborted animals and the **associated** placenta should be buried or burned. Keep other animals and humans from touching it.
- If milk is not pasteurized, it should be at least boiled before a person drinks it to kill *Brucella,* as well as other harmful organisms.

22.7 PORK TAPEWORM

Pork tapeworm was covered in Chapter 27. This disease is called cysticercosis.
See page 339.

Review: The adult of this tapeworm lives in the intestine of humans (host animal) and
may cause diarrhea and abdominal discomfort. Whole sections of the tapeworm break
off and pass out in the feces. Each of these tapeworm sections can contain many tapeworm
eggs. If a pig (intermediate host) eats human feces infected with tapeworm eggs, the eggs
hatch in the stomach and intestine of the pig to become larvae. These larvae travel to
various muscles in the pig's body and form small "blisters" or "cysts" which can remain
for many years. Later, when the pig is killed for meat, these cysts are eaten by humans.
If the meat is cooked well, the cysts are killed and nothing happens. However, if the meat
is only partially cooked or eaten raw, then these cysts break open and mature tapeworms
develop inside the digestive system of the human. Then the cycle starts all over again.

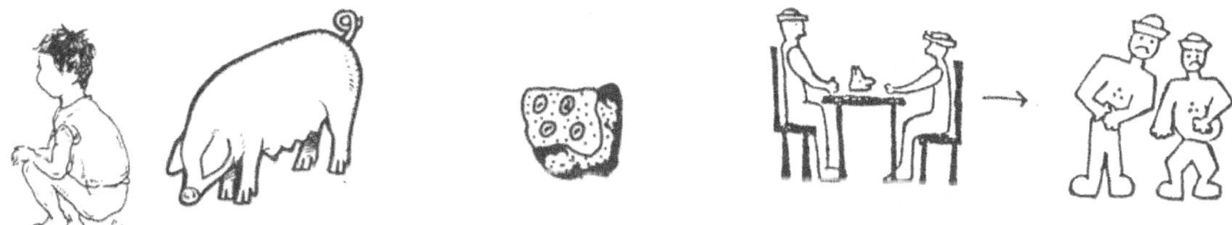

Pig eats human feces with   **Pig meat with cysts.**   **Humans eat pig meat with**
tape worm segments.   **Cysts and become infected.**

Treatment
- Treat infected humans with worm medicines effective against tapeworms.

Control / Prevention
- Do not allow pigs to eat human fecal material. Ensure that people use latrines and pigs
  do not run loose (to eat human feces).

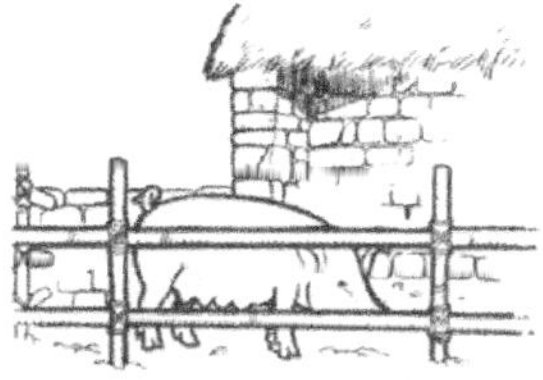

Don't let pigs run loose

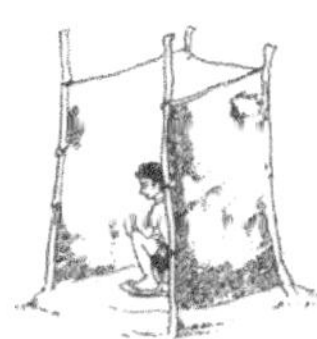

Use latrines

- Thoroughly cook pig meat before eating. Heating the meat to about 50 degrees C
  will kill the cysts in the meat. Before cooking the meat, cut the meat into small
  pieces to ensure thorough cooking.

23.0 Laboratory Procedures

AHA's may collect samples to send to a laboratory or perform simple laboratory procedures themselves. Using a laboratory can help to confirm a diagnosis, which better guides the choice of treatments for animals that are already sick. It also helps in the development of preventive measures for animals that might be exposed to the same illness, but are not yet sick. If possible, always communicate with a laboratory beforehand to determine which samples to take, how to take them, how to send them to the laboratory, as well as to tell the laboratory when the samples might arrive.

23.1   REPORTS

A report should always accompany a sample sent to the laboratory or an animal sent for post mortem examination.   The report should include the following information:

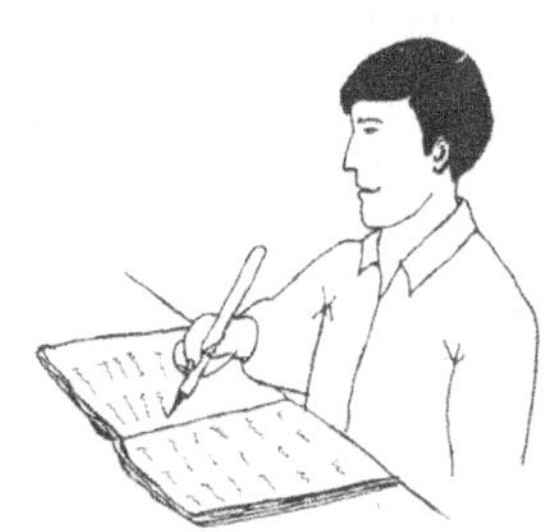

- species, breed, age, and sex
- complete history of the case
- vaccinations
- main findings from the physical examination
- main findings from examining the animal's environment (e.g. type of care, possible exposure to toxic plants or substances)
- location of the animal when symptoms first began
- location of the animal during the past month (to determine possible exposures)
- number and type of other animals affected with similar symptoms
- any treatment (when, what, and how much), and response to treatment

23.2   POST MORTEM EXAMINATIONS

A post mortem, also called a "necropsy", is the examination and dissection of an animal after it dies. The purpose of the post mortem is to try to determine the cause of death. During a necropsy, samples might be taken for the laboratory.

Caution: First of all, remember that an animal may have died from a zoonotic disease (a disease that can spread to humans). Wear plastic or rubber gloves (or plastic bags) on your hands when performing   a necropsy, particularly when brucellosis or rabies is suspected.

If **anthrax** is suspected (e.g. the animal suddenly died and had black blood coming from its mouth), do not perform a post mortem! Instead, bury the animal at least 1 meter deep. Blood contaminated with anthrax that has been exposed to air will cause the anthrax organism to form spores that will indefinitely contaminate the soil. Anthrax spores in the soil will pose a risk to people and other animals in the future.

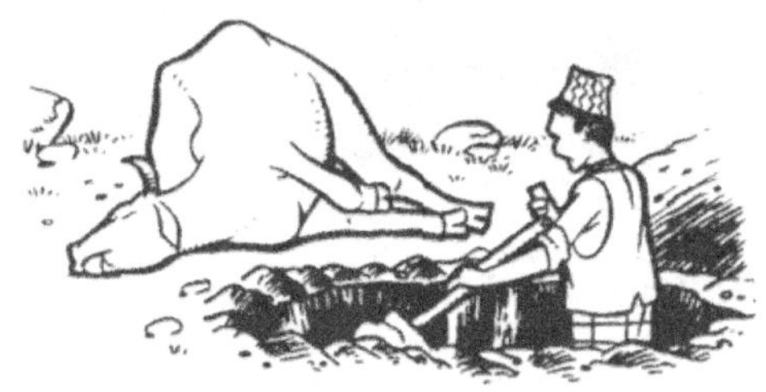

23.2.1 Performing a Post Mortem (for all livestock except poultry):

1. Take a complete history.

2. Examine the outside of the animal carefully (e.g. for wounds, diarrhea, external parasites).

Preparing the animal

3. Position the animal on its right side.

4. Cut through the skin of the animal in a line down the middle of its belly, from the sternum to the groin. Be careful not to cut through the muscles and into the internal organs. Carefully separate the skin from the muscles underneath it (a knife may be necessary for this).

5. Cut the skin and muscles which hold the left front leg close to the body in its normal position, and lay the front leg back, away from the ribs.

6. Similarly, cut into the groin and hip joint, and also lay back the hind leg.

7. Make a sort of shelf on top of the animal using the skin that has been pealed back as well as the front and back left legs. This "shelf" can be used to place organs and tissues for examination.

8. Cut the belly muscles from the sternum to the groin, being careful not to cut into the intestines or stomach.

9. Insert a knife between the ribs and cut from near the backbone to the sternum. Then cut along the cartilage which connects the ribs to the sternum.

10. Separate the ribs from each other and push them up and back, causing them to break near the backbone.

Examination of the animal's insides

11. Examine the spleen first. If it is enlarged, soft, bloody purple color, and the animal died suddenly, it may have been anthrax. Stop the post mortem immediately. Take a blood smear and bury the animal. Send the smear to the lab for examination. Begin taking antibiotics (e.g. penicillin or tetracycline) yourself.

12. Cut the tissues which hold the internal organs in place and remove them carefully. Place these organs on the shelf made with the skin and legs. Do not pierce the stomach.

13. Tie the esophagus at the stomach and cut above the tie.

14. Tie the rectum at the level of the pelvic bones and cut it below the tie.

15. Remove the stomach and intestines and lay them to one side.

16.   Remove liver, kidneys and any lymph nodes which look swollen.

- Also look at the testes or ovaries & uterus, and the urinary bladder.

- Examine the liver for flukes near the bile ducts. Cut the liver into strips and see if it is hard. (Normal liver is not hard and can be easily crushed with fingers.)

- In all of these organs, look for bleeding (hemorrhage).

17.   Remove and observe the diaphragm, heart and lungs. Cut open the trachea and the main bronchi and observe. Are there worms in the bronchi, etc.?

18.   Fresh samples of any organ or lymph node which looks abnormal can be cut off and sent to the lab. See below.

19.   Normal lungs are pink in color. Bad lungs will be a dark color (like the color of the liver). Test the lungs by cutting a small piece and putting it into water. Good lungs will float; bad lungs will sink.

20.   For circling disease (gid) open the skull and look for cysts.

21.   For rabies, the skull should be opened and the brain removed. Be careful and wear gloves or plastic bags on your hands. If near to the laboratory, one half of the brain should be packed in ice and sent to the laboratory; the other half in 10% formalin and also sent.

22.   Cut open the rumen, stomach, and the intestines and observe for worms.

- Sometimes the worms look like tiny pieces of thread in the abomasum or intestines. They can be seen on the surface of the abomasum if one looks closely.

- Also, one can take some stomach contents from the surface of the abomasum and put them on a window screen. They can be washed with water and examined for worms.

- Any presence of blood on the lining of digestive system, or in the digestive system itself, should be noted.

23.   If the joints are swollen, they should also be cut open and examined. Is there pus or fluid in them?

24.   Bury the animal.

25.   Clean all other instruments with water and then disinfectant.

26.   Wash your hands thoroughly and carefully.

27.   All abnormal findings should be carefully recorded, along with the history, in a report.

23.2.2 Performing a Post Mortem for Poultry

1. Remove the feathers from the abdominal side of the body and lay the body on its back with the wings spread slightly.

2. Cut the carcass open by making an incision through the belly wall near the sternum.

3. Cut the ribs forward and downward on each side.

4. Lift and remove the sternum.

5. Grasp the abdominal organs and pull them up and out.

6. Firmly hold the digestive system near the gizzard, and cut it above the gizzard.

7. Observe the heart, lungs, liver and kidneys.

8. Cut open and observe the esophagus, crop, pharynx and larynx; also the trachea and mouth.

9. Cut open the whole digestive system and observe for parasites and hemorrhages.

10. Carefully note any enlarged lymph nodes or any other abnormal findings.

11. Clean up and report as above.

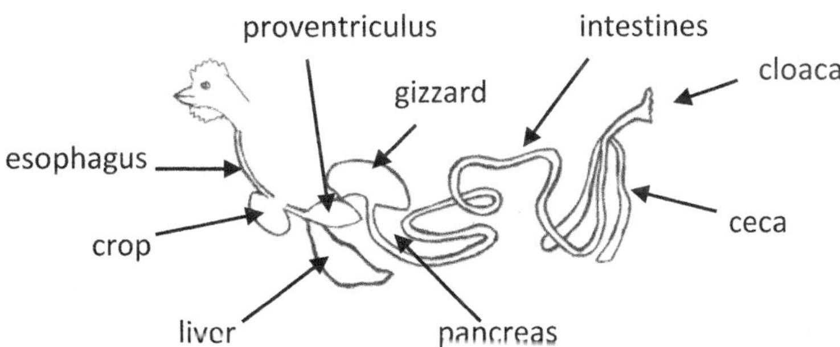

Digestive tract of poultry

23.3 TISSUE SAMPLES

Take a small piece of tissue (1 cm square only) and send it in ice to the lab. If this is not possible, **samples no thicker than 1 cm can be sent in 10% formalin.** There must be enough formalin to keep the samples from becoming rotten. Therefore, however much sample is added, 10 times more formalin must also be added. Formalin bottles must be sealed tightly or they will leak. A report should accompany all samples.

23.4   URINE SAMPLE

Hematuria is defined as blood in the urine.
Hemoglobinuria is defined as hemoglobin (color only) in the urine.

Both hematuria and hemoglobinuria make the urine red in color. However, it is very important to distinguish between these two in order to treat "Red Water" correctly. The following lab test does not require a centrifuge or anything else. You simply need an old medicine bottle or a tea glass.

Examination of Urine by Sedimentation for Hematuria and Hemoglobinuria

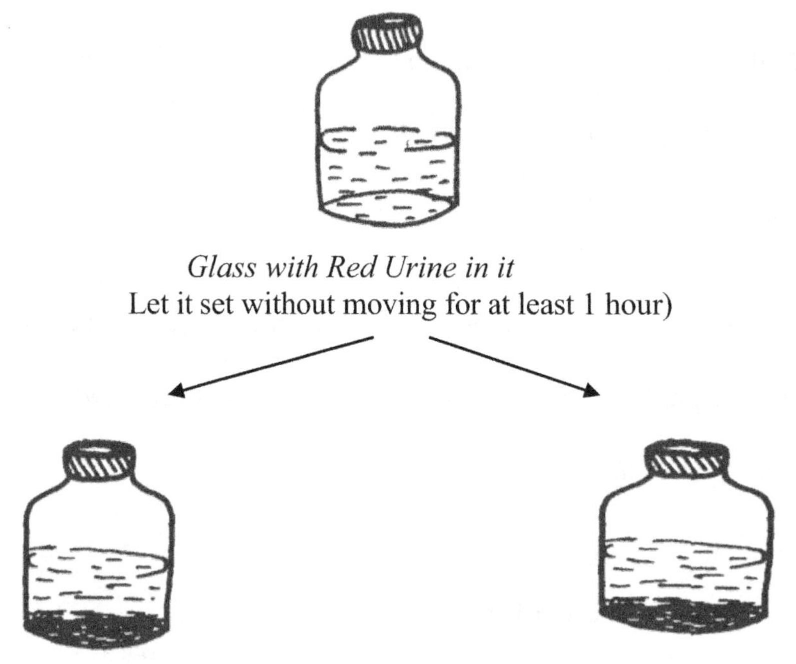

Glass with Red Urine in it
Let it set without moving for at least 1 hour)

Hematuria

Most of the red color has settled at the bottom of the glass as sediment. Urine is above the sediment.

This kind of urine comes from a wound or tumor in the urinary system. These wounds are caused by stones in the urinary system or by cancer (e.g. from eating bracken fern). If examined with a microscope, red blood cells will be seen in the sediment at the bottom.

Hemoglobinuria

The glass with red urine in it looks just like before. There is no settling of the red color in the bottom of the glass. This kind of urine comes from Babesiosis or from eating plants with red color in them. If examined with a microscope, no red blood cells are seen

23.5 FECAL SAMPLES

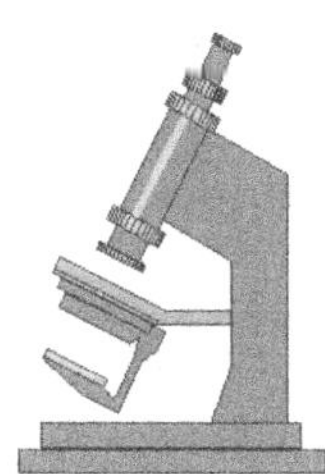

Many different parasites lay eggs that come out in the feces. By examining the feces with various procedures, it may be possible to tell the exact type of parasite which is living in the animal's body. This is called a **"fecal exam."** Most types of fecal exams require special equipment, including a microscope.

When is a Fecal Exam Necessary?

- A fecal sample is not necessary whenever an animal shows the signs of internal parasites. However, if an animal has already been treated for the most likely parasite in the last 3 weeks or so, and it still has diarrhea, etc., then it is best to perform a fecal exam.
- If the sample is positive, think about why it is positive. Was the correct medicine given? Was the dose of medicine enough? Was the medicine spilled when it was fed? Was some of the medicine left in the bottle when it was fed?

Types of Fecal Exams

There are many types of fecal exams, but only a few of them are appropriate for AHAs. This book will deal briefly with only 3 types of fecal exams:

- Direct smear
- Floatation
- Sedimentation

Fresh Samples Needed

Certain types of parasites are seen best with certain types of fecal tests. For all types of fecal exams, a fresh sample is essential. If the sample is old and dry, the results will not be accurate. In general, the feces should be examined within 12 hours after the feces pass out of the animal. (If the fecal sample is put in the refrigerator, then it can be kept longer.)

The best type of fecal exam for each type of parasite is listed below:

-Trematodes (flukes)	Sedimentation method
-Nematodes (roundworms)	Floatation method
-Cestodes (tapeworms)	Method varies with type of tapeworm
-Coccidia	Floatation method

23.5.1 Examples of Parasite Eggs

<u>**What Do You See?**</u> In general, the following rules are true (there are also many exceptions!)

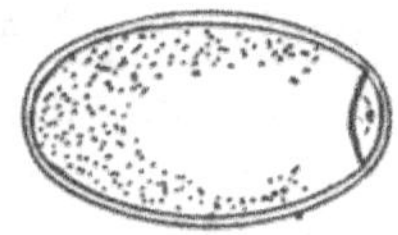

<u>Trematode</u> eggs are fairly large and have a "cap" (operculum) on one end of the egg. Liver fluke eggs are slightly smaller, and more of a brownish yellow color than are rumen fluke eggs.

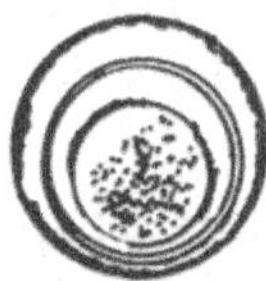

<u>Large Roundworm</u> eggs are fairly round in shape with a thick shell.

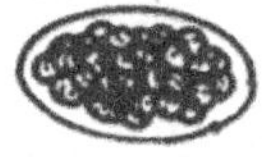

<u>Small Roundworm</u> eggs are usually smaller, have a thin shell, and are slightly elongated in shape.

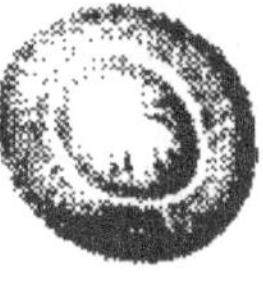

<u>Tapeworm</u> eggs are usually slightly bigger than small roundworm eggs. They are roughly round in shape and have a thick shell. Sometimes several "lines" within the egg itself are seen.

23.5.2 Direct Smear Method:

Direct smear is the easiest method. Most types of eggs can be seen using this method. However, it is not very accurate and can be confusing. Because only a tiny amount of feces is actually examined, often the results are negative even when there are eggs in the rest of the feces. Also, along with the parasite eggs, one sees all kinds of undigested pieces of grass, pieces of pollen, dirt, etc.; and it is all very confusing.

Procedure:
- A small amount of fresh feces (a drop) is mixed with several drops of water on a microscope slide.
- Examine under low power. If you think you see an egg, switch to a higher power and examine the egg more closely.

Results:
- If an egg is seen, the sample is positive. However, if an egg is not seen, you cannot say for sure that the sample was definitely negative. Instead, you can simply say that you did not see the egg. **If the sample is negative but the animal has all the signs of internal parasites, you should still treat the animal for internal parasites; or you should do a specific fecal sample (like sedimentation or floatation).**

23.5.3 Sedimentation Method:

This is a good method to use because it allows looking specifically for liver fluke eggs. It is also easy to do. It is based upon some eggs being heavier than water and sinking to the bottom of a solution of feces. If feces sit in a solution of water, fluke eggs and some tapeworm eggs will slowly settle to bottom of the sample.

Procedure:
- Place about 1 teaspoon of fresh feces in a clear tea glass.
- Fill the glass about 1/2 full with fresh water and stir with a clean stick.
- Filter this solution through an ordinary tea strainer (one layer only) into another clean tea glass.
- Rinse clean water through the strainer to fill the new glass.
- Let sit for 30 – 60 minutes so heavy things can settle to the bottom of the glass.
- Pour off clear water from the top of the glass. Sediment must remain.
- Fill glass again with water and allow to sit again for about 30 minutes. Pour off clear water from the top of the glass. Sediment must remain. Repeat again if time allows.
- Add New Methylene Blue to the sediment (not essential but aids in the identification of rumen fluke eggs).
- Mix several drops of sediment with clean water on a clean slide.
- Examine entire slide under medium power for liver/rumen fluke eggs.
- If negative (no eggs seen) then prepare a new slide and repeat 2 more times.

Note: It is not necessary to let the sample settle 3 times; it just makes for easier examination.

Results:
- 1 egg seen means the sample is positive. However, even if all 3 slides are negative, the animal could still have liver flukes. A bit of feces that was negative may have just been examined. If in doubt, go ahead and treat the animal for liver fluke according to the symptoms.

23.5.4 Floatation Method:

This method of fecal exam is based upon the fact that some eggs are very light and tend to float up to the top of a solution of feces. In order to help the eggs float even better, the water must be made thicker than usual, causing the light eggs to quickly float to the top. Roundworm eggs, coccidial oocysts and some tapeworm eggs are light, and they tend to float to the top of the solution easily.

Use ordinary salt, sugar or magnesium sulfate to make the concentrated "floatation solution." In general, use luke-warm water and continue to stir, adding salt or sugar until it no longer dissolves. (It takes about .35 kg sugar per half liter of water.) Some people think that sugar solution is better because it is sticky; and the eggs tend to stick to the microscope slide more easily.

Procedure:
- Prepare the saturated solution as mentioned above.
- Mix a small amount of fresh feces (1/4 – 1/2 teaspoonful) with several ml of saturated solution in the bottom of a 10-12 ml test tube.
- Add more saturated solution until the test tube is filled to the top and extends slightly over the lip of the test tube.
- Gently place a clean cover slip or microscope slide on top of the test tube. If air bubbles form while placing the slide on top of the tube, then remove it and try to place it more carefully the next time.
- Let sit for 30 – 45 minutes.
- Remove the slide or cover slip carefully from the top of the test tube. (If using a cover slip, place it on a clean microscope slide. If using a slide, place a cover slip over the sample on the slide.)
- Examine with a microscope. First use low power and then switch to higher power when you think you see an egg. You must examine the whole cover slip carefully; do not just examine in one place.

Results:
- If the sample is not fresh, or it was allowed to sit for too long, the eggs will burst and will not be seen. Also, coccidial oocysts (eggs) are very tiny and difficult to see. They often look like tiny air bubbles.

23.6 BLOOD SMEARS

Making a blood smear is the process of taking a drop of blood and "smearing" it out in a thin layer on a microscope slide. For diseases like Babesiosis and Trypanosomiasis, it is very important to take a blood smear and actually see the organism. Even if a microscope is not available, prepare a blood smear and send it into a laboratory for examination.

How to Make a Blood Smear:
- For Babesiosis and Trypanosomiasis, a fairly thick smear of blood is needed. For Anthrax and other diseases, a thin blood smear is best.
- <u>For live animals:</u> Only a tiny drop of blood is needed. Therefore, it is easiest to take a sample from an ear vein for a blood smear.
    - Identify an ear vein and puncture it with a sharp, sterile needle.
- <u>For dead animals:</u> Make a blood smear of blood from the ear. Be careful to wear gloves, and take only a tiny drop if anthrax is suspected.

Thin Blood Smears for Anthrax and Other Diseases:

- Remember – be careful if you suspect anthrax. A tiny drop of blood from the ear of the dead animal is enough. Protect your hands.
- A very small drop of blood is placed near the end of a clean glass slide.
- Quickly, another clean glass slide is taken and the drop of blood on the first slide is touched with an end of the second slide. This allows the blood to spread evenly along the edge.
- The top slide is held at an angle of about 45 degrees to the bottom slide which should be on a flat, level surface. 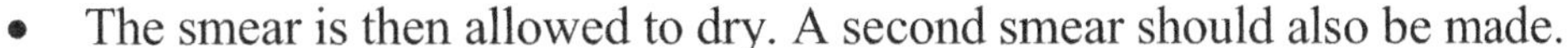
- The top slide is pushed gently and smoothly along to the end of the second slide, drawing the blood along behind it.
- The smear is then allowed to dry. A second smear should also be made.
- Do not make the smear too thick or it will be difficult to examine.
- After the second smear is made, the two slides are placed together, back to back, with the blood surfaces outward. They are wrapped in a thin piece of paper.

Thick Blood Smears e.g. for Babesiosis and Trypanosomiasis:

- A small drop of blood is placed near the center of a clean glass slide.
- Spread out the blood with a clean match stick (Rinse the match stick ahead of time and allow it to dry).
- Do not make it too thick or it cannot be examined.
- The blood is then allowed to dry.
- A second smear is also made and allowed to dry.
- After the second smear is made, the two slides are placed together, back to back, with the blood surfaces outward. They are wrapped in a thin piece of paper.
- These samples, along with the report which describes the case, are sent into the lab.

23.7   INSECT AND WORM / FLUKE SPECIMENS

When purchasing formalin in the market, it is usually a 40% solution. The glycerin purchased in the market is 100% glycerin. These need to be diluted according to the situation. To make a 10% solution of formalin, take 25 ml of 40% solution (from the market) and add 75 ml of water. This gives us 100 ml of a 10% solution.

Internal Parasites: (worms, flukes, maggots, cysts) Put into formalin. Nematodes: 3.5% solution; Cestodes: 5-10% solution; Trematodes: 10% solution. Do not put too many in one jar or they may spoil – there should always be 10 times more formalin than parasites in any bottle.

Large Insects: Catch insects carefully so as to cause no damage. Then pin through the thorax using a fine pin. Store in a special box, or in a bottle, in order to protect from dust, etc.

Small, Soft-bodied Insects: Store in 10% formalin.

Small, Hard-bodied Insects: Put in 5% glycerine. (If no glycerin is available, then use concentrated alcohol. Even local alcohol works.) All bottles should be well sealed and tape applied around the top to prevent evaporation.

Chapter 24.0 Poultry Health

INTRODUCTION

Poultry health is a difficult and complex subject. This section covers a few of the most common health problems of chickens in most countries. These include:

- Infectious diseases such as Newcastle Disease, fowl pox, Pullorum-Typhoid, chronic respiratory disease, coccidiosis and Gumboro Disease; as well as internal and external parasites such as worms and lice; and

- Nutritional deficiencies, because a well-balanced, well mixed feed may not be available. (The problem may be especially severe if the chickens are kept indoors.)

24.1 INFECTIOUS DISEASES

Many infectious diseases in poultry can be prevented by proper sanitation and hygiene. In general, flocks which are kept separate have fewer health problems than those that mix with other flocks. To prevent almost all infectious diseases in chickens, the following rules apply:
- **Prevent contact with other chickens.**
- **Never allow strangers/visitors inside the chicken house.**
- **Bury all dead chickens immediately, kill and remove weak, sick chickens from flock.**

Some infectious diseases are passed from generation to generation through the egg. These are called, "egg transmitted diseases." Even though the egg may look and taste normal, microorganisms may be there which can infect the chick. To prevent such diseases, it is necessary to test the hens. If the tests show that the hen is carrying the disease, even if she looks healthy, her eggs should not be saved for hatching.

24.1.1 Newcastle Disease

Newcastle Disease is an acute, deadly disease that affects chickens of all ages. It is caused by a virus. It spreads rapidly, and may kill most of the chickens in the area. The nervous and respiratory systems are usually affected.

Symptoms:
- Fever, depression and loss of appetite.
- Swollen head, and sometimes swollen wattles.
- Watery discharge from nostrils and eyes with difficult breathing.
- Nervous signs such as twisting of the head and neck, paralysis and walk as if drunk, wings relaxed and held away from body.
- Green diarrhea which is sometimes bloody.
- Sudden death.

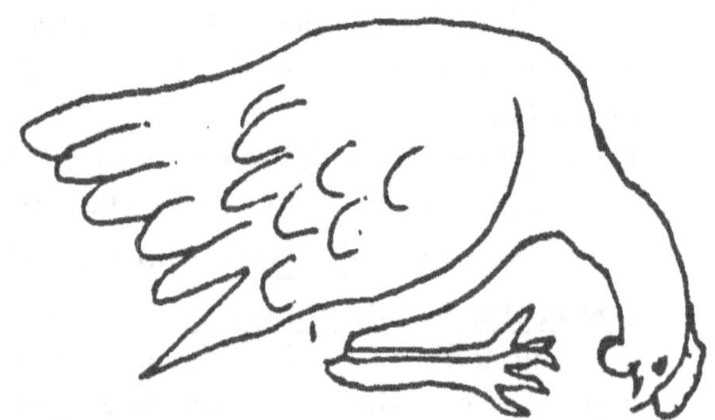

Postmortem findings:
* Hemorrhage (red spots) and swelling in the wall of the esophagus, proventriculus and any part of the intestines. Particularly typical of Newcastle disease, is hemorrhage at or near the junction of the esophagus and proventriculus.
* Necrotic patches (yellow spots), surrounded by inflamed (red) tissue in the intestinal wall.
* Hemorrhage in muscles, with fluid buildup in lungs (edema).
* Sometimes in a laying hen: broken egg in the abdominal cavity.

Diagnosis:
* Based on symptoms and postmortem findings.
* No history of Newcastle disease vaccination.

Treatment:
* No treatment is effective.
* Kill and bury all sick chickens.

Prevention/Control:
* Give Newcastle disease vaccine according to the vaccine manufacturer's instructions (usually at one to four days of age, and a second dose several days later):
    * $\Rightarrow$ by drops in the eyes or nostrils, or
    * $\Rightarrow$ in the drinking water, or by spray using special equipment
* Keep flocks isolated from other flocks. Never allow strangers/visitors inside the chicken house.
* Bury all dead chickens immediately and kill or remove weak, sick chickens from flock.

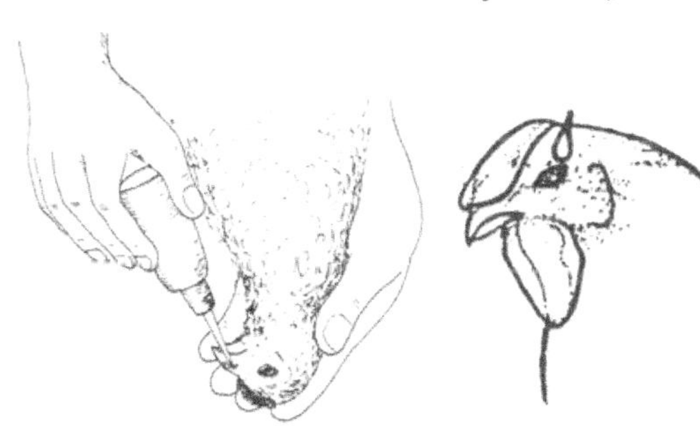

Notes: *Immediately* use all opened vials of Newcastle disease vaccine. Do not save an opened vial for later use. A vaccine for feed application may soon be available.

24.1.2 Fowl Pox

Fowl Pox is a disease of chickens that spreads slowly by mosquitoes. It is caused by a virus and affects chickens of all ages. It is seen in two forms: the dry form which causes skin sores (scabs), and the wet form which causes sores in the mouth and throat. The wet form may cause choking if the windpipe plugs.

Symptoms:
* Sores on the parts of the body without feathers (head, eyes, legs, vent) that may later form scabs and ooze pus.
* Sores on the tongue, in the mouth and trachea that may cause death from choking.
* Eyelids may be stuck together so that the affected chickens cannot see to eat or drink.
* Feet and legs may be affected and swollen.

Postmortem findings:
* Sores, especially scabs, on face or feet.
* Sores in mouth and throat area.

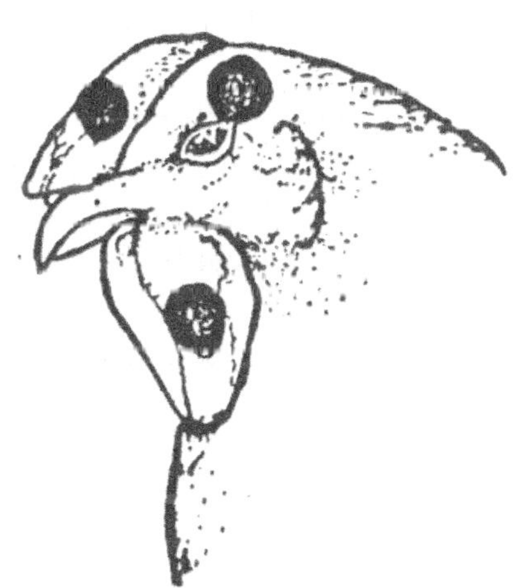

Diagnosis:
* Based on symptoms, post-mortem findings, and history.

Treatment:
* Separate all affected chickens from the flock.
* Give affected chickens special care:
    * provide easy access to food and water.
    * clean sores and apply antibiotic ointment or Gentian Violet.
    * apply antibiotic ointment *made for eyes* to the eyes. ***Do not put ordinary skin ointment in or near the eyes.***

Prevention / Control:
* Vitamins or antibiotics in the drinking water are helpful.
* Give Fowl Pox Vaccine according to the vaccine manufacturer's instructions (i.e. read the vaccine insert). Usually the vaccine is given at approximately six to eight weeks of age, with a booster dose six to eight weeks later.
* Reduce mosquitoes around poultry house by draining areas where mosquitoes breed. During an outbreak, it may be necessary to use mosquito spray inside and around the poultry house.

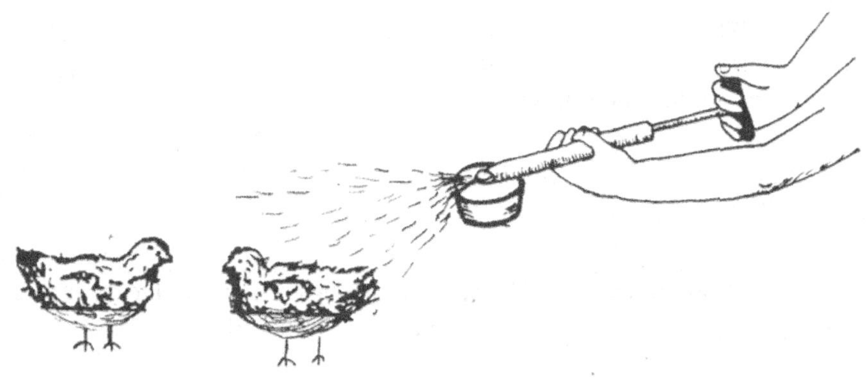

24.1.3 Pullorum (Bacillary White Diarrhea – BWD) and Fowl Typhoid

Pullorum and Fowl Typhoid are very similar diseases. In fact, the treatment and diagnosis are so similar that they will be discussed as one disease for this book.

Pullorum is also called "Bacillary White Diarrhea" (BWD). It is an acute or chronic infection caused by a bacteria called <u>Salmonella pullorum</u>. Fowl typhoid is also an infectious disease, caused by a closely related bacteria, <u>Salmonella gallinarum</u>. Both diseases are egg-transmitted diseases. This means that birds which survive the infection remain carriers and transmit the disease to the next generation through the eggs. Carrier hens can be detected by a blood test. The eggs of carrier hens should not be hatched.

Symptoms of Pullorum:
- Chickens are listless (sleepy) and often have white diarrhea.
- Many chicks die in the first two or three weeks of life.
- Sick birds appear to be cold. They crowd together and do not eat.

Symptoms of Fowl Typhoid:
- Depression and lack of appetite.
- Increased thirst – probably from fever.
- Diarrhea, yellow-green in color.
- Pale comb and ruffled feathers.

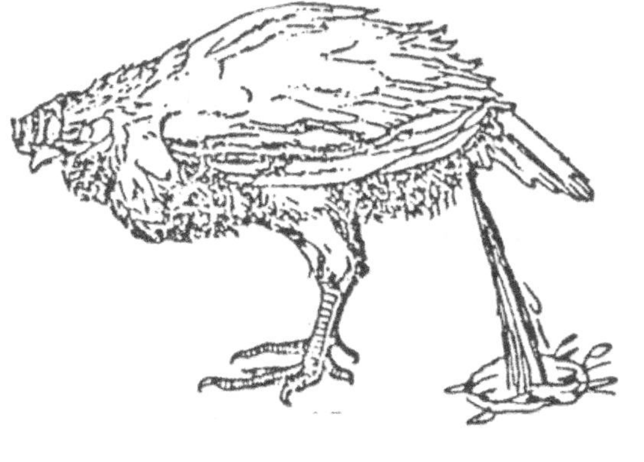

Postmortem findings of Pullorum:
- Inflammation (redness) of the intestines.
- Small yellow spots on the heart, lungs and liver.

Postmortem findings of Fowl Typhoid:
- Enlarged liver with green discoloration.
- Enlarged spleen and kidneys.
- Enlarged small intestine with "watery" contents.

Diagnosis for both Pullorum and Fowl Typhoid:
- Based on symptoms and postmortem findings.

Treatment for both Pullorum and Fowl Typhoid
- Give the chickens "sulfa drugs" or "furacin"
    - ⇒ Sulfa drugs can be given in drinking water or a sulfa tablet can be given by inserting it deep inside the chickens mouth. Use an appropriate dose found in the medicine table.

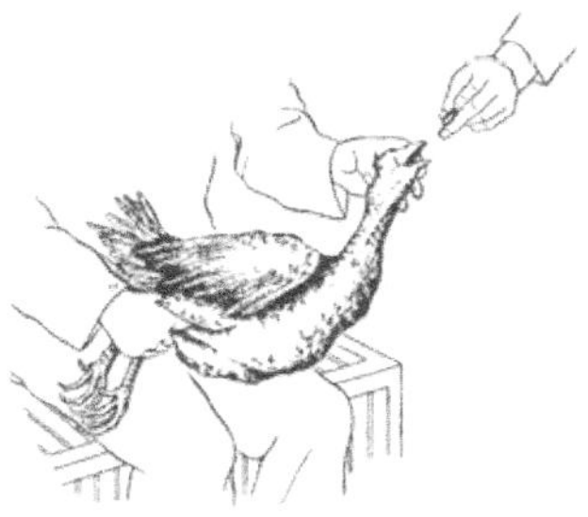

Sulfa by tablet

    - ⇒ Furacin can be dissolved in the drinking water. Follow the instructions on the label which usually indicate 0.5 grams Furacin powder per liter of water. Give for 5 to 10 days

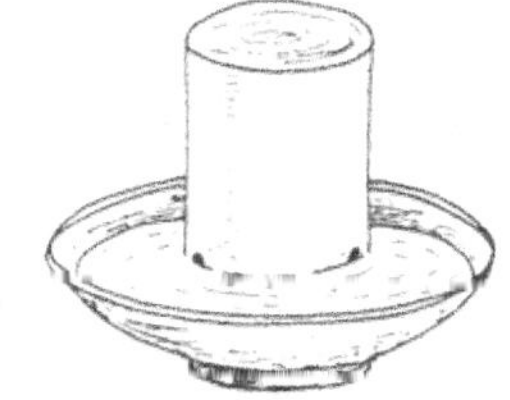

Furacin by drinking water

- Important: Provide clean, fresh water that is easily accessible to encourage affected chickens to drink.

Prevention / Control:
- Start baby chicks on drinking water containing Furacin.
- Select hatching eggs from hens that test negative by the "rapid plate blood test." Hens that test positive or had BWD should be butchered. Do not save their eggs for hatching.
- Sanitation.

24.1.4 Chronic Respiratory Disease (C.R.D.)

Chronic respiratory disease is an egg-transmitted disease caused by an organism called "Mycoplasma gallisepticum. Moving, overcrowding, or stressing chickens in any way may trigger an outbreak of CRD. The disease is complex because three or more conditions are needed for the disease to develop. One condition is the presence of mycoplasma organisms. The second condition is stress. The third condition is presence of another bacteria, such as E. coli.

Symptoms:
- Discharge from the eyes or nostrils.
- Difficult breathing.
- Lack of appetite for feed and water.
- Listless and appear chilled.
- Failure to grow properly.

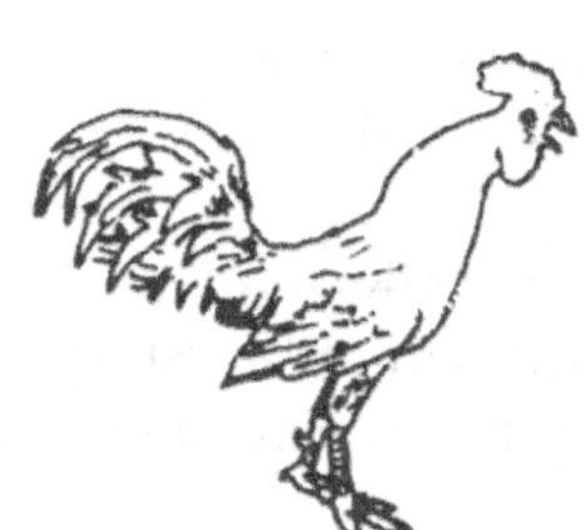

Postmortem findings:
- Thick, yellow pus (cheese-like) around heart, in lungs and air sacs.
- Trachea or wind pipe is inflamed (red in color).
- Sinuses inflamed (reddened in color) and contain mucus.

Diagnosis:
- Based on symptoms.

Treatment:
- Antibiotics
    - Tylosin injections (the best choice, if available and affordable).
    - Tetracycline in feed or water.
    - Penicillin injections.
    - Erythromycin or Furazolidone.

Control:
- For broilers: raise only one age group at a time (called an "all-in, all-out program"). Clean and disinfect between each group of broilers.
- Buy chicks from good hatcheries that are guaranteed to have no mycoplasma. Chicks from these hatcheries may cost more.
- Blood test hens. Use eggs for hatching only from those hens that test negative.

24.1.5 Coccidiosis

This disease was covered in the parasite section but will be discussed here also since it is a common and deadly infectious disease of poultry. Coccidiosis is caused by protozoa called occidian. One particular form of the disease occurs when the occidian live in the cecum (large intestine). This cecal form causes bloody diarrhea and sudden death, especially in growing chickens. Coccidia spread when healthy birds come in contact with manure from infected birds.

Symptoms:

* Red-tinged diarrhea (bloody) and death especially in young chickens.
* Depression and decreased appetite.
* Poor weight gain and egg production loss.
* The comb may look pale.

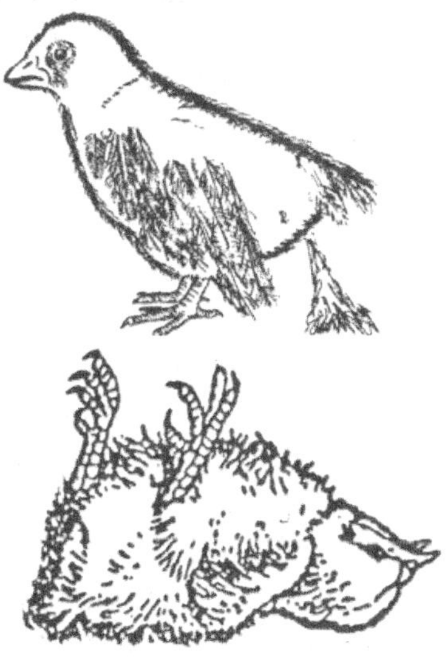

Postmortem Findings:

* Enlarged cecum containing blood.
* Intestine near the cecum appears enlarged and rotten
* White spots or lines on the intestinal wall.
* Microscopic examination of intestinal scrapings show coccidial oocysts (eggs).

Diagnosis:

* Based on symptoms and postmortem

Treatment/Prevention:

* There are several drugs that treat coccidiosis. These include *amprolium*, sulfaquinoxaline (SQ), and sulfamethazine (*Sulmet*). Find out which drugs are available in your area and follow label instructions from the manufacturer.
* A vaccine called *Cocci-Vac* may be available in the near future to prevent coccidiosis.
* There are several drugs that can be put in the feed or water to prevent or control coccidiosis. These drugs include monensin, lasalocid, and salinomycin.
* For broilers: raise only one age group at a time (called an "all-in, all-out program") and clean and disinfect between each group of broilers.
* It may be necessary to grow chickens in cages off the ground, on slat or wire floors to reduce coccidiosis infection. Such cages permanently separate the chickens from their manure.

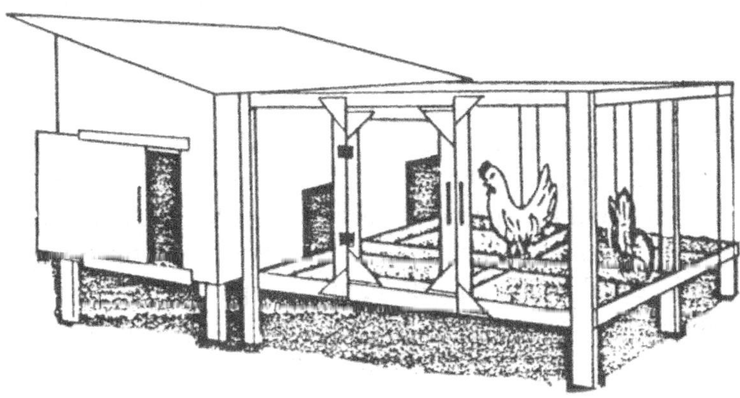

Chickens raised on slat or wire floors, separated from their manure.

24.1.6 Gumboro disease / Infectious Bursal Disease

(A Disease of Young Chickens)

This is a very infectious disease that spreads quickly among young chickens. It is caused by a virus that is easily carried from one chicken house to another on people's clothes, by insects and other methods. Sometimes the virus seems to be stronger than other times, and more animals will die in an outbreak.

- Chickens less than three weeks of age do not usually die from this disease. However, this disease destroys a chicken's ability to resist other diseases. Chickens which survive this disease may later die from other diseases – even if they are properly vaccinated and treated.
- Chickens 3 – 6 weeks of age often die quickly after becoming sick.
- Chickens 6 – 18 weeks of age may become sick, but it is quite rare.

Symptoms:
- Chickens become uncoordinated.
- Watery diarrhea is common, along with soiled feathers around the vent.
- Often more than 20% of the chickens die, but the others recover in less than one week.

Postmortem Findings:
- The cloacal bursa is swollen and may have red spots in it.
- The chest muscles and leg muscles often are swollen and may have bloody spots in them.

Diagnosis:
- Based on symptoms and postmortem.

Treatment / Prevention:
- There is no treatment.
- Various vaccines are available. Some are stronger than others and it is quite confusing. Please seek advice from local authorities regarding which vaccines are best in your area.
- Breeder flocks should be vaccinated 1 or more times during their growing period. If they have resistance, then their chicks will be more able to gain resistance to this disease.
- Occasional blood tests from breeder flocks will help to determine whether or not they have been vaccinated.
- After an outbreak of this disease, the chicken house must be disinfected very carefully. Then it should be left vacant for several months to be sure that the virus is killed. Only after that should new chickens be put back into the chicken house.

24.1.7 Internal parasites

Common internal parasites of chickens include small and large roundworms, and tapeworms. Cecal worms, small worms in the cecum, can also be a problem because they carry the organism causing "blackhead" in turkeys. To prevent the spread of cecal worms to chickens, turkeys should not be raised together with chickens. Many worms are spread when healthy birds come in contact with egg-containing manure from infected birds. Therefore, internal parasite problems are more common in chickens raised on the ground than those housed off the ground on slat or wire floors.

Symptoms:
- Chickens are thin, and fail to gain weight or lay eggs properly.
- Chickens may have diarrhea.
- When slaughtering chickens, worms can be seen if One checks the inside of the intestines.

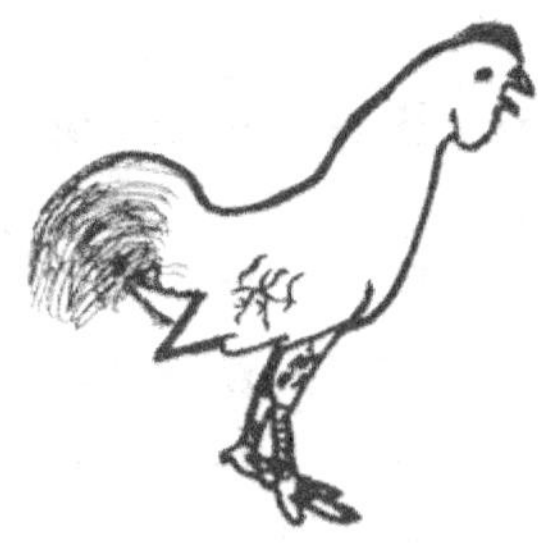

Diagnosis:
Based on symptoms and postmortem
findings of worms in the intestines.

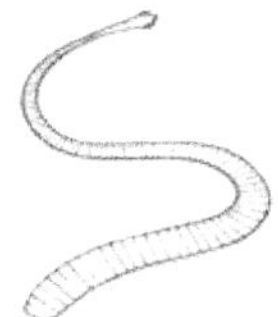

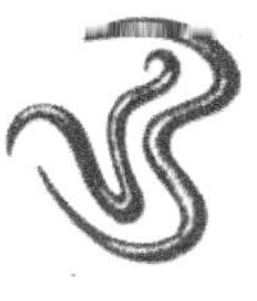

Cestode   *roundworm or cecal worms*
(tapeworm)

Treatment:
- For roundworms, treat chickens every 2 or 3 months with piperazine.
- For tapeworms, cecal worms, and roundworms: several herbal medicines, such as *Wormal* pills, can be given every 2 or 3 months. *Wormal* kills roundworms, tapeworms, and cecal worms. Note: Piperazine is not needed if *Wormal* is used.

Prevention / Control:
- As with coccidiosis, most worms can be controlled by growing chickens in cages off the ground, on slat or wire floors. This prevents contact with the infected manure from other chickens.

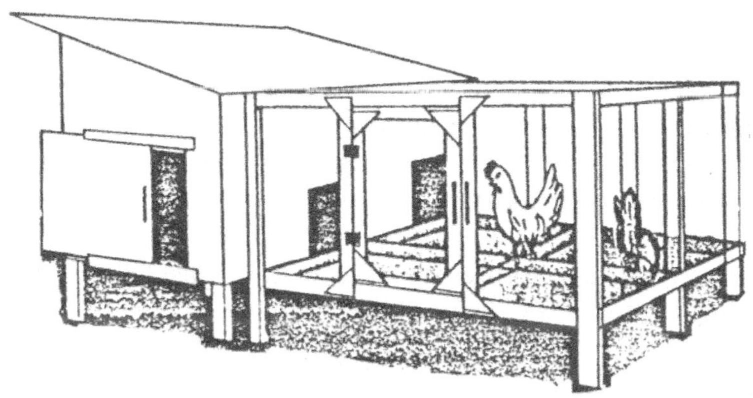

24.1.8 External parasites

Lice, mites, ticks, and fleas are common external parasites of chickens. Lice and mites bite and damage the skin. Mites, ticks, and fleas suck the blood and cause anemia (thin blood) and poor egg production. Certain external parasites can carry other diseases, such as fowl pox and spirochetosis.

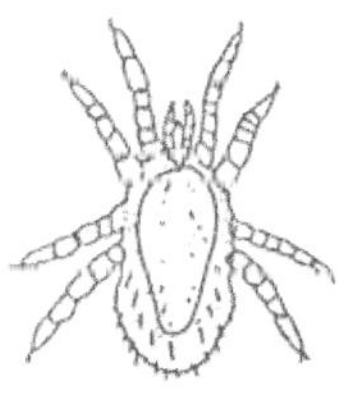

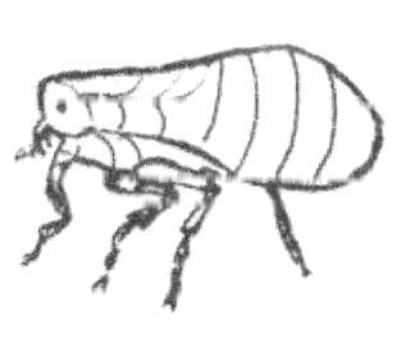

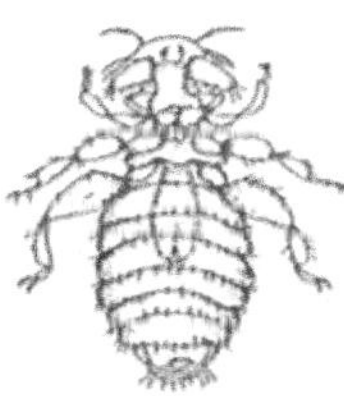

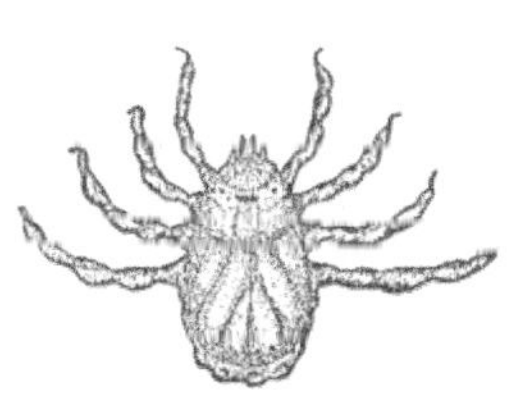

Mite   Flea   Louse   Tick

Symptoms:

- Lice cause scaly, damaged skin and are often visible to the human eye.

  - Scaly-leg mites cause crusty, thickened, unsightly legs. Red mites
    (also called nocturnal mites) attack during the night and can
    cause severe anemia which make the birds weak and poor egg
    producers. Feather mites produce scabs and anemia resulting in
    poor egg production. Feather mites tend to look like moving
    dust particles.

- Fleas can burrow in the skin and cause ulcers

- Mosquitoes can suck the blood of birds and cause poor egg
  production, or even death. Mosquitoes also carry several viral
  diseases such as Fowl Pox.

Fleas on the wattle and comb

- Ticks attack at night and suck blood resulting in anemia and poor egg production.
  Often red spots can be seen where the ticks have fed. Ticks can also carry a disease
  called "spirochetosis."

Treatment:

Dust with powder insecticides such as malathion five percent (5%) or Coumaphos five
percent (5%) according to label instructions. Dusting should be repeated according to
the label instructions (usually every 4 weeks).

For leg mites, the legs can be dipped in kerosene. However, care must be taken
not to let the kerosene touch the feathers or skin.

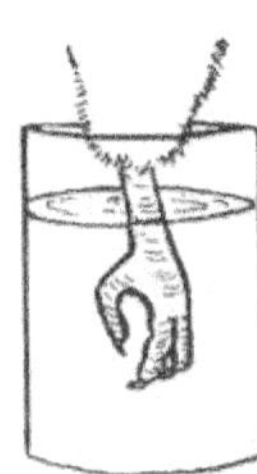

Warning: Insecticides can be poisonous if used improperly. Liquid malathion
57% should first be mixed with water *according to instructions* (usually 30 cc in
four liters of water) as it is too strong to apply directly.

24.2 NUTRITIONAL DEFICIENCIES

Poultry generally grow very rapidly and have specific nutritional requirements. Due to
their rapid growth, nutritional deficiencies usually become evident quickly. This occurs
when poor quality ingredients have been used, when an error has occurred at the feed factory,
or when the feed has been stored for more than one month in a hot warehouse and has lost its
vitamins. (The quality of feed begins to deteriorate after only two weeks.) Nutritional
deficiencies in poultry may affect fertility, hatchability, feathering, and growth. To avoid
deficiencies, good quality feed ingredients, including a vitamin premix, should be properly
mixed and fed before the feed loses its vitamins. It is therefore   best to purchase from a
reliable and honest feed mill operator who has access to high quality ingredients.

24.2.1 Calcium and Phosphorus Deficiencies

Calcium and phosphorus deficiencies usually occur together with a deficiency of
Vitamin D. If these three ingredients are not in the diet in correct amounts, the chickens
will fail to grow properly. The bones are affected, resulting in "rickets." Laying hens are
unable to stand up, and they lay soft shelled eggs. Hens in cages are especially sensitive to
calcium and phosphorus deficiencies.

Symptoms:
- Weak, soft bones (rubbery), lameness, stiff-
  legged walking, swollen joints, and soft
  beaks.

- Inability to stand, especially in caged hens
  (called "cage fatigue.")

- Ruffled feathers, poor growth, poor egg
  production, thin or soft-shelled eggs.

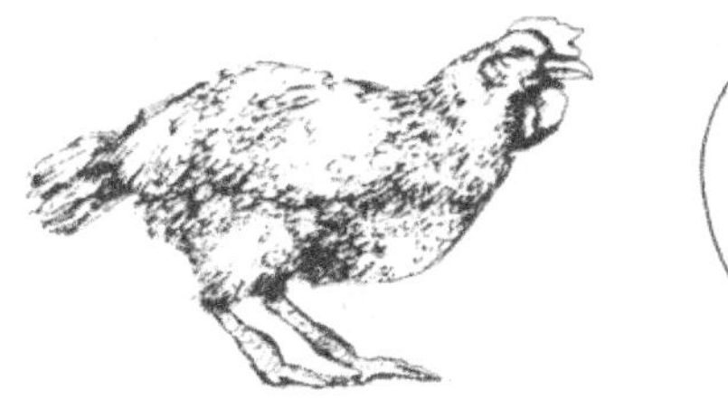 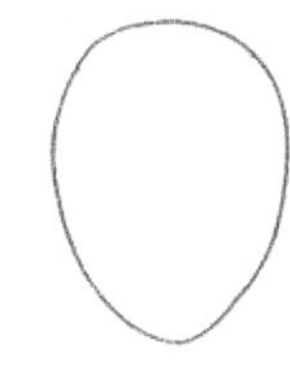

Hen with weak legs   *Soft-shelled egg*

Diagnosis:
- Based on symptoms, postmortem findings and feed analysis (if available).

Treatment / Prevention:
- Remove paralyzed hens from wire cages and put them on the ground or floor; or
  place cardboard insert on floor of cage until the hens recover.
- Buy feed from a reliable dealer who adds proper amounts of vitamin and mineral
  premixes to the ration.
- Add water soluble vitamin D_3 to the drinking water.
- Oyster shells are a good source of calcium. It can be fed free choice in a separate
  feeder; or sprinkled on the feed at the rate of one pound (one-half kg) per 100 adult
  chickens.

Warning: If feed has to be stored for more than one month in a hot environment, it is best to
put poultry vitamins in the water following label instructions until fresh feed is available.

Chapter 25.0 Nutrition Appendix
More Details of Basic Nutrition

25.1 CLASSES OF LIVESTOCK

Review: An important first step in understanding the details of animal nutrition is to divide livestock into two major groups:

Grass-eaters

These are animals that have digestive systems adapted to eating large quantities of forage and other rough feeds. They have bacteria and protozoa in their stomachs and intestines to help them digest this type of food. Grass-eaters include cattle, buffalo, sheep, goats, llamas, alpacas, horses, mules and burros. In addition to eating forages, these animals are also able to digest grains and other more expensive feeds.

Note: AHAs must be careful not to give medicines (such as antibiotics) by mouth that may harm the beneficial bacteria and protozoa in the stomach and intestines of grass-eaters.

Non-grass eaters

These animals may eat small quantities of tender, green grass and vegetables but they mainly require other kinds of food. These include pigs, chickens, dogs, cats and most birds (people   are also in this group.) Non-grass eaters cannot digest rough feeds like mature grasses. Instead, they require grains, vegetables or meat to survive.

25.2 COMPOSITION OF FOOD

Food can be divided into two categories based on the amount of water in the feed.

Water

All foods have some water in them.

Dry Matter

In the laboratory, after the water is removed from the food, only "dry matter" is left. The dry matter contains the other four nutrients: protein, energy, minerals and vitamins, as well as substances the body cannot use (waste). The waste passes out of the body as manure.

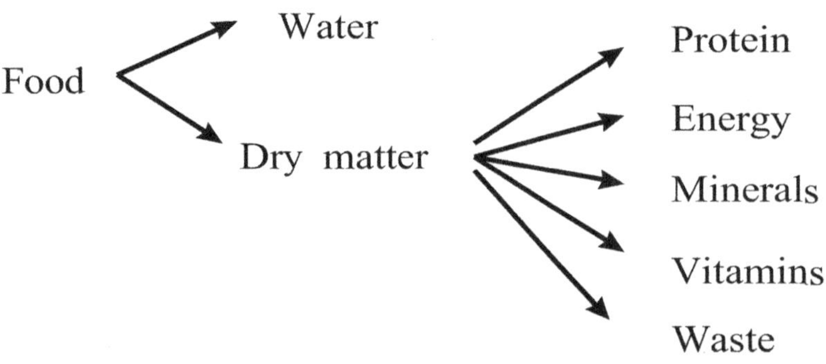

25.3 DRY MATTER

The amount of "dry matter" varies according to
the food. For example, fresh, green forage
contains about 70 percent water and 30 percent
dry matter. Dried kernels of maize contain only
15 percent water and 85 percent dry matter. Even
maize or corn flour that appears dry contains 10
percent water and 90 percent dry matter. Straw
also contains about 10 percent water and 90 percent
dry matter.

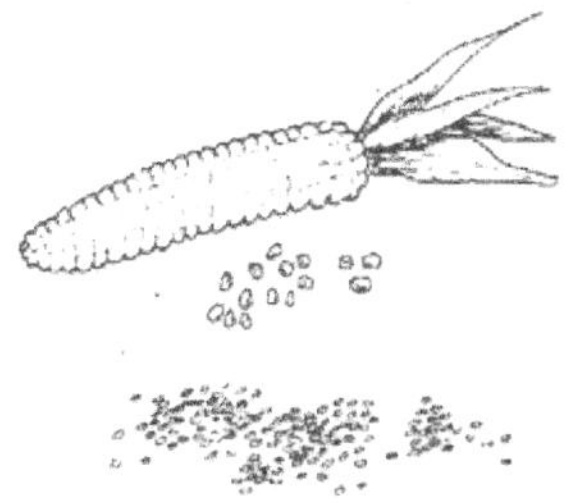
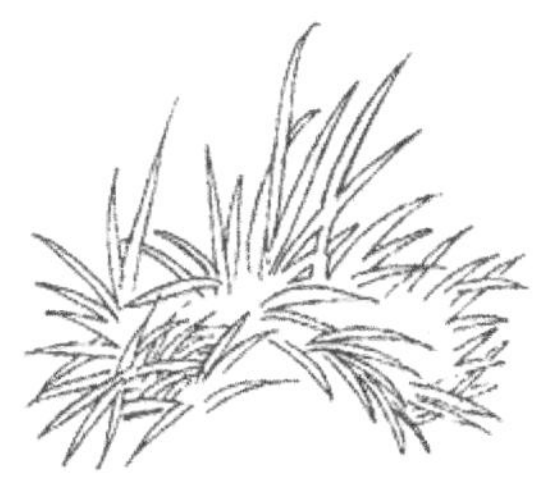

85% dry matter   *30% dry matter*

Why is this important to know? The more dry matter in a food, the more an animal must
drink. If an animal lacks water, it will lose its appetite and become malnourished, <u>even if food
is available</u>. This is especially true when food is dry, like straw or cereal grains.

Some farmers do not give water to their animals, believing they get enough from forage.
However, <u>livestock must receive enough fresh water daily to be healthy and productive</u>!

25.4 DIGESTIBILITY

Digestion is when the body breaks food down into smaller particles, which are taken into the
blood and sent throughout the body. These substances contain the five major nutrients used
by the body for growth, maintenance, and production.

Some feeds are difficult to break down into smaller particles, while other feeds are more easily
broken down. The technical word for this concept is **digestibility**. The more digestible a food
is, the more easily it is broken down into basic nutrients that the body can use. Food with much
fiber, such as old, dry forage or straw, is less digestible.

Why is this important to know? An animal might eat a large quantity of food but continue
to lose weight. This may be because the food is rough, old forage that is not very **digestible**.
Most of it is not used, and instead passes out of the animal's body as manure.

Digestibility of Grasses: In general, **forage is most nutritious
and digestible if it is cut for food before, or just when, it
begins to flower.** Before grass flowers, it is easily digestible by
grass-eaters and has more vitamins. However, after it flowers, the
plant begins to dry up, becomes less digestible and loses its
vitamins. The easily digestible components are replaced by less
digestible substances, such as "lignin."

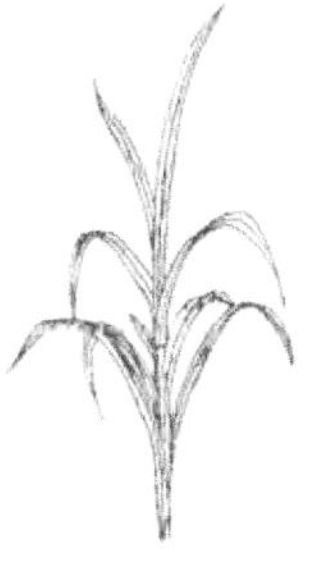
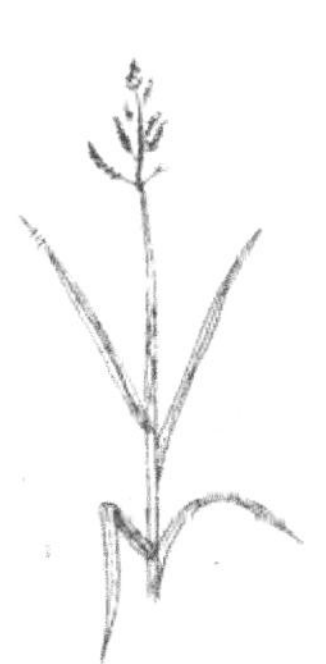

> **Forages are most digestible if they are cut before, or just when, they begin to flower.**

Therefore, forages should be fed before becoming too mature. If fed at the proper time, they provide most nutrients (except for salt) needed by a grass-eating animal. **Note: Even <u>for making hay</u>, forages should be cut when still green and tender to make the most nutritious and tasty hay.**

25.4.1 Roughages and Concentrates

Some animal nutrition workers divide animal feeds into two general kinds: **roughages** and **concentrates**.

Roughages are bulky foods that contain lots of fiber and small amounts of nutrients. Roughages are important for grass-eating livestock to stimulate the digestive system and keep it functioning properly. Some roughage (like tender, green forage and well-made hay) are quite nutritious because they are digestible. Roughages from mature dry plants are mostly fiber and are not very digestible or nutritious. These poorly digested roughages include straw, very mature grass, corn stalks, poor rice bran and poor silage.

Concentrates contain large amounts of nutrients in a small amount of food. There are energy concentrates - (containing a high quantity of energy) such as cereal grains or cereal by-products, high quality rice bran, or mustard seed cake. There are also protein concentrates (containing a high quantity of protein) such as soybean meal, fish meal, or blood meal. Concentrates often have vitamins and minerals mixed in them. Non-grass eaters (like pigs, birds, dogs, cats, and people) require concentrates in their diet.

> **Concentrates should be purchased only from a trustworthy source. The ingredients and amounts of all concentrates should be clearly marked on the label!**

Summary of Digestibility

1. Grass-eating animals can digest more roughage because of the bacteria and protozoa in their stomachs and intestines. Animal health agents must be careful not to give medicines by mouth that may harm these beneficial bacteria and protozoa.

2. Non-grass eating, simple-stomached animals (like man, chickens and pigs) cannot digest roughage feeds. They require more concentrates to stay healthy.

3. The more young and tender a grass is, the more nutritious and digestible it is. Young, tender, green, **digestible** forages supply most of the nutrients needed by grass-eating livestock (except for salt).

Review: Any time livestock do not have enough of a certain nutrient, they are <u>deficient</u> in that nutrient. For example, if they do not have enough minerals, they have a "<u>mineral deficiency</u>." If they do not have enough protein, they have a "<u>protein deficiency.</u>" Animals deficient in one nutrient are often deficient in other nutrients also.

25.5.1 Protein Deficiency

This is the most common deficiency, particularly among young, growing animals. To prevent protein deficiency, feed extra "protein foods" to young animals from the time of weaning until they approach mature size. Females need more protein during the last 1/3 of pregnancy and while they are giving milk.

25.5.2 Energy Deficiency

Nursing mothers will become energy deficient (and thin) if they do not receive <u>more</u> food while they are lactating, particularly food rich in energy. Sows that become energy deficient are often infertile for several months after weaning their piglets. Cows that don't get enough energy will not become pregnant until after their calves are weaned.

In young animals, protein and energy deficiencies often occur together, and become worse with parasite problems. It may be difficult to tell which is the main problem. However, experience shows that if a grass-eating animal is fed enough tender, green grass (and given medicine for parasites regularly), it often improves rapidly.

25.5.3 Mineral Deficiencies

General principles: Soils may be deficient in some essential minerals. Animals eating forages from these soils may also become deficient in the same minerals. In tropical areas, the soil is often deficient in phosphorous. Sometimes minerals are present in the soil, but they are not in a form that can be used by the animal. In some areas, the soil has been analyzed to know what deficiencies it has.

Warning! Shopkeepers often try to sell unnecessary vitamin and mineral supplements, particularly injections, since farmers often believe that injections are more effective than something given in the mouth is. Injections of most vitamins and minerals last for only a short time. They may be useful to get animals with severe deficiency signs started back to health. However it is almost always less expensive and better over long time periods to provide vitamins and minerals as part of an animal's regular diet.

Often the more important problem is that the animal lacks energy and protein. This problem will not be solved by an injection! Instead the animal needs more food that has energy and protein! Once this problem is solved, a chronic mineral deficiency can be solved, not by injections, but by <u>feeding</u> a local source of minerals.

What to do? Before spending money on expensive mineral mixes, do the following:

Seek advice from a trustworthy person who knows about livestock nutrition (and possibly human nutrition) and is not employed by a company selling mineral mixes.

Try to obtain information from the Ministry of Agriculture regarding the types of soil in your particular area, and any known mineral deficiencies.

Seek local, inexpensive sources of minerals that can be fed to the animal. Remember, most mineral deficiencies do not require expensive injections!

Exception: Specific deficiencies require emergency injections in order to save an animal's life, such as calcium deficiency after giving birth. See Milk Fever, page 270.

Preventing Mineral Deficiencies

The following mineral mixes are not expensive and help prevent deficiencies. Feeding these mixtures may be especially beneficial for **growing animals**, **pregnant** and **milking females.**

Mineral mixes may be fed **"free choice,"** or mixed in appropriate amounts in the grain or silage, if animals are fed these feeds frequently. "Free choice" means that the animal can eat it anytime according to its own "free choice." Animals receiving minerals free choice have fewer problems with mineral deficiencies or excesses. Mineral mixes should be placed in boxes or other containers, available to the animal, but protected from the rain. When feeding minerals "free choice", fresh water should always be available.

1. "Trace mineralized salt"
In areas where mineral deficiencies are common, it may be worthwhile to feed "trace mineralized salt." This salt has various minerals, including iodine, added to it, but usually does not include phosphorus and calcium. This special salt is sometimes available from the government livestock services at a

very reasonable price. Trace mineralized salt, iodized salt, or plain salt should be fed regularly at a   rate of one-half kg per 100 kg of food; or it can be given "free choice." Don't forget to give plenty of water at the same time!

2. "Make it yourself" mineral mixes

The following mineral-mixes, which may be made at home, may be useful – especially if phosphorus deficiencies are suspected. The following mixtures can be made at home and fed to livestock to reduce mineral deficiency problems.

Mix #1 (Best):   - 1 part   defluorinated rock phosphate
                     - 2 parts crushed bones (or steamed bone meal)
                     - 2 parts iodized (or trace mineralized) salt

Mix #2 (Better): - 1 part bone meal
                      - 1 part iodized, trace mineralized or regular salt

Mix #3 (Good):   - 1 part iodized, trace mineralized or regular salt
                     - 4 parts wood ash

Of the three mixes above, number one is the best; number two is the second best; and number three is third best. However, number three is easy to make and it is better than not feeding any minerals at all.

- In areas where no minerals are available, wood ashes can be mixed in the feed at a rate of one spoonful (five ml) per 40 kg body weight, per day. Be careful not to use ashes from trees that are known to be poisonous.

25.5.4 Most Common Mineral Deficiencies

Calcium & Phosphorus Deficiency

Calcium and phosphorus are important for bones and teeth and for proper functioning of muscles and nerves. They are especially important in the diet of pregnant, lactating and growing animals. Since milk is a good source of calcium and phosphorus, nursing animals rarely experience deficiencies of these minerals. Calcium and phosphorous are usually discussed together because the ratio of the two minerals in a diet is important.

Calcium Deficiency: Calcium deficiency is found most often in pigs or chickens fed only cereal grains. These grains are high in phosphorous but low in calcium. Sows with this deficiency "dog sit" (their back legs do not work), and sometimes can't stand up at all. Calcium deficiency in chickens causes difficulty or inability to walk, soft bones, big joints, poor growth, ruffled feathers, and production of eggs with soft shells. Rarely calcium deficiency can occur as an acute paralysis in high producing dairy cows around the time of calving.

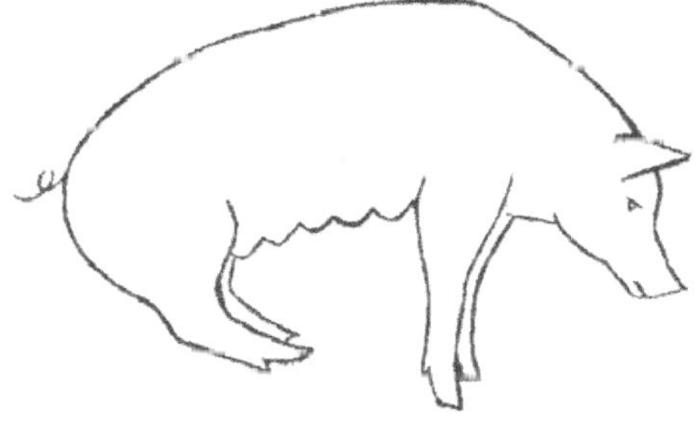

*Sow with paralyzed hind legs
due to calcium deficiency*

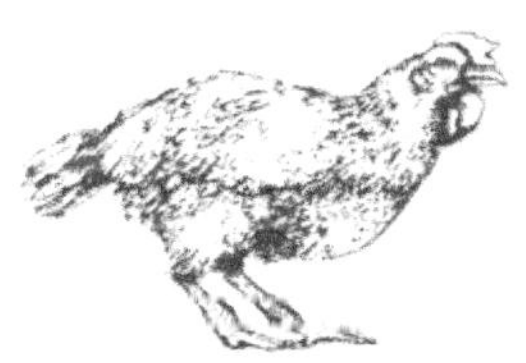

*Hen with weak legs and
swollen joints due to calcium
deficiency*

Phosphorus deficiency is seen more often. Many tropical soils are deficient in phosphorus. Phosphorus deficiency is usually a chronic problem.

Symptoms / Diagnosis
1. Loss of appetite
2. Weakness and paralysis in the hind legs, reproductive failure, and poor milk production
3. Chewing of wood, bones and other things in an effort to find phosphorous
4. Lameness, and in young animals, sore and swollen joints (called, "rickets")

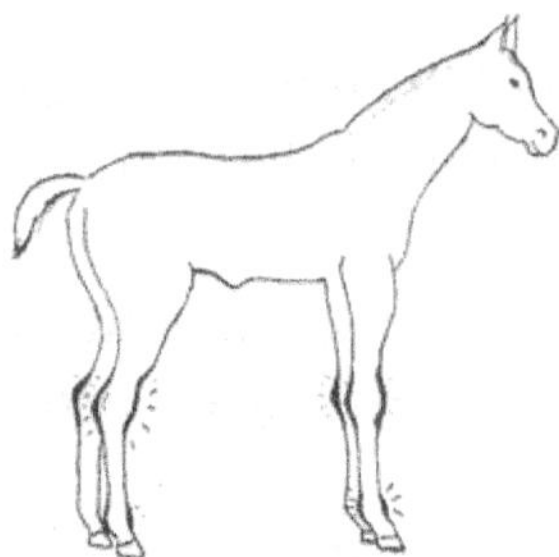

Treatment of Calcium/Phosphorus Deficiency
Phosphorus deficiency is treated by feeding mineral mixtures that contain phosphorus. Dicalcium phosphate and defluorinated rock phosphate are good sources of phosphorus.

Salt Deficiency
All livestock and people regularly need salt in their diet. Salt is made up of two main minerals, **sodium** and **chloride**. Salt is necessary for muscles and nerves to work properly.

Salt Deficiency may occur when animals work hard and sweat extensively, or when animals do not have enough salt in their diets.

Symptoms/Diagnosis: Salt deficient animals are very hungry for salt, and will chew and lick various objects in an effort to find it. They lose their appetite, become thin, and shiver and shake. Eventually they will die.

Treatment of Salt Deficiency can easily be accomplished by using mineral mixes, or by allowing animals to eat plain salt. An animal is very unlikely to eat too much salt if adequate water is always available.

Iodine Deficiency
A small amount of iodine is needed in an animal's diet for normal development. It is
especially important in the diet of pregnant females.

Iodine deficiency seems to occur only in certain areas. The Ministry of Health or Agriculture
may know where the iodine deficient areas in your country are, and may have established a
prevention program (at least for people).

Symptoms/Diagnosis
1.   Goiters: If the people in an area have large lumps on the sides of their necks (goiters),
        then the area is probably deficient in iodine.
2.   Pregnant female animal's that are iodine deficient often give birth to weak or dead
        babies. If the dead baby is cut open, the thyroid gland may appear red and enlarged.

Treatment of Iodine Deficiency
In iodine deficient areas, it may be possible to buy salt with iodine added to it (called "iodized
salt"); or one can feed "trace-mineralized salt." If iodized salt is unavailable, and if baby
animals appear to be iodine deficient, add potassium iodide to regular salt at a rate of 2.2
grams of potassium iodide per 10 kg of salt

Magnesium Deficiency
Magnesium, like calcium, is needed for proper functioning of muscles and nerves.

Magnesium deficiency is most often seen in high producing ewes, goats and cows when they
change from mature forage to **lush green pasture**. It is commonly called "grass tetany" or
"grass staggers."

Symptoms/Diagnosis
Some animals are found suddenly dead with no previous symptoms. Other animals may act
strange and nervous for several days, then suddenly fall down, convulse, and die within hours.
The convulsions involve shaking of the body and frantic movements of the legs.

Treatment
Give calcium/magnesium in the vein with a preparation made for this purpose. Follow the
label instructions carefully. This IV medicine must be given slowly while monitoring the
animal's heartbeat. If the heartbeat becomes erratic, stop the IV until the heartbeat is normal
again, then continue giving it even more slowly. Animals that are not gravely ill can receive
an injection of calcium/magnesium under the skin (sub-cutaneous).

Prevention
Include magnesium in the mineral mix, or fertilize pastures with magnesium.

SIGNS OF THE MOST COMMON VITAMIN DEFICIENCIES

Vitamin A deficiency
- blindness, cloudy eyes, excess tearing
- tilted head
- uncoordinated, staggering, fainting
- infertility
- deformed hooves & rough skin or hair
- animals born malformed, without eyes, blind, weak or dead
- respiratory disease & diarrhea

Vitamin B deficiency
(Vitamin B deficiencies are rare in ruminants & horses, but occur in chickens & pigs.)
<u>Biotin</u>
-In pigs: foot sores, small litters
-In chickens: ruffled feathers, deformed legs, crusty skin on the feet, & around the beak & eyes.
<u>Choline</u>
-In pigs: uncoordinated behavior, abnormal shoulders
<u>Niacin</u>
-In pigs: diarrhea, weight loss, rough skin and hair
<u>Pantothenic Acid</u>
-In pigs: "goose-stepping" and bloody diarrhea
-In chickens: thickened feet pads, ragged or missing feathers, eyelids sticking together, scabs around the mouth
<u>Riboflavin</u>
-In pigs: poor growth, infertility, no appetite, rough skin, or piglets born dead
-In chickens: paralysis with curled toes
<u>Thiamin</u>
-In ruminants which have been fed grain or silage: circling and / or blindness

Vitamin C deficiency
-Does not occur except in guinea pigs

Vitamin D deficiency
-Very rare if livestock are exposed to sunlight and/or eat forage
-In chickens: weak bones and eggs with soft shells

Vitamin E deficiency
-muscle stiffness, weak or dead newborn
-high number of cows with retained placentas (normally 5% or less have retained placentas)
-staggering in chickens
-sudden death in fast growing pigs

Vitamin K deficiency
-very rare; occasionally seen in animals grazing on sweet clover, causes failure of the blood to clot and excessive bleeding

Vitamin A deficiency
Vitamin A deficiency is **the most common vitamin deficiency of livestock.** This
vitamin is necessary for normal bones, reproduction, disease protection and sight.
Normally, vitamin A is found in <u>young,</u> <u>green</u> <u>fresh</u> forages, or foods that are yellow or
orange in color, such as various fruits and vegetables. There is little vitamin A in <u>old</u>
forages. Feed that has been stored for a long period of time, particularly in hot weather,
may lose vitamin A.

Symptoms/Diagnosis: Vitamin A deficient animals often have eye problems. They
might not see at night, or their eyes may form tears, become cloudy, or become
completely blind. They may also be infertile or have diarrhea, respiratory problems,
deformed hooves, dry skin and hair. Animals born from mothers that are deficient in
Vitamin A may be eyeless, blind, malformed, weak or dead. Vitamin A deficient pigs
may have a tilted head. Cattle may stagger and faint.

Treatment of Vitamin A Deficiency: The long-term treatment is to feed <u>fresh,</u> <u>young,</u>
<u>green</u> forage or fruits and vegetables that have normal yellow-green color. For example,
overripe fruit or vegetables can be fed to livestock. For severely affected animals, a
single injection of vitamin A at ~2000 IU/100 pounds (45 kg) is effective as a short-term
solution.

Vitamin B deficiency
Vitamin B deficiencies are rare in grass-eating animals because the micro-organisms in their
digestive tract make these vitamins. Vitamin B injections may be useful to stimulate
appetites in animals not eating. However, the underlying problem must still be identified and
treated. Ruminants eating silage may suffer from thiamin deficiency resulting in circling and
blindness. These animals should receive an injection of thiamin. In pigs and chickens,
vitamin B deficiencies can occur especially if they are receiving a <u>single source of feed</u>
lacking these vitamins. It is less likely if they are fed a variety of food. The animal's feed or
water can be supplemented with vitamin B sources to treat and prevent this problem.

Vitamin E deficiency
Vitamin E is normally found in most natural feeds. However, old hay, straw and cereal
grains may be deficient in vitamin E. Feeds that are stored for a long period of time may
lose their vitamin E. The functions of vitamin E, and selenium (a mineral), are closely
related to each other and are often discussed together.

Symptoms/Diagnosis: Vitamin E deficiency affects the muscles of young, nursing
animals. The muscles develop white-colored areas and cannot function properly, making
the animal stiff and unable to stand. Sometimes, the heart muscle of baby animals does
not work properly and the baby may be born weak or die suddenly.

Treatment of Vitamin E Deficiency: Short-term treatment requires several daily
injections of a combination of vitamin E and Selenium. The dose written on the label
must be followed carefully. In addition, and for long-term treatment, foods rich in
vitamin E should be fed. High-quality green grass is a good source of vitamin E.

> *Remember: Vitamin injections are never a long-term solution for a poor diet!*

25.5.5 Mineral Excesses

Mineral excesses occur when an animal eats too much of a certain mineral and becomes ill. The most common problem involves **salt**.

"Salt Poisoning" or "Salt Toxicity"
<u>Salt poisoning due to lack of water</u>
An animal can eat salty food with no problems - <u>if it has enough water to drink</u>. Even if too much salt is mixed in the feed mixture, a normal animal will not be harmed because it tends to drink enough water for the amount of salt eaten. **"Salt poisoning" occurs when livestock are given salt and do not have enough water to drink.** The problem is not really an excess of salt, but a lack of water.

<u>Salt Poisoning due to forced feeding of salt</u>
According to local customs, animals in some areas are not fed salt in their food on a regular basis, nor are they given it "free choice." Instead, each animal is fed a handful of salt about once per month. The salt is forced into the animal's mouth. This causes problems, particularly in working animals or those with inadequate water.

Symptoms
General symptoms include no appetite and abnormal behavior.

Pigs with Salt Poisoning
Pigs with salt poisoning appear blind and deaf. They sit in funny positions, jerk their heads, and fall down. Eventually, they lie on their sides, tremble, convulse, move their legs back and forth, and die.

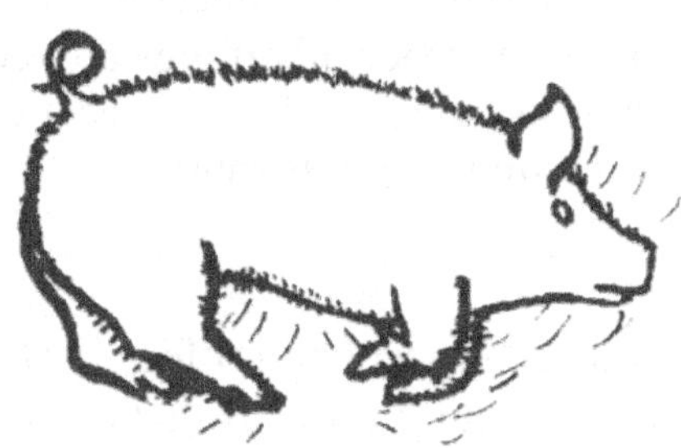

Pig trembling and convulsing due to salt toxicity

Cattle with Salt Poisoning
Cattle may vomit, have diarrhea and urinate continuously. They may stagger, stumble or drag their hind feet. Working animals, after being force fed, may collapse and not be able to work.

Diagnosis of Salt Poisoning
Diagnosis is based on the symptoms, and a history that the animals were receiving salt without enough water; or a history that the animals were force fed salt over the last few days.

Treatment of Salt Excess / Salt Poisoning
Give the affected animals fresh water to drink. However, do not give them all the water they want at once, since this may make the symptoms worse. Instead, give small amounts frequently. For example, give a liter of water to an oxen every half hour until the animal is no longer thirsty. Animals with severe symptoms tend to die despite treatment.

Prevention of Salt Excess (and other mineral excesses)
Always provide fresh, clean water "free choice." That is, have water available at all times
for the animal to drink; or provide the animal with as much water as it wants several times
daily. Explain to livestock owners the dangers of force feeding salt or restricting water.
Owners usually understand if you explain that people do not eat salt all at once; and
people are thirsty after eating salt. Livestock are the same.

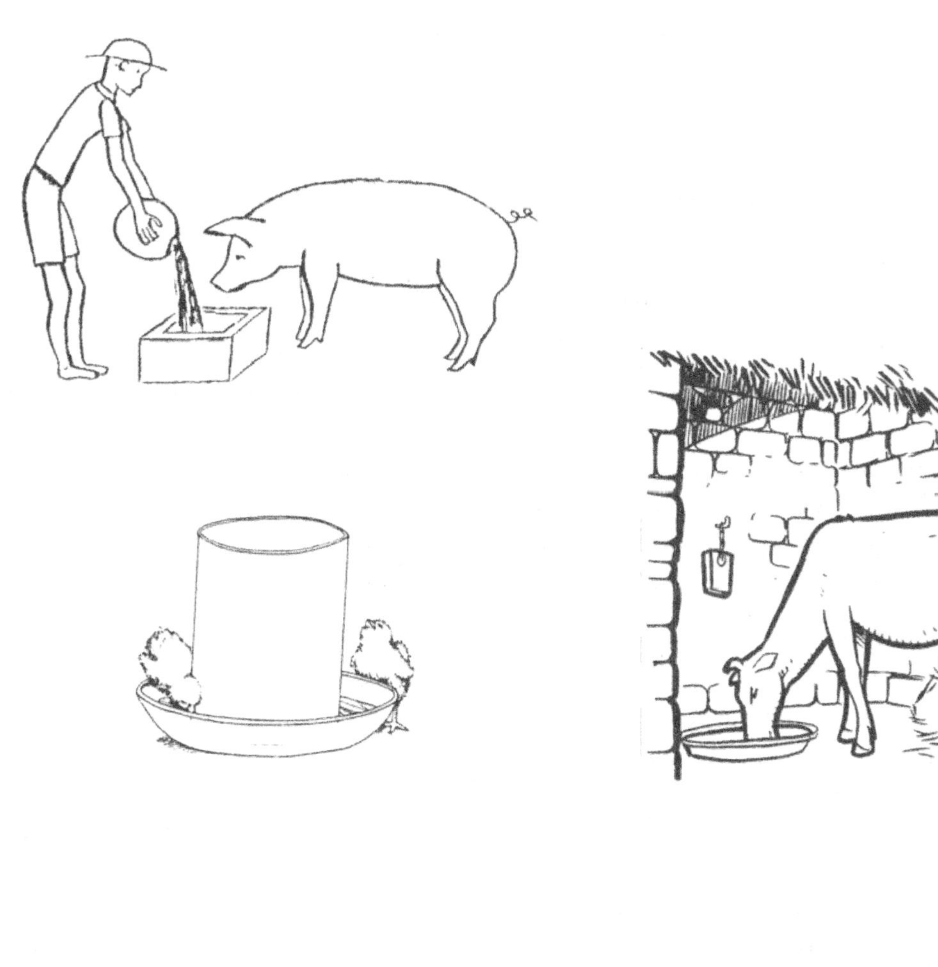

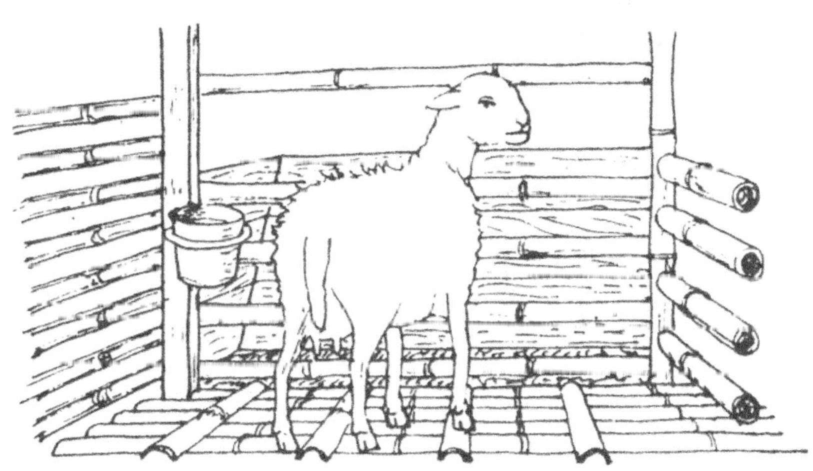

Chapter 26: Appendix –
Insecticide Use for Control of External Parasites

A GOOD EXAMPLE OF PESTICIDE USE: CONTROLLING TICKS

There are several major methods of applying acaricides (tick medicines) and other pesticides:

1. **Spraying:** Using special equipment, some pesticides are mixed with a water solution and sprayed onto the animals.
2. **Dust / Dust bags:** Some pesticides are applied directly as dusts or put into bags that the animals rub against.
3. **Backrubbers:** Some dusts or liquids are mixed with oils and placed in backrubbers that the animals rub against.
4. **Direct Applications:** Using a cloth, sponge, or brush, some pesticides are directly applied to the area of skin where the parasites are present.
5. **Pour-On**: These insecticides can be poured on the back of the animal in small amounts. They are absorbed into the blood, and then kill external parasites located almost anywhere in, or feeding on, the body.
6. **Dips:** Some medicines are put into a water solution and the animals are bathed or dipped into the solution. This method requires a special tank in which to dip the animals.
7. **Injections:** There are injections like ivermectin that kill most internal and external parasites.

26.1 Spraying of Pesticides

Spraying utilizes equipment which turns liquid pesticide into a fine spray or mist.

Advantages: It is preferable for horses because they are easily injured in a dip. Spraying is more gentle than dipping, and recommended for valuable stock, heavily pregnant cows, cows with big udders, and weak animals. Because the necessary equipment costs less than a dip vat, and smaller volumes of pesticide are used, spraying is more cost effective when small numbers of animals need to be treated.

Disadvantages: Because spraying takes time for each animal, it is difficult to use for large herds or flocks. In addition, it is easy to miss some spots on an animal during the spraying process. Approximately ten liters of spray is needed per animal for large cattle and horses to completely wet the coat.

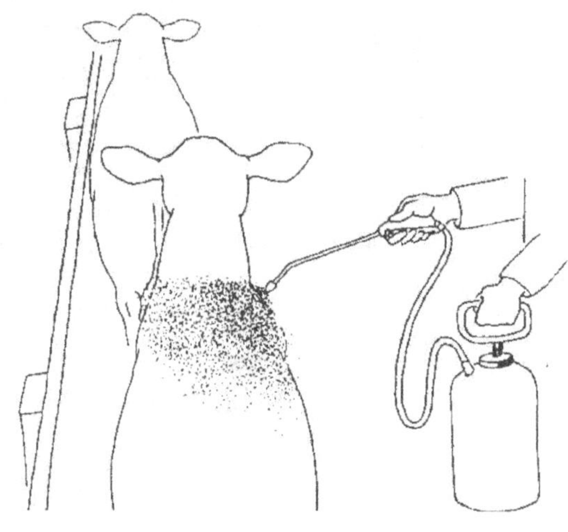

26.2 Dust / Dust bags

Some pesticides are applied directly as dusts or put into bags that the animals rub against.

26.3 Direct application of Pesticides

This method involves the use of a cloth, sponge, or brush, to directly apply pesticides to the area of skin where the parasites are present.

> **Advantages:** Sometimes it is necessary to apply pesticides directly to the area where parasites are located on the animal. For instance, two-host and three-host ticks tend to cluster in the ears or around the scrotum, udder, tail, and vulva where animals cannot easily rub the ticks off. These types of ticks often spread tick-borne diseases. Sometimes, even after dipping or spraying, these ticks do not come off. Direct application of acaracides kills the ticks and protects against re-infestation.
>
> Note: <u>acaricides based in oil or grease</u> kill the ticks and protect longer against re-infestation than water-based acaricides.
>
> **Disadvantages:** This process is time-consuming. Also, before applying to the ears or skin, it is preferable to trim long hair (with <u>round-ended</u> scissors) so acaricide is placed directly on the ticks.

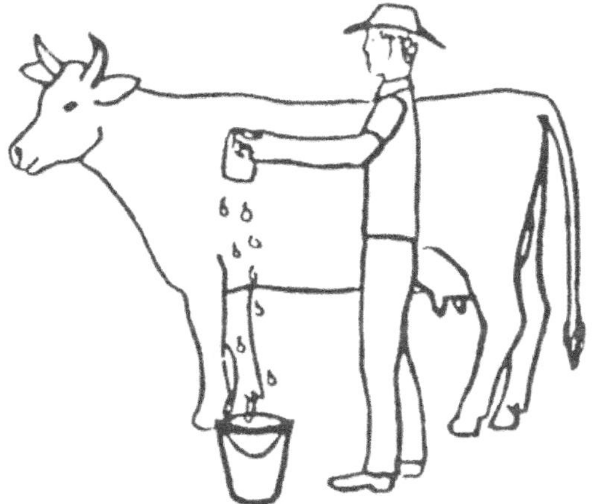

Direct Application of Pesticides

26.4 Backrubbers

Some dusts or liquids are mixed with oils and placed in backrubbers that the animals rub against. See page 116, Chapter 8 for more details.

26.5 Ear Tags

Some ear tags have pesticide in them, and slowly release the chemicals into the animal's body.

26.6 "Pour-on" Pesticides

"Pour-on" refers to the process of pouring a small amount of an <u>acaracide made especially for this purpose</u> on the back of the animal. The acaricide is subsequently absorbed into the animal's body and will kill ticks even in hidden places such as in the ears, around the tail and vulva, or between the legs. Remember to carefully follow the instructions and verify that the product is indeed for use as a "pour-on." Also make sure that it is safe for the species of animal you wish to treat. Most pour-ons are prepared for cattle.

Disadvantages:
- The animal must be individually restrained to apply the pour-on.
- Pour-on medicines are more expensive than other acaricide preparations.

Advantages:
- There is no need to buy a sprayer or build a dip tank.
- The acaricide is easily brought to the animal instead of bringing the animal to a dip.
- No water is needed to mix with the pour-on.

Picture of Pour-On Medicine Application

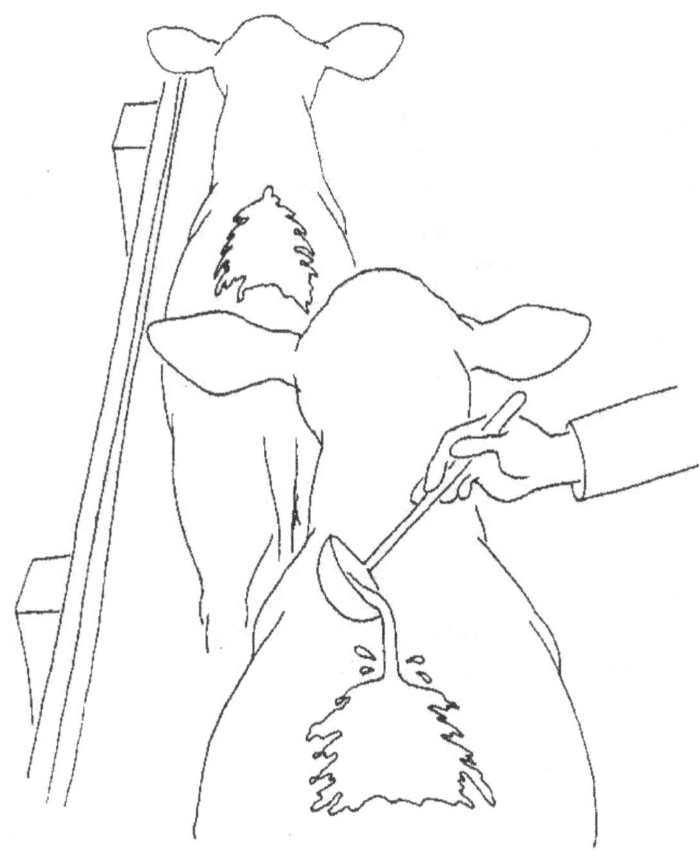

26.7 Dipping

Dips are useful when a large number of animals, particularly cattle, sheep, llamas and alpacas, are treated. Dips are also quite efficient. However initial costs are high because a dip tank must be constructed.

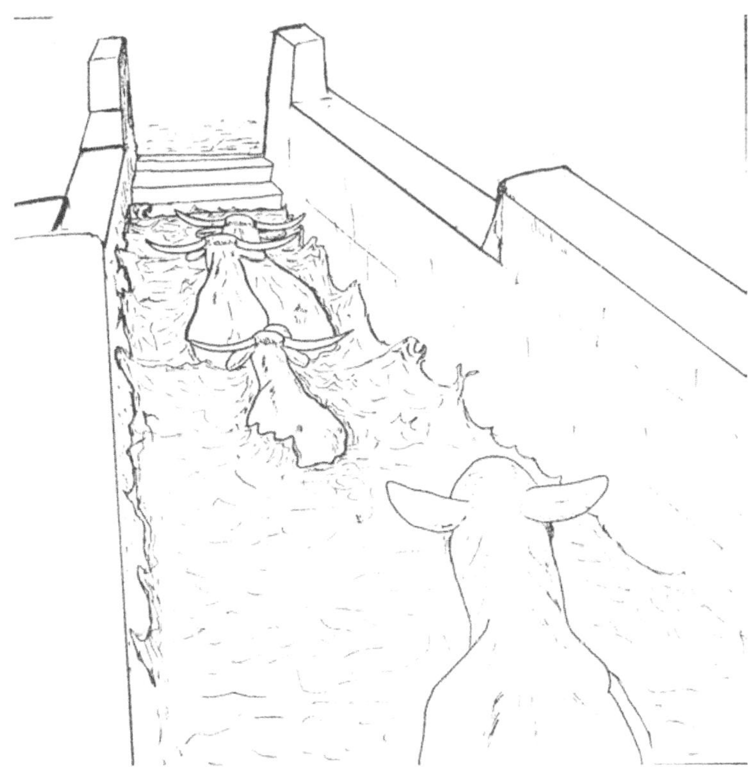

26.7.1 Well constructed dip tanks

- Should be located so that draining does not contaminate drinking water.
- Should be located so that animals don't have to swim to or from the dip.
- Should be covered to prevent dilution by rainwater and to reduce evaporation (as much as 500 liters per week may be lost in hot, windy, or dry areas).
- Should be long and deep enough to allow complete immersion of the animal, and only wide enough to comfortably allow one animal through at a time. Typical well-constructed tanks hold between 9,000 to 14,000 liters.
- Should have access along its entire length so handlers can assist an animal in distress. Ropes and pronged sticks 3 meters in length should be readily available along the tank for this purpose.
- Should have a collecting pen with a hard surface (for cleanliness) leading to the entrance of the tank.
- Should have a foot-bath ramp about 8 meters long leading into the tank. Shallow lengthwise grooves should be made in the floor of the foot-bath to spread open the claws of the hoof. This ramp should be cleaned after each use.
- Should have a safe, non-slippery "jump-off" point to the tank from the collecting pen.
- Should have a ramp the width of one animal leading out of the dip. This ramp should drain the dip solution from the animal back into the tank and allow for any needed individual treatment.

Modification for Small Herds: For small herds, a modified method is available which uses less dip solution. A more shallow tank is constructed which contains approximately 2250 liters and submerges the animal only up to its flanks. The animal is yoked while standing in the bath and buckets of the dipping solution are scooped from the dip and poured over the animal's body to complete the treatment. This method has been used successfully in East Africa.

26.7.2 Dip Tanks For cattle and buffalo

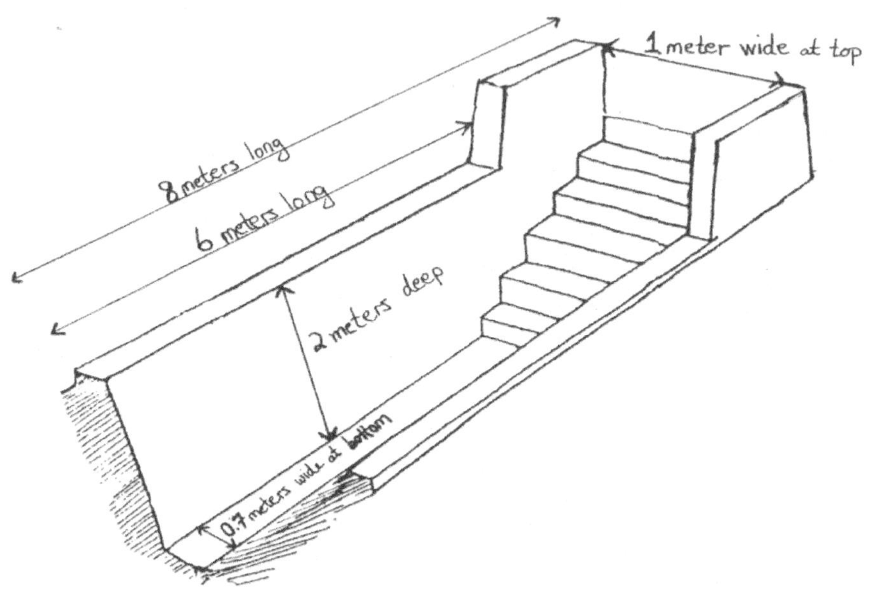

26.7.3 Alternative Dip Tanks For sheep and goats

Similar principals are used to construct and manage sheep and goat dips, except the dips are smaller. As an alternative, a simple dip tank can be made by cutting an oil drum in half length-wise, and building a stand to firmly stabilize the half-drum. The animals are then dipped by hand in the half-drum. As with cattle dips, mixing instructions must be meticulously followed. Sheep and goats are more sensitive to toxicity from acaricides than cattle and horses. Verify the volume of the tank or drum. For example, a "200-liter drum" cut in half usually should hold about 100 liters solution. However, <u>this must be verified</u> before mixing the dip solution to be sure pesticide concentration is accurate.

200 liters

170 liters

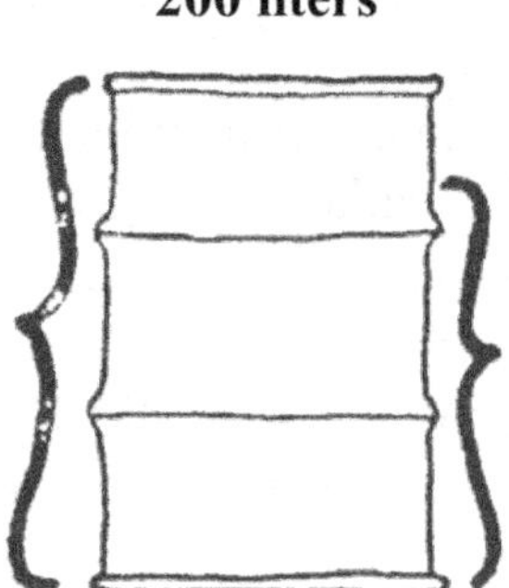

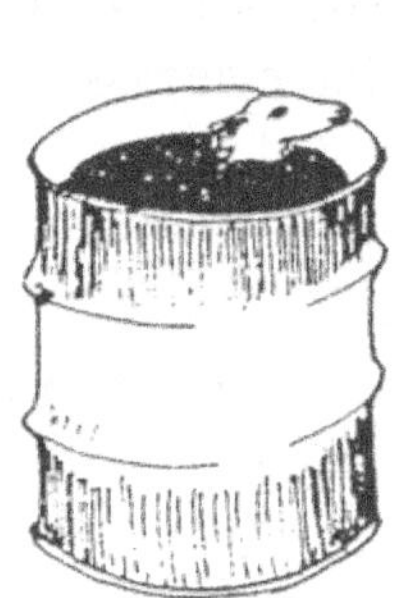

26.7.4 Regular, Smaller Dip Tanks for Sheep and Goats

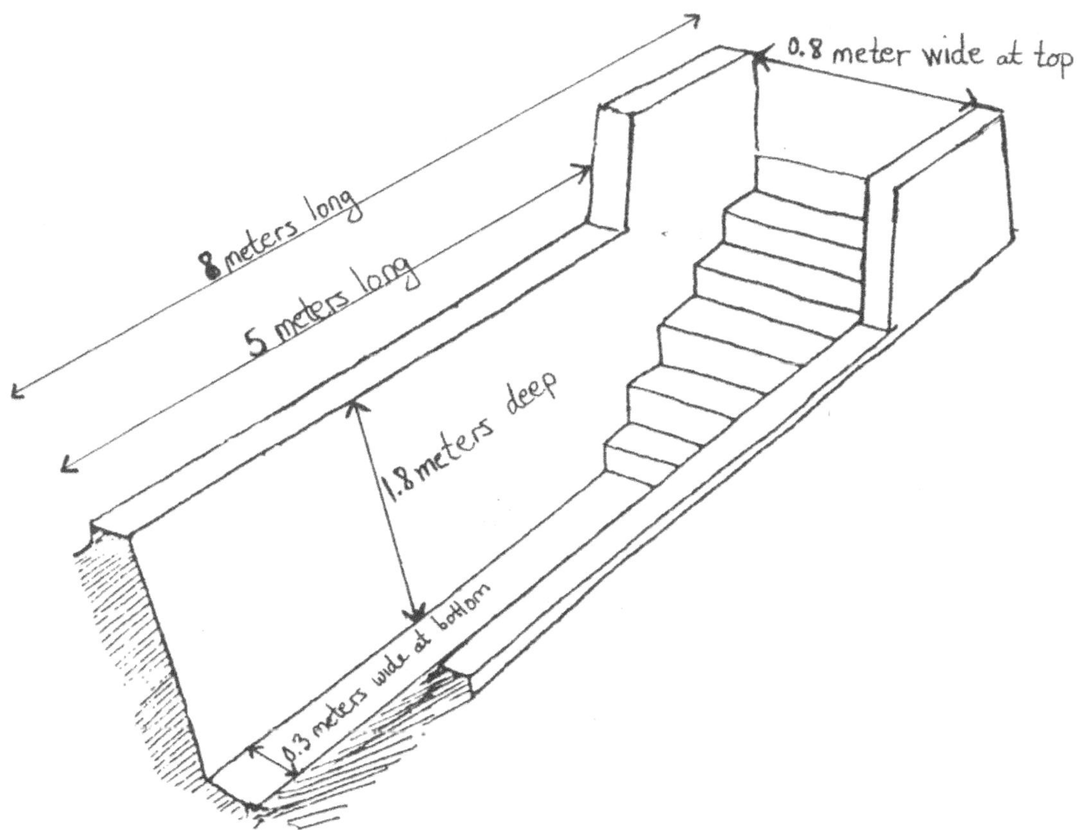

26.7.5 Management of the dip tank

Dip solution can be TOXIC if mixed incorrectly!

It is extremely important that the correct amount of dip concentrate be mixed with the correct amount of water. This is important for two reasons:

- If there is too much acaricide for the amount of water, the solution may be toxic and animals might be poisoned.
- If there is not enough acaricide for the amount of water, the solution will not kill the ticks and the whole dipping process will be a waste of time, money and energy.

How is this done?

1.   Verify the approximate volume of the dip.
    Remember: volume = length x width x height
        Because this tank is an abnormal shape, it is easiest to:
- assume an average width of 0.85 meters (1 meter + 0.7 meter)
- assume that the exit ramp occupies half the volume for 2 meters

Example: Volume =   length x   width   x   height

Volume = 6.0 meters x 0.85 meters x 2 meters = 10.2 meters^3 (body of the tank)

$$\frac{2.0 \text{ meters} \ x \ 0.85 \text{ meters} \ x \ 2 \text{ meters}}{2} = 1.7 \text{ meters}^3 \text{ (ramp area)}$$

11.9 meters^3

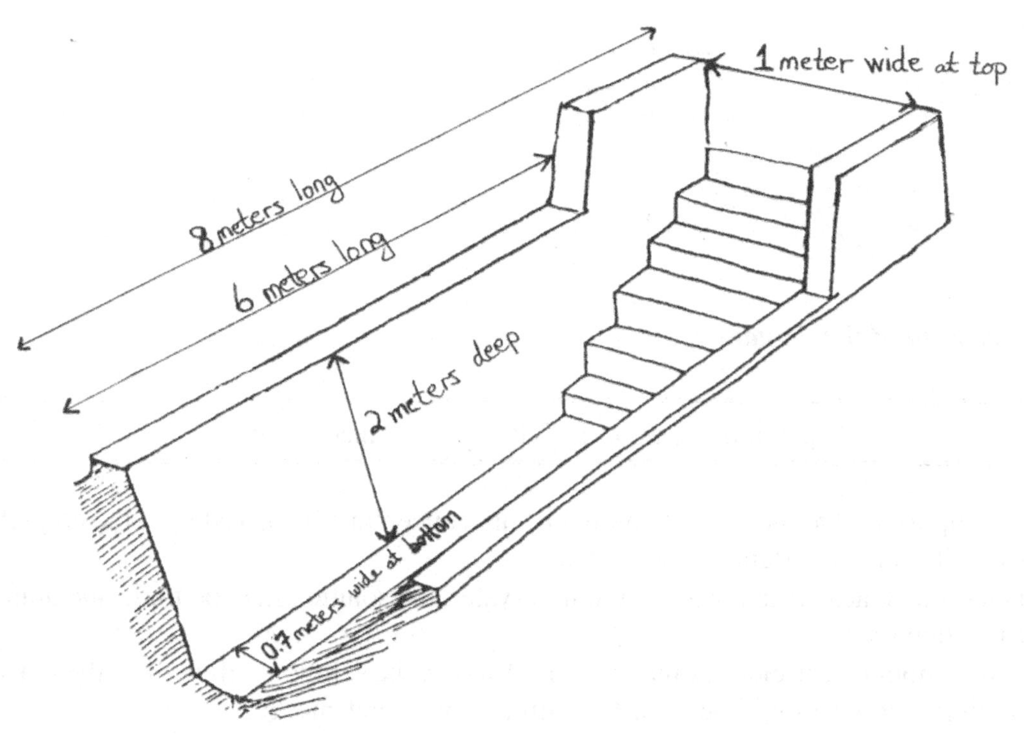

2. Permanently mark the volume level for every 5000 liters on the side of the tank or on a measuring stick. The last 5000 liters to normal dipping levels should be indicated more precisely with marks every 500 to 1000 liters. In areas where flooding is a problem, 500 liter marks should be indicated from above the normal dipping level to overflow levels.

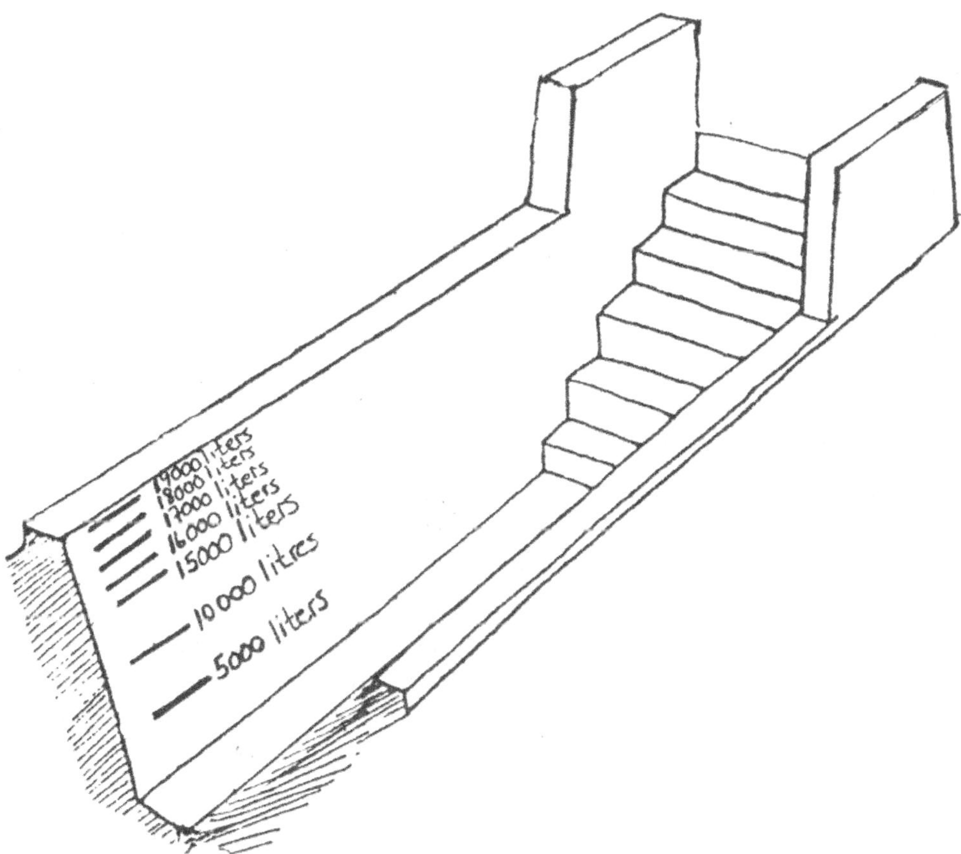

3. Clean the tank of debris.

4. Select and purchase a suitable dip concentrate based on those which are known to be effective in your area, availability, cost, and environmental safety.

5. Read and follow carefully the instructions for mixing and use.

6. Fill the tank with the correct amount of water.

7. Add the correct amount of dip concentrate. Spread it evenly over the surface of the bath water and stir it until well mixed.

DO NOT USE ANIMALS TO MIX OR STIR THE DIP SOLUTION

8. Maintain a register of the date and number of cattle dipped, the date and amount of dip concentrate used for partial replenishment, the date of complete drainage and refilling, the name of dip concentrate used each time, and any other important observations or problems.

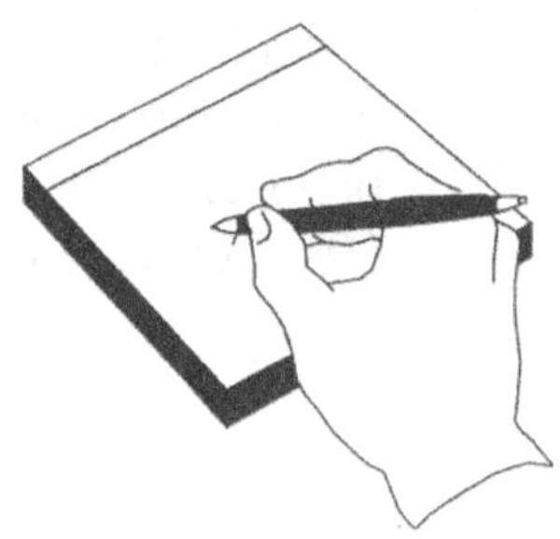

26.7.6 Refilling the dip tank

Since acaricides are less effective in dirty water, dips should be periodically drained (or pumped out) and refilled when the dip solution becomes "dirty." How frequently the dip solution is changed depends on the size of the tank, soil type, rainfall and the measures taken to keep the dip solution clean. Areas with clay soil and/or heavy rainfall will soil the dip much more rapidly than sandy soil and/or dry climates.

Here is a general guide:
- Dips with a volume of 9,000 up to 13,000 liters should be drained and refilled with fresh solution after 20,000 to 25,000 head of cattle.
- Dips with a volume of 13,000 up to 18,000 liters should be drained and refilled with fresh solution after 30,000 to 35,000 head of cattle.

26.7.7 Dip replenishment - the head count system

Occasionally it is necessary to partially replenish the dip tank due to water loss from use and evaporation. How does one calculate how much water and how much dip concentrate to add for replenishment? One method is called the "head count method" and is based on 2.83 liters of water removed per head of cattle dipped. It is necessary to have the following information for this calculation:

- The number of cattle treated since the last replenishment or complete refill of the tank.

- The "replenishment rate" listed on the label of the dip concentrate.

- The formula is:

$$\frac{2.83 \text{ liters X number of cattle dipped}}{\text{replenishment rate on label}} = \text{liters of dip concentrate required}$$

26.7.8 Principles of good stock management during dipping

- **Early morning, no rain:** Dipping is best done early in the morning in hot climates, and, if possible, not during rainy weather.

- **Not thirsty:** The animals should be brought quietly and gently to the collecting pen and watered before entering the dip. Otherwise, they will quench their thirst with the dip solution.

- **Quietly and gently:** To minimize the stress of dipping, they should always be handled quietly and gently, being allowed to enter the foot-bath in single file and dip at their own pace.

- **Immerse the heads:** Since many animals learn to enter the dip without immersing their heads, a person with protective clothing should be stationed with a dipping crutch at the side of the dip to gently immerse the heads of animals.

- **Simultaneous treatment:** For optimal tick control, all animals on the same farm or sharing the same grazing areas should be treated simultaneously.

- **Spray pregnant & weak animals:** Unhealthy or debilitated animals should be sprayed and not dipped. Similarly, animals within one month of giving birth should be sprayed and not dipped. This will help to avoid rupture of the uterus and/or abortion.

Interval between treatment with acaricides

- For optimal tick control, the tick breeding cycle must be broken. It is, therefore, best to apply acaricides before the adult female ticks engorge and drop their eggs.

- If the predominant species is the one-host ticks (e.g. <u>Boophilus</u>), the interval between two treatments should be 12 days for excellent control, or 21 days for good control.

- If the predominant species is a two-host or three-host tick, the interval between two treatments should be seven days. If the infestation is heavy, it is better to give four treatments at an interval of three, four and three days respectively. This should be complemented by direct application to the inside of the ears, as well as the areas around the scrotum, udder, tail, anus and vulva.

Chapter 27.0 Internal Parasite Appendix
A Detailed Approach to Treatment & Control of Internal Parasites

27.1 SOME DEFINITIONS

Definitive host
- The organism in which an adult parasite lives and reproduces is called the definitive host.

Intermediate Host
- The organism in which immature parasites develop is called an intermediate host. Except for tapeworms, the parasite does not usually cause serious illness in the intermediate host.

Larvae
- Immature forms of various parasites are also called larvae. Larvae often cause damage to internal organs if they travel through the body.

27.2 HOW PARASITES AFFECT THE BODY

The effects of internal parasites may include anemia, diarrhea, and poor growth. These effects are especially serious in young animals but can affect all ages.

27.3 INTERNAL PARASITES AND RESISTANCE

An animal may have parasites yet remain healthy because it has developed resistance to the parasites. The animal's resistance depends on its age, nutritional status and general health as well as the presence of antibodies due to previous exposure to the parasites.

27.4 TYPES OF INTERNAL PARASITES

General name	Category	Location in the host's body
Large roundworm	Nematode	small intestines
Small roundworm	Nematode	stomach and small intestines
Lungworms (small roundworm)	Nematode	Lung
Liver fluke	Trematode	Liver
Rumen fluke	Trematode	Rumen
Tapeworm	Cestode	small intestines[1]; organs and tissues[2]
Coccidia	Protozoa	small and large intestines
Babesiosis	Protozoa	Blood
Trypanosomiasis	Protozoa	Blood

[1] in the definitive host
[2] in the intermediate host

27.5 LARGE AND SMALL ROUNDWORMS - GENERALITIES

Large and small roundworms irritate and damage the lining of the stomach and the intestine, resulting in poor food absorption and growth. Some roundworms damage the liver and lungs as their larvae migrate throughout the body. Large roundworms may block the intestines. Lungworms (a type of small roundworm) irritates the animal's airways, cause coughing, increased risk of lung infection, and a general unhealthy appearance. All of these effects are especially serious in young animals.

27.5.1 Large Roundworms in the Small Intestines

Horses, pigs, chickens, young cattle and buffalo, dogs and cats can have large roundworms, which live in the small intestines. Sheep and goats do <u>not</u> have large roundworms.

Life Cycle of Large Roundworms

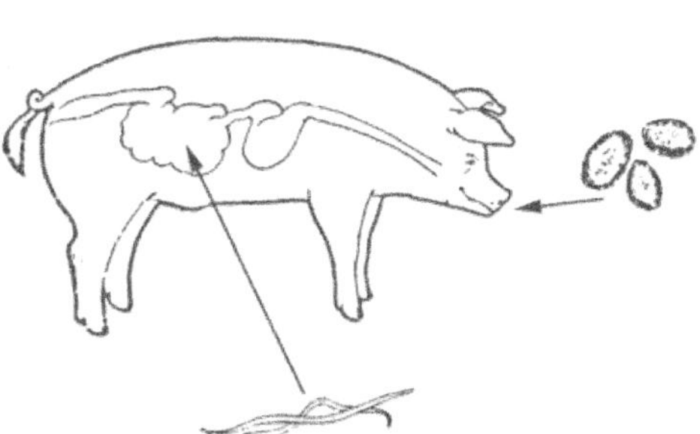

1. The adult worms in the small intestines lay eggs, which are passed in the feces. These eggs must remain in the environment for several weeks and develop to a more mature stage before they can infect another animal. Under certain conditions, the eggs can survive for several years in the environment.

2. The eggs are eaten by another animal and, if at the right stage, hatch into larvae in the small intestine.

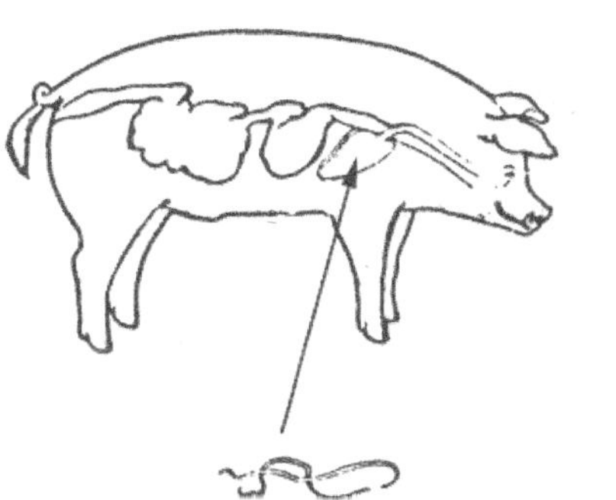

3. The larvae pass through the intestinal wall, into the bloodstream and then through various organs such as the liver and lung, damaging each organ through which it passes.

4. Finally, the larvae return to the lungs, are coughed up, and swallowed. They larvae mature to become adults in the small intestines.

The life cycle takes one to three months.

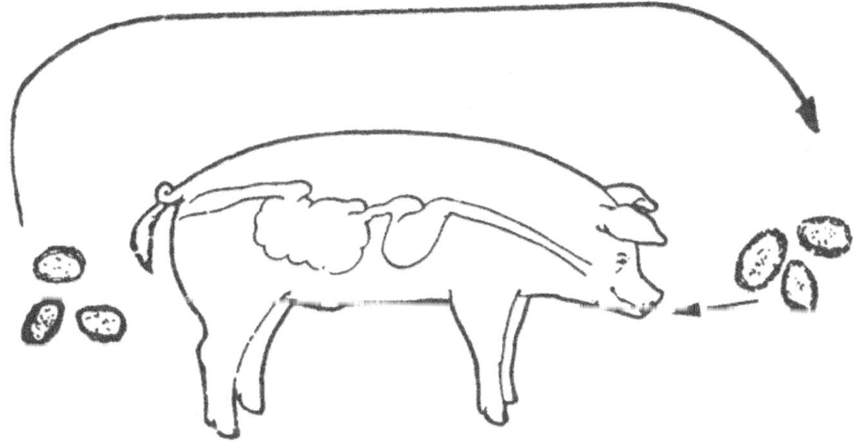

<u>**Symptoms**</u>

* Mostly young animals are affected. They have poor growth, appear unhealthy, may cough, and may have diarrhea *or* constipation as well as a complete blockage of the intestines.

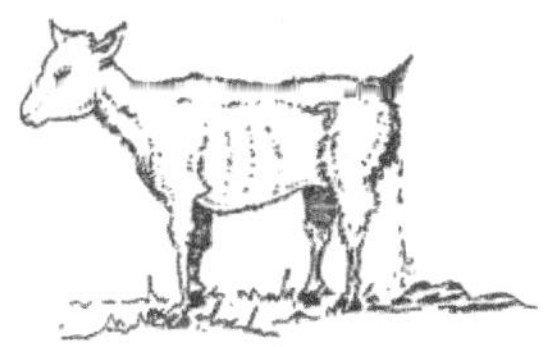

<u>**Diagnosis**</u>

- Diagnosis is usually based on symptoms, a history of not having received parasite medicine recently, and knowledge that large roundworms are a problem in your area.

- *Necropsy:* In a dead animal, white spots may be observed on the liver. These spots are scars due to the worms moving through the liver.

- *Laboratory:* Using a microscope, large roundworm eggs might be observed in the feces. However, sometimes the animals may be ill due to the larvae, and no eggs may be observed in the feces.

<u>**Treatment**</u>

- The least expensive treatment is piperazine, which is usually available. Other medicines work well on small roundworms but do not work well for large roundworms and are quite expensive. Animals should be wormed regularly every 3-6 months according to the situation.

<u>**Control**</u>

- These eggs can survive for months to years in a moist, cool environment. Direct sunlight and certain disinfectants kill the eggs. All animals at risk should be wormed regularly. All new animals should be wormed before they are mixed with the other animals. In addition, pregnant mothers should be wormed to reduce infection in their babies.

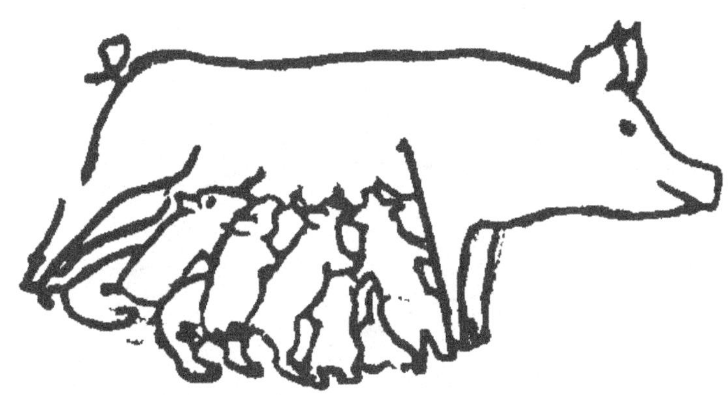

- To prevent large roundworm infection in her piglets, a pregnant sow should receive roundworm medicine during the last month before giving birth.

Specifics about Large Roundworms in the Animals They Affect

Large Roundworms in Buffalo and Cattle
<u>Neoascaris</u> <u>vitulorum</u> is the large roundworm (up to 25 centimeters long) found in cattle and buffalo calves. Adult buffalo and cattle are resistant to *Neoascaris* but calves may get sick from this large roundworm until about 6 months of age. Calves can become infected before birth.

Note: Some people withhold the first milk called "colostrum" from calves thinking that this will prevent infection with large roundworms. However, this will not prevent infection and is very risky since colostrum *protects* the newborn from many diseases.

- Give piperazine to calves and repeat the treatment 4 weeks later. Dose according to label.

Control
- Regular treatment of young, infected animals will control the disease.

Large Roundworms in Sheep and Goats
Large roundworms are not normally found in sheep and goats.

Large Roundworms in Pigs
Ascaris suum is the large roundworm commonly found in the small intestines of young and adult pigs. The larvae damage the liver and lungs, and make the lungs more susceptible to infections. Unlike the roundworm in cattle and buffalo, Ascaris suum does not infect baby pigs before they are born.

Treatment
- Piperazine is the least expensive treatment. Dose according to label. Do not wait for a positive fecal exam to treat for Ascaris suum. All animals (young and old) should be treated at least every six months. Pregnant sows should receive piperazine during the month before giving birth. Remember, prevention is better than cure!

Control
- Eggs can survive for years in moist conditions but will die within several weeks in direct sunlight. A farrowing crate should be left clean, empty and exposed to sunlight for a few weeks before putting a sow into it. Baby pigs and their mothers should be kept separate from other pigs and in a clean, dry environment. Again, pregnant mothers should also be wormed during the month before farrowing.

Large Roundworms Horses
Parascaris equorum is the large roundworm of horses. Its life cycle is similar to that of pigs. It is a problem only in young horses, sometimes giving them colic or blocking their intestines.

Treatment
- Piperazine is the least expensive. Dose according to label. Other medicines may be available which treat roundworms as well as other parasites.

Control
- Keep mothers and babies in clean pens, and treat foals (baby horses) with medicines against roundworms during their first year of life (beginning at one month of age).

Large Roundworms in Birds

<u>Ascaridia</u> <u>galli</u> is the large roundworm of many domestic birds. This worm is smaller than other common large roundworms. Compared to healthy birds, young birds with lowered resistance, due to illness or a nutritional deficiency, are more likely to get ill from this worm.

Treatment
- Treat all chickens at least every 6 months depending upon the severity of the problem. Dose according to label.

Control/Prevention
- Good sanitation and regular worming can control this problem.

Large Roundworms in Dogs

<u>Toxacara</u> <u>canis</u> is the large roundworm of dogs and is of **public health** importance. Its life cycle is similar to that of the large roundworm in cattle and buffalo. Puppies suffer most and can be infected before they are born. Children in contact with puppies can become infected with <u>Toxacara</u> <u>canis</u> and may suffer from damage to their liver, brain, lungs and eyes.

Treatment
- Piperazine is the most inexpensive treatment although other medicines are effective as well (e.g. thiabendazole, pyrantel pamoate, mebendazole). Dose according to label.

Control
- To prevent the passing of eggs in the feces (and possible infection of humans), puppies *and* their mothers should be treated when the puppy is two weeks old and then every three weeks until the puppy is three months old. Treatment should continue on a regular basis (e.g. every 3-6 months) depending on the severity of the problem.

27.5.2 Small Roundworms in the stomach and intestines

There are many small roundworms that live in the stomach and intestines.

Life cycle of small roundworms in the stomach and intestines:
1. The adult worms live in the stomach or intestines, and lay eggs.
2. The eggs pass out with the manure and, in warm weather, hatch.
3. The larvae are eaten when the animal is eating contaminated food or water, or sucking on a dirty udder. Animals kept in crowded, dirty, wet conditions get more roundworms.
4. The larvae inside the animal's intestines develop into adults and begin laying eggs.

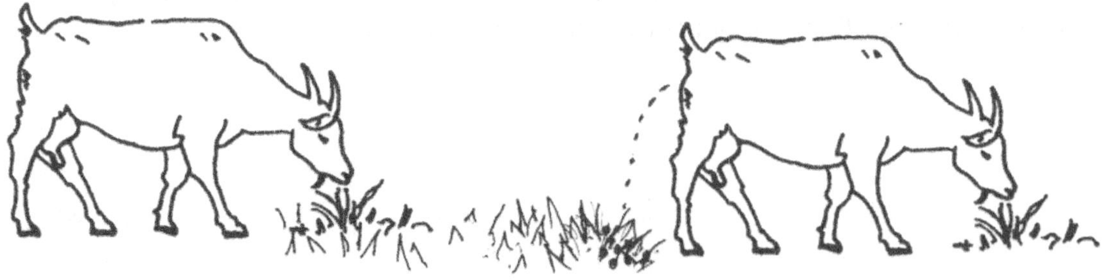

Symptoms:

- Most roundworms suck blood, making an infected animal "anemic" (i.e. thin and watery blood). In anemic animals, the normally pink tissue under the eyelid becomes white. Anemia may result in extra fluid collecting under the lower jaw of the animals and is sometimes called "bottle jaw" or "big-head." Roundworms may also cause diarrhea and a poor appetite particularly in young animals.

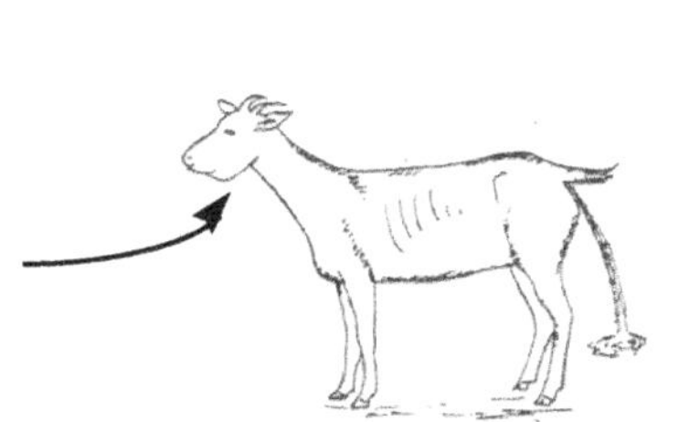

Bottle jaw

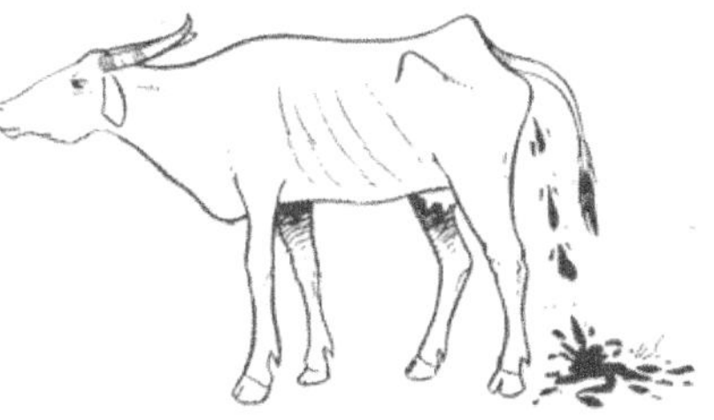

Diarrhea

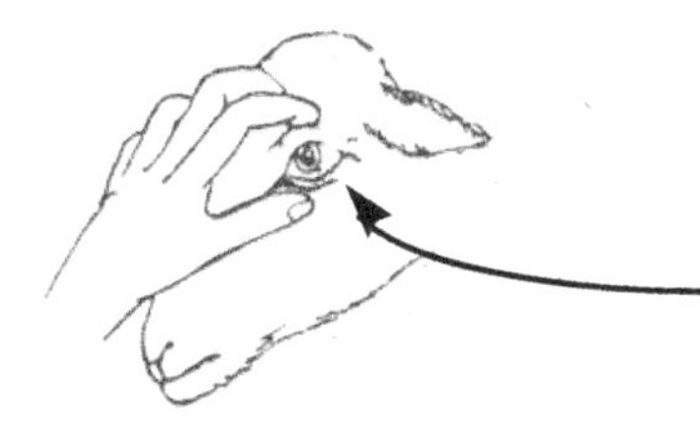

Pale under the eyelids (anemia)

Diagnosis:

- *Symptoms:* Diagnosis is usually based on symptoms: particularly anemia and diarrhea; a history of not having received parasite medicine recently; and knowledge that small roundworms are a very common problem in livestock kept in dirty, wet conditions and where no pasture rotation is practiced. Response to treatment will confirm the diagnosis.

- *Necropsy:* Small roundworms can also be found in the digestive tract of dead animals, particularly if you wash the stomach contents on a screen.

- *Laboratory:* Using a microscope, small roundworm eggs can often be found in the feces.

Treatment:

- You will probably have access to various medicines that treat small roundworms. Read the label and choose the least expensive medicine that is available and known to be effective against small roundworms in your area. Generally, animals should be treated at least every 6 months but the frequency may vary depending upon local conditions. There may be a certain time of year (springtime in most temperate climates) when parasites are most severe; and treatment should be more frequent during this period. Repeated treatment with the same medicines may cause the worms to become resistant to treatment. When this happens, a different medicine should be used.

Control:

Small roundworms can be controlled by:

Good sanitation
- Keeping feed in mangers where animals cannot defecate.
- Keeping water in troughs where animals cannot defecate.
- Cleaning pens regularly and leaving them empty to dry, preferably in the sun.

Pasture Rotation
- Moving animals to a new pen or pasture every few months, and leaving previously grazed pastures free for at least 3 months.
- Note: It's best move animals to a new pen or pasture on the same day of treatment against internal parasites.

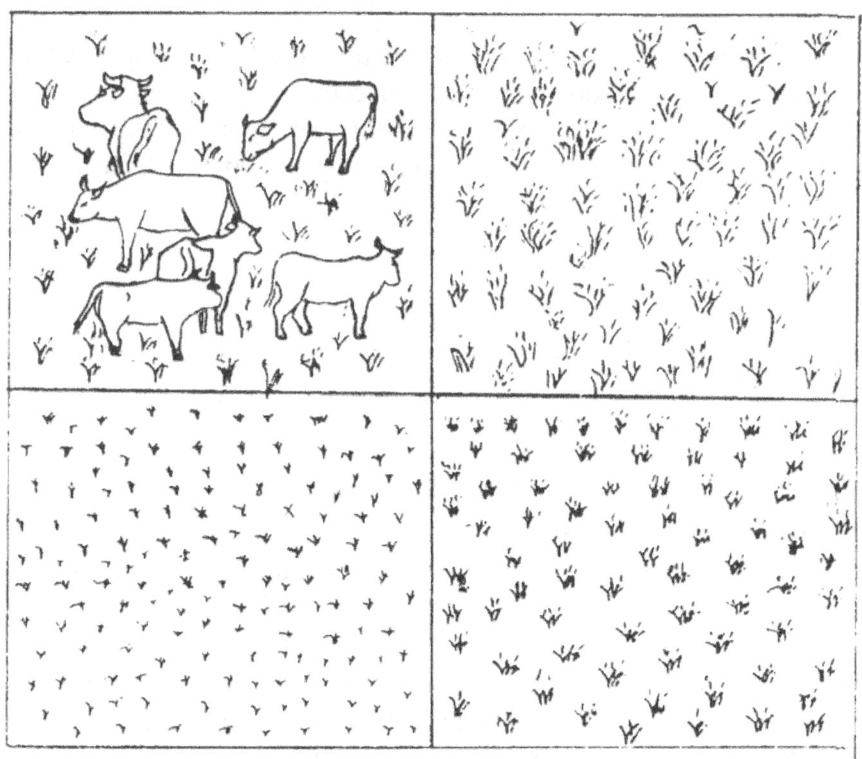

Pasture rotation

- Animals graze on one pasture for a period of time (e.g. 1 month). They are then moved to a second pasture while the previously grazed pasture is allowed to "rest." They are then moved to a third pasture and fourth pasture allowing the previously grazed pastures to "rest." During the rest period, parasites are exposed to sunlight and drying, and they die. Then grazing animals are not exposed to the parasites once they are rotated back onto the pastures.

Examples of Common Small Roundworms

In the stomach

<u>Haemonchus</u> (large stomach worm or wire worm) is red or red-striped in color, 1-3 centimeters long, and easily seen in the stomach of dead animals. It occurs in almost all ruminant animals.

<u>Ostertagia</u> (medium or brown stomach worm) is about 1 centimetre long and brown in color.

<u>Trichostrongylus</u> (small stomach worm, bankrupt worm) is the smallest roundworm worm in the stomach (about 0.5 centimeter long).

In the small intestines

<u>Cooperia</u> (bankrupt worm) is just less than 1 centimeter in length and difficult to see.

<u>Ancylostoma</u>, and <u>Bunostomum</u> (hookworm).

<u>Ancylostoma</u> is seen in man and meat-eating animals. <u>Bunostomum</u> is found in ruminants. These worms are easily recognized because of their hook-shaped head. The larvae can infect an animal by entering through the skin or mouth. The adults live in the intestine and can rapidly cause severe anemia.

Examples of Small Roundworms (continued)

Nematodirus (long necked worm) looks like hookworm but causes a lack of appetite and more severe diarrhea than hookworms.

In the large intestines:
Trichuris (Whipworm) is found in the cecum, and is easily recognized by its long tail. It is usually not harmful.

Chabertia (largemouth worm) is 2 centimeters long with a large mouth. It destroys the wall of the intestine and causes bloody diarrhea.

Oesophagostomum (nodular worm) is white in color and about 2 centimeters long. The larvae cause small abscesses in the wall of the large and small intestines. These abscesses may break open and cause severe infections and diarrhea.

27.5.3 Lungworms

Lungworms are a problem mostly in young animals. They develop in the small air passages of the lungs and damage the tissue, resulting in poor growth of the animal. This damage can also lead to pneumonia. The following list indicates the scientific name of various lungworms and the animals they affect:

> Dictyocaulus (cattle, sheep and goats)
> Protostrongylus (sheep and goats)
> Meullerius (sheep and goats)
> Metastrongylus (pigs)
> Aelurostrongylus (cats)

Life cycle of lungworms:

1. Although the life cycle varies depending upon the type of lungworm, in general, the adult lungworms live in the lungs and lay eggs.
2. The eggs are then coughed up and then swallowed.
3. With some types of lungworms, the eggs hatch into larvae while in the intestines and then pass out with the manure, contaminating the ground or forage. The larvae pass through various stages in the environment. With other types of lungworms, the eggs themselves pass out of the animal in the manure and hatch into larvae. The larvae are then eaten by "intermediate hosts" such as earthworms, slugs or snails.
4. Grazing animals are infected when they eat the larvae in the environment (for some types of roundworms) or when they eat intermediate hosts (for other types of larvae).
5. The larvae then move from the intestines to the lungs.

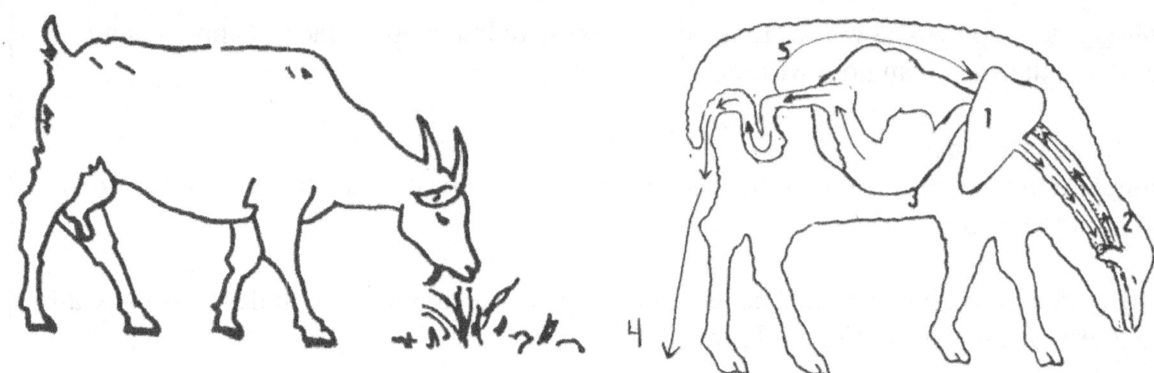

- Lungworms may cause coughing, difficult breathing, and poor weight gain. Lungworms also make an animal more susceptible to pneumonia caused by other organisms (i.e. bacteria or viruses).

Diagnosis:
- *Symptoms:* Lungworms can be diagnosed on the basis of general symptoms, knowledge that lungworms are a problem in your area, and response to treatment.

- *Necropsy:* In dead animals, lungworms can be observed in the lungs. The worms are white and up to 8 centimeters in length.

- *Laboratory:* Using a microscope, lungworm eggs can be observed in the feces if specimens are prepared using a special technique (called "Baerman" technique).

Treatment:
- Common roundworm medicines, such as tetramisole, thiabendole and albendazole, are effective against lungworms (check the label). Use that which is available, least expensive, and known to be effective in your area. Always follow label instructions.

Control:
- Treat for lungworms at least every 6 months. The frequency depends on the severity of the problem in you area. In some countries, a lungworm vaccine is also available. Information about it can usually be obtained from your ministry of agriculture. Adult animals may recover without treatment.

27.6 FLUKES (TREMATODES)

27.6.1 Liver Flukes (Fasciola)

Liver flukes are a serious problem of livestock in many countries. The two most common liver flukes have the scientific names "<u>Fasciola</u> <u>hepatica</u>" and "<u>Fasciola</u> <u>gigantica</u>." Flukes can be a problem wherever there exists a certain species of snails and wet conditions such as rice paddies. Even if animals are not grazed on rice paddies, they can be fed rice straw contaminated with liver fluke cysts called "metacercariae." Liver flukes damage the liver tissue and can block the liver ducts.

Life cycle of liver fluke

1. Adult liver flukes lay eggs in the bile ducts. The eggs pass into the small intestine and out of the animal with the manure.
2. In wet environments, the eggs hatch into larvae called "miracidium."
3. These larvae burrow into snails which are "intermediate hosts," and develop into "cercariae" another stage of larvae.
4. The cercariae burrow out of the snail and onto blades of grass or straw. They make protective shell and become "metacercariae" which is about the size of a grain of dust.
5. Animals eat the metacercariae while grazing. In the intestines, the metacercariae lose their shell, become young flukes and travel to the liver where they become adults. The cycle usually takes about 2 months.

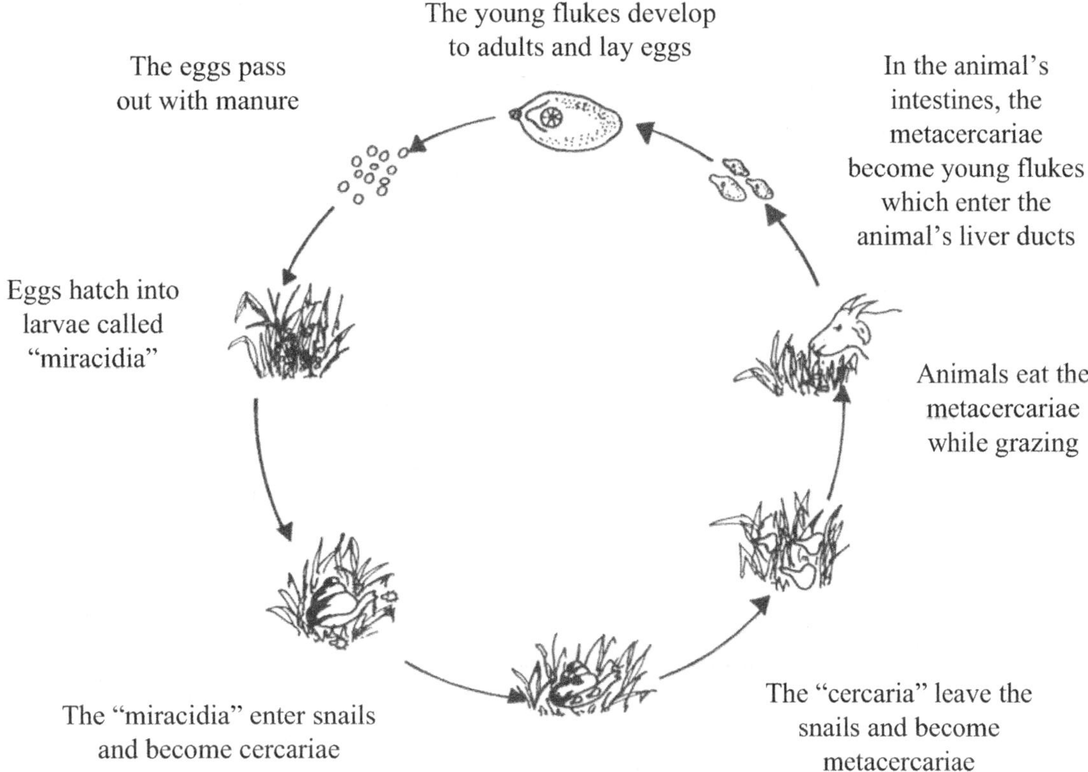

Symptoms of liver fluke:

- The symptoms of liver fluke are loss of appetite, diarrhea, poor condition, and anemia. If the anemia is severe, fluid may collect under the lower jaw. A severe liver fluke infection damages the liver, which may result in "jaundice," a condition which turns the tissue yellow, and is a sign that the animal may die. Symptoms often become more severe when food is scarce, for example, during the dry season.

Diagnosis of liver fluke:

- *Symptoms:* Liver flukes can be diagnosed on the basis of general symptoms, knowledge that liver flukes are a problem in your area, and response to treatment.

- *Necropsy:* In dead animals, liver flukes may be seen in the liver ducts. They are flat like a leaf and up to five centimeters in length. Liver flukes also damage the liver tissue, giving it a hard texture. Examining livers of dead animals is one of the best ways to verify whether liver flukes are a problem in your area.

- *Laboratory:* Examining fecal specimens for liver fluke eggs is useful, however infected animals may have a negative result (i.e. no fluke eggs found).

Treatment of liver fluke:
- There are several good medicines for liver flukes. Use the label to verify whether a certain medication is effective against liver flukes. Use that which is least expensive and known to be effective in your area.
- **Caution:** The older liver fluke medications like carbon tetrachloride, and hexachloroethane are less expensive, but generally less effective and have many side effects, particularly on weak and pregnant animals. The authors recommend the use of the newer medicines such as oxyclozanide, and albendazole. Some of the newer medicines kill not only adult flukes, but also the immature ones, before they cause damage to the liver.
- If the animal is not eating well, treatment with appetite stimulants, such as vitamin B, may help the animal recover more rapidly.

Control:
The following three methods can help control liver flukes:

1. Treat animals with liver fluke medicines at least 3 times annually. The frequency may vary depending on local conditions and the severity of the problem.
2. Eliminate the snails (i.e. the intermediate host) although the methods used should not endanger other animals, poison the drinking water, or damage the environment. Ducks can help reduce the snail population.
3. If feeding rice straw, ensure that it is well dried because drying will kill some metacercariae. If possible, feed tree fodder since it is less likely to be contaminated with metaceraria than forage or rice straw.

27.6.2 Flukes in the Rumen (<u>Paramphistomum</u>)

The rumen fluke, whose scientific name is "<u>Paramphistomum</u>," can be a problem wherever there exists a certain species of snails and wet conditions such as rice paddies. Even if animals are not grazed on rice paddies, they can be fed rice straw contaminated with the rumen fluke cysts called "metacercariae."

Life cycle:
- The life cycle is similar to that of liver flukes except the young flukes that emerge from the metacercariae in the intestines travel to the rumen instead of the liver.

Symptoms:
- Rumen flukes may cause diarrhea and poor condition, especially in young animals.

Diagnosis:
- *Symptoms:* Rumen flukes can be diagnosed on the basis of general symptoms, knowledge that rumen flukes are a problem in your area, and response to treatment.

- *Necropsy:* Adult rumen flukes are easily seen attached to the rumen wall and look like red kernels of rice.

- *Laboratory:* Examining fecal specimens for rumen fluke eggs is useful, however infected animals may have a negative result (i.e. no fluke eggs found).

Treatment/Control:
- Killing the rumen fluke larvae will help stop the symptoms of diarrhea. Killing the adult rumen flukes will help decrease contamination of pastures and rice paddies with fluke eggs.
- The medicine niclosamide will treat rumen fluke larvae. The medicines oxyclozanide, and albendazole kill adult rumen flukes.

27.7 TAPEWORMS (CESTODES)

Tapeworms are long, flat, white worms that live in the small intestine. These worms have a segmented body, and a head with a sucking mouth part.

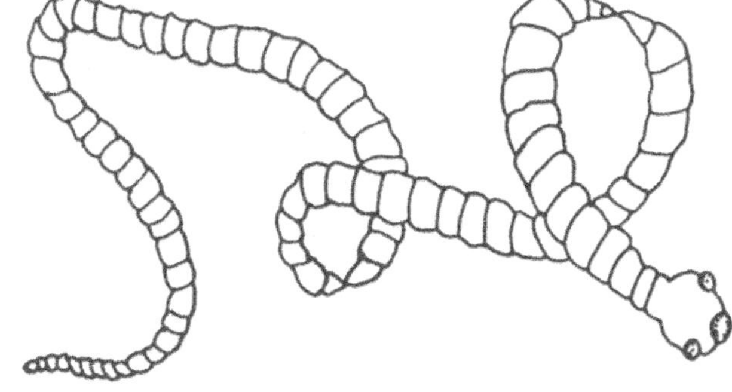

Tapeworms require two different animals to complete their life cycle. The immature tapeworm makes a cyst in an "intermediate host" and can cause illness in animals and people.
The adult tapeworm lives in a "definitive host" and does not usually cause serious illness.

<u>**General Lifecycle:**</u> See pages 338, 339 and 340.
1. A definitive host animal eats the cyst often by eating the meat of an infected intermediate host. In the intestines, the cyst (immature tapeworm) leaves its shell and develops into an adult. The adult consists of many segments each containing eggs. The segments break off, pass out in the feces, and release eggs.
2. The eggs are eaten by an intermediate host and hatch into larvae. The larvae move throughout the body of the intermediate host and form cysts.

Diagnosis:
- *Symptoms:* In the definitive host, there are few clinical symptoms, except possibly some diarrhea. However, tapeworm segments, resembling rice, may be seen in the feces.

- In the intermediate host, the cysts can cause various symptoms depending upon their location, . but are difficult to diagnose except by special laboratory tests.

- *Laboratory:* If the segments from an infected definitive host are squashed, then the tapeworm eggs can be seen with a microscope. Diagnosing cysts in an infected intermediate host requires specialized tests.

Treatment:
- In livestock, treatment of the cysts is usually difficult or unfeasible. In people, some cysts can be removed surgically or treated with special medicines.
- Treatment of the adult tapeworm breaks the cycle of the tapeworm.

<u>**Control:**</u>

- In general, preventing the definitive host from eating the raw meat of intermediate host can help break the cycle of most tapeworms.
- Use of latrines by humans, and cooking pig meat very well before eating it can help control the pig-human tapeworm.

Specific examples of tapeworms -

Their definitive hosts, and intermediate hosts

Humans

As definitive hosts, humans can have digestive upsets from the pork tapeworm "<u>Taenia</u> <u>solium</u>" and beef tapeworm "<u>Taenia</u> <u>saginata</u>."

As intermediate hosts, humans can be seriously ill by the cysts of "<u>Taenia solium,</u>" and "<u>Ecchinococcus granulosa.</u>"

Cattle and Buffalo

As definitive hosts, cattle and buffalo are not usually affected by adult tapeworms.

As intermediate hosts, cattle can be sick from the cysts of <u>Echinococcus</u>. They are may have cysts from "<u>Taenia</u> <u>saginata</u>" which can ruin their meat.

Sheep and Goats

As definitive hosts, young sheep and goats can be affected by the adult tapeworm <u>Monezia</u>. Adult sheep and goats are not usually affected by adult tapeworms.

As intermediate definitive hosts, sheep and goats have cysts from the species "<u>Taenia</u>" and "<u>Ecchinococcus</u>" resulting in **"circling disease" or "Gid"**

Pigs

As definitive hosts, pigs are not usually affected by adult tapeworms.

As intermediate hosts, pigs have cysts of <u>Ecchinococcus</u> <u>granulosa</u> and <u>Taenia</u> <u>solium</u> which may ruin the meat, but the pigs do not get sick.

Dogs

As definitive hosts, dogs may be infected by the adults of <u>Dipylidium</u>, <u>Ecchinococcus</u> and <u>Taenia</u> species.

As intermediate hosts, dogs can have cysts of <u>Taenia</u> <u>solium</u> and <u>Ecchinococcus</u>, but do not show symptoms.

Poultry

As definitive hosts, poultry can have diarrhea and lack of appetite due to the adult tapeworms of <u>Davinia</u> and other species.

As intermediate hosts, they are not important.

Horses

As definitive hosts, horses can be affected by the adults of <u>Anoplocephala</u>. Large numbers of these may cause diarrhea and weight loss.

As intermediate hosts, this is not significant.

27.7.1 "Gid" or "Circling Disease" (<u>Taenia</u> <u>multiceps</u> or <u>Taenia</u> <u>pisiformis</u>)

Life cycle:
1. The adult tapeworm lives in the intestine of dogs, wolves, jackals and foxes. The eggs are passed in the feces and eaten by sheep and goats as they graze.

2. The eggs hatch into larvae in the intestines of sheep and goats. The larvae migrate through the animal's tissue and form a cyst. Cysts that form in the brain cause "Gid."

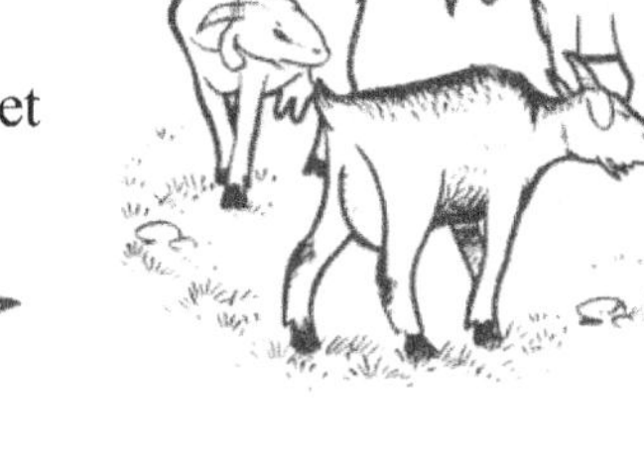

Symptoms:
When the cysts of <u>Taenia</u> <u>multiceps</u> or <u>Taenia</u> <u>pisiformis</u> form in the brain of sheep or goats, they may circle, tilt their head, lose their appetite, appear very tired, cry out, or act strangely. They slowly get worse and eventually die.

Diagnosis:
Diagnosis is based on general symptoms and necropsy when one can find the cyst in the brain.

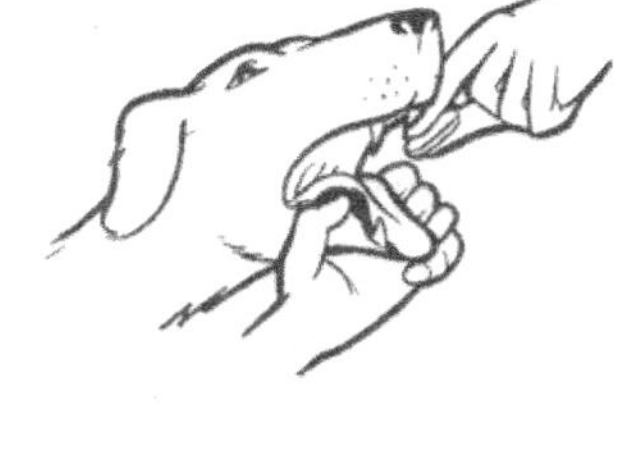

Treatment:
Generally, there is no treatment and affected animals should be slaughtered. However, some vets and farmers locate a soft, swollen area on the skull of the sick animal and puncture it to relieve the pressure. This sometimes causes some improvement.

Control:
The cycle can be broken by two methods:
1. Treat all dogs in an area with tapeworm medicine.

2. Do not allow dogs to eat raw meat. Instead, burn the offal of slaughtered animals.

27.7.2 *Monezia*
Monezia is a tapeworm that lives in the small intestine of ruminants.

Cattle and Buffalo: *Monezia* does not usually cause illness in cattle and buffalo. Therefore, it is not recommended to treat cattle and buffalo for tapeworms. However, the presence of tapeworm segments in the feces of cattle or buffalo, may indicate that the animals are also infected with small roundworms and need treatment.

Sheep and Goats: *Monezia* may cause some digestion problems in young sheep and goats, but rarely in adults. However, in adult sheep and goats, it is rare to see tapeworm segments in their feces unless they are already sick from small roundworms.

<u>**Life cycle:**</u>
1. The adult tapeworm lives in the small intestines of the host (sheep, goats, cattle, and buffalo).
2. Segments containing eggs break off from the adult and pass out with the feces.
3. Mites eat the eggs, which hatch and develop into "cysticercoids."
4. The host eats the mites. The cysticercoids are released from the mites and become adults in the small intestines of the host.

<u>**Symptoms:**</u>
* Young sheep and goats are thin and malnourished looking. They may show signs of anemia.

<u>**Diagnosis:**</u>
* Tapeworm segments may be visible in feces. Other signs of anemia such as pale gums may also be seen.

<u>**Treatment:**</u>
* Young sheep and goats with tapeworms should be treated for *both* tapeworms and small roundworms. Cattle, buffalo, adult sheep and adult goats need to be treated for small roundworms only.

<u>**Control:**</u>
* Treat regularly for small roundworms. Practice pen/pasture rotation. Treat the animals with worm medicine the same day they are being rotated to a new pen/pasture. Clean pens and let them dry for several days in the sun before moving animals into them.

27.7.3 Pork Tapeworm caused by <u>Taenia solium</u> – cysticercosis

This tapeworm causes public health problems. The adult of this tapeworm lives in the intestines of humans and might cause digestive upset and some diarrhea. More importantly, <u>Taenia solium</u> can form cysts in the tissues of humans and cause serious disease depending on where the cyst develops (such as in the brain). <u>Taenia solium</u> also forms in the meat of pigs and ruins their meat. The cystic form of this disease is called "**cysticercosis.**"

<u>**Life cycle**</u>
1. From an infected person, tapeworm segments pass into the feces and release their eggs.

2. Pigs eat infected human feces and become infected. The eggs become larvae in the pig's intestines. The larvae move to various muscles in the pig's body and form cysts.

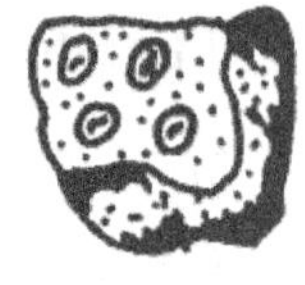

Cysts in meat

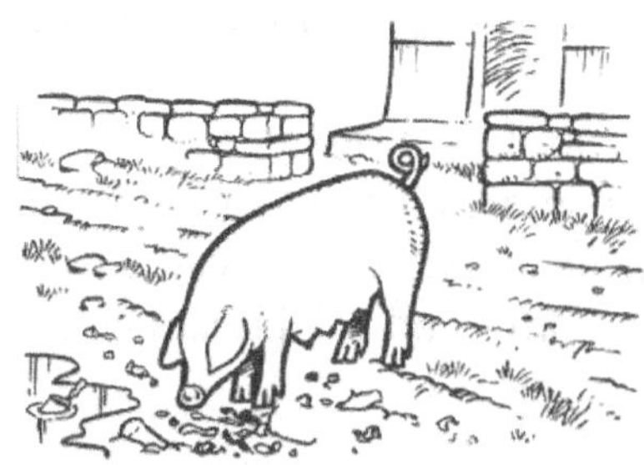

3. Humans who eat poorly cooked pig
    meat or who ingest the <u>Taenia</u> eggs
    (due to poor hygiene or eating
    something contaminated with the
    eggs) become infected.

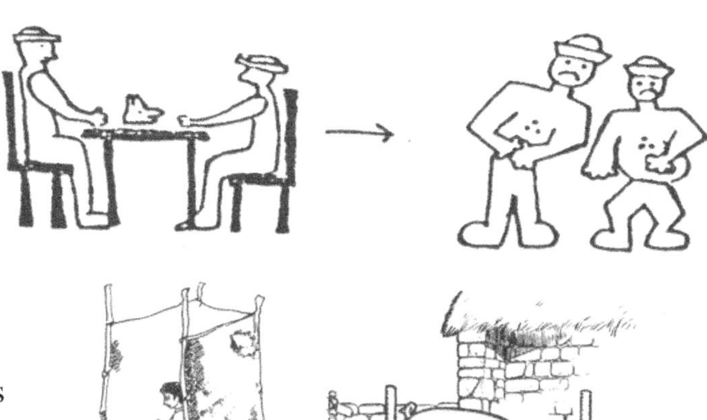

Control:

Cysticercosis can be controlled by two
methods:

1. Keep pigs from eating human feces. This
    may be difficult because it requires latrine
    use by humans and/or not allowing pigs to
    run loose.

2. Cook all pig meat well before eating. The cysts die when cooked at temperatures of at least 53
    centigrade or 120 Fahrenheit for at least one minute. Cut the meat into small pieces before cooking
    to ensure that all parts of the meat are well cooked.

27.7.4 Hydatid tapeworm caused by <u>Echinococcus</u> <u>granulosus</u> - Hydatidosis

<u>Echinococcus</u> <u>granulosus</u> is a tapeworm of dogs that causes cysts in humans, goats, pigs, buffalo,
and cattle (as intermediate hosts). The cystic form of this disease is called "hydatidosis."

Life cycle:

1. The adult tapeworm lives in the dog's intestines and lays eggs, which pass out in the feces.

2. Goats, pigs, buffalo, cattle, or humans (as intermediate hosts) may eat these eggs in contaminated
    food or pastures. The eggs hatch into larvae which then migrate through the animal's or person's
    body and can form large cysts called "hydatid cysts." The condition is called "**hydatidosis.**" In
    some places this is a severe public health problem.

3. A dog eats raw meat contaminated with cysts. In the dog's intestines, the cysts release larvae,
    which become adult tapeworms.

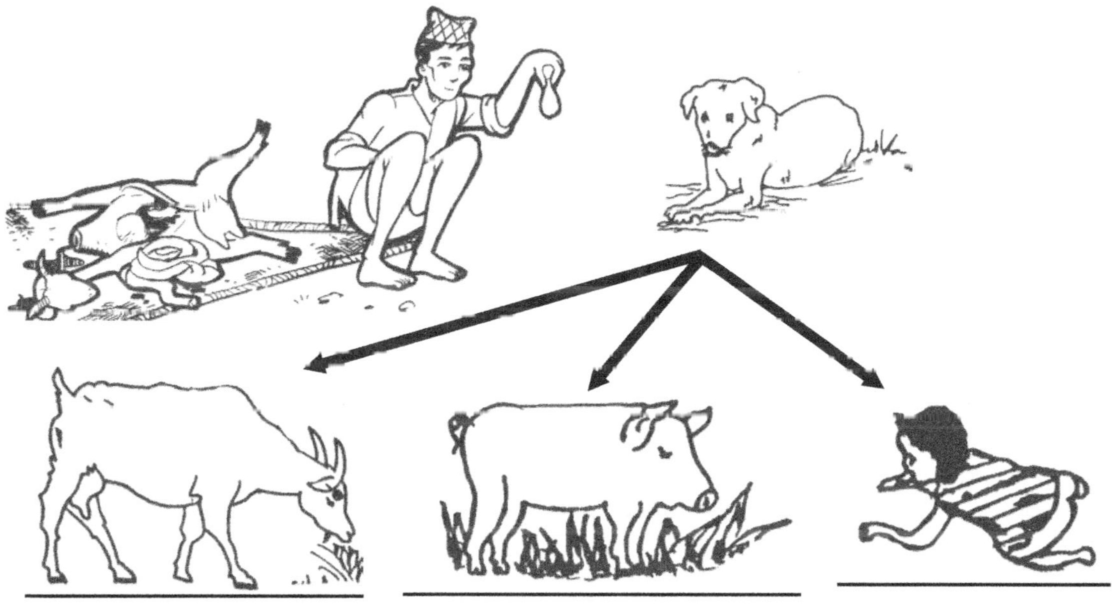

Treatment:

There is no feasible treatment in livestock. In humans, hydatid cysts are removed surgically and some medicines are used.

Control:

The disease cycle can be broken by the following two methods:

1. Feed all dogs tapeworm medicine regularly. The frequency of treatment depends on the severity of the problem.
2. Never feed raw meat to dogs. Instead, burn the offal of slaughtered animals.

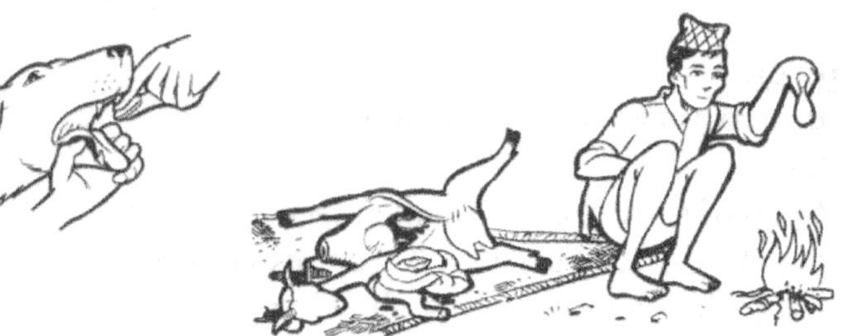

27.8 COCCIDIA

Coccidia are an important cause of disease, particularly in young livestock. Animals most severely affected are sheep, goats, cattle, buffalo, pigs, rabbits and poultry. Generally, each animal species has its own type of coccidia, except for sheep and goats, which can share the same type. Coccidia damage the lining of the small and large intestines. Infection with coccidia is more likely if animals are crowded, or if sanitation is poor.

Life cycle:

1. The adult coccidia live in the intestine and lay eggs (oocysts) which pass out in the feces.

2. If the moisture and temperature is correct, the oocysts change form and become "infective."

3. The infective eggs are eaten and become adults in the intestines.

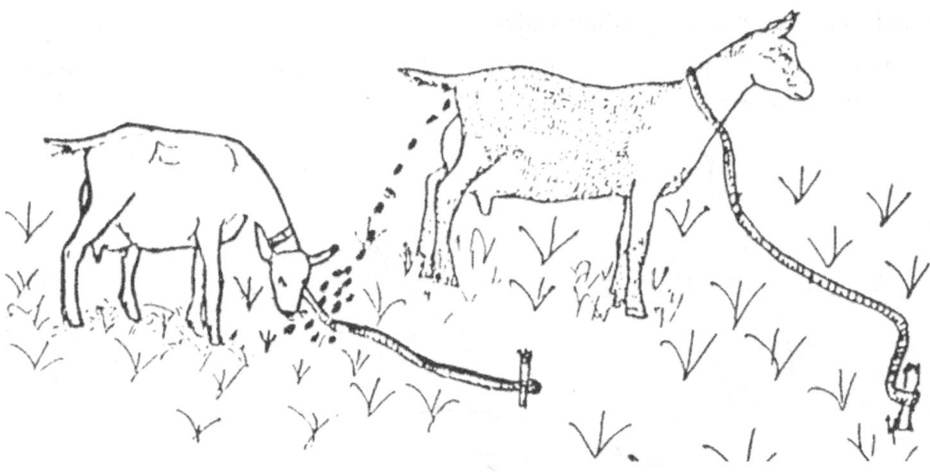

Symptoms:

- Diarrhea, which is often bloody, and weight loss are the most common symptoms. Animals that do not die from the effects of diarrhea, may develop resistance to that particular species of coccidia. However the resistance may diminish over time if the animal is not re-exposed to coccidia. In rabbits, coccidia attack the liver and may cause rapid death.

<u>**Diagnosis:**</u>
- *Symptoms:* Coccidia can be diagnosed on the basis of general symptoms, knowledge that coccidian is a problem in your area, and response to treatment.

- *Necropsy:* The lining of the intestines is bloody. In rabbits, white spots may be seen in the liver.

- *Laboratory:* Using a microscope, oocysts may be observed in the feces. However, infected animals may have a negative fecal exam.

<u>**Treatment:**</u>
- There are several drugs that treat coccidia such as "sulfa drugs" and amprolium. Use the least expensive product that is available and known to be effective in your area. Carefully follow the label instructions.

- Animals weakened by coccidiosis need a clean, dry, protected pen, as well as access to clean water and fresh food to recover more rapidly.

<u>**Control:**</u>
- The eggs can survive for a long time in dirty, moist environments. Therefore, good sanitation is important in the control of coccidia.

- *Pens:* Pens for young animals should be kept clean and dry, and should not be overcrowded. Periodically, pens should be cleaned, disinfected and left empty (preferably in the sun) for several days.   Strong disinfectant and even extreme heat (using a torch) are sometimes needed to rid an animal pen of coccidia eggs.

- *Pastures:* Practicing pasture rotation, and avoiding overstocking of pastures can help control coccidia of grazing animals. Also, coccidia eggs do not survive well if exposed to drying and sunlight.

- There are some products such as amprolium and monensin that can be put in the feed or water to prevent coccidia. Monensin is often put in the feed of chickens to prevent coccidia (however, it is very toxic for horses!).

Trypanosomes: See Page 275.

Babesiosis: See Urinary System / Red Water, page 245.

28.0 Using Medicines Safely and Effectively

28.1   MEDICINE BY ITSELF IS NOT ENOUGH

No medicine works alone to combat disease. The body must also work and, therefore, needs strength and support to fight the disease and repair body tissues. This strength comes from receiving **clean water**, **fresh air, energy** (from food), and **a dry, protected environment,** which are called "supportive treatment." Every sick animal should receive supportive treatment to minimize its suffering and increase its chances of recovery.

28.2   HUMAN MEDICINES VERSUS VETERINARY MEDICINES

Medicines made for people are usually safe for animals. However, the reverse is not true.

> **A medicine made for animals should not be used for people.**

For instance, it is safe to give to an animal penicillin bought at a human pharmacy. However, a person should not receive penicillin labeled "for veterinary use."

28.3   SELECTING THE RIGHT MEDICINE

Refer also to Chapter 4. See page 61.

The treatment chosen depends on several things:
- diagnosis
- number of animals involved
- medicines available
- price of medicine
- value of the animals
- probability that animals will survive and become productive again
- ability of the owner or AHA to use the medicines properly
- ability of the owner to pay
- preferences of the owner

The AHA must explain to the owner the treatment options, price, work involved, and likelihood for recovery. Only then can the owner make the best decision, taking into account the situation and the value of the animal.

It is often impossible to give the best or most complete treatment. For example, the best treatment may require daily injections, and this may be impossible for an owner living far away (unless someone nearby can give the injections). Perhaps another medicine must be chosen. Or the owner may not have enough money for full treatment. The AHA must help the owner decide which treatment will be best for each situation.

There may also be certain pressures placed on the AHA. Some farmers <u>expect</u> an AHA to give injections, even if unnecessary! **Some medicines, such as antibiotics, may lose their effectiveness when overused or used needlessly!** Moreover, medicines cost money and are sometimes in limited supply.

28.3.1 Keeping Records and Writing Prescriptions

It is important to keep a notebook with information regarding animals examined and treatments given. This information will be useful for sharing with other AHAs and veterinary doctors regarding your work and the most common animal health diseases in your area.

In addition, it is important to write down a "prescription" so that medicine is given in the proper manner, at the proper time, and to the proper animal. Also, when sending an owner to purchase medicine in the market, a prescription is necessary so that the correct medicine is purchased.

Prescription Information and information for notebook:
1. Owner's name.
2. Date.
3. Name of medicine.
4. Animal to which it is given (age, breed, etc.).
5. Illness (mention main symptoms, temperature, respiration, etc.).
6. Dose (amount to be given).
7. How often to give the medicine.
8. For how many days should the medicine be given.
9. How to give the medicine.
10. Precautions.
11. For your own records: record whether the animal recovered and any other comments such as cost of the medicine, fees charged, etc.

For all owners, even those who can read and write, you must explain the following information. If you doubt whether they understand or not, then have them repeat it back to you: Dose (amount to be given). How often to give it. For how long. How to give it. Explain the precautions (if any).

28.4   CARE AND STORAGE OF MEDICINES

Store medicines in secure places inaccessible to children and animals.

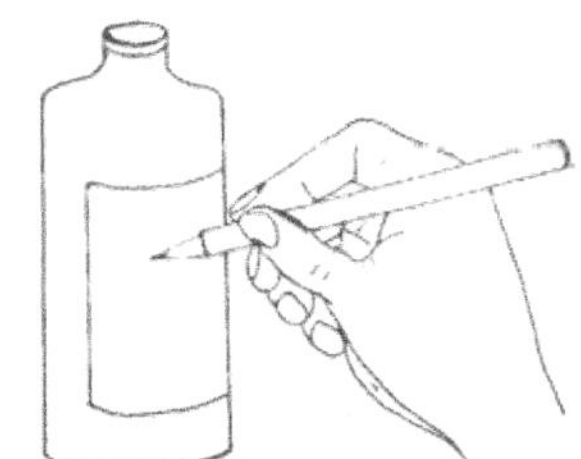

All containers of medicines should be labeled with the name, strength and expiration date. If the label is fading or has been erased or washed off, relabel it. DO NOT use unlabeled medicines.

Store medicines in clean, dry, fresh places. Direct sunlight or excessive heat can damage medicines.

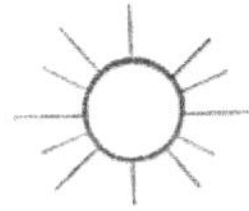

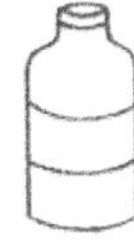

Never freeze medicines unless otherwise indicated on the label. Freezing can damage some medicines.

Always follow the instructions on the label of the medication regarding how to use and store it. Most labels include instructions.

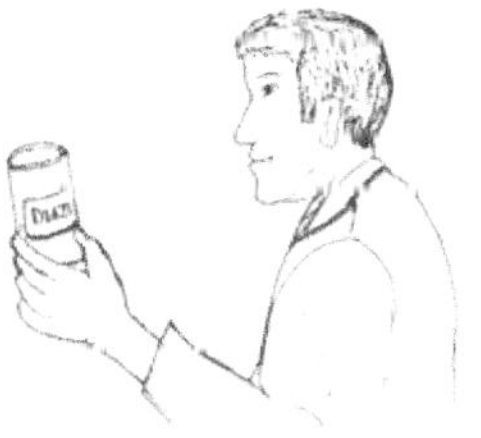

28.5   DISPOSAL OF MEDICINES

Medicines, vaccines, syringes, needles and other materials that could be harmful to humans or animals should be burned, buried or disposed of in such a manner that people and animals can't find them.

A good AHA **NEVER** throws needles, razor blades or other sharp instruments on the ground after use. This is especially important in places where people walk barefoot.

Do not leave your garbage behind! Leaving your garbage behind is sloppy, makes a bad impression, and may be dangerous to the community. **Carry garbage containers with you!** AHAs should carry a container for miscellaneous garbage and a closed jar for used needles, razor blades and other sharp items. **AHAs should take their garbage <u>with them</u> and dispose of it safely**. If someone is injured by the garbage of an AHA, it is the AHAs fault!

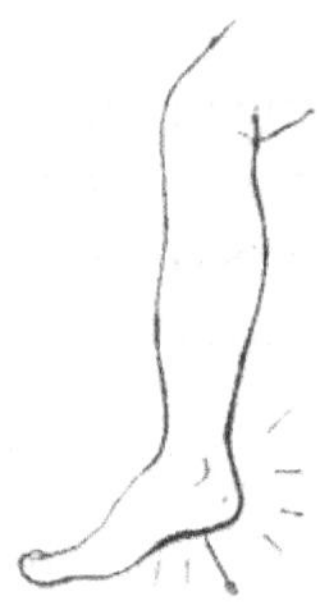

28.6   MEDICINES - NAMES, FORMS & STRENGTHS

> **The same medicine:**
>
> Can have different brand names!
>
> Can come in different forms!
>
> Can have different strengths!

28.6.1 Same Medicine - Different Names

Generic Name versus Brand (Trade) Name

The names of medicines are sometimes confusing, because there can be various names for the same medicine. On one label, there are usually two names:

- **Generic name**: The generic name is the chemical name of the medicine. It is often written in <u>small letters</u> on the label. The generic name is recognized throughout the world. It is like one common language. An example of a generic name is **levamisole.**
- **Brand name:** The brand name (or trade name) is a name given by the company or manufacturer and is often written in <u>big letters</u> on the label. Each company has its own name for a certain drug. For example, levamisole (the generic name) has many brand names, such as *Levasole, Citarin, Ripercol, and Tramisol* depending on the manufacturer and the country where it is manufactured.

The same drug with different brand names

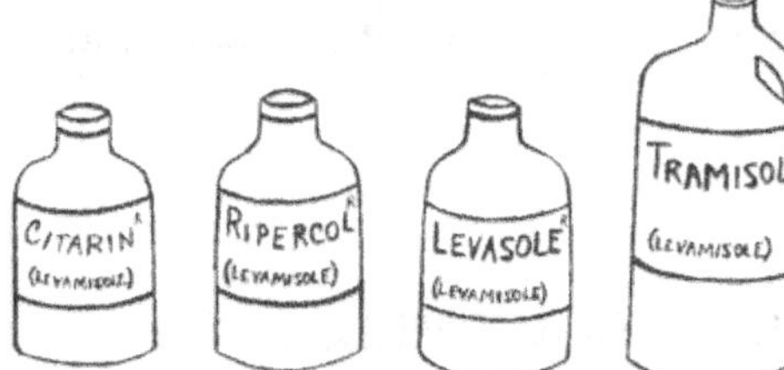

Why is this important? It is important because sometimes the same product may be available under a different brand name. In this book **generic names** are used most commonly but the brand name is also included at times. The brand name is written in *italics* and begins with a capital letter. For instance, one common name for oxytetracycline is *Terramycin*.

28.6.2 Same medicine - Different forms

The same medicine can come in different forms. For example, medicines can be:

powder, liquid, capsules or pills	to be given in the mouth
liquid	to inject
liquid, ointment, cream, powder	to put on the skin or a wound
ointment	to put in the eye or up a teat

Why is this important to know? Sometimes a medicine can be easier to administer or less expensive in a different form. For example, giving medicine in the mouth does not require syringes and needles, or someone who knows how to give injections.

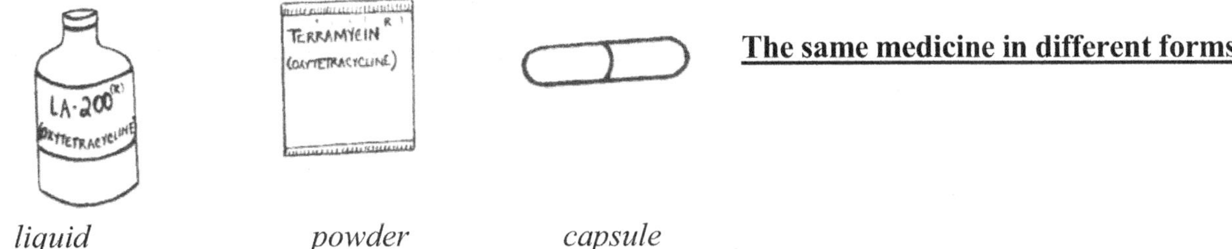

The same medicine in different forms

liquid   *powder*   *capsule*

28.6.3 Same medicine - Different strengths

The strength of the medicine is the amount of active ingredient in a certain volume of medicine.

A cubic centimeter or "cc" is a measure of volume. One cc is also equal to one milliliter or "ml."

> 1 cc = 1 cubic centimeter = 1 ml = 1 milliliter

Amounts of the active ingredient in the medicine are often expressed in milligrams or "mg."

Therefore, the strength of a medicine is often expressed as:
"milligrams per milliliters" or "mg/ml" or "mg/cc."

For example, 50 mg/ml means there are 50 milligrams of active ingredient in each milliliter (or cc) of medicine.

Why is it important to know? The strength of the medicine makes a difference in the price of the medicine, and the amount given to the animal. These capsules of tetracycline are in different strengths.

50 mg   100 mg   250 mg

28.7   MEDICINE LABELS – READ THEM CAREFULLY

After a choice has been made to use a certain medicine, the label on the medicine must be read very carefully. Because there are many different kinds and sizes of animals, it is very important to read the label of veterinary drugs. Also, it is important to always carefully label a medicine before you give it to owners for treating their own livestock.

**Medicines can be USEFUL but...
they can also be DANGEROUS.**

Medicines can be dangerous if not used properly. To prevent mistakes, carefully read the label with the following questions in mind:

- Is the **generic name** correct?

- Is this medicine **dangerous** for the **intended use** or **specific animal** (e.g. pregnant or young animals)?

- Is this medicine **dangerous** for the **AHA** (e.g. pesticides, allergies)?

- Is the medicine **expired**? (Check the expiry date.)

- What is the correct **dosage**? (Look in this book or sometimes on the label or package insert.)

- What is the correct **manner** to give the medicine (injection, in the mouth, on the skin, in the teat)?

- How **often** should the medicine be given?

28.7.1 Expiry Dates

There may be two dates written on the medicine container:

1. The **manufacturing (mfg) date** is the date the medicine was made, usually indicated by month and year (using a western calendar). For instance, 1/99 (or Jan 99) means that the medicine was made in January 1999.

2. The **expiry date (exp)** is the last day the medicine should be used. After this date the medicine may not be as effective or change so that it is not safe anymore.

Some medicines only indicate the expiry date.

28.7.2 Other Terms found on Labels

The following terms may also be on the label:

Recommended Dose:

The effective, safe dose for a specific animal.

Maximum Dose:

The maximum dose which should be given regardless of the weight of the animal.

Administration:

How to give the medicine. The following abbreviations may be used:

IM = intramuscular (in the muscle)
SC or SQ = subcutaneous (under the skin)
IV = intravenous (in the vein)
Orally, Per Os, PO = in the mouth
Topically = on the skin or wound

Frequency:

How often to give the medicine. The following abbreviations might be used:

SID = once per day
BID = twice per day
TID = three times per day
QID = four times per day
"q" means "every." For example, "q12 hours" means "every twelve hours"

Protection/Caution/Warning:

Special instructions for special situations (e.g. pregnancy, lactation) or animals
(e.g. young animals, certain species of animal).

Withdrawal Time:

The amount of time needed to rid the body of the medicine or its residues.
Withdrawal times can be indicated for slaughter of the animal, or for its milk.

Examples of Withdrawal Time:

If the milk withdrawal time is 72 hours, the animal's milk is not safe to drink for the first 72 hours after the medicine was given, because the milk may contain harmful medicine residues. After 72 hours, the cow's milk is safe to drunk by humans.

If the meat withdrawal time is 1 week, then the animal should not be slaughtered for at least 1 week after the medicine was given.

Species:

Some medicines should only be used on certain species of animals.

Liveweight or Bodyweight:

This refers to the weight of the animal and is often abbreviated as "l.w" or b.w.."
The term is used when indicating doses.

Toxic Dose:

The toxic dose is usually the maximum dose which can be given safely. If the toxic dose is exceeded, the animal may die.

28.8   ADMINISTRATION OF MEDICINES

Feeding medicines, injections, etc, were covered in Chapter 4, Principles of Treatment. See pages 63 - 75.

28.9   MEASURING MEDICINES

<u>Solid</u> medicines and powders are usually measured in:
- milligrams (mg) or in grams (gm)
  Remember: 1000mg = 1 gm
- IU or U (international units or units). This is how penicillin is often measured.

<u>Liquid</u> medicines are measured in:
- milliliters (ml) or in liters (l)
  Remember: 1000ml = 1 liter

If there is no scale to weigh or measure medicines, find some containers and spoons commonly available in your area and measure various amounts of commonly used medicines in them. Then show the farmers how to use these containers or spoons to measure medicines without special equipment.

For example:
- some teaspoons holds about 5 ml of liquid
- some tablespoons hold about 15 ml of liquid
- some tobacco tins hold about 25 gm of Magnesium Sulfate

28.10 CALCULATING DOSES OF MEDICINES

The **dose** of a medicine refers to **how much**, **how often,** and **how many days** a medicine is given. Use the following steps to calculate the **amount** of medicine to give.

<u>Step 1</u>
Determine the **body weight** of the animal. See Pages 36-41.

<u>Step 2</u>
Find out the **dose** of the medicine. If the dose is given in **mg**/kg (milligrams per kilogram), use step 3. If the dose is given in **ml**/kg, then skip to step 4.

<u>Step 3</u>
Calculate the **weight** of medicine needed for that dose.

> Dose (mg/kg) X weight (kg) = total number of mg of medicine needed for that dose.

For example: if the dose is 20 mg/kg, and the goat weighs 20 kg, then:

20 mg/kg X 20 kg = 400 mg of medicine needed for that dose.

This means that a 20kg goat needs 400 mg of medicine.

If the medicine is in powder (solid) form, your calculation is finished. Simply give the 400 mg of medicine (usually mixed in the feed or water) to the goat at the specified frequency and number of doses.

If the medicine is in liquid form, an additional calculation is necessary to know the **volume** of medicine to give. For this additional calculation, you will need to know the strength of the medicine.

Calculate the **volume** needed using the following information:
-        **weight** (mg) of medicine needed and
-        **strength** of the medicine. This is always listed on the bottle of medicine and is usually listed in mg/ml. To include the strength as a factor in the formula, simply invert the fraction. For example, if the bottle of oxytetracycline has a strength of 100 mg/ml, invert it to 1 ml/100 mg when calculating the volume needed below.

Volume needed in ml = (Total number of mgs needed) X (strength in ml/mg)

For example: the 20kg goat in the previous example needed 400 mg of medicine. If the strength of our liquid medicine is 100 mg/ml, the volume of medicine needed is:

400 mg   X   1ml/100 mg   =   4 ml of medicine needed

Therefore, give the goat 4ml or 4cc of medicine.

Step 4

If the dose is given as **ml/kg**, all you need is the weight of the animal to calculate the **volume** of medicine needed with the following formula:

Dose (ml/kg) X weight (kg) = ml medicine required

For example, if the dose is 2 ml/kg and the a pig weighs 30 kg, then:

2ml/kg X 30kg = 60ml or 60cc of medicine needed

Simply give the pig 60cc of the medicine.

Note: If it is an injection, it should be divided up and given in at least three different sites on the pig. Don't give more than 20 cc of medicine in any injection site.

28.10.1 Actual Examples Dose Calculation

1. Label on a container of powdered worm medicine
Protection of consumers: Animal should not be slaughtered within seven days and milk should not be used for human consumption within 24 hours of feeding the medicine.

Route: Drenching for cattle, sheep and goat; mix with food for pig; mix with water for poultry.

M.F.G: May 94.

Expiry: 48 months after the M.F.G. date.

Recommended dosage: 45 mg/kg l.w. for cattle, sheep, goat and pig.

For Poultry: Dissolve 10 gram of powder in 4 liter of water for 100 birds.

Maximum doses for cattle and sheep: 15 grams for cattle; 2 grams for sheep and goats

Species: Cattle, sheep/goat/pig/poultry.

<u>Using the information on the label:</u>
For a 30 kg goat:
45 mg/kg X 30 kg = 1350 mg = 1.35 gm

For a 50 kg goat:
45 mg/kg X 50 kg = 2250 mg = 2.25 gm

However, the maximum dose is 2 gm! Therefore we can give only 2.0 gram to the 50 kg goat.

2. Giving a tetracycline injection:

Dosage on label or in textbook: 4 mg/kg for IM injection

Weight of a buffalo that needs the medicine: 400kg

Calculation: 4 mg/kg x 400 kg = 1,600 mg medicine for the 400 kg buffalo
But the tetracycline is in liquid form, therefore the following calculation is needed using the strength of the medicine.

Strength of tetracycline (from bottle): 50 mg/ml

Calculation: 1,600 mg X 1 ml/50 mg = 32 ml for a 400 kg buffalo

Therefore, give the 400 kg buffalo an IM injection of 32 ml of tetracycline.

29.0 Common Medicines and their Doses

INTRODUCTION

It is very important that medicines are handled properly, and that the correct amounts are given. It is also important that treatment records are carefully written down. This information should include clear identification of the animal treated, the major symptoms, clinical observations (temperature, pulse, respiration, etc.), the name of the medicine, the dose of the medicine, how often the medicine was given, the cost of the medicine, and any comments regarding whether the animal recovered, etc. For a review of this, see page 344.

29.1 INJECTIONS

29.1.1 Antibiotics

- The function of antibiotics is to kill, or prevent the growth of, the bacteria that cause various diseases. However, antibiotics work effectively against only certain types of bacteria. It is the AHA's responsibility to select the correct antibiotic for a certain disease problem.

- If antibiotics are not used properly, then the bacteria get stronger and stronger until the antibiotic no longer works against that particular bacteria. This is called, "antibiotic resistance," and is a growing problem in the world. Some antibiotics which used to work very well against certain diseases are no longer effective.

- In general, **do not feed antibiotics to adult grass-eating animals** because antibiotics also kill the beneficial microorganisms located in the stomach. Instead use injectable antibiotics. However, if no one is available to give an injection, it may be necessary to feed antibiotics to an adult grass-eating animal (like cattle, buffalo, etc.).

- Do not use antibiotics to fight against diseases that are caused by viruses. An exception to this is when a disease starts out with a virus and then a bacteria causes problems. For instance an animal may get wounds on its feet from Foot and Mouth Disease (a virus). Later, these wounds become infected (a bacteria). Penicillin does nothing against the FMD virus but will help to kill the bacteria that caused the wound to become infected.

- There are 6 different groups of antibiotics in this book. Each group works differently in the body and each works differently against various microorganisms. Each type of antibiotic remains in the body for a different length of time. The correct "withdrawal" time must be observed, or the antibiotics may be harmful to any people that may eat the meat or drink the milk from animals that have been treated with antibiotics. See page 348. The five groups of antibiotics are -
  The penicillin and cephalosporin group,
  The tetracycline group,
  The aminoglycoside group,
  The sulfa group, and
  The chloramphenicol and miscellaneous group.

Penicillin and Cephalosporin Group

This group includes penicillin , amoxicillin, ampicillin, cephalexin, ceftiofur and others. Penicillin is still a very useful antibiotic for many infections in livestock. It is especially good for the types of infections that produce pus. Penicillin is also very safe. Too much will not kill an animal, but if too little is used, it causes **antibiotic resistance**.

Some animals have an allergy to penicillin and may develop red, itchy skin. Other animals may develop an allergic reaction that interferes with normal breathing. Such animals can die very quickly. See Page 85. Such a reaction can be treated with **epinephrine**. If an animal has ever had an allergic reaction to penicillin, that animal should never be given any type of penicillin again. (The same is true for any medicine that has produced an allergic reaction - that particular animal should never receive any form of that medicine again or it may die.)

As the following tables show, penicillin is very effective different types of infections in livestock, especially for preventing tetanus when an animal has a deep wound. Penicillins and cephalosporins are often the first antibiotics used if the type of bacteria is unknown. They work especially well when combined with aminoglycoside antibiotic drugs. They should not be combined with tetracyclines, sulfas or chloramphenicol. Penicillins are rather inexpensive but cephalosporins can be quite expensive.

Aminoglycoside Group

This group includes streptomycin, gentamicin, kanamycin, neomycin and others. Aminoglycosides kill bacteria by disturbing the chemical machinery inside the bacteria. They are very effective against some common bacteria but they must be used with caution because of toxic side effects to the hearing and kidneys. In general, if they are given in the gut, they stay in the gut; if injected, they stay in the internal tissues. They often work well for treating diarrhea in baby animals. Injectable aminoglycosides have very long withdrawal periods. Aminoglycosides should not be combined with tetracyclines, sulfas, or chloramphenicol.

Tetracycline Group

This group includes tetracycline, oxytetracycline, chlortetracycline and others. They inhibit bacteria so the bacteria can't grow properly. They work well in the liver, respiratory tract and skin. Tetracyclines can be given by mouth, injection or externally (topically) to the eye. *Do not give them to horses because horses can die from a strange reaction to tetracyclines.* They are inexpensive and easily available. Do not combine with any other antibiotics.

Sulfa Group

This group includes many antibiotics that start with the name "sulfa" like sulfamethazine and sulfadimidine. This class of antibiotics has been around since the 1930s. Sulfas can be given by mouth, injection, or externally when treating wounds. Do not give sulfas with any other antibiotics.

Deciding Which Antibiotic to Use – Some Practical Tables

- The large number of diseases, and the problem of antibiotic resistance, make the selection of the right antibiotic a difficult decision. However, the following rules should help to select an effective antibiotic. If the first choice does not seem to work after 3-5 days, then move to another in the list. When switching to another antibiotic, it is probably better to choose an antibiotic from a different group. For example if the penicillin is not working,

it is probably better to try an antibiotic from another group. (Drugs and Their Usage, CVM
Publications)

(Note: Pen = penicillin and cephalosporin group, Tet = tetracycline group,
Amin = aminoglycoside group, Sulf – sulfa group, Chlor = chloramphenicol
Genitourinary = condition affecting the reproductive or urinary system)

Table of Antibiotics for Horses and Donkeys

Condition (Problem)	First Choice	Second Choice
Pneumonia	Pen, Amin	Sulfa
Diarrhea	Pen, Amin (oral)	Sulfa
Genitourinary	Pen	Amino
Other Soft Tissues	Pen	Sulfa

Table of Antibiotics for Cattle and Buffalo

Condition (Problem)	First Choice	Second Choice
Pneumonia	Pen, Tet	Sulfa, Amin
Diarrhea	Amin (oral)	Sulfa
Genitourinary	Pen	Amin, Sulfa
Mastitis	Pen	Tet, Sulfa
Other Soft Tissues	Pen	Tet

Table of Antibiotics for Swine

Condition (Problem)	First Choice	Second Choice
Pneumonia	Pen	Tet
Diarrhea	Amin (oral)	Sulfa, Tylosin
Genitourinary	Pen	Tet
Skin	Pen	Amin

Table of Antibiotics for Sheep and Goats

Condition (Problem)	First Choice	Second Choice
Pneumonia	Tet	Sulfa, Tylosin
Diarrhea	Amin	Sulfa
Genitourinary	Tet	Pen, Amin, Sulfa
Mastitis	Pen	Amin
Other Soft Tissues	Pen	Tet

Table of Antibiotics for Dogs and Cats

Condition (Problem)	First Choice	Second Choice
Pneumonia	Pen, Sulfa	Amin, Tet
Diarrhea	Pen, Amin (oral)	Sulfa, Chlor
Genitourinary	Pen	Sulfa
Other Soft Tissues	Pen	Sulfa
Skin	Chlor	Erythro, Sulfa

Using Penicillins and Cephalosporins

Different Kinds of Penicillin Injections: Some kinds of penicillin start to work quickly but then are able to kill bacteria for only a short period of time. These are called *short-acting* or *intermediate-acting* penicillin. Other types of penicillin take longer to start working (almost a whole day) but then they work for several days.These are called *long-acting* penicillin.

Summary: Penicillin is the drug of choice for most infections of the skin, muscle and uterus. It especially works well for tetanus. Never give procaine or benzathine penicillin IV. Always give it IM or SC. Penicillin may be found in powder form in a vial (glass bottle) and should be mixed with distilled water or with boiled (and cooled) water. Or it may be pre-mixed and available as a liquid. After mixing the powder with water, it loses its strength in 7 days and should be thrown away.

PENICILLIN G (benzathine)
Indications: See "penicillin and cephalosporin group" above.
Dosage and Route:
        Horses- 10,000-40,000 IU/kg, IM, every 2-3 days
        Cattle- 40,000 IU/kg, IM, every 2-3 days
        Swine- 40,000 IU/kg, IM, every 2-3 days
        Sheep- 15,000 IU/kg, IM, every 4-5 days
        Dogs- 40,000 IU/kg, IM, every 5 days
        Cats- 40,000 IU/kg, IM, every 5 days
        Rabbit- 40,000 IU/kg, IM, every other day
Withdrawal Period: Note: effective doses greatly exceed the labeled dose, therefore the label withdrawal period must be longer than the label requires.
Cattle- IM dosing, meat 21 days, milk 13 days, SC dosing, meat 42 days
Precautions: This is a long acting penicillin preparation, take special note of the long time between doses.

PENICILLIN G (procaine)
Indications: See "penicillin and cephalosporin group" above.
Dosage and Route:
        Horses- 20,000-50,000 IU/kg, IM, 2-3 times daily
        Cattle- 20,000-54,000 IU/kg, IM, SC 1-2 times daily
        Swine- 20,000-54,000 IU/kg, IM, SC 1-2 times daily
        Sheep- 6-16 mg/kg, IM, 1-2 times daily
        Llama- 40,000 IU/kg, SC, daily
        Dogs- 20,000 IU/kg, IM, SC 1-2 times daily
        Cats- 20,000 IU/kg, IM, SC 1-2 times daily
        Rabbit- 50,000-100,000 IU/kg, IM, 2 times daily
Withdrawal Period: Note: effective doses greatly exceed the label dose, therefore the withdrawal period must be longer than the label specifies.
Cattle- IM dosing, meat 21 days SC dosing, meat 42 days

AMPICILLIN (*Polyflex, Albipen*)
Indications: See "penicillin and cephalosporin group" above.
Dosage and Route:
        Horses- 11-22 mg/kg, IM, IV, 2-3 times daily
        Cattle- 5-12 mg/kg IM once daily
        Swine- 5-12 mg/kg IM once daily

Llama- 11 mg/kg IV, 3 times daily
Dogs- 22 mg/kg, by mouth, 3 times daily; or
       11-22 mg/kg, SC, IM, 3-4 times daily
Cats- 22 mg/kg, by mouth, 3 times daily; or
       11-22 mg/kg, SC, IM, 3-4 times daily
Ferret- 10 mg/kg IM, 2 times daily, or
       20 mg/kg SC, 2 times daily, or
       20 mg/kg by mouth, 2 times daily
<u>Withdrawal Period</u>: Cattle- meat 6 days, milk 2 days

CEPHALEXIN (*Keflex*)

<u>Indications</u>: See "penicillin and cephalosporin group" above.
<u>Dosage and Route</u>:
    Horses- 10-30 mg/kg by mouth, 3-4 times daily
    Goats- 30 mg/kg. SC
    Dogs- 10-30 mg/kg by mouth, 2-4 times daily
    Cats- 10-30 mg/kg by mouth, 2-4 times daily
    Rabbit- 15 mg/kg, SC, 2 times daily
    Guinea Pig- 15 mg/kg, IM, 2 times daily
    Chicken- 55-110 mg/kg by mouth, 2 times daily

CLOXACILLIN (*Orbenin, Dariclox, Dri-clox*)

<u>Indications</u>: See "penicillin and cephalosporin group" above.
<u>Dosage and Route</u>:
    Cattle-500 mg of cephapirin <u>benzathine</u>; or
       200 mg of cephapirin <u>sodium </u>by intramammary
       infusion into each quarter
    Dogs- 10-40 mg/kg by mouth or IM 3-4 times daily
    Cats- 10-40 mg/kg by mouth or IM 3-4 times daily
<u>Withdrawal Period</u>:
    Cattle- Cephapirin <u>benzathine</u>; meat & milk 30 days,
       Cephapirin <u>sodium</u>; meat 10 days, milk
       discarded for 2 days (2.5 days Canada).
<u>Precautions</u>: The <u>benzathine</u> infusion should only be used in dry cows.

PEN/STREP (Penicillin G Procaine + Dihydrostreptomycin)

<u>Indications</u>: See "penicillin and cephalosporin group" above.
Usually formulated to give 400,000 IU of Pen G Procaine + 0.5 g
Dihydrostreptomycin per 2 ml.
<u>Dosage and Route</u>:
    Horses- 10-12 ml IM, 1-2 times daily
    Foals- 1 ml/22 kg, 1-3 times daily
    Cattle- 10-12 ml IM, 1-2 times daily
    Calves- 1 ml/22 kg, 1-3 times daily
    Swine- 1 ml/22 kg, 1-3 times daily
    Sheep- 1 ml/22 kg, 1-3 times daily
<u>Withdrawal Period</u>: Food animals - meat 30 days, milk 3 days

Using Aminoglycosides

GENTAMYCIN (*Gentocin, Garamycin*)

Indications: See " aminoglycoside group" above. Gentamicin is a readily available and affordable aminoglycide which is commonly given by mouth for scours (diarrhea), by injection for generalized infections, in ophthalmic preparations for treatment of eye infections, and in otic preparations for treatment of ear infections in dogs and cats. Note the long withdrawal periods when injected in cattle and pigs. It is not absorbed from the gut when given orally.

Dosage and Route:

        Horses- 2-4 mg/kg, IM, SC, IV, 1 time daily
        Cattle- 2.2 mg/kg, IM, IV, 3 times daily
        Swine- 5 mg, IM in 1-3 day old piglets, or
                5 mg by mouth in 1-3 day old piglets; or
                25 g/gallon of drinking water for 3 days
        Llama- 2 mg/kg IM, 3 times daily
        Dogs- 2 mg/kg, SC, IM, 3 times daily
        Cats- 2 mg/kg, SC, IM, 3 times daily
        Chicken- 0.2-1 mg total dose, SC, 1 time daily
        Rabbit- 4 mg/kg, IM, 1 time daily
        Ferret- 5 mg/kg, IM, 1 time daily
        Gerbil- 5 mg/kg, IM, 1 time daily
        Guinea Pig- 5 mg/kg, IM, 1 time daily
        Hamster- 5 mg/kg, IM, 1 time daily

Withdrawal:

        Cattle-meat 180-360 days, milk 5 days
        Swine-if injected, meat 40 days; if oral, meat 3-14 days

Precautions: Possible kidney damage with high doses for prolonged periods. Do not use in combination with other drugs in the aminoglycoside group.

Using Tetracyclines

These also are broad-spectrum antibiotics because they kill many different kinds of bacteria. They are found in the market with many different names such as *Terramcycin, Oxysteclin, Hostacycline, etc.* In the market, they come in different strengths such as 50mg/ml or 100mg/ml. Most commonly they start to work quickly but need to be given every day (daily). There is a *long-acting* tetracycline that is available sometimes. Some kinds can be given IV, others cannot. Therefore, read the label carefully!

Precautions: **Never use in horses, donkeys, or mules** because it damages the microorganisms of the cecum. Do not use orally in ruminants if possible. It is found in the form of tablets, powder, liquid, injection, bolus, etc. Oral tetracycline can be used in dogs and cats with no problems. However it should not be used in ruminants unless there is no one available to give an injection.

OXYTETRACYCLINE)

Indications: See "tetracycline group" above.

Dosage and Route:

        Cattle- 4-11 mg/kg IM, IV daily; or
                10-20 mg/kg by mouth, 4 times daily
        Cattle- Long acting injection (LA-200)

20 mg/kg IM once
Swine- 6-11 mg/kg IM, IV daily; or
        10-20 mg/kg by mouth, 4 times daily
Swine-Long acting injection (LA-200)
        20 mg/kg every 2 days
Sheep- 10-20 mg/kg by mouth, 4 times daily; or
        6-11 mg/kg IM, IV, 1 time daily
Sheep-Long acting injection (LA-200)
        20 mg/kg every 3 days

Goats- 10-20 mg/kg by mouth, 4 times daily; or
        6-11 mg/kg IM, IV, 1 time daily
Goats- Long acting injection (LA-200)
        20 mg/kg every 3 days
Llamas- 11 mg/kg IV, once daily
Llamas-Long acting injection (LA-200)
        20 mg/kg every 3 days
Dogs- 7-12 mg/kg IM, IV 2 times daily; or
        22 mg/kg by mouth, 3 times daily
Cats- 7-12 mg/kg IM, IV 2 times daily; or
        22 mg/kg by mouth, 3 times daily

Withdrawal Period: Cattle by mouth- meat 5 days, milk 4 days
        Cattle IM, IV- meat 18 days, milk 3 days
        Cattle Long Acting IM- meat 28 days
        Swine- Meat 21 days
        Sheep-meat 21 days

Precautions: Do not use in horses. Do not give with milk, or any other antibiotics. It may cause
stomach upset. If the injection is a large volume divide it into several sites.

Using Sulfas

These drugs are usually sold as oral medicines but occasionally they are available as
injections. Even though they work similarly to antibiotics, they seem to have fewer bad effects on
the beneficial microorganisms in the rumen. Therefore these drugs are often used as oral medicines
to treat infections in ruminants. They are commonly used to treat diarrhea, urinary infections and
some kinds of wound and hoof infections.

These drugs must be given with lots of water. If the animal is not drinking water, then do not
give these drugs or they may damage the kidney.

SULFADIAZINE + TRIMETHOPRIM (*Tribrissen*)
Indications: See "sulfa group" above. This medicine is a combination of sulfamethoxazole and
trimethoprim. It works like a *broad-spectrum* antibiotic and is less expensive than ampicillin.
Dosage and Route:
        Horses-30 mg/kg by mouth, 2-3 times daily, or
                15 mg/kg IV, 2 times daily
        Cattle- 30 mg/kg by mouth, one time daily
        Swine- 48 mg/kg IM daily
        Sheep - 75 mg/kg by mouth daily; or
                13-20 mg/kg IM, SC, IV daily
        Dogs- 15-30 mg/kg by mouth 1-2 times daily

Cats- 30 mg/kg by mouth 2 times daily
Withdrawal Period: Cattle-meat 3 days, milk 7 days
                       Swine-meat 10 days
                       Sheep-meat 14 days

SULFADIMIDINE (*Sulfamez*)
Indications: See "sulfa group" above.
Dosage and Route:
        Cattle- 110 mg/kg by mouth daily; or
               150 mg/kg SC daily
        Swine- 110 mg/kg by mouth daily 150 mg/kg SC daily
        Sheep- 110 mg/kg by mouth daily 215 mg/kg SC daily
        Goats- 110 mg/kg by mouth daily 215 mg/kg SC daily
Withdrawal Period: Cattle- meat 15 days, milk 3 days
        Swine-meat 15 days
        Sheep-meat 15 days
        Goats-meat 15 days, milk 3 days

SULFAMETHAZINE
Indications: See "sulfa group" above.
Dosage and Route:
        Cattle- 200 mg/kg by mouth for one day, then
               100 mg/kg one time daily
        Swine- 200 mg/kg by mouth for one day, then
               100 mg/kg one time daily
        Sheep- 30 ml of 12.5% solution by mouth for one day, then 15 ml daily
        Dogs- 50 mg/kg by mouth 2 times daily
        Cats- 50 mg/kg by mouth 2 times daily
        Rabbit - 2 g/L drinking water
        Chicken- 1 g/L drinking water
Withdrawal Period: Cattle- meat 10 days, milk 4 days
        Swine-meat 14 days

29.1.2 Antihistamines

(Pheniramine maleate, Chlorpheniramine maleate, Promethazine)

These drugs are useful in some cases of poisoning, particularly if part of the body is swollen.
It is also useful for insect bites and stings. Antihistamines are only useful if given to the animal
very soon after it becomes ill. If the animal was bitten or stung several days ago, this medicine
will probably be of no use. See allergies, Chapter 5, page 84.

Follow the label for dosage and instructions.
If one injection does no good, there is no point in repeating it. If the first injection helps, then
injections should be given twice a day until the animal is better.

29.1.3 Anti-Inflammatory Drugs

Inflammation is the body's response to microbial, chemical or physical injury. Inflammation
causes heat (fever), redness, pain, swelling, and loss of function. A good example of this process
is a bee sting. In most cases inflammation is the body's way of fighting the attack,

controlling damage and beginning the process of repair. In some cases the inflammatory process can become a long-term problem. In these cases it may be helpful to decrease the inflammation by giving anti-inflammatory drugs. These drugs come in two large groups "steroids" and "non-steroids." "Steroids" resemble hormones made in the body like cortisone that normally limit inflammation. "Non-steroids" are synthetic drugs like aspirin that block the signs of inflammation. Each group has its own set of good and bad effects. "Steroids" decrease the body's defense against infectious disease and produce excessive appetite, weight gain, water consumption and urination. "Non-steroids" can irritate, and cause ulcers in the gastrointestinal system. The following list of anti-inflammatory drugs includes those that are most commonly available for use in animals.

Steroids

Warning:

1.   Steroids should not be given to pregnant animals unless it is necessary to save the mother's life. If they are given, especially in the last few months of pregnancy, the baby will most likely be aborted (die and be born early) 2-4 days after the injection is given.
2.   If the animal has a wound, it must never be given steroids without an antibiotic injection at the same time, or the animal may die from an infection.

DEXAMETHASONE

Indications: Dexamethasone is a potent and long lasting steroid anti-inflammatory. It is useful in the treatment of arthritis, lameness, and muscular injuries.

Dosage and Route:

      Horses- 0.02-0.2 mg/kg by mouth, IM, IV, daily

      Cattle- 5-10 mg/kg IM, IV, daily

      Swine- 1-10 mg IM, IV, daily

      Dogs- 0.25-1.25 mg by mouth, daily for 3-5 days; or

            0.5-1 mg IM, IV, daily for 3-5 days

      Cats- 0.125-0.5 by mouth, IM, IV, daily for 3-5 days

      Rabbit- 2.6-4 mg/kg IM, as needed

Withdrawal Period: Unknown

Precautions: See warning above.

PREDNISOLONE

Indications: Prednisolone is a medium duration steroid that is useful in the treatment of arthritis, lameness, and muscular injuries. It is almost identical to prednisone.

Dosage and Route:

      Horses- 0.25-1.0 mg/kg IM daily

      Cattle- 0.2-1.0 mg/kg IM daily

      Swine- 0.2-1.0 mg/kg IM daily

      Dogs- 0.5 mg/kg by mouth, every 1-2 days

      Cats- 1.2 mg/kg by mouth, every 1-2 days

Withdrawal Period. Unknown

Precautions: See warning above

Non-Steroids

ASPIRIN – See Oral medicines, 29.2.5 in this chapter.

FLUNIXIN MEGLUMINE (*Banamine, Finadyne*)

<u>Indications:</u> Flunixin meglumine is a very potent (aspirin-like) anti-inflammatory which is used primarily in horses and cattle to treat lameness, colic, and calf scours (diarrhea).
<u>Dosage and Route:</u>
    Horses- 1.1 mg/kg by mouth, IM, IV, 1-3 times daily
    Cattle- 2.2 mg/kg IV every 12 hours if needed for a total of 3 doses
    Swine- 2.2 mg/kg by deep IM injection every 12 hours
        if needed for a total of 3 doses (according to Australian Package insert)
    Llama- 0.5-1 mg/kg IV 1-2 times daily
    Dogs- 0.5-1.0 mg/kg IV only once or twice.
<u>Withdrawal Period:</u> Cattle- meat 14 days, milk 4 days
<u>Warning:</u> Do not use in cats. Use with caution in pregnant animals. High doses for prolonged periods **will cause** gastrointestinal ulcers. The drug relieves pain so well that it has also been accused of masking the severity of colic and therefore delaying more effective treatment like surgery. Do not use in combination with any one anti-inflammatory drugs.

PHENYLBUTAZONE (*Bute, Butazolidin*) See Oral Medicines in this chapter, 29.2.5.

29.1.4 Diuretics (Furosemide, *Lasix, Ridema):*

Diuretics cause the body to make more urine and get rid of extra, unwanted water (edema). Sometimes after a difficult birth, swelling around the vulva can be helped to go away with a diuretic injection. Swollen teats and udder may become less swollen and painful after a diuretic injection. Warning: Diuretics must NEVER BE USED FOR AN ANIMAL WHICH IS NOT PRODUCING URINE. Diuretics are expensive and can be very dangerous. They are used more than they should be.

Dosage: Varies with the diuretic. Read the label.

29.1.5 Supplements / Supportives (Vitamins & Minerals)

Nutritional insufficiency is common in developing countries due to short supplies of affordable high quality feeds, and parasite infections. Vitamin and mineral deficiencies are especially common. The best treatment for these conditions is to provide a good diet – **not to** use expensive injections. However in some situations, injections are also given to help the animal recover its appetite and health quickly. See page 106 for more details on good diets.

IRON DEXTRAN
<u>Indications:</u>   Iron dextran is most often needed for piglets. It may also be needed for animals that have lost a large amount of blood from an injury, or from severe parasite infestations.
<u>Warning:</u> Calculate the dose carefully and keep away from children.
<u>Dosage and Route:</u>
    Horses- 500-1,000 mg IM (Split into 2-3 sites) every 7 days
    Swine- 100-200 mg IM, 1-4 day old pigs; or 50-100 mg IM, every 7 days
    Dogs- 10-20 mg IM once
    Cats- 50 mg IM once
<u>Withdrawal Period:</u> None required

VITAMIN A & D INJECTION
Indications: Vitamins A & D may be deficient when feed quality is lacking. The concentration and directions for use may vary from country to country. The doses listed are a guide for the U.S. products which contain 500,000 IU vitamin A and 75,000 IU vitamin D3 per ml.
Precautions: The injection can be quite painful, make certain the animal is properly restrained.
Dosage and Route:

      Cattle- Adult 2-4 ml IM
            Yearlings 1-2 ml IM
            Calves 0.5 - 1.0 ml IM
      Swine- Adult 1-2 ml IM
            Growing 0.5 - 1.0 ml IM
            Baby Pigs 0.25-0.5 ml IM
      Sheep Adult 1-2 ml IM
            Fattening Lambs 0.5-1.0 ml IM
            Lambs 0.25-0.5 ml IM

Note: They can also be given orally. Follow the label directions, do not exceed label directions, these vitamins can be toxic if given too long.
Withdrawal Period: Meat 60 days

VITAMIN B-COMPLEX INJECTION
Indications: The B-complex vitamins are an assortment of closely related B and other vitamins. The concentration and directions may vary from country to country. The doses listed are a guide.
Precautions: Protect from light, sunlight and heat, which can destroy these vitamins. The products may stain if spilled on skin or clothing. The injection can be quite painful, make certain the animal is properly restrained.
Dosage and Route: Read label carefully.
Withdrawal Period: None required

CALCIUM INJECTIONS (*Calboral, Mifex,* etc.)
Needed for high producing animals which collapse (e.g. Milk Fever, See page 270.)   This is rarely needed except in high-producing dairy cows. Chronically malnourished animals should be treated orally. If needed for Milk Fever, be careful to follow labels on bottle carefully. Never give calcium too quickly IV. Instead give slowly, drop by drop.

29.1.6 ANTIDOTES

ATROPINE (Atropino Sulfato)
Indications: Atropine is used as an antidote for organophosphate insecticide poisoning. See page 83. Doses listed are a guide. Atropine should be given in high enough doses and often enough to control the signs of organophosphate poisoning.
Warning: High doses can cause excitement, dry mouth, vomiting, constipation, seizures, rapid heart rate and shock.
Dosage and Route:

      Horses- 0.22 mg/kg, IM, SC
      Cattle- 0.5 mg/kg, IM, SC
      Swine- 0.22 mg/kg, IM, SC
      Sheep- 0.5 mg/kg, IM, SC

        Goats- 0.5 mg/kg, IM, SC
        Dogs- 0.2-2.0 mg/kg, IM, SC
        Cats- 0.2-2.0 mg/kg, IM, SC
<u>Withdrawal Period</u>: not known

EPINEPHRINE (Adrenaline)
<u>Indications</u>: Epinephrine is used as an emergency drug to treat extreme allergic reaction (anaphylaxis). These sudden, severe, sudden, life threatening allergic reactions may be caused by insect stings, vaccination reaction, or exposure to penicillin.
<u>Precautions</u>: Epinephrine can cause fear, excitement, vomiting, increased heart rate and irregular heart rate. The effects of epinephrine only last for a few minutes but usually the dose does not need to be repeated.
<u>Dosage and Route</u>: For the 1:1,000 solution (1mg/ml)
        Horses- 0.3-0.5 ml per 45 kg IM, SC
        Cattle- 0.5-1.0 ml per 45 kg IM, SC
        Swine- 0.5-1.0 ml per 45 kg IM, SC
        Sheep- 0.5-1.0 ml per 45 kg IM, SC
        Goats- 0.5-1.0 ml per 45 kg IM, SC
        Dogs- 0.1-0.2 ml per 10 kg IV, IM, SC
        Cats- 0.1ml IV, SC
(For the 1:10,000 solution, give 10 times the volume listed above because it contains 0.1 mg/ml)

29.1.7 Injectable Sedatives, Tranquilizers, Analgesics and Anesthetics

Tranquilizers and sedatives help animals to temporarily become calmer and less reactive to noises, movement and pain.

Analgesics relieve pain.

Anesthetics fall into two categories: local and general.
-**Local anesthetics** are injected <u>around</u> the desired area or <u>into</u> the nerve that supplies the desired area Local anesthetics prevent the nerves from feeling pain.
-**General anesthetics** work on the brain. An animal under a general anesthetic will appear to be asleep to the extent that it cannot be awakened. The animal given a general anesthetic will not move when a painful procedure is performed on it. General anesthetics are used most often to perform major surgery. They are also potentially dangerous and should be given only by veterinary doctors or an AHA who has received some special training.

Using Tranquilizers and Sedatives
1. To quiet an unruly animal for examination, transport, or putting on a cast or splint.
2. Can be given along with local anesthetics in order to perform suturing.
<u>Warning</u>:
1. If the animal is depressed or very sick, the tranquilizer may affect the animal more than usual. If the liver is not working well, it will take longer for the animal to awaken. A smaller dose may be given to help lessen the effects.
2. If the animal is highly excited before the tranquilizer is given, the animal may become even more excited, or the tranquilizer may have no effect at all.

3. These are potentially dangerous and should be given only by an AHA who has received some special training.

XYLAZINE
<u>Indications</u>: See above.
<u>Warnings</u>: Do not use alone if working around the back legs in horses.
Do not use if animal has heart problems.
Do not use in late pregnancy in cows, sheep, or goats, as it may cause abortions.
Do not use in cats.
<u>Dosage and Route</u>: Sedation 10-15 minutes after IM administration, lasts 1-2 hours; analgesia lasts 15-30 minutes.
     Horse- Standing sedation 0.88-1.1 mg/kg IM.
     Foals- 0.88-1.1 mg/kg IM
     Cows- 0.11-0.22 mg/kg IM.
          Note: This dose will cause the cow to lie down. Give lower doses if standing tranquilization is desired. DO NOT GIVE IN LATE PREGNANCY.
     Sheep- 0.1-0.2 mg/kg IM.
          Note: Sheep are less sensitive to xylazine than cattle.
     Goats- 0.1-0.15 mg/kg IM.
          Note: Goats are more sensitive to xylazine than cattle.
     Pigs- 2.2 mg/kg IM.
          Note: Not reliably effective in pigs.
     Llamas- 0.1-0.25 mg/kg SQ before ketamine or alone
     Guinea Pigs- 5 mg/kg IM with ketamine at 20-40 mg/kg mixed in the same syringe.
          Lasts 15-35 minutes.
     Rabbits- 4.0-5.0 mg/kg IM.

ACEPROMAZINE MALEATE
Onset of action 15-20 minutes after injection, lasts 2 hours.
     Horse- 0.044-0.088 mg/kg IM
     Cows- 0.01-0.02 mg/kg IM
     Goats and Sheep- if weigh less than 50 kg, 0.1-0.2 mg/kg
               If weigh more than 50 kg, 0.05-0.10 mg/kg
     Pigs- 0.11-0.44 mg/kg IM, to a maximum of 15 mg.
     Dogs- 0.062-0.25 mg/kg IM, or SQ.
          May be given by mouth at 1.1-2.2 mg/kg.
     Cats- 0.062-0.25 mg/kg IM, or SQ.
          May be given by mouth at 1.1-2.2 mg/kg.

Using Analgesics (Pain Killers) *(Novalgin,* Paracetamol)
These are useful injections for animals with bad pain. It helps animals with foot and mouth disease to eat and move when their mouths and feet are painful. It helps animals after accidents, or with serious injuries like broken legs, to feel and eat better. Some analgesics are also used to lower fevers.
<u>Dosage:</u> See label for specific instructions
<u>Warning:</u> Aspirin and other non-steroidal anti-inflammatories may cause stomach ulcers, especially in young animals.

ANALGIN
Dosage: Give IM. See label for specific instructions.

ASPIRIN
See Oral Medicines, 29.2.5 in this chapter.
DYPYRONE
See Page 63. Use according to label to bring down fever.

PARACETAMOL *(Paracetol)*
Dosage: Give IM. See label for specific instructions

PHENYLBUTAZONE
See Oral Medicines

FLUNIXIN MEGLUMINE
<u>Indications</u>: Works well for relieving belly pain, lowering fevers and helping counteract the poisons of some bacteria.
>   Horse- 1.1 mg/kg IM every 12 hours
>   Warning: May get severe infection in the muscle when given IM. Use penicillin if the horse becomes infected in an injection spot. In young horses use one or two doses **only** as it may cause stomach ulcers.
>   Cow- 1.1 mg/kg IM. Give every other day.
>   Note: May cause stomach ulcers in young calves.
>   Llama- 1.1 mg/kg IM once daily

Using Local Anesthetics (lidocaine, novocaine, lignocaine, and bucaine)

This can be used in all animals for injection under the skin. These medicines make the injected area unable to feel pain. They are used to inject under the skin of a wound which needs to be sutured.

These local anesthetics are usually available in about 2% solutions. If they are more concentrated than this, then dilute them with distilled water to about 2%.

<u>Dosage and instructions</u>: See pages 217, 218.

Using General Anesthetics
These should be used only by a veterinary doctor or an AHA with special training.

29.1.8 Hormones

ESTROGEN
Synthetic estrogen is used to bring animal into heat. This is used for animals with chronic uterine infections (pyometra) and for other animals that never come into heat.
Heat appears about 3 days after injection. It is then best to wait until the next natural heat to breed (3 weeks later).
<u>Warning</u>: Estrogen injections cause abortions and may cause cystic ovaries. They are illegal in some countries.
<u>Dose</u>: Read the label!

OXYTOCIN
It causes the uterus to contract and makes milk come down into the udder.
This is used for retained placenta. See page 153.
This is used for treatment of dystocia in pigs. See page 138.
Dose: Read the label!

PROSTAGLANDIN
This drug is used to bring a female animal into heat. It is safer to use than estrogen and therefore in some countries this drug is legal but estrogens are not. However, it is usually more expensive.
Warning: This drug will also cause a pregnant female to abort. Therefore it must be used carefully.
Dose: Read the label!

29.1.9 Antiprotozoals *(Berenil, Babesan)*

These are used for Babesiosis and other protozoal diseases.
Dose: Read the label carefully because each medicine is different. Also, these medicines are expensive.

29.2 ORAL MEDICINES

Some oral medicines require combining different ingredients together. Others do not. The following medicines are simple and can be purchased in the local market.

Abbreviation:
1.   Animal: To which animal the drug is given.
2.   Dosage: How much to give for a particular species, and how often to give it.
3.   How: How to prepare the drugs, e.g. with water, drenching, with food, etc.

29.2.1 Bloat / Tympany

LOCAL HERBAL MIXTURES (*Timpol*))
Check the local market. In South Asia, some of these are quite effective and can be purchased in traditional medicine shops.
Timpol
a.   Animal: Buffalo, cow, ox, goat, sheep.
b.   Dosage: 100 grams, every 2-4 hours, until recovery
c.   How: Mix with water and drench.

MUSTARD OIL
a.   Animal: Cow, ox, buffalo, sheep, goat,
b.   Dosage: Cattle/buffalo .5 liter- 1.0 liter, sheep/goat ¼ liter, every 2-4 hours until recovery
c.   How: Drench or stomach tube.

MINERAL OIL
Effective to clear out the digestive system in cases of bloat. See laxatives, in 29.2.3 below.

MAGNESIUM SULFATE (EPSOM SALTS)
Effective to clear out the digestive system in cases of bloat. See laxatives, in 29.2.3.

29.2.2 Diarrhea

ORAL REHYDRATION SOLUTION See page 268.
a.	Animal:	An animal suffering from dehydration due to diarrhea, etc.
b.	Dosage:	Small amounts each, given frequently, every ½ hour or so.
c.	How:	Drenching.

KAOLIN
a.	Animal:	With Diarrhea. To make stools more thick.
b.	Dosage:	50 gram (cattle, buffalo), 2 times a day until recovery. 1 gram (sheep/goats), 2 times a day until recovery.
c.	How:	Mix with water and drench.

29.2.3 Laxatives

MAGNESIUM SULFATE (EPSOM SALTS)
Dissolve the salts in warm water and drench, or use a stomach tube. The animal must also have adequate water to drink, or the Epsom salts will not work effectively.
a.	Animal:	All animals (except last 2 months of pregnancy).
b.	Dosage:	Cattle/buffalo 200-300 gram. Sheep/goats 25-50 gram.
c.	Freq.:	Only once or twice in all.
d.	How:	Mix with warm water and feed orally. Magnesium sulfate will not work without water.

MINERAL OIL
Indications: Mineral oil is also known as white petrolatum, liquid petrolatum, liquid paraffin and white mineral oil. It is a tasteless, odorless, transparent, colorless, oily liquid that is insoluble in water. It is most commonly used in horses to treat constipation, and fecal impaction and is also used as a laxative in other species. Some people also it use to cause loose stools and move poison out of the intestinal tract as diarrhea.
Warning: Mineral oil must be given by stomach tube to prevent going into the lungs and causing pneumonia.

a.	Animal:	All animals
b.	Dosage:	Horse, cattle, buffalo 1-4 liters Sheep, goats, swine 100-500 ml.
c.	Freq.:	Only once or twice in all.
d.	How:	By stomach tube

29.2.4 Treatment of Poisoning

ACTIVATED CHARCOAL
See page 81.

NEW METHYLENE BLUE
For treatment of nitrate poisoning. See page 82.

SODIUM THIOSULFATE
For treatment of cyanide poisoning. See page 81.

29.2.5 Pain

ASPIRIN

<u>Indications</u>: Aspirin can be used to treat inflammation and swelling, fever and pain.
<u>Warning</u>:
- Aspirin can cause stomach upset and ulcers. It is best to give with a meal. At very high doses it can cause sickness and death. Use with great caution in cats. Do not use in pregnant animals. **Keep away from children!**
- Do not give to an animal that is dehydrated.
- Do not give to an animal that is bleeding or in shock.
- Do not give to an animal on which surgery is to be done.
- Discontinue treatment if the animal has black feces or blood in its feces.

<u>Dosage</u>:
      Horses- 15-100 mg/kg by mouth, 2-3 times daily
      Cattle- 15-100 mg/kg by mouth, 2-3 times daily
      Swine- 10 mg/kg by mouth, 4 times daily
      Dogs- 10 mg/kg by mouth, 2 times daily for fever; or
            25-35 mg/kg by mouth, 3 times daily for pain and joint swelling
      Cats- 6 mg/kg by mouth, every 2-3 days for fever; or
            10 mg/kg by mouth, every 2 days (48 hours) for pain (TOXIC IF GIVEN MORE OFTEN)

PHENYLBUTAZONE (*Bute, Butazolidin*)
<u>Indications</u>: Phenylbutazone is a strong aspirin-like drug that has been used successfully for many years. It fights inflammation, fever and pain. It is not effective in treating the pain of colic. Several days of treatment may be needed to see the full effect of the drug.
<u>Warning</u>: High doses over a long period of time can cause loss of appetite and ulcers in the mouth. Excessive doses can cause death. DO NOT USE IN CATS.
<u>Dosage and Route</u>:
      Horses- 2.4-4 mg/kg by mouth, 1-2 times daily
      Cattle- 4-8 mg/kg by mouth; or
      Swine- 4-8 mg/kg by mouth daily
      Llama- 2-4 mg/kg by mouth daily
      Dogs- 14 mg/kg by mouth, 3 times daily. maximum dose 800 mg/day
<u>Withdrawal Period</u>: Cattle-meat 14 days, milk 5 days

29.2.6 Oral Antibiotics

SULFADIAZINE + TRIMETHOPRIM (*Tribrissen*)
<u>Indications</u>: See "sulfa group" above. This medicine is a combination of sulfamethoxazole and trimethoprim. It works like a *broad-spectrum* antibiotic and is less-expensive than ampicillin.

<u>Dosage and Route</u>:
        Horses-30 mg/kg by mouth, 2-3 times daily
        Cattle- 30 mg/kg by mouth, one time daily
        Sheep - 75 mg/kg by mouth daily
        Dogs- 15-30 mg/kg by mouth 1-2 times daily
        Cats- 30 mg/kg by mouth 2 times daily
<u>Withdrawal Period</u>: Cattle-meat 3 days, milk 7 days
        Swine-meat 10 days
        Sheep-meat 14 days

SULFADIMIDINE *(Sulfamez)*

<u>Indications</u>: See "sulfa group" above.
<u>Dosage and Route</u>:
        Cattle- 110 mg/kg by mouth daily
        Swine- 110 mg/kg by mouth daily
        Sheep- 110 mg/kg by mouth daily
        Goats- 110 mg/kg by mouth daily
<u>Withdrawal Period</u> Cattle- meat 15 days, milk 3 days
        Swine-meat 15 days
        Sheep-meat 15 days
        Goats-meat 15 days, milk 3 days

SULFAMETHAZINE

<u>Indications</u>: See "sulfa group" above.
<u>Dosage and Route</u>:
        Cattle- 200 mg/kg by mouth for one day, then
            100 mg/kg one time daily
        Swine- 200 mg/kg by mouth for one day, then
            100 mg/kg one time daily
        Sheep- 30 ml of 12.5% solution by mouth for one day, then 15 ml daily
        Dogs- 50 mg/kg by mouth 2 times daily
        Cats- 50 mg/kg by mouth 2 times daily
        Rabbit - 2 g/L drinking water
        Chicken- 1 g/L drinking water
<u>Withdrawal Period</u>: Cattle- meat 10 days, milk 4 days
        Swine-meat 14 days

OXYTETRACYCLINE

<u>Indications</u>: See "tetracycline group" above.
<u>Dosage and Route</u>:
        Cattle- 10-20 mg/kg by mouth, 4 times daily
        Swine- 10-20 mg/kg by mouth, 4 times daily
        Sheep- 10-20 mg/kg by mouth, 4 times daily
        Goats- 10-20 mg/kg by mouth, 4 times daily
        Dogs- 22 mg/kg by mouth, 3 times daily
        Cats-   22 mg/kg by mouth, 3 times daily
<u>Withdrawal Period</u>: Cattle by mouth- meat 5 days, milk 4 days
        Swine- meat 21 days
        Sheep-meat 21 days

Precautions: Do not use in horses. Do not give with milk, or any other antibiotics.It may cause stomach upset. If the injection is a large volume, divide it into several sites.

NITROFURANS

Used as antibiotics and to slow the reproduction of coccidia. It is found in the market in the form of a liquid, a powder, ointment, or bolus. It is useful in non-specific diarrhea and protozoal bloody diarrhea.

a.	Animal:	Non-ruminants with diarrhea.
b.	Dosage:	Furazolidone 2g/kg of ration for 2-4 wk.
		Nitrofurazone 10mg/kg b.w. orally for 3 days.
c.	Freq.:	Once daily (for nitrofurazone)
d.	How:	Mix in feed (furazolidone) or drench.

POULTRY ANTIDIARRHEAL MEDICINES

Many forms of medicines (often sulfas or amprolium) are available in the market for diarrhea in chickens. Use the dose on the label or look in these notes for the specific disease conditions.

29.2.7 Pregnancy Toxemia Treatment

PROPYLENE GLYCOL

Cattle – 250 - 500 ml by mouth, once daily for 5-10 days for treatment.

Sheep – 60 - 120 mls twice daily for 5-10 days.

29.2.8 Oral Diuretics

LOCAL HERBAL MIXTURES (*Stonil*)

Sometimes available. Their efficacy is really unknown.

Stonil

a.	Animal:	Large and small.
b.	Dosage:	50 gram (cattle/buffalo)
		15 gram (sheep/goat)
c.	Freq.:	2 times a day.
d.	How:	With water by drench

29.2.9 Stomach Stimulant

LOCALLY-MADE TABLETS, POWDERS & MIXTURES (*Himalayan Batisa / Herminsa*)

These are available in the market. Some are effective and some are not.

Himalayan Batisa / Herminsa :

a.	Animal:	Ruminant
b.	Dosage:	Cattle/buffalo 50 gram
		Sheep/goats 5 gram
c.	Freq.:	Every 6-12 hours.
d.	How:	Drenching with water.

VITAMIN B TABLETS

Many are available. Sometimes they are helpful and sometimes they are not. Use according to label.

29.2.10 Internal Parasite Medicines (Anthelminthics)

Some people do not feed these medicines immediately after breeding (first 2 months of pregnancy); nor during the last month of pregnancy. However, many of them are safe and cause no problems.

For Coccidia

AMPROLIUM (*Amprol, Corid*)
Indications: Amprolium is used to treat coccidiosis.
Warning: High doses or prolonged administration can produce nerve damage. Administration of thiamine can counteract the effectiveness of amprolium. Do not use for more than 12 days in puppies.
Dosage & Route:
> Cattle- 5-10 mg/kg/day by mouth for 5 days
> Swine- 25-65 mg/kg by mouth, 1-2 times daily for 3-4 days, or
> > 100 mg/kg/day in food or water
> Sheep- 55 mg/kg by mouth daily for 19 days
> Goats- 55 mg/kg by mouth daily for 19 days
> Llama- 5 mg/kg by mouth for 3 weeks
> Dog- 100-200 mg/kg per day orally, 7-10 days

Withdrawal period: Cattle: 24 hours

Broad Spectrum Anthelminthic (effective against worms and flukes)

These are quite effective but also expensive.

ALBENDAZOLE (*Valbazen, Albomar*)
Easy to carry (light tablets); easy to feed. It is very effective and should be fed two or three times per year. It can be fed with leaves, bread or other food.
Indications: Albendazole kills liver flukes, tapeworms, stomach worms, intestinal worms and lungworms. It is also used as a general dewormer in horses, dogs and cats.
Warning: Do not give to female cattle in the first 45 days of pregnancy or within 45 days of breeding.
Dosage & Route:
> Horses- 50 mg/kg by mouth for 2 days
> Cattle- 10 mg/kg by mouth
> Swine- 5-10 mg/kg by mouth
> Sheep- 7.5-15 mg/kg by mouth for adult liver flukes
> > 3 mg/kg by mouth for 35 days for prevention of liver flukes
> Goats- 7.5-15 mg/kg by mouth for adult liver flukes
> > 3 mg/kg by mouth for 35 days for prevention of liver flukes
>
> Llama- 6.5 mg/kg by mouth
> Dogs- 25-50 mg/kg by mouth for 5 days
> Cats- 30 mg/kg by mouth for 6 days

Withdrawal period:
> Cattle- meat 27 days, do not use in milking cows

IVERMECTIN
Indications: This is a paste which is put into the mouth, and which the animal eats. It is expensive but kills almost all internal and external parasites. It is safe. It is approved for use in more species of animals than any other antiparasite drug. The only disadvantage is cost.

Warning: Do not give Collie dogs more than the 0.006 mg/kg dose as a fatal reaction may result. Do not give to dogs with heartworms.

Dosage and Route:
> Horses- 0.2 mg/kg by mouth
> Cattle- 0.2 mg/kg by mouth or SC
>> 0.5 mg/kg pour-on (only use pour-on product for this route of application)
> Swine- 0.3 mg/kg SC or IM
> Sheep- 0.2 mg/kg by mouth
> Goat-   0.2 mg/kg SC
> Llamas- 0.2 mg/kg by mouth or injection
> African Buffalo- 0.2 mg/kg SC
> Camel- 0.2 mg/kg SC
> Dogs- 0.006 mg/kg by mouth monthly for heartworms.
>> 0.05 mg/kg by mouth for removal of heartworm microfilariae.
>> 0.2 mg/kg by mouth or by injection for intestinal worms
> Cats- 0.2 mg/kg by injection for ear mites
>> 0.3 mg/kg by mouth or injection for intestinal worms
> Guinea Pig- 0.2-0.3 mg/kg SC
> Rabbit- 0.2-0.4 by mouth, IM, SC

Withdrawal Period:
> Cattle- Meat 49 days. Do not use in milking cows
> Sheep- Meat 11 days.
> Pigs- Meat 18 days.

TETRAMISOLE AND OXYCLOSANIDE (*Nilzan*) (Vallchlra)

Indications: For the treatment of worms and flukes in cattle, buffalo, sheep and goats. It is very effective but difficult to carry. Administer by drench two or three times per year, depending on the area.

Warning:

Dosage and Route:
> Cattle, Buffalo
>
> | | |
> | --- | --- |
> | Up to 50 kg | 16.5 ml |
> | 50-100 kg | 33 ml |
> | 150-200 kg | 66 ml |
> | 300 kg and above | 100 ml |
>
> Sheep and Goat
>
> | | |
> | --- | --- |
> | Up to 15 kg | 5 ml |
> | 15-30 kg | 10 ml |
> | 30-45 kg | 15 ml |
> | 45 kg and above | 20 ml |

Withdrawal Period: Read label

Broad Spectrum Anthelminthic (effective against many different worms)

FENBENDAZOLE (*Panacur, Fencur*)

Indications: Effective against all kinds of gastrointestinal roundworms, immature and adult worms, eliminates tapeworms in sheep. It is one of the most popular anthelminthics because it is safe and effective. It is also available in many different forms, including oral paste and powders.

Warning: Dogs, cats, and pigs must get the drug daily for three days in a row to be effective.

<u>Dosage and Route</u>:

        Horse- 5 mg/kg by mouth; or 10 mg/kg by mouth for <u>Parascaris equorum</u>,
                or 50 mg/kg by mouth for <u>Stongyloides westeri.</u>
        Cattle- 5 mg/kg by mouth; or 10 mg/kg by mouth for <u>Moniezia</u> and <u>Ostertagia.</u>
        Swine- 3 mg/kg by mouth for 3 consecutive days; or 5-10 mg/kg by mouth
        Sheep- 5 mg/kg by mouth for 3 days
        Camel- 4.5-15 mg/kg by mouth
        Llamas-10-15 mg/kg by mouth
        Goats- 5 mg/kg by mouth for 3 days
        Dogs- 50 mg/kg by mouth daily for 3 days
        Cats- 50 mg/kg by mouth daily for 5 days
        Rabbit- 10 mg/kg by mouth every 14 days for 2 doses

<u>Withdrawal Period</u>:

        Cattle- meat 14 days, milk 4 days
        Sheep- meat 14 days
        Goats- meat 14 days, milk 1 day

LEVAMISOLE

<u>Indications</u>: Levamisole is one of the standard anthelmintics that has been used effectively for many years. It is a broad spectrum drug that is commonly given by mouth, but special formulations are available for injection or pour-on.

<u>Warning</u>: Do not use at the same time as chloramphenicol. Toxic doses may produce signs similar to organophosphate toxicity; diarrhea, salivation, tremors, and foaming at the mouth. Atropine is somewhat helpful in treating an overdose.

<u>Dosage and Route</u>:

        Horses- 8 mg/kg by mouth
        Cattle- 8 mg/kg by mouth
             10 mg/kg using special pour-on product
             6 mg/kg by SC
        Swine- 8 mg/kg in water or feed
        Sheep- 8 mg/kg by mouth
        Goats- 8 mg/kg by mouth
        Llamas- 5-8 mg/kg by mouth
        Camels- 5-8 mg/kg by mouth
        Dogs- 10 mg/kg by mouth daily for 10 days for heartworm microfilaria; or
             7-12 mg/kg by mouth daily for 3-7 days for lungworm
        Cats- 20-40 mg/kg by mouth every other days for 6 treatments

<u>Withdrawal Period</u>:

        Cattle- meat 9 days, do not use in milking cows
        Sheep- meat 3 days
        Swine- meat 9 days

MEBENDAZOLE (*Benzicare, Equiverm, Telmin*)

<u>Indications</u>: Mebendazole is most commonly used in horses, dogs, cats, sheep and swine. It is used to treat lungworms and other worms. It is quite effective.

<u>Dosage and Route</u>:

        Horses- 10-15 mg/kg by mouth; or
             15-20 mg/kg by mouth for 5 days against lungworms
        Cattle- 15 mg/kg by mouth
        Sheep- 15 mg/kg by mouth

Llamas- 22 mg/kg by mouth for 3 days
Camels- 22 mg/kg by mouth
Dogs- 22 mg/kg by mouth for 3 days
Cats- 22 mg/kg by mouth for 3 days
Ferret- 50 mg/kg by mouth twice a day for 2 days

Withdrawal: Sheep- meat 7 days
Precautions: Mebendazole must be given daily for 3 days in a row to be effective in pigs, dogs, and cats.

THIABENDAZOLE
Indications: It is very effective against a wide range of worms, including lungworms.

Dosage and Route
 Horses- 50-100 mg/kg by mouth
 Cattle- 50-100 mg/kg by mouth
 Swine- 50-75 mg/kg by mouth
 Sheep- 50-100 mg/kg by mouth
 Goats- 66 mg/kg by mouth
 Llamas- 50-100 mg/kg by mouth daily for 1-3 days
 Camels- 66 mg/kg by mouth
 Dogs- 50 mg/kg by mouth daily for 3 days
 Rabbits- 100-200 mg/kg by mouth
Withdrawal Period: Cattle- meat 3 days, milk 4 days
 Sheep- meat 30 days
 Goats- meat 30 days

Narrow Spectrum (kills only flukes)

HEXACHLOROETHANE (*Hexathane*) (Vallachira)
Indications: This drug is bitter tasting but it is cheap and effective for flukes in ruminants. It is fed as a drench but tends to stick in the dosing bottle. Administer 2 or 3 times per year, depending on the need in the area.
Warning:
Dosage and Route:
 Cattle, Buffalo
  Give from 15-100 gms/animal, at a rate of 10 gm/50kg of body weight.
 Sheep, Goat
  Feed 8 – 15 gm per animal, at a rate of 2 gm / 10 kg body weight.
Withdrawal Period: Read label

HEXACHLOROPHENE (*Distodin, Flukin*) (Vallachira)
Indications: This drug comes at 100 mg tablets or 1000mg (1 gram) bolus. It is cheap and effective for flukes in ruminants. The tablets are fed, or they are crushed and fed as a drench. Administer 2 or 3 times per year, depending on the need in the area.
Warning:
Dosage and Route: The general dose is 10-15 mg/kg body weight.
 Cattle, Buffalo (use large bolus), 1 – 2 tablets depending on size of animal
 Calves – ½ bolus
 Sheep, Goat (use small tablet), 1 - 2 tablets depending on size of animal
 Lambs – ½ bolus
Withdrawal Period: Read label

OXYCLOSANIDE

<u>Indications</u>: Oxyclozanide kills adult liver flukes in cattle and sheep.
<u>Warning</u>: Calculate the dose carefully because the toxic dose is only 4 times the
recommended dose.
<u>Dosage and Route</u>:
      Cattle- 10-15 mg/kg by mouth
      Sheep- 10-15 mg/kg by mouth
<u>Withdrawal Period</u>: Cattle- meat 14 days, milk 0 days

Narrow Spectrum (kills only certain worms)

NICLOSAMIDE

<u>Indications</u>: Niclosamide kills tapeworms in dogs, cats and sheep.
<u>Dosage and Route</u>:
      Sheep- 52 mg/kg by mouth
      Dogs- 150 mg/kg by mouth
      Cats- 150 mg/kg by mouth
      Rabbit- 100 mg/kg by mouth, 2 doses one week apart

PIPERAZINE

<u>Indications</u>: Piperazine is a very effective against large roundworms in large and small animals,
and has been used for many years. It is not broad spectrum. In some areas, it is not
recommended in cattle, sheep and goats due to resistance of parasites in these species.
<u>Dose is calculated based upon the amount of piperazine base.</u>
<u>Warning</u>: Toxic doses may cause tremors, seizures and weakness. Do not give to animals
with liver or kidney disease.
<u>Dosage and Route</u>:
      Buffalo calves-25-300mg/Kg repeat in four weeks
      Horses- 88-110 mg/kg of piperazine base by mouth
      Swine- 110 mg/kg of piperazine base by mouth
      Dogs- 45-65 mg/kg of piperazine base by mouth
      Cats- 45-65 mg/kg of piperazine base by mouth
      Gerbil- 2-3 g/L drinking water for one week
      Guinea Pig- 2-5 g/L drinking water for one week
      Hamster- 10 g/L drinking water
      Rabbit- 200 mg/kg by mouth
      Chicken- 250 mg/kg by mouth, or
          1 g/L drinking water for three days

29.3 EXTERNAL MEDICINE FOR SKIN USE

SOAP
- For cleaning wounds and washing hands.

MAGGOCIDE CREAM
- Used for all animals to prevent infection and maggot infestation.
- After cleaning wounds, apply a little around the wound.

GENTIAN VIOLET
- For all animals, use a 2% solution as a disinfectant. After cleaning wounds, apply around wound as required. Use daily until wound heals. Good for helping to dry out wounds.

IODINE
- It is used as a disinfectant for fresh wounds. It is can cause irritation.

POVODINE-IODINE (*Betadine*)
- It is a disinfectant, use at 0.5% - 2% for cleaning wounds

SULFUR POWDER
- For mange on all animals, mix with animal fat, vegetable oil, or petroleum jelly (Vaseline). One part sulphur and 10 parts animal fat, vegetable fat, or Vaseline. Rub the affected area once a week for 3-6 weeks. (Wounds should be cleaned first).

BENZYL BENZOATE
- For Rabbit ear mange: scaly wounds, blood and pus inside ears. Put $^1/_2$ teaspoonful inside the ear and rub gently. Apply once a week for 4 weeks.

ANTIBIOTIC OINTMENT
- For surface wounds on all animals; 2-3 time daily, after cleaning.

MALATHION POWDER
- For all animals, for external parasites. Mix powder with ashes: 1 part Malathion (dust) for 10 part ashes. Rub into hair and skin, all over body if needed. Use once a week for 3-6 weeks.

TURPENTINE
- Used for maggots. Use as much as needed (burns badly).

CAMPHOR BALLS (Mothballs)
- Crush and mix with water for maggots.

POTASSIUM PERMANGANATE
- To stop bleeding (use crystals).
- 1:1000 for washing wounds

HYDROGEN PEROXIDE
- For cleaning ears and wounds. Use weak concentration

29.4 SPECIAL PURPOSE MEDICINES

EYE WASH
- Boric Acid with boiled, cool water at 1:100.

EYE OINTMENT
- **Only special medicines can be used in eyes because eyes are extra-sensitive.** Medicine made for eyes usually says, "for eyes" or "ophthalmic" on it. (Ophthalmic means "eye".)

- Tetracycline group. For all animals. Specially made for eyes and eye wounds. Dose as needed: apply twice daily after cleaning the eye.

- Penicillin ointment for eyes: For eye infections. Use for 7 - 10 days, after cleaning of eye.

EYE DROPS
- Also used for eye infections. Must be applied more frequently than eye ointment, probably 5-10 times daily. Not practical for livestock. <u>Never use eye ointment containing steroid in horses' eyes.</u>

EAR OINTMENT
- Some ointments are made specifically for use in ears. These are labeled "Otic (Ear) Ointment," or "for use in ears." Apply in ear after washing.

INTRA-MAMMARY
- Used for mammary disease (mastitis). Use 1 tube daily for 3-5 days in teat. Check the label for specific instructions. See page 157 for proper use.
- (*Pendistrin, Mastalone,* etc.). Do not use steroids on pregnant cows! Check the tube first.

INTRA-UTERINE
- Sulphadimidine - For all animals. After removing retained placenta or dead baby, wash out uterus and place as far into the uterus as possible.
    - 10 gm for cattle/buffalo
    - 2.5 gm for sheep/goats

- Tetracycline bolus - For all animals. Use 1-2 tablets after washing out the uterus.

- Nitrofurazone - Use as per label

29.5 VACCINES

For a complete discussion of infectious diseases, resistance, immunity, and disease prevention and control, see Chapter 6, page 91. Proper handling of vaccines is also covered in Chapter 6.

Different methods of vaccine production are used throughout the world. Therefore each vaccine must be used carefully according to the specific instructions for that vaccine. This book will not cover those details. Rather, seek out advice about the vaccines available in your area. Use available vaccines according to the instructions given by the government veterinary officers and vaccine producers in your area.

29.5.1 General Guidelines For Vaccine Administration
- For many vaccines, the cold chain must be carefully maintained or the vaccine will be ineffective. See page 91.
- The withdrawal period is usually 21 days, but some require 60 days. Check the label.
- DO NOT chemically disinfect syringes and needles used to administer vaccines. Chemical residue could render the vaccine ineffective.

- Vaccinate pregnant animals 2-4 weeks prior to expected birthing.
- Vaccinate only healthy animals.
- READ THE LABEL INSTRUCTIONS COMPLETELY PRIOR TO USE.

29.5.2 Listing of Possible Vaccines for Diseases Covered in this Book

The following is a list of vaccines used for diseases covered in this book. Not all of these vaccines may be available in your area.

Avian Vaccines (Vaccines for Birds)

CHRONIC RESPIRATORY DISEASE (Mycoplasma gallisepticum)
COCCIDIOSIS (Eimeria species)
FOWL CHOLERA (Pasturella multocida)
FOWL POX VIRUS (Pox virus)
INFECTIOUS BURSAL DISEASE (Gumboro Disease)
NEWCASTLE DISEASE (Avian pneumoencephalitis)

Bovine Vaccines (Vaccines for Cattle and Buffalo)

ANTHRAX (Bacillus anthracis, Splenic Fever, Charbon, Milzbrand)
BLACKLEG (Clostridium chauvoei)
BRUCELLOSIS (Brucella abortus, Bang's Disease, Contagious Abortion)
FOOT AND MOUTH DISEASE
HEMMORHAGIC SEPTICEMIA (Shipping Fever, Pasturella hemolytica), Pasturella multocida)
LEPTOSPIROSIS (Leptospira pomona, etc.).
RABIES (Rabies virus)
RINDERPEST (Cattle plague, peste bovina)
TETANUS (Lockjaw, Clostridium tetani)
WARTS (Papilloma virus)

Canine Vaccines (Vaccines for Dogs)

DISTEMPER VIRUS
LEPTOSPIROSIS (Leptospira canicola, etc.).
RABIES

Caprine Vaccines (Vaccines for Goats)

BLACKLEG (Blackquarter, Big head, Clostridium chauvoei)
ENTEROTOXEMIA (Overeating Disease, Pulpy Kidney Disease, Clostridium perfringens)
POX (Goat and Sheep Pox Virus)
SOREMOUTH (Contagious Ecthyma)
TETANUS (Lockjaw, Clostridium tetani)

Equine Vaccines (Vaccines for Horses)

ANTHRAX (Bacillus anthracis)
STRANGLES (Distemper, Barn fever, Streptococcus equi)

Feline Vaccines (Vaccines for Cats)

RABIES

Llama Vaccines (Vaccines for Llamas)
ENTEROTOXEMIA (<u>Clostridium perfringens</u>)
RABIES
SOREMOUTH (Ecthyma)
TETANUS (<u>Clostridium tetani</u>)

Ovine Vaccines (Vaccines for Sheep)
ANTHRAX (<u>Bacillus anthracis</u>)
BLACKLEG (<u>Clostridium chauvoei</u>, Big head)
HEMMORHAGIC SEPTICEMIA (Shipping Fever, <u>Pasturella hemolytica and multocida</u>)
POX VIRUS
RABIES
RINDERPEST
SOREMOUTH (Ecthyma)
TETANUS (<u>Clostridium tetani</u>)

Porcine Vaccines (Vaccines for Pigs)
ANTHRAX (<u>Bacillus anthracis</u>)
ATROPHIC RHINITIS (<u>Pasturella multocida</u>)
HOG CHOLERA
LEPTOSPIROSIS (<u>Leptospira canicola, etc.</u>)
TETANUS (<u>Clostridium tetani</u>)

29.6 ANTISEPTICS AND DISINFECTANTS

By definition, a **disinfectant** kills microorganisms.
By definition, an **antiseptic** slows or stops the growth of organisms but does not kill them.

Antiseptics and disinfectants are used for cleaning wounds and for killing microorganisms in the environment. Some disinfectants are very irritating and actually damage living tissue when applied to wounds. Therefore it is very important to classify disinfectants and antiseptics as to whether they are "irritating" or "non-irritating".

Below is a list of some common disinfectants and antiseptics; what they are used for; and the concentration used.

Common Disinfectants
ACRIFLAVINE
Non-irritating disinfectant used for cleaning wounds in a concentration of 1:1000.

ALCOHOL
Alcohol may be used on skin or equipment, but should not be used in open wounds. Soak instruments, suture and cotton wool for about 20 minutes in concentrated (70% ethyl alcohol or drinking alcohol).

CHLORHEXIDINE (*Nolvasan, Virosan*)
Chlorhexidine is one of the safest and most effective antiseptics available. It has very good activity against bacteria, molds, yeasts and viruses. It works rapidly. It is available as a plain solution, and as a scrub solution. The scrub solution contains a detergent and should be rinsed off after use. The plain solution is very good at rinsing and soaking open wounds.
Surgical Prep- 2.0-4.0%

Open Wounds- 0.05%
Disinfection- 0.5-2.0%
Do not use the strong solutions on open wounds.

CHLORINE BLEACH (Sodium Hypochlorite)

Chlorine bleach is readily available and is effective in killing viruses and bacteria. It can be used full strength for disinfection or diluted for use in wounds, but it can damage living tissues.
Open wounds- 0.125% (1/4 strength)
Disinfection- 0.5% (full strength)
Do not use on living tissue if better agents are available. Be careful when handling the solution because it will bleach fabrics and other materials. Do not mix with ammonia or any other cleaning or disinfection agents, as toxic fumes may result.

CRESOL

Cresol compounds are effective in killing bacteria but have less effect on bacterial spores, viruses or fungi. They are primarily used to disinfect non-living surfaces.
Use as directed to clean and disinfect non-living surfaces.
Cresol smells badly. Do not use or store around human food. It is poisonous and should be handled carefully.

DESSICATION

This means "drying out" and it is a very effective way to kill some bacteria and, especially, the immature forms of parasites. Some worm eggs can live a long time (several years) in damp dung and in dark places. However, they can live only a short time if the dung is removed and the area dries out.

FORMALIN

Irritating disinfectant purchased in the market as a 40% solution. Can be used in a foot bath for footrot at a concentration of 2%. Also used as a preservative for tissues as a 10% solution. Can also be mixed as follows and used to clean poultry houses: 40% formalin 35 ml; Potassium Permanganate 17.5 gm for 100 cubic feet.

GENTIAN VIOLET

Non-irritating disinfectant used for cleaning wounds in a 0.5 - 2% solution (5 - 20 gm per liter of water). G.V. is very good to apply to wounds that need to dry out. After cleaning the wound well, apply as needed.

HYDROGEN PEROXIDE

Hydrogen peroxide is a readily available solution usually prepared in a 3% solution. It readily foams and hisses when poured into an open wound. Hydrogen peroxide is very good at flushing out abscesses. It is also toxic to animal tissues and should only be used for initial cleaning and flushing of dirty wounds and abscesses. Repeated use may slow healing.
Use full strength 3% solution on wounds and abscesses.

IODINE

The standard "drug store" iodine tincture is a 2% solution that is painted directly on small cuts and scrapes. A stronger 7% iodine is sometimes used in veterinary medicine as a caustic and is used to treat the umbilical cords of newborn livestock.
Small cuts and scratches- 2% iodine

Umbilical cords- 7% iodine

Do not confuse the two different iodine solutions. The 7% solution is caustic and should not be used on burns and deep wounds. Keep both solutions away from eyes, and away from flames.

PHENOL
Irritating disinfectant, even in 0.2% solutions. It is used especially for environment cleaning at 1:32 - 1:150.

POTASSIUM PERMANGANATE
Can be irritating in concentrations of 1:100. However, it is non-irritating in concentrations of 1:1000 or 1:5000. It can be used in more dilute solutions for washing wounds; and it can be used in concentrated solutions for cleaning the environment.

SAVLON
Non-irritating disinfectant used for cleaning wounds and for sterilizing instruments. Mix it at a rate of 1:200 for washing wounds. Mix it at a rate of 1:100 with water for instruments. Never soak instruments for more than 30 minutes because it can cause rust and damage. For long term storage of instruments use the following mixture: 4 gm of sodium nitrate; 1 liter of water; and 10 ml of Savlon.

ULTRAVIOLET RAYS (from sun)
Rays are used for cancer treatment. Ultraviolet rays help kill microorganisms in the environment, especially in a dry environment. Sunlight, plus cleaning of dung, etc., is an excellent form of sterilizing the environment (e.g. pasture rotation).

WATER (BOILED)
Used for equipment sterilizing; also use boiled, cooled water to wash wounds.

Common Antiseptics:

ALUM
Non-irritating antiseptic used for cleaning wounds (especially the mouth in FMD). Mouth washing is done with alum-water at a very low concentration (1%) solution.

BORAX
Non-irritating antiseptic used for hot compresses of wounds at a concentration of 2 - 3%.

LIME
Used for environmental cleaning; and for decaying of dead animals.

BORIC ACID
Non-irritating antiseptic used to wash wounds. Especially safe for washing out eyes at a concentration of 1:100. Can be made into an ointment for wounds at 1:40 in Vaseline.

29.7 PESTICIDES TO USE AND WAYS TO APPLY THEM

These are names of possible pesticides. Contact your nearest extension agent for details regarding the most effective, cheapest pesticide for your area. After identifying the correct medicine, follow the instructions carefully for mixing and application.

PESTS	Sprays	Dusts/ Dustbags	Backrubbers Facerubbers	Eartags	Direct Application	Pour - on	Dip	Injection
Ticks	Coumaphos, Malathion, Amitraz, Tetra-chlorvinphos, Stirofos – Dichlorvos, Permethrin	Coumaphos (ear ticks) Malathion		Cypermethrin, Diazinon, Stirofos/tetra-dichlorvinphos ,			Coumaphos	
Fleas	Malathion, Permethrin, Stirofos, Carbaryl (*Sevin*)	Malathion, Permethrin, Stirofos, Carbaryl (*Sevin*)						
Lice	Coumaphos, Malathion, Methoxychlor, Amitraz, Stirofox Stirofos + dichlorvos, Phosmet, Permethrin	Coumaphos[1], Malathion, Methoxychlor, Stirofos, Phosmet, Permethrin	Methoxychlor[2]	Cypermethrin,			Coumaphos	
Mites	Amitraz, Phosmet, Permethrin	Malathion Cythion			Sulfur powder mixed 1:10 in vegetable oil. Used motor oil	Ivermectin	Coumaphos	Ivermectin

[1] Dust Bags: For example, a 1-% Coumaphos powder can be used. Apply 4 to 10 pounds in doubled burlap bags. Hang the bags where animals treat themselves daily, such as near mineral or salt blocks and in the exit of the milking barn. Bags should hang 4 to 6 inches so they rest on the animal's back as it walks by. Protect the bags from weather. Do not hang the bags over feed, mineral or water troughs.

[2] Backrubber oil: For example, mix 1 liter of 24% EC in 4 liters of diesel fuel. Apply 4 liters per 20 feet of cable regularly.

PESTS	Sprays	Dusts/ Dustbags	Backrubbers Facerubbers	Eartags	Direct Application	Pour - on	Dip	Injection
Black flies, mosquitoe	Pyrethrins, Dichlorvos, Permethrin					Permethrin		
Horn flies	Coumaphos, Malathion, Pyrethrins Methoxychlor, Dichlorvos	Coumaphos 1%, Malathion 4 or 5% Methoxychlor Stirofos, Permethrin	Coumaphos, Malathion[3]	Cypermethrin, Diazinon, Many others		Ivermectin, Fenthion,		Coumaphos
House flies	Pyrethrins Dichlorvos, Permethrin			Cypermethrin Diazinon, Many others		Permethrin		
Stable flies	Pyrethrins Dichlorvos Permethrin			Cypermethrin, Diazinon, Many others		Permethrin		
Horse flies	Pyrethrins, Dichlorvos Permethrin					Permethrin		
Tsetse flies	See local extension agent for details to make traps							
Maggots	Prevention is important. Apply insecticides around wounds to prevent maggots. For treatment, apply local treatment to kill maggots. Pick them out. Clean well. See text for details, page 118							
Cattle grub (warble)	Coumaphos					Ivermectin Coumaphos Trichlorfon Famfur Fenthion,		Ivermectin

[3] 165 ml of 57% EC in 4 liters of diesel fuel. Soak the backrubbers in this.

Vocabulary

A

Abdomen- The part of the body that contains the stomach, kidneys, liver, and intestines.

Abortion- Death of the baby in the uterus.

Abscess- A localized collection of pus.

Absorption- The uptake of substances into or across tissues such as skin, intestine, and kidney tubes.

Acute- Sudden and short lived. An acute illness is one that starts suddenly and lasts a short time.

Allergy (allergic reaction)- A problem such as itching, rash, hives, sneezing, and sometimes difficult breathing or shock that affects certain animals when specific things are breathed in, eaten, injected, or touched. Some drugs like penicillin may also cause an allergic reaction.

Analgesic- Medicine to calm pain.

Anatomy- The science of the structure of an animal body.

Anemia- A disease in which the blood gets thin for lack of red blood cells. Signs include tiredness, pale skin, lack of energy, and a swelling under the jaw.

Anthelmintic- A chemical substance which destroys worms.

Antibiotic- A chemical substance which inhibits the growth of, or kills, bacteria. Antibiotics are not affective against viruses.

Antihistamine- Medicine used to fight allergies.

Antiparasitic- An agent which is destructive to parasites.

Antiseptic- A chemical substance which will stop or slow the growth of microorganisms.

Artery- A vessel carrying blood from the heart through the body. Arteries have a pulse. Veins, which return blood to the heart, have no pulse.

B

Bacteria- One-celled microorganisms that can be seen only with a microscope. Some bacteria cause disease, others do not.

Bladder stones- See Kidney Stones.

Bolus- A very large tablet made to be swallowed by horses, cattle, sheep, and goats.

Booster- A repeat vaccination to renew the effect of an earlier series of vaccinations.

Brand name- Trade name. The name a company gives to its product. A brand name medicine is sold under a special name and is often more expensive than the same generic medicine.

Breech delivery- A birth in which the baby starts to come out tail first. The AHA must correct the position so that the hind legs and tail come out together.

C
Cancer- A growth of highly abnormal cells which spread locally and/or to other parts of the body through the blood or lymph. The natural course of this growth is often fatal.

Carbohydrates- Energy foods like maize, wheat, rice, cassava, potatoes, and squash.

Centigrade (C.)- A measure or scale of heat and cold.

Cervix- The opening or neck of the womb at the back of the vagina.

Chronic- Long term or frequently recurring. A chronic disease is one that lasts a long time.

Circulation- The flow of the blood through the veins and arteries by the pumping of the heart.

Colic- Sharp abdominal pains caused by spasms or cramping of the gut.

Colostrum- The mother animal's first milk. It looks watery but it is rich in protein and helps to protect the young from infection.

Conjunctiva- A thin, protective layer that covers the white of the eye, and the inner side of the eyelids.

Constipation- Dry, hard, difficult stools (bowel movements) that do not come often.

Contagious disease- A sickness that can be spread easily from one animal to another.

Contractions- Tightening or shortening of muscles. The strong contractions of the womb when a mother is in labor help to push the young out of the womb.

Contraindication- A situation or condition when a particular medicine should not be taken. (Many medicines are a contraindication in pregnancy).

Cubic Centimeter (cc.)- A unit of volume in the metric system equal to a milliliter (ml).

D
Deficiency- Not having enough of something; a lack.

Dehydration- A condition in which the body loses more liquid than it takes in. This lack of water is especially dangerous in young animals.

Diarrhea- Frequent or runny stools. Diarrhea often leads to dehydration.

Diet- The kinds and amounts of certain foods that an animal should or should not eat.

Discharge- A release or flowing out of fluid, mucus, blood, or pus.

Disinfectant- A chemical which frees objects from infective microorganisms. Usually used on non-living objects.

Dislocations- Bones that have slipped out of place at the joint.

Drench- A liquid mixture of a medicine, given by pouring into the back of the mouth

Drug- Any chemical compound that may be used or administered as an aid in the diagnosis, treatment or prevention of disease or other abnormal conditions, for the relief of pain or suffering, or to control or improve any disease condition.

E
Ectoparasite- A parasite that lives on the outside of the body of its host.

Edema- Accumulation of excessive fluid in the subcutaneous tissues.

Endoparasite- A parasite which lives in the body of its host.

Embryo- The beginnings of an unborn animal when it is still very small.

Epidemic- An outbreak of disease affecting many livestock in a community or village at the same time.

Expiration date- The month and year marked on a medicine that tells when it will no longer be good. Throw away most medicines after this date.

F
Fahrenheit (F.)- A measure or scale of heat and cold. Water freezes at 32 degrees F, and boils at 212 degrees F.

Fetus (fetus)- The developing of a baby animal inside the uterus.

Fever- A body temperature higher than normal.

First Aid- Emergency care or treatment for an animal that is sick or injured.

Flukes- Flat worms that infect the liver, blood, or other parts of the body and cause different diseases.

Fracture- A broken bone.

Fungus- A parasitic microorganism that causes diseases like ringworm.

G

Generic name- The scientific name of a medicine, as distinct from the brand (trade) names given to it by the different companies that make it.

Germs- Very small organisms that can grow in the body and cause some infectious diseases (microorganisms).

Goiter- A swelling on the lower front of the neck (enlargement of the thyroid gland) caused by lack of iodine in the diet.

Gram (gm.)- A metric unit of weight. There are about 28 grams in an ounce. There are 1000 grams in one kilogram.

Gut thread or gut suture material- A special thread for sewing or stitching tears. The gut thread is slowly absorbed (disappears) so that the stitches do not need to be taken out.

H

Heart (girth) - Measurements of the distance around the body just behind the forelimbs; used in many weight estimation calculations. Hemorrhage- Severe or dangerous bleeding.

Herb- A plant, especially one valued for its medicinal or healing qualities.

Hereditary- Passed on from parent to offspring.

Hernia (rupture) - An opening or tear in the muscles covering the abdomen that allows a loop of the gutto push through and form a ball or lump under the skin.

History- An account of information concerning the animal. It includes but is not limited to breed, sex, age, previous illnesses, previous vaccinations, housing, food, and major symptoms of illness.

Hives- Hard, thick, raised spots on the skin that itch severely. They may come and go all at once, or move from one place to another. It is a form of an allergic reaction.

Hormones- Chemical made in parts of the body to do a special job. For example, estrogen and progesterone are hormones that regulate heat and pregnancy.

I

Immunity- It is when an animal develops its own protection against a specific organism. When the white blood cells protect the body against invading substances (antigens) by attacking and killing infectious organisms.

Immunizations (vaccinations)- Medicines that give protection against specific diseases, for example, rabies.

Infection- A sickness caused by bacteria or other germs. Infections may affect part of the body only (such as an infected foot), or all of it (such as HS).

Infectious disease- Caused by living organisms such as bacteria, viruses, and parasites. The organisms enter the body through an opening in the skin, or a body opening, and cause damage.

Inflammation- A localized protective response caused by injury or death of tissues. It is characterized in the acute form by signs of 1. Pain 2. Heat 3. Redness 4. Swelling.

Insecticide- A poison that kills insects.

Intramammary- Within the mammary gland or udder.

Intestines- the guts or tube-like part of the food canal that carries food and finally waste from the stomach to the rectum.

Intramuscular- In the muscle.

Intramuscular (IM) injection- An injection put into a muscle (usually the neck or leg muscles).

Intravenous- In the vein.

J
Jaundice- A yellow color of the eyes and skin. It is a sign of disease in the liver, gallbladder, pancreas, or blood.

K
Kidneys- Large, bean-shaped organs in the abdomen that form urine.

Kidney stones- Small stones that form in the kidneys and pass down the ureter to the bladder, and out the urethra. They may block the ureter or the urethra and make urination painful or impossible.

Kilogram (kg)- One thousand grams. A kilo is equal to a little over two pounds.

L
Larva (larvae)- The young worm-like form that comes from the egg of many insects or parasites. It changes form when it becomes an adult.

Laxative- A medicine used for constipation that makes stools softer and more frequent.

Liter (l.)- A metric measure equal to about one quart. A liter of water weighs one kilogram.

Liver- A large organ in the abdominal cavity. It is important in digestion.

Lubricant- An oil or soap used to make surfaces slippery.

Lymph nodes /glands- Small lumps under the skin which are located in different parts of the body, including the neck, between the legs, the chest, and the abdomen. These glands act like traps for germs. When they are infected, they become painful and swollen.

M

Malnutrition- Health problems caused by lack of the nutrients the animal needs.

Mastitis- An infection of the udder, often in the first weeks or months after giving birth. It causes the udder to become hot, swollen, and red.

Microorganism- A minute organism. Those of interest are bacteria, fungi, viruses, and protozoa. They cannot be seen without the help of a microscope.

Microscope- An instrument with lenses that make very tiny objects look larger.

Milligram (mg.)- A unit of weight in the metric system; one thousandth of a gram.

Milliliter (ml.)- A unit of volume in the metric system; one one-thousandth of a liter.

Minerals- Simple metals or other things the body needs, such as iron, calcium, iodine, and phosphorus.

Mucus- A thick slippery liquid that moistens and protects the nose, throat, stomach, guts, and the female reproductive tract.

N

Navel- Umbilicus; the place in the middle of the abdomen where the umbilical cord was attached.

Necropsy- Examination of a body after death (also known as a post mortem).

Nerves- Thin threads or strings that run from the brain to every part of the body and carry messages for feeling and movement.

Non-infectious diseases- a disease that does not spread from animal to animal (e.g. malnutrition, bladder cancer, bloat, etc.

Normal- Usual, natural, or average. Something that is normal has nothing wrong with it.

Nutritious- nourishing. Nutritious foods are those that have the things the body needs to grow, be healthy, and fight off disease

O

Obstruction- A condition of being blocked or clogged. An obstructed gut is a medical emergency.

Ointment- A salve or lotion to use on the skin.

Ophthalmic- Pertaining to the eye.

Oral- Pertaining to the mouth.

Oral rehydration solution (ORS)- A drink to correct dehydration; which you can make with boiled water, sugar, salt, and sodium carbonate. It can also be made with rice flour instead of sugar.

Organ- A part of the body that is more or less complete in itself and does a specific job. For example the lungs are for breathing.

Otic- Having to do with the ears.

Ounce- A measure of weight equal to about 28 grams. There are 16 ounces in one pound.

P
Paralysis- Loss of the ability to move part or all of the animal's body.

Parasites- Worms and tiny animals that live in, or on, another animal or person, and cause harm. Fleas, intestinal worms, and protozoa are parasites.

Parenteral- Not by mouth but by injection.

Pasteurization- The process of heating milk or other liquids to a certain temperature (60 degrees) C for about 30 minutes in order to kill harmful bacteria.

Pelvis- Hip bones.

Pesticide- A poison that kills pests such as ticks and insects.

Petroleum jelly (petrolatum, Vaseline)- A grease-like jelly used in preparing skin ointments.

Placenta (after birth)- The dark and spongy lining inside the womb where the fetus joins the mother's body. The placenta usually comes out within several hours, after the young animal is born.

Prevention- Action taken to stop sickness before it starts.

Prolapse- The slipping outside of a part of the body from its normal position; for example a prolapsed uterus or rectum.

Proteins- Body building foods necessary for proper growth and strength.

Protozoa- Microorganisms that may cause disease (e.g. coccidia).

Pulse- The rhythmic expansion of an artery which may be felt with a finger and corresponds to each beat of the heart. The pulse rate is the number of pulsation's of an artery per minute.

Pupil- The round opening or black center of the iris of the eye. It gets smaller in bright light and larger in the dark.

Pus- A liquid product of infection made up of cells and body fluid.

R
Rate- The number of times something happens in a given amount of time; for example the pulse.

Rectum- The end of the large intestine close to the opening from the body.

Resistance- The ability of something to defend itself against something that would normally harm or kill it. Many bacteria become resistant to the effects of certain antibiotics.

Respiration- Breathing. The respiratory system includes the bronchi, lungs, and other organs used in breathing. The respiration rate is the number of times an animal breathes in one minute.

S
Sanitation- Public cleanliness involving community efforts in disease prevention, promoting hygiene, and keeping public places free of waste.

Scrotum- The bag between a male animals legs that holds his testicles or balls.

Sedative- A chemical agent which decreases excitement.

Shock- A dangerous condition with severe weakness or unconsciousness, cold, sweat, and fast or weak, pulse. It is caused by dehydration, hemorrhage, injury, burns, or a severe illness.

Seroma- A collection in the tissues of serum and blood.

Side effects- Problems caused by using a medicine.

Sterilization- (1) to kill microorganisms on instruments, bottles, and other things by boiling or heating in an oven. (2) Also, a permanent way of making a male or female unable to reproduce.

Stethoscope- An instrument used to listen to sounds in the body, such as the heartbeat.

Subcutaneous (SQ or SC)- Beneath the skin.

Symptoms- The feelings or conditions related to a disease.

T
Tablespoon- A measuring spoon that holds 3 teaspoons or 15 ml.

Teaspoon- A measuring spoon that holds 5 ml. Three teaspoons equal one tablespoon.

Temperature- The degree of heat in a living body.

Thermometer- An instrument used to measure how hot the body temperature is.

Tick- A crawling insect-like bug that buries its head under the skin and sucks blood.

Topical- For the skin. A topical medicine is to be put on the skin.

Toxemia- A sickness resulting from certain poisons (toxins) in the body; for example, pregnancy toxemia.

Toxic- Poisonous.

Toxicity- The quality of being poisonous.

Toxin- A substance which is highly poisonous for other living animals.

Transmit- To pass on, transfer, or allow spreading from one animal to another.

Tumor- An abnormal mass of tissue. Some tumors are due to cancer.

U
Ulcer- A hole in the skin that can be shallow or deep. A popped vesicle can cause them.
Deep ulcers can become chronic and take a long time to heal.

Umbilical cord- The cord that connects a baby from its navel to the placenta on the inside of its
mother's womb.

Umbilical hernia- A large, outward bulge of the navel- caused by a loop of the intestine that has
pushed through the muscles holding the guts.

Umbilicus- See *Navel.*

Urethra- Urinary tube or canal. The tube that runs from the bladder to the vagina or penis.

Urinary tract- The system of organs concerned with the formation and getting rid of urine-such as
kidneys, bladder, and urinary tube *(urethra)*

Urine- Liquid waste from the body; made by the kidneys.

Uterus- Womb.

V
Vaccinations- See *Immunizations.*

Vagina- The tube or canal in females that connects the cervix (the door to the uterus) to the
outside of the female's body.

Vessels- Tubes. Blood vessels are the veins and arteries that carry the blood through the body.

Virus- A group of very small microorganisms that cause disease. Viruses are not killed by
antibiotics.

Vitamins- Protective foods that our bodies need to work properly.

Vomiting- Throwing up the contents out of the stomach through the mouth.

W
Welts- Lumps or ridges raised on the body, usually caused by a blow or an allergy (hives).

Withdrawal period- the amount of time for a removal of a medicine from the body to allow
safe consumption of the meat, milk, or the eggs.

Womb (uterus)- The sac inside a female's abdomen where a baby is made.

General Index
Things in this book are listed in the order of the alphabet.

A B C D E F G H I J K L M N O P Q R S T U V W X Y Z

Capacity, space or volume refers to the measurement of liquid.
1 teaspoon = 5 cm or 5 milliliters (ml)
3 teaspoons = 1 tablespoon
1 tablespoon = 15 cc or 15 ml
2 tablespoons = 30 cc or 30 ml = 1 fluid ounce

8 fluid ounces = 1 cup = 240 cc or 240 ml
2 cups = 1 pint = 480 cc or 480 ml
2 pints = 1 quart = 32 fluid ounces
1 quart is just less than 1 liter

1 liter = 1000 cc or ml)
4 quarts = 1 gallon = nearly 4000 cc, ml

Weight refers to the weight of material
16 ounce (oz) = 1 pound (1 lb)
1 pound = 454 grams (gm)
1000 g = 1 kg (kilo, kg)
1 kg = 2.2 lbs

1 ounce = 28 grams
1 gram (gm) = 1000 milligrams (mg)
1 Green (gr) = 65 mg

Metric system
1 milliliter (ml) = 1 cc
1000 ml = 1 liter
1 gram (gm) = 1000 milligrams (mg)
1 kg (kilo, kg) = 2.2 pounds (1bs)

About the Authors

Peter N. Quesenberry
Email: pmqberry@gmail.com

BS   1976 University of California, Davis
DVM   1978 University of California, Davis
MPVM (Public Health)   1991 University of California, Davis

Following graduation from veterinary school, Dr. Quesenberry joined the Chino Valley Veterinary Group and practiced there as a dairy vet for 2 years before he and his wife Mary went to Nepal in 1980. In Nepal he worked to further establish a clinic and an animal health training program for farmers. In addition, he helped train veterinary technicians for the government of Nepal and wrote curricula and textbooks. In 1990 Dr. Quesenberry returned to the States and completed his masters before returning to Asia in 1991. Dr. Quesenberry is currently serving as an advisor to local foundation and lives in the very northern tip of Thailand, in Chiang Rai.

Peter and his wife Mary have 3 children. Nat and Cheri were born in Nepal, and Wynn was born in Thailand. The whole family was actively involved with the "Where There Is No Animal Doctor" / "Handbook of Animal Health" project and sincerely hopes it will impact many peoples' lives in a positive way.

Maureen Birmingham

BS 1981   University of Illinois, Urbana DVM
1983   University of Illinois, Urbana MPH 1990
Harvard University, Boston
Prev Med Res U.S. Centers for Disease Control and Prevention, Atlanta

Dr. Birmingham worked as a large animal veterinarian for 2 1/2 years at Paradise Veterinary Practice in Upstate New York. She then worked in Haiti for ~4 years. There she worked with an indigenous NGO to develop training on animal husbandry and health for farmers and animal health agents. She was also seconded to the International Institute for Cooperation in Agriculture to help with the African Swine Fever Eradication effort in Haiti. She then worked in Bolivia for ~1.3 years with an indigenous NGO to train animal health agents. After subsequent post-graduate training in public health and epidemiology and a preventive medicine residency, she worked for the US Centers for Disease Control and Prevention as an epidemiologist, detailed to the World Health Organization in Geneva, Switzerland from 1993-2004 on polio eradication and surveillance of vaccine preventable diseases. She then worked for WHO in the   South East Asia Region on emerging diseases. At the time of this printing she is currently the WHO representative in Argentina.

Maureen and her husband Dan have 3 children: Erika, Evelyn and Zoe.

References

Animal Health Improvement Program, **How to Make Livestock Healthy**, the UMN, Kathmandu, Nepal, 1989.

Bell, John C., Palmer, Stephen R., Payne, Jack M., **The Zoonoses**, Edward Arnold, A Division of Hodder and Stoughton, London, 1988.

Bruner, D.W., Gillespie, J.H., **Hagan's Infectious Diseases of Domestic Animals**, Comstock Publishing Associates, Cornell University Press, Ithaca NY, 1973.

Carlson, James, **Raising Healthy Cattle Under Primitive Conditions**, CVM, World Concern, Seattle, WA.

Craven, Alison, **Animal Health,** Animal Health Improvement Program, UMN.

Dunn, Angus M., **Veterinary Helminthology**, William Heinemann Medical Books LTD, London, 1969.

Goodman, Earl, **Raising Healthy Pigs Under Primitive Conditions**, CVM, World Concern, 1990.

Grimley, Will; Lynn, Randy; Robinson, Beth, **Drugs and Their Usage,** CVM, World Concern, 1998.

Hart, B. and Mitchell, G.L., **Aus.Vet.Journal,** 41,305.

Hendersen, Judy, **Auxiliary Health Workers Teaching Manual,** Karnali Technical School.

Laboratory Aids to Clinical Diagnosis, 36 Gordon Square, London, WCI

Leman, Glock, et al, **Diseases of Swine**, 5th Edition, The Iowa State University Press, Ames, Iowa, USA, Philippine Copyright, 1982.

Manual for Animal Health Auxiliary Personnel, Food and Agriculture Organization of the United Nations, 1983.

Manual of Veterinary Parasitological Laboratory Techniques, London, Her Majesty's Stationery Office

Merck Veterinary Manual, 4th and 6th Editions, Merck and Co., Inc., Rahway, NJ, USA, 1973, 1986

Oehme, Frederick W., Prier, James E., 1980, **Text book of Large Animal Surgery**, Williams and Wilkins, Baltimore, 1974.

Prasad, B., **Veterinary Pharmaceuticals**, Satish Kumar Jain, College Book Store, 1701, Nai Sarak, Delhi 10006

Quesenberry, P.N., **Raising Healthy Pigs in the Hills of Nepal**, the UMN. Quesenberry, P.N., **The JTA Handbook on Animal Health,** the UMN.

Roberts, Stephen J., **Veterinary Obstetrics and Genital Diseases**, Published by the author, Ithaca, New York, 1971.

Schwartz, L. Dwight, **Pennsylvania Poultry Health Handbook**, Pennsylvania State University, College of Agriculture, University Park, Pennsylvania. Slowinski, Annette, Class notes on Animal Health, 1990.

Soulsby, E.J.L., **Helminths, Arthropods & Protozoa of Domesticated Animals**, Williams and Wilkins Company, Baltimore, 1976.

South Carolina **Agriculture Chemical Handbook** published by Clemson University.

University of Georgia Agriculture Extension Service: various publications on parasitology. Vallachira, Aravindan, **Veterinarians Drug Index**, Third Edition, Jaypee Brothers Medical Publishers, New Delhi, India, 1995.

Werner, David, **Where There is No Doctor**, Hesperian Health Guides, Berkeley, CA, 1977, 2019.

Made in the USA
Monee, IL
07 July 2026

56552029R00236